The Dementias

The Dementias
Early Diagnosis and Evaluation

edited by

Karl Herholz
Wolfson Molecular Imaging Centre
University of Manchester
Manchester, U.K.

Daniela Perani
Vita-Salute San Raffaele University
San Raffaele Scientific Institute
Milan, Italy

Chris Morris
Wolfson Unit of Clinical Pharmacology
University of Newcastle upon Tyne
Newcastle upon Tyne, U.K.

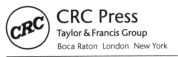

CRC Press is an imprint of the
Taylor & Francis Group, an **informa** business

CRC Press
Taylor & Francis Group
6000 Broken Sound Parkway NW, Suite 300
Boca Raton, FL 33487-2742

First issued in paperback 2017

© 2006 by Taylor & Francis Group, LLC
CRC Press is an imprint of Taylor & Francis Group, an Informa business

No claim to original U.S. Government works

ISBN-13: 978-0-8247-2897-7 (hbk)
ISBN-13: 978-0-367-39073-0 (pbk)

Visit the Taylor & Francis Web site at
http://www.taylorandfrancis.com

and the CRC Press Web site at
http://www.crcpress.com

Preface

Our motivation to compile this book stems from our exposure to a number of issues that are difficult to reconcile. Most people probably welcome the increase in longevity that is observed in many countries today, but this also brings with it a substantial increase in dementia with prevalence and incidence rising steeply beyond 70 years of age. It is widely acknowledged that this imposes severe stress on families and caregivers and risks the failure of social welfare systems. Dementia may therefore become one of the most difficult challenges for societies in this century. Yet, we are far away from a medical solution. Even if a drug that could slow or halt the progression of dementing diseases was made available tomorrow, it probably would have only limited effect since too much brain function has been lost to degenerative brain disease once the clinical symptoms of dementia become clearly evident. Restoration of normal cognition will therefore remain an elusive goal. Thus, there is the danger that any available drug would either be given too late to prevent dementia and its consequences, or it would be given indiscriminately to people with nonspecific complaints or even without any symptoms. Since only a small proportion of these individuals are likely to develop dementia within the next few years, precious medical resources would be wasted. Early and accurate diagnosis of dementing diseases before the onset of dementia therefore becomes of paramount importance if we are to avoid such a situation and use preventative treatment strategies efficiently once they become available.

Over the past few years, many new methods and techniques have been developed to improve early diagnosis. Most of these require special training and expert knowledge for application and an understanding of their potential and limitations. In this book, active researchers who are experts in their respective fields present and evaluate these methods to provide a guide to their use in early dementia diagnosis and assessment. It is, however, quite clear that no single method can cover all aspects that are relevant for early diagnosis. With this overview we hope to provide comprehensive information to clinicians, researchers, and the pharmaceutical industry about which methods are the most effective ones for screening, early diagnosis of symptomatic subjects, and distinguishing between different dementing diseases. While we cannot yet provide definitive answers to all these questions, we hope that the evaluation will provide guidance for further research.

Clinical evaluation and care are the basis of dementia diagnosis and treatment, and we therefore put the chapter on clinical issues at the beginning. Neuropsychology provides methods for the objective and quantitative assessment of symptoms and behavioral and cognitive deficits, and therefore this naturally takes its place close to clinical evaluation. Next comes cerebrospinal fluid and blood biomarkers that hold promise in complementing symptom-based diagnosis by adding biochemical information on the underlying disease process. Chapters on genetics and novel molecular targets provide the latest information on risk factors and molecular mechanisms with their perspectives for early diagnosis. After that we enter the wide arena of in vivo imaging methods, which have undergone rapid development and bewildering diversification in recent years, ranging from structural imaging with computed tomography and magnetic resonance imaging to functional and molecular imaging with functional magnetic resonance imaging, magnetic resonance spectroscopy, single-photon emission computed tomography, and positron emission tomography. Most of these are ready to be applied in the clinical arena, but quite often their actual value and efficacy is still under dispute. Authors therefore explain the techniques and provide information on diagnostic sensitivity and specificity when available. The methods chapters are then concluded with a view from neuropathology, which still provides the most detailed methods for tissue examination and therefore sets the diagnostic gold standard, although the significance of post-mortem studies in early dementia is limited because of the lack of clinical follow-up data, for obvious reasons. We did not want to leave our readers with just a compilation of methods and data but felt that an overview and final evaluation, although necessarily somewhat subjective, should conclude the book. We also address some of the wider implications of improved early diagnosis that need consideration when we enter this extremely important clinical field, which may hold dangers, but hopefully many surprises as well.

Karl Herholz
Daniela Perani
Chris Morris

Acknowledgments

We are very grateful to the authors, who are all busy researchers but dedicated a significant amount of their time to the book. Their contribution cannot be overestimated. This interdisciplinary project would probably not have been possible without previous scientific collaboration of the editors and some of the authors, which was supported by the European Commission in their framework programs 4 to 6. Last but not least, we thank the publisher's editorial and production team, especially Geoff Greenwood and Dana Bigelow, for their continuous encouragement and support. The publication of this book was generously supported by an educational grant from GE Healthcare.

Contents

3. Biomarkers in Blood and Cerebrospinal Fluid *73*

Harald Hampel and Katharina Buerger

4. Genetics: Facts and Perspectives *109*

*Sandro Sorbi, Paolo Forleo, Francesca Massaro,
and Andrea Ginestroni*

Contributors

Katharina Buerger   Alzheimer Memorial Center and Geriatric Psychiatry Branch, Department of Psychiatry, Ludwig-Maximilian University, Munich, Germany

Steven T. DeKosky   Departments of Psychiatry and Neurology, University of Pittsburgh, Pittsburgh, Pennsylvania, U.S.A.

Nadine J. Dougall   Division of Psychiatry, Gordon Small Center for Research in Old Age Psychiatry, University of Edinburgh, Edinburgh, U.K.

Klaus P. Ebmeier   Division of Psychiatry, Gordon Small Center for Research in Old Age Psychiatry, University of Edinburgh, Edinburgh, U.K.

Nicola Filippini   Laboratory of Epidemiology Neuroimaging and Telemedicine (LENITEM), IRCCS San Giovanni di Dio FBF—The National Center for Research and Care of Alzheimer's Disease, Brescia, Italy

Paolo Forleo   Department of Neurological and Psychiatric Sciences, University of Florence, Florence, Italy

Norman L. Foster   Imaging and Research, Center for Alzheimer's Care, and Department of Neurology and The Brain Institute, University of Utah, Salt Lake City, Utah, U.S.A.

Giovanni B. Frisoni   Laboratory of Epidemiology Neuroimaging and Telemedicine (LENITEM), IRCCS San Giovanni di Dio FBF—The National Center for Research and Care of Alzheimer's Disease, Brescia, Italy

Andrea Ginestroni   Department of Neurological and Psychiatric Sciences, University of Florence, Florence, Italy

Harald Hampel   Alzheimer Memorial Center and Geriatric Psychiatry Branch, Department of Psychiatry, Ludwig-Maximilian University, Munich, Germany

Steen G. Hasselbalch   Neurobiology Research Unit and Memory Disorders Research Group, Copenhagen University Hospital, Rigshospitalet, Copenhagen, Denmark

Karl Herholz   Wolfson Molecular Imaging Centre, University of Manchester, Manchester, U.K., and Department of Neurology, University of Cologne, Cologne, Germany

Kurt A. Jellinger   Institute of Clinical Neurobiology, Vienna, Austria

William E. Klunk   Department of Psychiatry, University of Pittsburgh, Pittsburgh, Pennsylvania, U.S.A.

Gitte M. Knudsen   Neurobiology Research Unit, Copenhagen University Hospital, Rigshospitalet, Copenhagen, Denmark

Brian J. Lopresti   Department of Radiology, University of Pittsburgh, Pittsburgh, Pennsylvania, U.S.A.

Francesca Massaro   Department of Neurological and Psychiatric Sciences, University of Florence, Florence, Italy

Chester A. Mathis   Departments of Radiology, Pharmacology, and Pharmaceutical Sciences, University of Pittsburgh, Pittsburgh, Pennsylvania, U.S.A.

Chris Morris   Wolfson Unit of Clinical Pharmacology, Chemical Hazards and Poisons Division–Newcastle, Health Protection Agency, and School of Neurology, Neurobiology, and Psychiatry, The Medical School, University of Newcastle upon Tyne, Newcastle upon Tyne, Tyne and Wear, U.K.

Robert D. Nebes   Department of Psychiatry, University of Pittsburgh, Pittsburgh, Pennsylvania, U.S.A.

Daniela Perani   Departments of Neuroscience and Nuclear Medicine, Vita-Salute San Raffaele University and San Raffaele Scientific Institute, Milan, Italy

Julie C. Price   Department of Radiology, University of Pittsburgh, Pittsburgh, Pennsylvania, U.S.A.

Sandro Sorbi   Department of Neurological and Psychiatric Sciences, University of Florence, Florence, Italy

Nicholas Tsopelas   Department of Psychiatry, University of Pittsburgh, Pittsburgh, Pennsylvania, U.S.A.

Kate E. Wilson   Institute for Ageing and Health, University of Newcastle, Newcastle General Hospital, Newcastle upon Tyne, Tyne and Wear, U.K.

1

The Clinical Issues

Norman L. Foster

*Imaging and Research, Center for Alzheimer's Care, and Department
of Neurology and The Brain Institute, University of Utah, Salt Lake City,
Utah, U.S.A.*

INTRODUCTION

The diagnosis and management of dementia will be a major challenge for health care systems in the coming decades. As the world's population ages, the prevalence of dementia will grow dramatically (1). Alzheimer's disease (AD), the most common cause of dementia, accounts for much of the increasing prevalence of dementia with age (2). However, many other causes of dementia, such as stroke and Parkinson's disease, also increase dramatically as people become older. The care of those with dementia causes great burdens on caregivers and society. The number of individuals with dementia will grow most rapidly in the developing world, but dementing diseases will have their greatest social impact in Japan, Europe, and North America, where their proportion of the population will be highest. Prevention and improved diagnosis and treatment of cognitive impairment and dementia offer the only hope to alter this grim equation.

Fortunately, there has been an explosion of information about neurodegenerative diseases, and dementia has moved from being a backwater to the vanguard of neuroscience research. New insights and conceptual breakthroughs have led to improved detection and evaluation of dementia, and there are many more new approaches now in development. There is every reason to expect these advances will continue and be translated into clinical practice. Awareness and application of these recent developments provide great opportunities for physicians to help patients and society.

DEMENTIA EVALUATION

The Role of Dementia Evaluation

Patients and families have many reasons for seeking a physician's advice when memory loss or cognitive impairments appear (Table 1). The hope of treatment that improves symptoms is a major motivation, but other important concerns also should be addressed. Physicians too often focus solely on treatment and fail to recognize the great value patients and families place on accurate diagnosis. There is comfort in understanding the cause of symptoms and in knowing that everything that should be done has been done. An accurate and specific diagnosis also empowers physicians. Once the cause of dementia is determined, the physicians can use their specialized knowledge of the disease to guide management and coordinate care. It becomes possible to develop a rational and evidence-based care plan appropriate for that disease. Family members also may be seeking help for themselves. An authoritative dementia evaluation can resolve conflicting opinions among family members and clarify their role in care. With a detailed management plan and prognostic information, patients, families, and physicians can plan for the future together.

Physicians often are reluctant to evaluate dementia because it opens a "Pandora's box" of concerns they aren't prepared to address (3). Many physicians lack the experience and confidence to perform an evaluation. Even if an evaluation is performed, physicians may be reluctant to inform patients and families of their diagnosis (4). Information about prognosis also may be withheld, even though it greatly benefits patients and their families (5). Usually patients and families aren't satisfied until they learn the specific cause of cognitive impairment; generalities, platitudes, and nostrums aren't sufficient. In one study, caregivers reported that a correct diagnosis of AD was provided in only 38% of initial physician consultations, causing them to seek care from someone else (6). Most recognize the limits of medicine, and appreciate a definitive diagnosis, even when few drug treatments can be offered. Patients with suspected neurological disease have less distress about their symptoms and less anxiety when they receive a definitive diagnosis (7). Physicians therefore should use whatever effective means are available to accurately determine the cause of dementia.

Table 1 Motivations for Seeking a Dementia Evaluation

Determine whether perceived memory loss or cognitive decline is truly present
Seek a specific medical explanation for the cause of symptoms
Find a treatment that can improve symptoms
Understand what can be expected in the future and how to prepare for it now
Learn whether other family members are at risk of developing similar problems
Know when and how to obtain help
Hope for continued support and better treatments in the future

Dementia evaluations require complex medical decision-making. There are no shortcuts or easy simplifications. Dozens of diseases that cause dementia must be distinguished (8). Clinical medicine offers no more difficult exercise in differential diagnosis. It is important not to underestimate the effort required for an accurate assessment. One must provide adequate time to obtain a detailed history and to perform a comprehensive mental status and neurological examination. Although daunting, physicians can find great satisfaction and intellectual reward in uncovering and treating cognitive impairment.

The evaluation of cognitive impairment and dementia consists of three distinct steps: (1) the recognition of cognitive deficits, (2) an initial assessment to decide whether dementia is present, and (3) when impairment is confirmed, the determination of its cause. Physicians often claim to have "diagnosed" dementia after completing only one of these steps. However, diagnosis is incomplete until all three are accomplished. Each step has distinct challenges and requires considerable clinical judgment.

Recognizing Impairment in Cognition

It is relatively easy to recognize sudden or severe cognitive loss, but substantial effort can be required when deficits are subtle or gradually progressive. Patients and families may identify explicit cognitive problems, but at least as often complaints are nonspecific or symptoms become evident to the physician only indirectly. Health professionals should be alert to "triggers" that suggest cognitive impairment (Table 2). This is necessary because patients often fail to mention that they have cognitive symptoms. This may be out of fear that they will lose their independence. Some patients are unable to recognize deficits as a result of their disease (anosognosia). Others may find it embarrassing to discuss

Table 2 Situations that Should Trigger a Dementia Evaluation

Patient complaints or concerns of others
   Persistent and progressive memory loss
   Inability to learn and retain new information
   Difficulty handling complex tasks
   Poor reasoning ability
   Trouble with spatial ability and orientation
   Difficulty with language
   Change in behavior
Observations during medical care
   Difficulty following directions
   Inability to provide an accurate medical history
   Vague or evasive responses to direct questions
   Appearing dependent on others for information or financial assistance
   Non-compliance or confusion about appointments and treatment
   Irritable or indifferent when asked direct questions

cognitive complaints, particularly since for many there continues to be a considerable social stigma attached to mental problems. Family members also may fail to reveal their concerns about a patient's cognitive problems, either out of respect for their relative's dignity or reluctance to interfere. To overcome these barriers, physicians must establish rapport and be compassionate and sensitive to these issues. Often a simple and direct question, such as "Any trouble with memory?", is sufficient to identify a subtle cognitive impairment.

Current methods of screening for cognitive impairment are too imprecise and time-consuming to apply to the general population, or even to all elderly people (9). However, elderly individuals seeking medical care have a much higher prevalence of dementia, and the routine use of a brief cognitive screen in the physician's office may be appropriate. When there are complaints or "triggers" suggesting cognitive problems, an initial assessment for dementia is essential (10).

The evaluation of dementia must consider different factors in each individual. A change in cognitive abilities can be determined only when a patient's literacy, education level, occupation, and usual activities are considered. Once concern about cognitive impairment is raised, a careful history from the patient and at least one collateral source (family member, friend or employer) is needed to determine whether there truly has been a change and whether it is progressive. A collateral source is necessary since patients may not be able to recognize their problems or report them accurately or with sufficient detail. When the reliability of patient responses appears uncertain, it often is prudent to defer a medical history until another source is available to confirm facts and to avoid basing judgments on misinformation. Interpreting a history of cognitive impairment requires considerable clinical skill. Depressed patients often perceive more memory loss than they truly have (11). Unrecognized visual problems or hearing loss may cause inaccurate responses that are mistaken for cognitive impairment. Confirming cognitive impairment can be particularly difficult in patients with legal or financial motives for initiating an assessment. A single visit may be insufficient, and serial examination may be required to confirm that the clinical course is stable or progressive.

Deciding Whether Dementia Is Present

After identifying cognitive impairment, the second step in evaluation is to determine whether dementia is present. Dementia is defined as a decline in two or more cognitive domains, such as memory, language, visuospatial processing, abstraction, and judgment, that is sufficient to cause impairments in everyday activities. The requirement for functional impairment means that dementia represents a more severe change in cognition and is more certain to be due to a true brain disease. Furthermore, the standard of functional impairment caused by cognition provides an independent measure of significant decline with face validity. By requiring impairment in at least two cognitive domains, the definition of dementia implies an extensive involvement of brain function. Deficits in a single cognitive domain, such as aphasia, apraxia or alexia, can be caused by damage in discrete areas in a single cerebral hemisphere, and alone do not constitute dementia. Memory loss is a particularly important sign in dementia. Although amnesia alone is insufficient to establish dementia, it is an indication that several brain regions may be affected, since memory loss is not localizable to a single cerebral hemisphere.

A careful mental status assessment is needed to be certain that symptoms cannot be explained by damage in a single anatomical region or a single cognitive domain. Intellectual function is multifaceted, and occasionally the physician and patient are so drawn to a single component of cognition that they miss the full extent of impairment. Several methods of assessing each cognitive domain should be used. For example, one should test both verbal and non-verbal stimuli to make sure that memory problems can't be attributed solely to aphasia.

Determining whether there truly is functional impairment and if it can be explained by cognitive loss require astute clinical judgment. Since cognitive difficulties usually develop insidiously, patients and their families often adapt to them easily. As a result, they may not recognize the loss in performance, or they may attribute it to factors other than dementia. For example, spouses may gradually take over cooking or family finances without considering that this was necessitated by changes in their mate. Likewise, inability to shop independently may be misattributed to arthritis, depression, or simply disinterest, rather than to cognitive loss. The physician faces the challenge of analyzing the evidence without simply accepting explanations patients and families provide, and of deciding whether functional decline is due to cognitive disability, physical disability, or both. It is important to consider typical daily activities and occupation throughout life to assess whether current deficiencies truly represent a change in abilities sufficient for dementia.

Cognitive impairment can be clinically significant, yet insufficient to cause functional limitation or represent dementia. Patients with problems in a single cognitive domain often avoid functional impairments by compensating with strengths in other cognitive areas. Stroke is a common cause of circumscribed cognitive deficits. For example, patients with Broca's aphasia due to a left hemisphere stroke may have severe aphasia, yet remain independent. Difficulties compensating for deficits that seem limited to a single cognitive domain suggest that problems are actually more pervasive than suspected; the patient may have dementia.

It is logical to expect that patients developing dementia initially would have impairment only in a single cognitive domain. Likewise, impairments insufficient to affect everyday activities should occur before dementia develops. These precepts underlie recent efforts to recognize prodromal dementia. There have been many attempts to define characteristics that might identify individuals who will eventually develop dementia. Currently, the terms most widely accepted for this situation are mild cognitive impairment (MCI) (often used in a clinical context) and cognitive impairment, not demented (CIND) (frequently used in epidemiological studies). Criteria for these conditions are not consistent from report to report, and their use should be scrutinized carefully. The prevalence of cognitive impairment insufficient to cause functional impairment appears to be greater than the prevalence of dementia, but more studies are needed (12). Despite the difficulties of definition, recognizing these conditions has more than heuristic value. They represent a group of patients with a significantly increased risk of developing dementia over subsequent years and are an appropriate target for new therapies (13).

It may be helpful to distinguish different kinds of cognitive impairment insufficient to be classified as dementia. Since different dementing diseases have predominant deficits in different cognitive domains, it is logical to assume that their initial symptoms also differ. For example, isolated memory impairment would be expected to precede the development of dementia in AD, where memory loss usually is the most prominent symptom. Likewise, progressive aphasia may precede frontotemporal dementia (FTD) (14). Thus individuals with amnestic MCI and predominant or isolated memory loss are believed to be more likely to progress to dementia caused by AD, and those with non-amnestic MCI may precede other forms of dementia (15). It also may be useful to classify patients by presumed etiology, since this can have prognostic significance (16,17).

Deriving reliable criteria to identify prodromal dementia based purely upon clinical grounds turns out to be more difficult than it might first appear. Not only must multiple areas of cognition be considered, but boundaries of both normal cognition for age and impaired cognition sufficient to represent dementia also must be defined. Detailed neuropsychological testing provides age-appropriate norms to guide clinical judgment and explicit operational criteria for clinical trials. MCI differs from CIND by requiring a voiced complaint of impairment. An expressed memory complaint is important because it is a strong predictor of AD and a face valid criterion for a change in ability (18). Individuals categorized as having MCI are more likely than those with CIND to progress to unequivocal dementia (13,19). In a diverse clinical population where diagnosis and management must be provided to everyone, the early recognition of prodromal dementia must rely on physician judgment and interpretation, rather than solely on neuropsychological test results or strict application of criteria.

Determining the Cause of Cognitive Impairment and Dementia

The final and critical step in a dementia evaluation is to determine the specific cause of significant cognitive impairment. This is valuable for many reasons (Table 3). There are a large number of potential causes to consider. Neurodegenerative diseases are the most common, but systemic medical illnesses and many other neurological disorders also can alter brain function and lead to dementia. A complete review of all dementing diseases is beyond the scope of this chapter, but the physician must consider all categories of disease during a dementia

Table 3 Benefits of Determining the Specific Cause of Dementia

Choose drugs that are known to be effective in that particular disease
Avoid drugs that are not appropriate for that disease, known to be ineffective, or are
  contraindicated
Know what disease complications to expect
Avoid unnecessary evaluations when a new symptom consistent with the disease develops
Plan for future care based upon the known clinical course of the specific disease
Educate caregivers about the cause of the disease, its symptoms, and recent research
  advances
Answer (sometimes unspoken) questions about family risk based upon genetics of the
  disease

evaluation, including genetic, metabolic, infectious, neoplastic, and vascular disorders (8).

There is a great opportunity and need to improve the methods used to recognize specific causes of cognitive impairment. Currently, we must rely on the clinical approaches of evaluating the medical history and examination and a few informative laboratory studies. The medical history is used to reconstruct the clinical course of the illness, noting the appearance and timing of symptoms. Physical and mental status examinations then are used to confirm and expand the character of the illness. Finally, this information and the results of laboratory testing and brain imaging are compared to typical clinical features of specific dementing illnesses (Table 4). The best match between a patient's findings and the characteristic features of a disease identifies the specific diagnosis, with the degree of congruence generally indicating the level of diagnostic certainty. Consensus diagnostic criteria and clinical guidelines are available for MCI and the most common dementing disorders and can be very helpful. Criteria are particularly valuable in communicating diagnostic information among health providers and in establishing a defined, homogeneous group of patients for research studies. However, clinical criteria provide only guidelines and are not applicable in all situations; clinical judgment is still necessary.

Some dementing diseases cause such distinctive abnormalities that they markedly assist diagnosis (Table 5). Other physical abnormalities are less specific. However, performance of a detailed neurological examination is critical, because it can identify subtle and asymmetric motor signs and gait abnormalities that suggest focal lesions or limit the disorders under consideration. Some routine laboratory tests should be obtained in every patient with dementia (28). This testing is warranted because it easily can identify common medical illnesses that cause or amplify dementia (Table 6). Particularly in the elderly, medical illnesses can cause cognitive impairment before physical symptoms are evident. When there is reason for clinical suspicion, further laboratory testing can help identify less common dementing disorders (Table 7).

The routine use of structural brain imaging for the evaluation of dementia has been more controversial, but is now generally accepted (28). It is indisputable

Table 4 Characteristic Presentation and Course of Mild Cognitive Impairment and the Most Common Dementing Diseases

Disease	Usual features	Diagnostic guidelines
Mild cognitive impairment	Insidious onset of progressive decline in cognitive abilities insufficient to cause impairment in everyday activities; must be associated with a complaint; several subtypes have been proposed: the amnestic form in which memory loss is predominant appears to be most likely to progress to Alzheimer's disease	ADCS criteria (13); International Workshop criteria (20)
Alzheimer's disease	Insidious onset of gradually progressive memory loss; memory loss remains the most prominent feature as aphasia, apraxia, impaired judgment, and behavior change develop; seizures and incontinence late in the disease	NINCDS-ADRDA criteria (21)
Vascular dementia	Sudden onset, stepwise progression of dementia associated with ischemic stroke; usually with focal motor and sensory deficits, although these deficits may resolve; cognitive deficits variable and correspond to the location of strokes; frontal lobe impairment may be most obvious with subcortical stroke; seizures and incontinence may occur early in the course	NINDS-AIREN criteria (22); Modified Hachinski Ischemic Score (23)

Dementia with Lewy bodies	Insidious onset of gradually progressive dementia with parkinsonism (either within a year of developing Parkinson's disease or alternatively the development of parkinsonism concurrent with dementia or soon thereafter); spontaneous visual hallucinations, unexplained fluctuations in symptom severity; visuo-spatial deficits and memory loss prominent	Consensus second workshop criteria (24)
Parkinson's disease with dementia	Idiopathic Parkinson's disease, followed by the insidious onset of progressive dementia more than a year later	Consensus workshop criteria (25)
Frontotemporal dementia	Insidious onset of progressive language or behavior disturbance, often with personality change; relative preservation of functional abilities at first; subsequently more pervasive progressive dementia with memory loss while language and behavior changes remain most prominent; often progresses to mutism; later development of parkinsonism common; may be associated with motor neuron disease	Consensus criteria (26); work group criteria (27)

Abbreviations: ADCS, Alzheimer's Disease Cooperative Study; NINCDS-ADRDA, National Institute of Neurological and Communicative Disorders and Stroke–Alzheimer's Disease and Related Disorders Association; NINDS-AIREN, National Institute of Neurological Disorders and Stroke–Association Internationale pour la Recherche et l'Enseignement en Neurosciences.

Table 5   Distinctive Features on Examination that Suggest a Specific Cause of Dementia

Abnormality	Disease most likely
Supranuclear gaze palsy	Progressive supranuclear palsy
Alien hand	Corticobasal degeneration
Chorea	Huntington's disease
Tendon xanthomas	Cerebrotendinous xanthomatosis
Dystonia	Wilson's disease
Keyser–Fleisher ring	Wilson's disease
Asterixis	Liver or renal failure
Icterus, ascites, hepatomegaly	Liver failure
Muscle fasciculations and atrophy	Frontotemporal dementia with motor neuron
Pupils nonreactive to light	disease
	Neurosyphilis

that computed tomography (CT) and magnetic resonance imaging (MRI) aid the recognition of many neurological illnesses causing dementia (Table 8). Although many of these diseases often cause focal abnormalities, the neurological examination alone may be insensitive for early detection or when patients are unable to adequately participate in a detailed assessment.

Simply identifying an abnormal laboratory test or brain scan is insufficient; one must interpret the results and their clinical significance. It is important to realize that "Occam's razor," or the search for a single unifying diagnosis to explain symptoms and signs, is not always appropriate when evaluating older patients (29). Since it is common for a medical illness to exacerbate an underlying dementing illness or for dementing diseases to co-exist and interact, the principle of parsimony of diagnosis may lead one astray (30,31). It is more appropriate to consider the possibility that multiple pathologies are causing cognitive decline.

It can be very difficult to be sure when two or more conditions are contributing to a patient's dementia, yet this has major implications for deciding on treatment and assessing response. Serial examinations may help disentangle

Table 6   Laboratory Studies Appropriate for Routine Use in Dementia Evaluations

Test	Causes of dementia detected
Complete blood count	Severe anemia, systemic infection, leukemia
Electrolyte panel	Electrolyte disturbances
Glucose and calcium	Hypoglycemia, hypocalcemia, hypercalcemia
Chemistry panel	Hepatic or renal disease
Thyroid function tests	Hypothyroidism or hyperthyroidism
Vitamin B_{12} level	B_{12} deficiency, pernicious anemia

Table 7 Ancillary Laboratory Studies for Dementia Evaluations

Test	Rationale and indications
Tests for syphilis	Neurosyphilis (in endemic areas, exposure, unreactive pupils)
HIV	AIDS (risk factors identified)
Urinalysis	Urinary tract infection (incontinence or urinary complaints)
Sedimentation rate	Vasculitis, temporal arteritis, chronic infection
Blood gases	Hypoxia, hypercarbia (lung disease, carbon monoxide exposure)
Drug screen	Alcohol, prescription and recreational drugs (exposure)
Heavy metals	Lead and arsenic poisoning (exposure, peripheral neuropathy)
Hu antibody	Paraneoplastic limbic encephalitis (history of relevant cancer)
Ceruloplasmin	Wilson's disease (liver disease, young age, dystonia)
Homocysteine	Risk factor for vascular dementia and perhaps Alzheimer's disease
Carbohydrate deficient transferrin	Clinically unapparent alcoholism
Apolipoprotein E genotype	Genetic risk factor for Alzheimer's disease
Presenilin 1 genotype	Familial early-onset Alzheimer's disease
Folate	Nutritional deficiency

symptoms and reveal which of several conditions is the predominant cause of the dementia. For instance, in a patient with mixed dementia due to AD and stroke, gradual progression of dementia without further strokes on MRI suggests that AD has caused the worsening of symptoms. By contrast, if there is sudden worsening

Table 8 Causes of Dementia that Can Be Detected Early with Structural Brain Imaging

Primary and metastatic brain tumors
Ischemic stroke
Intracerebral hemorrhage
Subarachnoid hemorrhage
Subdural hematoma
Multiple sclerosis
Brain abscess
Progressive multifocal leukoencephalopathy
Traumatic brain injury
Normal pressure hydrocephalus
Creutzfeldt–Jakob disease (diffusion-weighted and FLAIR MRI only)

Abbreviation: FLAIR MRI, fluid attenuated inversion recovery magnetic resonance imaging.

of dementia associated with new focal deficits, stroke is implicated as the cause of worsening and is likely to be more important. Unfortunately, awaiting serial observations entails delaying diagnosis and appropriate interventions.

In most cases, the cause of dementia currently can be determined with a high degree of accuracy, but not complete certainty. Consensus diagnostic criteria are available for several dementing diseases and can help, but they cannot address all clinical situations. Physicians must approach diagnosis with conviction and humility, recognizing the limits of current knowledge. The cause of cognitive impairment always should be considered open to review and possible revision until it is confirmed by pathologic examination (usually impossible during life) or the identification of a causative genetic mutation (relevant only in early-onset familial dementia). It is appropriate for physicians to recommend that families always obtain a postmortem examination to confirm clinical diagnoses, particularly because the results may have substantial implications for other family members.

The Rationale for Early Recognition and Evaluation

It is an accepted principle in medicine that early treatment is more effective than waiting and trying to treat the complications and full ravages of a disease. Of course, this assumes that the disease and its appropriate treatment are known. Otherwise, there is a risk that treatments will cause more harm than benefit. As already outlined, it is not easy to recognize cognitive impairment early and determine its cause. Consequently, some have argued that the evaluation and diagnosis of dementia should be delayed as long as possible to minimize diagnostic errors and avoid the adverse social consequences of labeling a person with dementia (32). It is true that the diagnosis of a dementing disease can lead to unwarranted rationing of medical care, unnecessary restrictions in activities, social stigma, discrimination by insurance companies, and altered perception of family and friends. Nevertheless, early recognition and treatment of dementia has many benefits that more than offset these disadvantages (Table 9). These benefits are particularly compelling when the rights of patient autonomy are considered and treatments become more effective. Medical paternalism has lost favor; we increasingly recognize that patients have the right to know what their physicians know about their condition, and the right to be involved in decisions that affect them (4). Societal misunderstanding and discrimination against people with cognitive impairment need to be addressed, but it is spurious to believe that the best medical response is to delay diagnosis or interventions. Individuals seeking medical attention for cognitive impairment already may have great distress, and there are social consequences of cognitive impairment regardless of medical care. Furthermore, unless early evaluation of dementia is undertaken, patients risk unnecessary disease complications and may lose the support of family and friends who misinterpret problems as volitional.

Table 9   Benefits of Early Recognition and Evaluation of Cognitive Impairment

Drug treatments are more effective if begun early
Permanent neuronal damage can be prevented in reversible dementias
Coexisting illnesses that may amplify symptoms can be treated
Complications of inappropriate treatments can be avoided
Disease complications can be prevented or identified and treated early
Home and driving safety can be assessed to prevent problems
Social supports can be provided to assist family members and permit patient to remain
   at home
Patients can participate in decision making and plan for their own future care

Utilizing New Diagnostic Technologies

New biomarkers and technology will develop as we learn more about the biochemical and anatomic pathology of specific dementing disorders. These advances will provide a great opportunity to improve diagnostic accuracy. It will be a significant challenge to determine how to use this new diagnostic technology most effectively. Diagnostic testing can be extremely valuable, but it also can be misused (Table 10). The proper application of new technology to dementia care always must involve individualized clinical assessment and treatment.

There is concern that new technology and preferential reimbursement for procedures have undervalued and damaged the therapeutic relationship patients develop with their physicians. Clinicians will need to integrate new diagnostic methods without losing the traditional humanistic values of clinical medicine. The professional relationship that develops with a patient is especially important in dementia care, because dementia alters even a patient's unique intellect and personality. To provide optimal dementia care, a physician must know very personal information about daily habits, and inner thoughts and feelings. The astute physician also must expand the professional relationship, which is traditionally with the patient alone, to include family members and caregivers (3). Such a therapeutic triad is a major asset during evaluation to provide a knowledgeable informant and to help explain the purpose and results of diagnostic

Table 10   Potential Misuses of Diagnostic Technology

Overuse—cost of needlessly repeated studies
Overdependence—using test results to decide whether there is dementia when clinical
   assessment is reliable; using test results to make a diagnosis without utilizing other
   relevant clinical data
Overinterpretation—assigning cause of dementia to clinically insignificant test results
Misinterpretation—failing to recognize the presence of clinically significant abnormal-
   ities, or mistaking a result as abnormal when it is not
Omission—failure to incorporate significant imaging findings in diagnosis

testing. Good communication between physician and caregivers also is critical to the success of ongoing care as symptoms continue to evolve.

Incorporating new diagnostic techniques will add greater complexity to the already intellectually demanding task of dementia evaluation. Test results cannot be considered in isolation. Instead, they have to be considered along with other evidence to decide the cause of symptoms. Sensitivity, specificity, predictive value, and the circumstances of testing must be taken into account following the principles of evidence-based medicine (33). Genetic testing, which can be more definitive than most diagnostic tests, adds further complexity to a dementia evaluation since ethical and legal implications for family members must be considered (34).

In addition to threatening traditional values and increasing the complexity of evaluations, new diagnostic tests will increase the costs of a dementia evaluation. Furthermore, invasive tests could cause physical harm. We should use new diagnostic methods wisely. The best strategy is to know their benefits and limitations, and use them only when clinical history and examination fail tests seem unlikely to be of much provide a highly confidant, accurate, and specific diagnosis. Technological advances that overcome current limitations will improve care and simultaneously justify their expense and burden for patients.

DIFFICULT DIAGNOSTIC CROSSROADS AND DECISION POINTS

The assessment of cognitive impairment and dementia requires a series of difficult decisions (Table 11). Some decision points will benefit from new technologies, others will not. New diagnostic tests seem unlikely to be of much benefit when deciding whether to initiate a dementia evaluation. Cognitive complaints, especially of memory lapses, are almost universal, and physicians will need to continue to rely upon their clinical judgment that further investigations are warranted. Patient and family complaints will continue to be important indicators of a significant problem, because medical advice about

Table 11   Difficult Diagnostic Crossroads and Decision Points

Identifying prodromal dementia in patients with cognitive impairment
Distinguishing single and multiple domain cognitive deficits
Distinguishing neurodegenerative disease from psychiatric illness
Identifying coexisting neurodegenerative disease
Identifying the cause of rapidly progressive dementia
Distinguishing AD and mimics of AD
Distinguishing dementias with parkinsonism
Recognizing mixed dementia
Selection and monitoring of treatment

Abbreviation: AD, Alzheimer's disease.

cognitive complaints is usually sought only when symptoms seem unusual, persistent, or severe. Deciding whether a patient has dementia or not also appears unlikely to benefit from new diagnostic technology. The threshold for determining that cognitive impairments are sufficient to impair everyday activities will continue to require much clinical information that must be judged based upon individual circumstances. The limitations of laboratory tests for this purpose are easily demonstrated. A brain scan can identify a stroke, but cannot tell whether it is causing symptoms. Likewise, while the genetic test for Huntington's disease can be definitive, it cannot be used to decide whether a person has chorea.

There is also a risk of overdependence on new diagnostic technology. Conventional laboratory testing and neuroimaging are already very good at identifying focal mass lesions, medical illnesses, and most dementing disorders that begin suddenly. Cognitive impairment caused by medication is also readily discernible and easily remedied without further diagnostic studies. As new methods become available, we should not overlook or abandon these already successful components of the dementia evaluation.

Several inevitable diagnostic decision points or crossroads are reached that would benefit significantly from new diagnostic approaches and biomarkers. Some reflect the challenges of diagnosing an illness well before its full extent is evident. Others involve the difficulty in unambiguously identifying common dementing diseases that lack distinctive clinical, laboratory, or imaging features or when multiple conditions are occurring simultaneously. Each of these decision points presents its own challenges and demands a different solution.

Identifying Prodromal Dementia in Patients with Cognitive Impairment

The earliest possible clinical recognition of dementing diseases requires identifying individuals currently without functional deficits whose cognitive impairment later will progress to frank dementia. Such individuals could be categorized as having MCI, CIND, or might be judged to be performing as expected for their age or for their background. Our current ability to recognize patients with prodromal dementia is unknown and varies immensely depending upon physician expertise and interest. Individual characteristics of patients and families undoubtedly play a crucial role in whether such individuals are recognized or brought to clinical attention. Even when cognitive complaints do not appear to be significant, it is appropriate to reassess patients later since they may be aware of changes that have not yet become clinically evident (10).

As currently constituted, MCI and CIND both include a heterogeneous group of disorders, some progressive and others stable. Not everyone with MCI or CIND has prodromal dementia, although everyone with progressive dementia that began insidiously first must have had cognitive impairment insufficient to interfere with everyday function. There is no easy solution for dealing with the issue of prodromal dementia. Some have suggested that physicians should assume that cognitive impairment represents early dementia to avoid delaying treatment (35). This approach is attractive for its simplicity and practicality, but it ignores the reality of a complex situation. Some individuals with MCI, and up to 5% to 10% of individuals with CIND, are found to revert to normal on re-examination (19). Thus, there would be many serious diagnostic errors with potential adverse consequences to patients and families if everyone classified as MCI or CIND were presumed to have prodromal dementia. The preferable alternative is to indicate the increased risk of a dementing disease and recommend close observation (36). However, this approach is unsatisfying to physician and patient alike and brings with it other problems. Patients and families must endure uncertainty and are unable to plan for the future. We already know from people at-risk for Huntington's disease that the uncertainty of having a serious illness in the future has its own morbidity and burden (37). Serial examinations raise issues of their own. What represents a significant change? When is test variability explained by normal fluctuations in performance? Our current inability to recognize when cognitive impairment alone represents a dementing disease delays diagnosis and treatment. We urgently need new diagnostic methods to address this important clinical decision point.

Distinguishing Single and Multiple Domain Cognitive Deficits

Impairment in only a single cognitive domain has special diagnostic and prognostic implications. A mild deficit in a single cognitive area can be benign and represent a previously unsuspected learning disability or a normal variation in ability. On the other hand, some neurodegenerative disorders characteristically have a focal onset. In these cases, demonstration of a circumscribed cognitive deficit can be helpful in early diagnosis. For example, FTD often begins as a progressive aphasia or semantic dementia, and corticobasal degeneration often starts with a strongly lateralized apraxia and motor disturbance (26,38). Deficit in a single cognitive domain also justifies a careful search for an explanatory small stroke or mass lesion.

By contrast, multiple domain cognitive deficits are more likely to represent prodromal dementia. MCI patients with cognitive deficits in multiple domains are more likely to progress to dementia over two years than those with only memory impairment (39). Neurodegenerative diseases typically cause pervasive deficits, even if there is a single predominant symptom. For example, patients with AD may have predominant language deficits or visuospatial deficits (40).

It often is not obvious whether cognitive impairment involves a single or multiple cognitive domains. An adept mental status examination, the skills of a speech pathologist, and standardized neuropsychological assessment can help, but may not be definitive. Clinical findings are not always reliable because they can be highly subjective and must be interpreted. Several functional brain imaging techniques offer the potential to more objectively assess whether there are abnormalities in brain areas serving specific cognitive domains. These imaging methods and objective biomarkers could significantly aid the difficult clinical decision crossroad of characterizing the extent of brain dysfunction.

Identifying When Cognitive Impairment Is Due to Psychiatric Illness

Mood and behavior disturbance often leads to a diagnostic conundrum. Both psychiatric disease and dementing disorders frequently cause cognitive impairment with behavioral symptoms. Families commonly report that behavior changes were an early symptom of what later clearly became a dementing disease. Many people find personality and behavior changes especially disturbing and they may be more likely to motivate an evaluation than memory problems. Many behavioral symptoms commonly are seen in AD (41). Apathy is probably the most common behavioral symptom, which often leads physicians and families to misinterpret symptoms as being due to depression. Furthermore, mood clearly can be affected when individuals recognize progressive problems with their memory. Since major depression can develop de novo in the course of AD, it should also be considered a complication of dementia (42).

It is characteristic for behavioral disturbance to be the initial and most prominent symptom in FTD. Behaviors may be so unusual that FTD is more likely to be misdiagnosed as a psychiatric disorder rather than as another dementing disorder. Symptoms like disinhibition, stereotypy, emotional shallowness, mental inflexibility, perseveration, and compulsions are sufficiently uncommon in dementing disorders that they are useful in diagnostic criteria and symptom checklists (26,43). Psychiatric disease is more common than dementia in younger age groups, and FTD often has an early age of onset. So it is no surprise that it is often difficult to distinguish FTD from psychiatric illness, until other cognitive deficits become apparent.

In psychiatric illness, there can be objective evidence of cognitive problems or they can be more perceived than real. There is increasing evidence that chronic schizophrenia can cause progressive dementia (44). Psychosis and mood disturbance due to any psychiatric disease sometimes are severe enough to interfere with cognitive performance and everyday activities, yet resolve when treated with psychotropic medication. Substance abuse also can cause memory loss and cognitive impairment, both when patients are under the influence of a drug, and as a long-term complication, such as Wernicke's disease (45). Depression is especially easily mistaken for a dementing disease because it, like neurodegenerative diseases, often develops late in life. Typical features of major depression also often are not expressed fully in the elderly (46). Depression frequently causes memory complaints. While patients with dementing diseases generally complain of less difficulty than family members, the reverse is typically the case for patients with depression. Distinguishing depression can be particularly difficult when cognitive complaints are accompanied by social withdrawal and lack of interest that alter everyday function. Diagnostic guidelines and criteria for depression may be helpful, but they still require the subjective and sometimes unreliable interpretation of symptoms.

The usual recommendation is to identify and treat depression and psychiatric illness before proceeding further with a dementia evaluation. This approach is appropriate given current options, but it may delay recognition and appropriate treatment of an underlying dementing disorder, especially if the response to antidepressant treatment is ambiguous. Since the biochemical and anatomic abnormalities in psychiatric and neurodegenerative diseases differ so markedly, it is reasonable to expect that future technologies will distinguish them.

Identifying Coexisting Neurodegenerative Disease

Even when an evaluation identifies a potential cause of cognitive impairment, there still is uncertainty that it accounts for a patient's symptoms. Laboratory studies may detect a medical illness, but treatment often does not completely reverse symptoms (47). This can be because the illness has already caused permanent neuronal injury, and stabilization of symptoms is the most that can be expected. Alternatively, the medical illness might persist despite the best treatment. For example, in some cases chronic renal failure and hepatic failure may be incurable, and symptoms would be expected to continue and fluctuate as the underlying illness varies. A final possible explanation is that there is a coexisting dementing disease. Currently, it is impossible to know which explanation is correct without serial assessments to see if impairments improve, are stable, fluctuate along with the medical condition, or are progressive. If symptoms are progressive despite effective treatment, there clearly is an additional dementing disorder whose diagnosis and treatment has been delayed greatly. In disorders where treatments are ineffective or only partially effective, recognition of an unrelated, clearly progressive dementing disorder often is delayed even longer until dementia is very severe.

Uncertainty in the outcome of delirium poses a similar problem and illustrates how common it is for causes of cognitive impairment to coexist. Medical care for dementia commonly begins with an episode of delirium. One study found that 40% of adults with dementia had a superimposed delirium on admission to the hospital. On the other hand, only 25% of those with delirium were found to have dementia, once their acute mental status changes had resolved (48). Usually a medical condition causing the delirium can be identified; nevertheless, a coexisting dementing disorder still must be considered. Patients with dementia are not only particularly prone to delirium, but also may have a prolonged period of recovery from delirium. This problem often appears in hospitalized patients. Pain medications, anesthetic agents, and sedatives frequently induce a protracted postoperative delirium in elderly patients. If not recognized and treated appropriately, delirium can cause either a misplaced presumption of dementia or delay the evaluation of an underlying dementing disease.

The possibility of medication induced cognitive impairment also can delay the recognition of a neurodegenerative disease. Medications commonly cause cognitive side effects, especially with aging that alters the metabolism of many drugs. The list of medications with potential to cause cognitive impairment is long. Some individual medications and classes of medications are particularly of concern (49). Psychotropic and sedative medications are common culprits, but drugs given primarily for systemic illnesses also can cause cognitive problems. Sometimes, it is possible to temporally relate the onset of symptoms with the first use of the medication. In other cases, the role of medication is proven when it is stopped and cognitive symptoms resolve. When discontinuance of medication cannot be medically justified, there may be little recourse except for serial observations. In any case, when medications are a potential factor, considerable clinical judgment is required and there is a delay in the final resolution of causality and treatment.

Even finding a serious neurological disease does not assure that the cause of cognitive impairment is established, and a progressive dementia may later be recognized. Brain atrophy caused by dementing diseases increases the risk of a subdural hematoma, and amyloid angiopathy of AD can cause intracerebral hemorrhage (50). Seizures beginning late in life also can be diagnostically ambiguous. Seizures cause memory lapses; in particular, partial complex seizures may be misdiagnosed as a dementing disease, especially because they also can cause behavioral changes. A suspected seizure disorder can be confirmed readily with an EEG. However, stroke and AD may explain the seizure disorder, making several explanations of dementia possible even when seizures appear to account for symptoms. The use of anticonvulsants adds another possible explanation. Clearly, we need diagnostic methods that can identify specific neurodegenerative diseases even when other causes of cognitive impairment are present.

Identifying the Cause of Rapidly Progressive Dementia

Dementia that becomes severe in less than a year requires urgent evaluation. Diseases that cause such rapidly progressive dementia differ from those with a more indolent course (Table 12). In addition to the clinical assessment and laboratory and imaging studies performed in a usual dementia evaluation, such cases warrant further testing, including a spinal fluid examination and an EEG. Many causes of rapidly progressive dementia are readily detected. Intracranial mass lesions are more likely, and delirium also must be considered. Bacterial, tuberculous, fungal, and viral infections can be identified with blood and spinal fluid cultures and testing for specific antigens. Paraneoplastic antibodies and spinal fluid cytology can help detect malignancies that are not identified on a physical examination or imaging studies. An EEG can identify non-convulsive

Table 12   Causes of Rapidly Progressive Dementia

Creutzfeldt–Jakob disease
Meningitis/encephalitis (including TB, fungal, herpes, carcinomatous, paraneoplastic)
Vasculitis
CNS lymphoma, primary and metastatic brain tumors
Subdural hematoma
Non-convulsive status epilepticus
Multi-infarct dementia (occasionally)
Alzheimer's disease (rarely)

Abbreviations: TB, tuberculosis; CNS, central nervous system.

status epilepticus. However, despite such extensive testing, it still may be difficult to determine the cause of rapidly progressive dementia.

It is particularly important to identify Creutzfeldt–Jakob disease (CJD) so proper precautions can be used to prevent the potential iatrogenic transmission (51). Definitively identifying CJD is difficult, but several clinical findings and laboratory tests often are abnormal in CJD and can aid diagnosis. Sequential EEGs may demonstrate the evolution of typical periodic discharges. MRI can reveal focal abnormalities in the cerebral cortex or striatum with diffusion-weighted or FLAIR sequences (52). High levels of the 14-3-3 protein usually can be detected in the spinal fluid (53). Clinical criteria for CJD have been developed incorporating these features (54).

Despite such clues, the diagnosis of CJD can remain elusive. Although diagnosis can often be made easily when typical features have evolved, early definitive identification of CJD is not easy, and a substantial group of patients have atypical features. CJD can have a surprising variety of clinical presentations. There can be initial memory loss that suggests AD, focal cognitive deficits that suggest a focal lesion, or a gait disorder that suggests a neurodegenerative disease. Some of these clinical phenotypes can be explained by variations in prion protein glycotype and its interaction with prion genotype, but this information currently is available only after a brain biopsy or autopsy (55). New variant CJD associated with bovine spongiform encephalopathy also has atypical features (56). Current laboratory testing for CJD is also fallible and cannot be relied upon when symptoms are atypical. While a spinal fluid 14-3-3 protein can be helpful if it is elevated, it is not always abnormal in CJD, and it can be elevated in several other disorders associated with rapid brain destruction (57). Brain biopsy is sometimes the only way to avoid the serious consequences of misdiagnosis or treatment delay.

Rapidly progressive dementia illustrates how clinical methods and diagnostic technology sometimes must be reconciled. The serious implications of a rapidly progressive dementia must be weighed against the costs and real risks of brain biopsy to the patient, surgical team, and pathology staff. The quandary of whether to perform this invasive testing is further complicated if there is difficulty in determining whether the illness really is progressing rapidly. There may not be informants, or their stories may differ. The physician then must consider all the evidence and judge its quality. Because of the need for urgent intervention, any suspicion must favor brain biopsy if no cause has been identified. However, if there is suspicion that historical information is inaccurate, it may be appropriate to defer brain biopsy until the rapid decline is confirmed by serial examinations. Such situations illustrate why there is still considerable need for practical biomarkers to identify disorders causing rapidly progressive dementia.

Distinguishing Alzheimer's Disease and Mimics of Alzheimer's Disease

AD was not recognized as the most common cause of dementia until systematic autopsy studies were performed in the 1960s and 1970s (58,59). Early investigations found that the clinical diagnosis of AD was frequently wrong. Subsequently, with the development of explicit criteria, comprehensive evaluation methods, and brain imaging, the clinical diagnosis of AD has become significantly more accurate, yet diagnostic errors remain (60,61). Today most errors are due to "AD mimics," illnesses that are clinically indistinguishable from AD (Table 13).

AD mimics can occur when there are atypical presentations of a dementing disorder that usually does not resemble AD. This may happen when such a disorder's typically distinctive features have not yet appeared. For example, familial CJD may have a course of many years that is very similar to AD and lack periodic EEG discharges (62). Likewise, progressive supranuclear palsy may lack its typical eye movement abnormalities (63).

Most AD mimics are disorders that ordinarily share so many characteristics with AD that they are difficult to distinguish. FTD and dementia with Lewy bodies (DLB) are the most important examples. Patients with FTD characteristically have particularly prominent behavioral or language disturbances, yet they frequently also meet diagnostic criteria for AD (64). Behavioral and language symptoms are common in both AD and FTD. Impaired judgment and insight is frequent in both AD and FTD, and probably reflects involvement of the

Table 13 Alzheimer's Disease and Its Mimics

Alzheimer's disease
Frontotemporal dementia, including Pick's disease
Dementia with Lewy bodies
Vascular dementia
Progressive supranuclear palsy
Familial Creutzfeldt–Jakob disease
Corticobasal degeneration

frontal association cortex. Aphasia also is not unique to FTD, and has long been considered a cardinal feature of AD as indicated in diagnostic criteria for AD (21). Diagnostic criteria suggest FTD can be distinguished from AD by the relatively early onset of behavioral and language symptoms, but this requires considerable subjective medical judgment. It also may be helpful to identify behavioral and language symptoms often seen in FTD but uncommon in AD, such as disinhibition, apathy, perseverative behavior, stereotypy of speech, echolalia, and mutism. However, their reliability and specificity for FTD are uncertain, and improvements in clinical criteria for FTD are still needed (65). Nevertheless, such differences in type, predominance, and evolution of symptoms are the basis for behavioral inventories meant to aid clinical diagnosis (43). Structural brain imaging may help distinguish AD and FTD by contrasting the severity of atrophy in involved brain regions (66). Probably the most frequent pathologic abnormality in FTD is nonspecific neuronal loss and gliosis with or without vacuolization. However, FTD sometimes is caused by distinctive abnormalities in tau, ubiquitin, or neurofilament protein (67,68). Eventually these should permit the development of biomarkers that identify histopathological subtypes of FTD.

DLB is another important AD mimic that now appears to be the second most common cause of dementia in the United States. It accounted for approximately 20% of all dementia cases in recent autopsy series (69). Although DLB always has pathologic changes characteristic of Parkinson's disease, it may not have noticeable motor signs or other distinctive features (70). DLB has the same biochemical signature of dopamine deficiency typical of Parkinson's disease and also has characteristic deposits of ubiquitin in cortical Lewy bodies; it is realistic to expect new diagnostic methods could exploit these features and aid in diagnosis.

Distinguishing the Cause of Dementia with Parkinsonism

Dementia is often accompanied by the same slowing of gait, rigidity, impaired balance, and bradykinesia usually associated with Parkinson's disease. Parkinsonism can precede the onset of dementia, develop concurrently, or appear only after many years of cognitive impairment. Clinicians now have considerable difficulty in distinguishing the several disorders causing dementia with parkinsonism (Table 14).

The thoughtful clinician faces a diagnostic quandary when confronting a demented patient with parkinsonism. With the exception of unusual cases where parkinsonism is caused by strategically placed cerebral infarcts, conventional laboratory studies and structural imaging provide little assistance. Unlike the pathologist who can identify, quantify, and localize neuronal loss and characteristic inclusions, the clinician is relegated to basing diagnostic judgments solely on clinical history and examination. In an admirable effort to achieve clarity and uniformity in diagnostic classification, consensus clinical criteria have been developed that are heavily dependent upon the relative timing of motor and

Table 14 Causes of Dementia with Parkinsonism

Dementia with Lewy bodies
Parkinson's disease
Alzheimer's disease
Frontotemporal dementia, including frontotemporal dementia with parkinsonism linked to chromosome 17 (FTDP-17)
Progressive supranuclear palsy
Corticobasal degeneration
Vascular dementia (rarely)

cognitive symptom onset (24). The criteria indicate that when spontaneous motor symptoms precede the onset of dementia, the cause is Parkinson's disease with dementia. If motor symptoms and dementia occur simultaneously early in the illness, the clinical diagnosis is DLB. However, if motor symptoms develop late in a progressive dementia, the cause is AD. Additional criteria address other symptoms and amplify these categories, but symptom onset remains critical to classification. Unfortunately, rules of symptom onset are arbitrary and require subjective interpretation of historical information that sometimes is limited or unreliable. These clinical criteria understandably have only modest ability to predict pathology (71). New technology to replicate biochemical and anatomic information used by pathologists for classification would aid diagnosis and development of more specific treatments enormously.

The challenges of clinical diagnosis of parkinsonism and dementia are understandable. Because continued use of drugs may be clinically necessary, it may be impossible to determine the onset of motor symptoms or whether they are spontaneous, as required by criteria. Extrapyramidal symptoms also are frequently seen in AD, although they usually begin later than in DLB. In one study that monitored motor symptoms prospectively, over half of patients with moderately severe AD develop new parkinsonian signs over two years (72). Consequently, many disorders causing parkinsonism also are AD mimics. For example, FTD may cause parkinsonism. This is particularly relevant in FTD with parkinsonism linked to chromosome 17 (FTDP-17), an early-onset, autosomal dominant disorder. In some families with FTDP-17, parkinsonism even may be the presenting symptom, and much more evident than dementia (73).

The consideration of additional symptoms considered in criteria for DLB may not resolve the difficulty with clinical diagnosis. For example, consensus criteria use visual hallucinations and fluctuations to distinguish DLB. However, medications and AD may cause visual hallucinations (74). Family reports of fluctuations can be difficult to interpret, and subjective clinical judgment is required to know when fluctuations are significant.

Pathologic studies also suggest why clinical diagnosis is so challenging. Cerebral Lewy bodies are accompanied by pathological changes of AD about two-thirds of the time (75). Thus some have called this "Lewy body variant of AD" (76). Much additional work will be needed to clarify these difficult clinical issues.

Recognizing Mixed Dementia

The dictum to avoid overdependence upon Occam's razor is amply demonstrated by the evidence that vascular and AD pathology frequently coexist. This co-occurrence of AD and vascular pathology is often termed "mixed dementia" (77). Mixed dementia is particularly frequent in the "oldest-old" (age 85 or older), the age group that will increase the most over the next several decades (2). We greatly need to improve our ability to diagnose mixed dementia. Current brain imaging often identifies vascular lesions, yet there is no easy way to determine how they contribute to patient symptoms. We know that vascular disease and AD interact in important ways to increase the likelihood of clinically significant cognitive decline (78,79). However, most reports on dementia focus on separate, "pure" clinical entities, and most effort has been focused on distinguishing vascular dementia from AD, rather than determining when both are present and clinically important.

Traditional approaches have suggested that the extent of vascular lesions on MRI scan might be useful, but recent studies have found this inaccurate (80). A requirement that dementia develop in association with a clinically recognized stroke has also been suggested by NINDS-AIREN criteria for vascular dementia (22). However, accurate historical information may be difficult, or cognitive changes may have been overlooked in the face of major motor deficits. Perhaps as a consequence, the requirement for time linkage appears to cause insensitivity for vascular dementia (80). The demonstration of focal motor or sensory deficits on the neurological examination might appear sufficient, but they may resolve, or strokes might affect areas of the brain associated with cognition without damaging motor or sensory pathways. In other cases, individual strokes may be too small to recognize clinically. Furthermore, subtle focal deficits may be difficult to elicit if the patient is evaluated only when severely demented.

Evidence of impairment of the cerebral cortex on functional imaging studies, rather than the number or location of subcortical infarcts, appears to be the best predictor of dementia (81). The effects of subcortical strokes can be mild, and the most prominent symptoms and metabolic abnormalities often reflect frontal lobe dysfunction (82). The cognitive deficits of strokes appear to be more than additive in their effects, and they may become noticeable only several months later (83,84).

Selection and Monitoring of Treatment

Although treatment is not the focus of this monograph, the selection and monitoring of treatment also can be a diagnostic decision point. A rational therapeutic plan can only be based upon a specific diagnosis. Otherwise, treatment is merely guesswork and outcomes are left to chance. Since imaging aids in identifying the specific cause of dementia, it plays an important role in the selection of initial treatment. Perhaps less well recognized is how the results of diagnostic brain imaging can be incorporated into subsequent treatment decisions. A specific diagnosis helps to predict treatment outcomes. When the response to appropriate disease specific therapy is unexpected, the accuracy of the clinical diagnosis should be questioned. For example, an explanation other than depression should be sought when severe apathy fails to improve with an anti-depressant. In this situation, FTD should be considered. Likewise, the motor symptoms of idiopathic Parkinson's disease almost always respond to treatment with dopaminergic agents. If they have never been beneficial, the diagnosis of Parkinson's disease with dementia is difficult to sustain, and another dementing disorder is more likely. In diagnostic reassessments like these, additional brain imaging methods can be considered or a repeat study that may reveal new or evolving abnormalities can help provide critical confirmatory information.

Since definitive diagnostic test results are usually lacking in dementing disorders, selection of treatment also is not definitive. Diagnostic confidence inevitably modifies physician judgments about treatment. The results of brain imaging can alter diagnostic confidence and influence therapy, particularly as the effects of initial treatments are monitored. For example, treatment with cholinesterase inhibitors might be aggressively pursued when clinical and imaging features are typical of AD, but discontinued if side effects develop when clinical and imaging findings are discordant for this diagnosis. Likewise, a therapeutic trial of drugs used to treat AD sometimes may be warranted when the diagnosis is uncertain. However, they might be avoided or discontinued if imaging finds predominant frontal abnormalities, since cholinesterase inhibitors provide little benefit and may worsen symptoms in FTD (85).

There is also great interest in using brain imaging to evaluate new drug therapies. There is evidence that longitudinal changes in MRI and glucose metabolism measured by positron emission tomography may permit more rapid and cost-effective clinical trials in dementia (86,87). However, validation of an imaging surrogate biomarker for disease progression is a major undertaking. Further investigations are needed before it is clear whether imaging results are reliable and can be appropriately interpreted in complex clinical trials. For example, one recent randomized trial of immunotherapy for AD found surprising imaging results that appear to be discordant with clinical outcomes (88). In the future, it may be possible with molecular imaging to design therapies for dementing diseases based upon individual biochemical profiles and disease staging, just as it is now starting to be used in clinical oncology (89,90).

SUMMARY

The evaluation of dementia is challenging, but worthwhile. Our ability to determine the cause of dementia has improved, but much remains to be done. There are many opportunities to refine our current methods at critical and difficult diagnostic decision points. The accuracy of early diagnosis is particularly important. Recent advances in knowledge about neurodegenerative disease and new technology offer the realistic hope that we will achieve significant progress in dementia diagnosis. However, we must carefully evaluate new imaging methods and biomarkers to assure that they are used appropriately, efficiently, and effectively.

ACKNOWLEDGMENTS

Supported in part by NIH grants RO1-AG22394 and P50-AG08671 (the Michigan AD Research Center), and the Donald W. Reynolds Foundation.

REFERENCES

1. Kawas CH, Katzman R. Epidemiology of dementia and Alzheimer's disease. In: Terry RD, Katzman R, Bick KL, Sisodia SS, eds. Alzheimer Disease. New York: Raven Press, 1999:95–116.
2. Brookmeyer R, Gray S, Kawas C. Projections of Alzheimer's disease in the United States and the public health impact of delaying disease onset. Am J Public Health 1998; 88:1337–1342.
3. Foster NL. Barriers to treatment: the unique challenges for physicians providing dementia care. J Geriatr Psychiatry Neurol 2001; 14:188–198.
4. Drickamer MA, Lachs MS. Should patients with Alzheimer's disease be told their diagnosis? N Engl J Med 1992; 326:947–951.
5. Christakis NA. Death Foretold: Prophecy and Prognosis in Medical Care. Chicago: University of Chicago Press, 1999.
6. Knopman D, Donohue JA, Gutterman EM. Patterns of care in the early stages of Alzheimer's disease: impediments to timely diagnosis. J Am Geriatr Soc 2000; 48:300–304.
7. Rochester-Toronto MRI Study Group. O'Connor P, Detsky AS, Tansey C, Kucharczyk W. Effect of diagnostic testing for multiple sclerosis on patient health perceptions. Arch Neurol 1994; 51:46–51.
8. Foster NL. Neuropsychiatry of dementing disorders. In: Fogel BS, Schiffer RB, Rao S, eds. Neuropsychiatry. New York: Lippincott, Williams and Wilkins, 2003:1034–1070.
9. U.S. Preventive Services Task Force. Screening for dementia: recommendation and rationale. Ann Intern Med 2003; 138:925–926.
10. Costa PT Jr., Williams TF, Somerfield M, et al. Recognition and Initial Assessment of Alzheimer's Disease and Related Dementias. Clinical Practice Guideline No. 19; Rockville, MD, U.S. Department of Health and Human Services, Public Health Service, Agency for Health Care Policy and Research. AHCPR Publication 1996 97-0702, 1996.
11. O'Connor DW, Pollitt PA, Roth M, Brook PB, Reiss BB. Memory complaints and impairment in normal, depressed, and demented elderly persons identified in a community survey. Arch Gen Psychiatry 1990; 47:224–227.

12. Graham JE, Rockwood K, Beattie BL, et al. Prevalence and severity of cognitive impairment with and without dementia in an elderly population. Lancet 1997; 349:1793–1796.

13. Grundman M, Petersen RC, Ferris SH, et al. Mild cognitive impairment can be distinguished from Alzheimer's disease and normal aging for clinical trials. Arch Neurol 2004; 61:59–66.

14. Mesulam M-M. Primary progressive aphasia. Ann Neurol 2001; 49:425–432.

15. Petersen RC. Mild cognitive impairment as a diagnostic entity. J Intern Med 2004; 256:183–194.

16. Jones S, Jonsson Laukka E, Small BJ, Fratiglioni L, Backman L. A preclinical phase in vascular dementia: cognitive impairment three years before diagnosis. Dement Geriatr Cogn Disord 2004; 18:233–239.

17. Luis CA, Barker WW, Loewenstein DA, et al. Conversion to dementia among two groups with cognitive impairment. A preliminary report. Dement Geriatr Cogn Disord 2004; 18:307–313.

18. Geerlings MI, Jonker C, Bouter LM, Ader HJ, Schmand B. Association between memory complaints and incident Alzheimer's disease in elderly people with normal baseline cognition. Am J Psychiatry 1999; 156:531–537.

19. Unverzagt FW, Gao S, Baiyewu O, et al. Prevalence of cognitive impairment: data from the Indianapolis study of health and aging. Neurology 2001; 57:1655–1662.

20. Winblad B, Palmer K, Kivipelto M, et al. Mild cognitive impairment—beyond controversies, towards a consensus: report of the international working group on mild cognitive impairment. J Intern Med 2004; 256:240–246.

21. McKhann G, Drachman D, Folstein M, Katzman R, Price D, Stadlan EM. Clinical diagnosis of Alzheimer's disease: report of the NINCDS-ADRDA work group under the auspices of department of health and human services task force on Alzheimer's disease. Neurology 1984; 34:939–944.

22. Román GC, Tatemichi TK, Erkinjuntti T, et al. Vascular dementia: diagnostic criteria for research studies. Report of the NINDS-AIREN International workshop. Neurology 1993; 43:250–260.

23. Rosen WG, Terry RD, Fuld PA, Katzman R, Peck A. Pathological verification of ischemic score in differentiation of dementia. Ann Neurol 1980; 7:486–488.

24. McKeith IG, Perry EK, Perry RH. For the consortium on dementia with Lewy bodies: report of the second dementia with Lewy body international workshop: diagnosis and treatment. Neurology 1999; 53:902–905.

25. McKeith IG, Galasko D, Kosaka K, et al. Consensus guidelines for the clinical and pathologic diagnosis of dementia with lewy bodies (DLB): report of the consortium on DLB international workshop. Neurology 1996; 47:1113–1124.

26. Neary D, Snowden JS, Gustafson L, et al. Frontotemporal lobar degeneration: a consensus on clinical diagnostic criteria. Neurology 1998; 51:1546–1554.

27. McKhann GM, Albert MS, Grossman M, Miller B, Dickson D, Trojanowski JQ. Clinical and pathological diagnosis of frontotemporal dementia: report of the work group on frontotemporal dementia and Pick's disease. Arch Neurol 2001; 58:1803–1809.

28. Knopman DS, DeKosky ST, Cummings JL, et al. Practice parameter: diagnosis of dementia (an evidence-based review). Report of the quality standards subcommittee of the American academy of neurology. Neurology 2001; 56:1143–1153.

29. Tangarorang G, Kerins G, Besdine R. Clinical approach to the older patient: an overview. In: Cassel C, Leipzig R, Cohen H et al., eds. Geriatric Medicine. New York: Springer-Verlag, 2003:149–162.

30. Drachman DA. Occam's razor, geriatric syndromes, and the dizzy patient. Ann Intern Med 2000; 132:403–404.

31. Hilliard AA, Weinberger SE, Tierney LM, Jr., Midthun DE, Saint S. Clinical problem-solving. Occam's razor versus saint's triad. N Engl J Med 2004; 350:599–603.

32. Connolly NK, Williams ME. Plaques and tangles in approaching dementia. Gerontologist 1993; 33:133–135.

33. Qizilabash N. Evidence-based diagnosis, in evidence-based dementia practice. In: Schneider LS, Chui H, Tariot P, Brodaty H, Kaye J, Erkinjuntti T, eds. Oxford, U.K.: Blackwell Science, 2002:18–25.

34. Hedera P. Ethical principles and pitfalls of genetic testing for dementia. J Geriatr Psychiatry Neurol 2001; 14:213–221.

35. Morris JC, Storandt M, Miller JP, et al. Mild cognitive impairment represents early-stage Alzheimer disease. Arch Neurol 2001; 58:397–405.

36. Petersen RC, Stevens JC, Ganguli M, Tangalos EG, Cummings JL, DeKosky ST. Practice parameter: early detection of dementia: mild cognitive impairment (an evidence-based review): report of the quality standards subcommittee of the American academy of neurology. Neurology 2001; 56:1133–1142.

37. Wiggins S, Whyte P, Huggins M, et al. The psychological consequences of predictive testing for Huntington's disease. N Engl J Med 1992; 327:1401–1405.

38. Litvan I, Bhatia KP, Burn DJ, et al. Movement disorders society scientific issues committee report: SIC task force appraisal of clinical diagnostic criteria for Parkinsonian disorders. Mov Disord 2003; 18:467–486.

39. Bozoki A, Giordani B, Heidebrink JL, Berent S, Foster NL. Mild cognitive impairments predict dementia in non-demented elderly with memory loss. Arch Neurol 2001; 58:411–416.

40. Martin A, Brouwers P, Lalonde F, et al. Towards a behavioral typology of Alzheimer's patients. J Clin Exp Neuropsychol 1986; 8:594–610.

41. Kaufer DI, Cummings JL, Christine D, et al. Assessing the impact of neuropsychiatric symptoms in Alzheimer's disease: the neuropsychiatric inventory caregiver distress scale. J Am Geriatr Soc 1998; 46:210–215.

42. Lyketsos CG, Lee HB. Diagnosis and treatment of depression in Alzheimer's disease. A practical update for the clinician. Dement Geriatr Cogn Disord 2004; 17:55–64.

43. Kertesz A, Davidson W, Fox H. Frontal behavioral inventory: diagnostic criteria for frontal lobe dementia. Can J Neurol Sci 1997; 24:29–36.

44. Friedman JI, Harvey PD, Coleman T, et al. Six-year follow-up study of cognitive and functional status across the lifespan in schizophrenia: a comparison with Alzheimer's disease and normal aging. Am J Psychiatry 2001; 158:1441–1448.

45. Victor M, Adams RD, Collins GH. The Wernicke-Korsakoff Syndrome and Related Neurologic Disorders Due to Alcoholism and Malnutrition. 2nd ed. Philadelphia: F.A. Davis Co., 1989.

46. Yesavage JA, Brink TL, Rose TL, et al. Development and validation of a geriatric depression screening scale: a preliminary report. J Psychiatr Res 1982-1983; 17:37–49.

47. Larson EB, Reifler BV, Featherstone HJ, English DR. Dementia in elderly outpatients: a prospective study. Ann Intern Med 1984; 100:417–423.
48. Lipowski ZJ. Delirium in the elderly patient. N Engl J Med 1989; 320:578–582.
49. Fick DM, Cooper JW, Wade WE, Waller JL, Maclean JR, Beers MH. Updating the Beers criteria for potentially inappropriate medication use in older adults: results of a U.S. consensus panel of experts. Arch Intern Med 2003; 163:2716–2724.
50. Greenberg SM, Rebeck GW, Vonsattel JP, Gomez-Isla T, Hyman BT. Apolipoprotein E epsilon 4 and cerebral hemorrhage associated with amyloid angiopathy. Ann Neurol 1995; 38:254–259.
51. Johnson RT, Gibbs CJ, Jr. Creutzfeldt-Jakob disease and related transmissible spongiform encephalopathies. N Engl J Med 1998; 339:1994–2004.
52. Bahn MM, Parchi P. Abnormal diffusion-weighted magnetic resonance images in Creutzfeldt-Jakob disease. Arch Neurol 1999; 56:577–583.
53. Huang N, Marie SK, Livramento JA, Chammas R, Nitrini R. 14-3-3 protein in the CSF of patients with rapidly progressive dementia. Neurology 2003; 61:354–357.
54. Brandel JP, Delasnerie-Laupretre N, Laplanche JL, Hauw JJ, Alperovitch A. Diagnosis of Creutzfeldt-Jakob disease: effect of clinical criteria on incidence estimates. Neurology 2000; 54:1095–1099.
55. Parchi P, Giese A, Capellari S, et al. Classification of sporadic Creutzfeldt-Jakob disease based on molecular and phenotypic analysis of 300 subjects. Ann Neurol 1999; 46:224–233.
56. Will RG, Zeidler M, Stewart GE, et al. Diagnosis of new variant Creutzfeldt-Jakob disease. Ann Neurol 2000; 47:575–582.
57. Burkhard PR, Sanchez JC, Landis T, Hochstrasser DF. CSF detection of the 14-3-3 protein in unselected patients with dementia. Neurology 2001; 56:1528–1533.
58. Blessed G, Tomlinson BE, Roth M. The association between quantitative measures of dementia and of senile change in the cerebral grey matter of elderly subjects. Br J Psychiatry 1968; 114:797–811.
59. Constantinidis J. Alzheimer's disease a major form of senile dementia? Clinical, anatomical, and genetic data. In: Katzman R, Terry RD, and Bick KL, eds. Alzheimer's Disease: Senile Dementia and Related Disorders. New York: Raven Press. 1978; 7:15–25.
60. Tierney MC, Fisher RH, Lewis AJ, et al. The NINCDS-ADRDA work group criteria for the clinical diagnosis of probable Alzheimer's disease: a clinicopathologic study of 57 cases. Neurology 1988; 38:359–364.
61. Becker JT, Boller F, Lopez OL, Saxton J, McGonigle KL. The natural history of Alzheimer's disease. Description of study cohort and accuracy of diagnosis. Arch Neurol 1994; 51:585–594.
62. Cochran EJ, Bennett DA, Cervenáková L, et al. Familial Creutzfeldt-Jakob disease with a five-repeat octapeptide insert mutation. Neurology 1996; 47:727–733.
63. Nuwer MR. Progressive supranuclear palsy despite normal eye movements. Arch Neurol 1981; 38:784.
64. Varma AR, Snowden JS, Lloyd JJ, Talbot PR, Mann DM, Neary D. Evaluation of the NINCDS-ADRDA criteria in the differentiation of Alzheimer's disease and frontotemporal dementia. J Neurol Neurosurg Psychiatry 1999; 66:184–188.
65. Mendez MF, Perryman KM. Neuropsychiatric features of frontotemporal dementia: evaluation of consensus criteria and review. J Neuropsychiatry Clin Neurosci 2002; 14:424–429.

66. Boccardi M, Laakso MP, Bresciani L, et al. The MRI pattern of frontal and temporal brain atrophy in fronto-temporal dementia. Neurobiol Aging 2003; 24:95–103.
67. Trojanowski JQ, Dickson D. Update on the neuropathological diagnosis of frontotemporal dementias. J Neuropathol Exp Neurol 2001; 60:1123–1126.
68. Josephs KA, Holton JL, Rossor MN, et al. Neurofilament inclusion body disease: a new proteinopathy? Brain 2003; 126:2291–2303.
69. Verghese J, Crystal HA, Dickson DW, Lipton RB. Validity of clinical criteria for the diagnosis of dementia with lewy bodies. Neurology 1999; 53:1974–1982.
70. Stern Y, Jacobs D, Goldman J, et al. An investigation of clinical correlates of Lewy bodies in autopsy-proven Alzheimer disease. Arch Neurol 2001; 58:460–465.
71. Papka M, Rubio A, Schiffer RB, Cox C. Lewy body disease: can we diagnose it? J Neuropsychiatry Clin Neurosci 1998; 10:405–412.
72. Sano M, Ernesto C, Thomas R, et al. For the members of the Alzheimer's disease cooperative study: a controlled trial of selegiline, alpha-tocopherol, or both as treatment for Alzheimer's disease. N Engl J Med 1997; 38:1216–1222.
73. Foster NL, Wilhelmsen K, Sima AAF, Jones MZ, D'Amato C, Gilman S. Participants in the conference: frontotemporal dementia and parkinsonism linked to chromosome 17: a consensus conference. Ann Neurol 1997; 41:706–715.
74. Paulsen JS, Salmon DP, Thal LJ, et al. Incidence of and risk factors for hallucinations and delusions in patients with probable AD. Neurology 2000; 54:1965–1971.
75. Samuel W, Alford M, Hofstetter CR, Hansen L. Dementia with lewy bodies versus pure Alzheimer disease: differences in cognition, neuropathology, cholinergic dysfunction, and synapse density. J Neuropathol Exp Neurol 1997; 56:499–508.
76. Sabbagh MN, Corey-Bloom J, Tiraboschi P, Thomas R, Masliah E, Thal LJ. Neurochemical markers do not correlate with cognitive decline in the lewy body variant of Alzheimer disease. Arch Neurol 1999; 56:1458–1461.
77. Langa KM, Foster NL, Larson EB. Mixed dementia: emerging concepts and therapeutic implications. JAMA 2004; 292:2901–2908.
78. Snowdon DA, Greiner LH, Mortimer JA, Riley KP, Greiner PA, Markesbery WR. Brain infarction and the clinical expression of Alzheimer disease. The nun study. JAMA 1997; 227:813–817.
79. de la Torre JC. Vascular basis of Alzheimer's pathogenesis. Ann NY Acad Sci 2002; 977:196–215.
80. Chui HC, Mack W, Jackson JE, et al. Clinical criteria for the diagnosis of vascular dementia: a multicenter study of comparability and interrater reliability. Arch Neurol 2000; 57:191–196.
81. Kwan LT, Reed BR, Eberling JL, et al. Effects of subcortical cerebral infarction on cortical glucose metabolism and cognitive function. Arch Neurol 1999; 56:809–814.
82. Tullberg M, Fletcher E, DeCarli C, et al. White matter lesions impair frontal lobe function regardless of their location. Neurology 2004; 63:246–253.
83. Wolfe N, Babikian VL, Linn RT, Knoefel JE, DEsposito M, Albert ML. Are multiple cerebral infarcts synergistic? Arch Neurol 1994; 51:211–215.
84. Tatemichi TK, Paik M, Bagiella E, et al. Risk of dementia after stroke in a hospitalized cohort: results of a longitudinal study. Neurology 1994; 44:1885–1891.

85. Chow TW, Mendez MF. Goals in symptomatic pharmacologic management of frontotemporal lobar degeneration. Am J Alzheimers Dis Other Demen 2002; 17:267–272.

86. Fox NC, Cousens S, Scahill R, Harvey RJ, Rossor MN. Using serial registered brain magnetic resonance imaging to measure disease progression in Alzheimer disease: power calculations and estimates of sample size to detect treatment effects. Arch Neurol 2000; 57:339–344.

87. Alexander GE, Chen K, Pietrini P, Rapoport SI, Reiman EM. Longitudinal PET evaluation of cerebral metabolic decline in dementia: a potential outcome measure in Alzheimer's disease treatment studies. Am J Psychiatry 2002; 159:738–745.

88. Fox NC, Black RS, Gilman S, et al. AN1792(QS-21)-201 study: effects of abeta immunization (AN1792) on MRI measures of cerebral volume in Alzheimer disease. Neurology 2005; 64:1563–1572.

89. Lardinois D, Weder W, Hany TF, et al. Staging of non-small-cell lung cancer with integrated positron-emission tomography and computed tomography. N Engl J Med 2003; 348:2500–2507.

90. Van Den Bossche B, Van de Wiele C. Receptor imaging in oncology by means of nuclear medicine: current status. J Clin Oncol 2004; 22:3593–3607.

2

Neuropsychological Screening and Advanced Neuropsychological Tests

Daniela Perani

Departments of Neuroscience and Nuclear Medicine, Vita-Salute San Raffaele University and San Raffaele Scientific Institute, Milan, Italy

Any supermarket cashier can make the diagnosis of Alzheimer's disease.
—Yearbook of Neurology and Neurosurgery (1990)

INTRODUCTION

Dementia is a syndrome characterized by the reduction of cognitive abilities (most often memory) to the point that impairment in daily activities occurs. Clinical assessment, supported by the results of neuropsychological tests, is at present the only in vivo non-invasive screening and diagnostic tool for Alzheimer's disease (AD) and other disorders associated with dementia. Dementia diagnosis, indeed, is based exclusively on clinical, behavioral, and neuropsychological findings according to DSM-IV (1). The same principle applies to the diagnosis of the most common causes of dementia: AD (2), vascular dementia (VaD) (3), and frontotemporal dementia (FTD) (4). According to NINCDS-ADRDA criteria, neuropsychological testing is required to confirm the presence of dementia, established on clinical grounds.

The recent development of symptomatic pharmacological treatment for AD and the possible introduction of new therapies in the near future make the assessment of dementia at its different stages a great scientific and public health challenge. Further, as dementia is a clinical diagnosis, there is no doubt that cognitive assessment plays a crucial role in the detection of early dementia in particular. Cognitive decline is not an inevitable outcome of aging, and can be the result of an incipient, unrecognized pathology. The term mild cognitive impairment (MCI) is reserved for patients whose impairment is documented by neuropsychological testing, but does not affect activities of daily living.

This chapter reviews the principles of neuropsychological assessment of dementia, including the application of standard batteries of neuropsychological tests and of short screening tests. It also analyzes the tests to be applied to detect and assess the specific deficits found in the different forms of dementia, and discusses the advantages and flaws of current screening and diagnostic tests of dementia. Not all patients with dementia evolve and decline in a similar fashion. On this ground, neuropsychological tests can provide a quantitative assessment of specific patients' profiles. Future research should determine the possible predictive value of these profiles.

NEUROPSYCHOLOGICAL ASSESSMENT

An ideal neuropsychological test should be psychometrically adequate. It should thus be reliable, valid, and have a high sensitivity and high specificity.

Reliability refers to the consistency of the information provided by the test, if administered to the same subject by two different examiners, or by the same examiner on two different occasions. An important issue, in particular for follow-up and therapeutic studies, is the availability of alternate forms, to avoid test-retest effects in the case of repeated examinations of the same subjects. The concept of validity is complex and has multiple facets. Validity refers to the function to be assessed in absolute terms (construct validity), or in relation to other tests, which are considered to be valid from the former point of view (concurrent validity). Moreover, diagnostic validity refers to the ability to correctly classify affected and unaffected subjects. The proportion of patients who are actually classified as demented by a test reflects its sensitivity. The sensitivity of a test decreases as a function of the proportion of cases of dementia, which the test is unable to classify (false negatives). The drawback of increasing the sensitivity of a test is the parallel increase of false positives, i.e., patients erroneously classified as demented. Therefore, a second index is crucial, i.e., specificity. Specificity reflects the proportion of non-demented subjects, which are correctly classified by the test. At present, the majority of diagnostic tests for dementia show very good sensitivity and specificity in the moderate stage of the disease, but not in the early stage. The Mini-Mental State Examination (MMSE) (5), for example, shows a sensitivity of 87% and a specificity of 92% for scores of 23–24 (6). Another issue is the need for tests with high sensitivity and specificity, not only in the very early, even "preclinical," and moderate stages of the disease, but also during the late stages (severe dementia).

A necessary step in order to fulfill the criteria for psychometric adequacy is the standardization of the testing procedures, and the availability of normative data, which allows to control for the effects of age, gender, and education. In principle, socioeconomic status and cultural background are also known to affect the performance on neuropsychological testing.

On practical grounds, there are a number of approaches to the cognitive assessment of dementia. A basic distinction is between clinical cognitive assessment, the application of intelligence tests, screening tests, and formal neuropsychological assessment, based on psychometric tests with normative values.

Clinical Assessment

The clinical evaluation of mental function is a part of the neurological and psychiatric examination. It consists of a series of "paper and pencil" tests that are aimed at investigating the main cognitive areas with only limited supportive material. The patient's performances are not measured quantitatively, but on the basis of the clinical experience of the examiner. There are several published guides to the neuropsychological examination at the "patient's bedside" (7–9). This kind of cognitive evaluation is the only level of assessment that is required by most diagnostic criteria, such as DSM-IV. It is, however, recommended to complete the assessment with brief quantitative screening tests. The clinical assessment can be standardized using rating scales, such as the Global Deterioration Scale (GDS) (10) and Clinical Dementia Rating (CDR) (11), which also include an assessment of functional status.

Medical history even in mildly affected patients should always include information from both patient and caregiver. In particular, the assessment of awareness of cognitive dysfunction might help in the distinction between AD and MCI. While most MCI patients tend to overestimate cognitive deficits when compared to their caregiver's assessment, AD patients in the early stages of disease underestimate cognitive dysfunction (12). Anosognosia can thus be regarded as a characteristic symptom at a stage of very mild AD, but not MCI.

Intelligence Tests

Tests that have been developed for the standardized evaluation of intelligence level in normal subjects have been traditionally used to assess cognitive decline due to neurological dysfunction. The intelligence quotient (IQ) provided, for example, by the Wechsler Adult Intelligence Scale (WAIS) battery has been used to diagnose and assess dementia. The IQ evaluates the multidimensionality of mental ability and provides a global score that characterizes an individual's performance as a whole, as well as a measure of aggregate intelligence that is composed of elements or abilities that are qualitatively differentiable (13). An early observation is that discrepancies between some verbal and performance tasks are evident in normal aging and accentuate in early dementia. Wechsler himself noticed that some subtests tend to "Hold" (Vocabulary, Information, Object Assembly, and Picture Completion) opposed to "Don't Hold" tests (Digit Span, Similarities, Digit Symbol, and Block Design). On this basis, he proposed a deterioration quotient (Hold–Don't Hold/Hold), which has been used as an index of dementia.

The length of the administration procedures, as well as the development of tests that are directly related to the cognitive impairments and that are specific to dementia, has progressively reduced the diffusion of the diagnostic application of intelligence tests. However, it should be noted that the use of the WAIS subtests with an emphasis on the quality of the responses rather than on the quantity is a source of interesting supplementary information for the clinician (14,15). There are abbreviated versions of the WAIS (16), which continue to be used in AD patients (17).

Screening Tests

These include a number of tests that can be administered in a limited amount of time and provide a brief examination of multiple aspects of cognition. Adequate psychometric information is available for some of these measures, such as the MMSE.

Mini-Mental State Examination

The MMSE is the most widely used short screening instrument for dementia. Since it has been translated into many languages, it represents an almost universal way of assessing the severity of dementia in individuals as well as in population samples. It tests a limited number of cognitive functions and can be administered in about 10 to 15 minutes. The score ranges from 0 to 30, and the "cut-off score" below which dementia can be suspected is 24. Normative data, which allow correction of raw values on the basis of age and education, are available for several languages. The test has good sensitivity at scores lower than 24, but it is influenced by age and educational variables, and shows less sensitivity in other neurological diseases such as Huntington's disease, multiple sclerosis, and Parkinson's disease. Huntington's disease patients showed distinct cognitive profiles in comparison to AD with better orientation for date and recall of words (18). The profile differences were independent of the severity of dementia and were able to classify patients as AD or Huntington's disease with 84% accuracy. A modified version of the MMSE has been proposed for patients with Parkinson's disease (19).

The Short Mental Status Test

This is another short screening test, including an improved memory test, which has been recently shown to increase sensitivity in comparison to MMSE in patients with MCI (20).

Clinical Dementia Rating Scale

Each patient with dementia presents with different progression rates. It might be important to obtain a clinical subdivision in dementia stages, without considering disease progression as a fixed and stereotyped model. CDR represents the most diffuse method of evaluation both in clinics and in research (21,22). CDR score is obtained by information provided by a caregiver or an operator and by a cognitive examination that assesses memory, judgment, abstract reasoning, and spatial and temporal orientation, plus evaluation of social and working activity, hobbies, and activities of daily living. The scores are 0 (normal), 0.5 (possible impairment), 1 (mild impairment), 2 (moderate impairment), and 3 (severe impairment). The scale has been extended to 4 and 5, in order to classify the most advanced stages of the disease (21).

Mattis Dementia Rating Scale

This scale assesses five cognitive domains: attention, initiation and perseveration, construction, conceptual thinking, and memory. The most difficult items are presented first, in contrast to many other tests in which items are presented in ascending order of difficulty. The total score clearly discriminates AD patients from normal control subjects. It also differentiates patients with dementia from patients whose cognitive functioning is compromised by psychiatric illness and from healthy community elderly subjects with limited education (23). The scale has been used with success in patients with conditions other than AD, including VaD (24) and AIDS (25). The subscales of the battery, however, might vary in sensitivity (26). In particular, attention and conceptual thinking do not discriminate controls from mildly impaired patients.

Other Tests

It must be stressed that even though these screening tests are frequently employed in clinical practice for the detection and diagnosis of dementia and AD, most of them lack sensitivity and specificity. Even if the MMSE is the most widely used by frontline physicians, difficulties with the MMSE in detecting early dementia have been reported, making it lengthy and potentially cumbersome to use (27). The main goal for future research in this domain is to provide clinicians with simple and brief tests, based on solid theoretical and experimental data, with high sensitivity and specificity.

The Blessed-Roth test, which includes an Information, Memory, and Orientation test (28), is largely used in dementia assessment.

The Clock Drawing test, widely appreciated for its simplicity and ease of administration, rendering it a popular tool in both clinical and research practices, is a brief measure used to detect cognitive decline associated with a variety of neurobehavioral disorders. It correlates highly with the MMSE and other measures of global cognitive decline. However, a challenging issue has been identifying the neuropsychological and neuroanatomic substrates underlying impaired performance on clock drawing in dementia (29). Cosentino and colleagues found that the drawing-on-command condition places high demands on executive control functioning, since patients are required to perform in a novel context, whereas the copy condition provides a purer measure of "visuoconstructional" ability. Their data suggest that heavy demands on executive control associated with the interruption of large-scale cortical–subcortical neural networks underlie impairment in clock drawing in mild dementia.

The 7 Minute Test (30) represents an attempt in that direction. Four brief tests (Enhanced Cued Recall, Temporal Orientation, Verbal Fluency, and Clock Drawing) are included, which showed a mean sensitivity of 92% and a mean specificity of 96%.

There are other promising new tools such as the Montreal Cognitive Assessment (MoCA), developed to screen patients who present with mild cognitive complaints and usually perform in the normal range on the MMSE (31). This study assessed the sensitivity and specificity of the MoCA in patients with MCI and AD and normal elderly controls. It showed sensitivities of 78% (MMSE) versus 100% (MoCA) in AD, and 18% (MMSE) versus 90% (MoCA) in MCI. The MoCA is a simple, stand-alone cognitive screening tool with superior sensitivity. It covers important cognitive domains, can be administered in 10 minutes, and fits on one page.

Another screening test aimed at identifying patients with MCI and patients with dementia in the early stages of the disease is the DemTect (32). It showed high sensitivities of 80% and 100% to detect MCI and mild AD, respectively. It is short (eight to 10 minutes), easy to administer, and its transformed total score (maximum 18) is independent of age and education. The DemTect helps in deciding whether cognitive performance is adequate for age (13–18 points), or whether MCI (9–12 points) or dementia (8 points or below) should be suspected.

Neuropsychological Batteries

Several batteries have been designed to test dementia. They comprise standardized, structured interviews, tests, and examinations for diagnosing common mental disorders in later life, with special reference to the dementias.

Their principal aim is to incorporate in a single instrument all the information required to make an accurate clinical diagnosis of dementia.

Cambridge Examination for Mental Disorders of the Elderly

The Cambridge Examination for Mental Disorders of the Elderly (CAMDEX) (33) is a standardized, structured interview and quantitative evaluation of a wide range of cognitive functions. The principal goal is to establish the type of dementia, e.g., AD type, VaD, dementia with Lewy bodies (DLB), FTD, or dementia secondary to physical disease. It can provide key features common to dementia and other psychiatric syndromes of later life that are likely to overlap with and cause difficulty in the differential diagnosis from dementia. The battery is also aimed to diagnose dementia at an early stage and to provide an estimate of the clinical severity of dementia. It is applicable to both clinical and community-based studies. CAMDEX incorporates several components to establish personal and family history, and concise neuropsychological tests to assess all the cognitive deficits specified in operational diagnostic criteria, i.e., memory impairment, aphasia, apraxia, agnosia, and disturbances in executive function. Items within a cognitive domain are graded in difficulty to permit assessment of the full range of cognitive ability. Scores can be calculated for each of these broad areas of cognitive function or added to give a total score.

Among several screening measures of CAMDEX, the CAMCOG is the only significant predictor for the clinical diagnosis of dementia. To gain efficiency, the screening measures of the CAMDEX protocol may be restricted to the CAMCOG (34).

A new version, CAMDEX-R, has been developed in order to increase its ability to diagnose different forms of dementia, including DLB and FTD, and to make clinical diagnoses based on DSM-IV and ICD-10 criteria.

Consortium to Establish a Registry for Alzheimer's Disease

The Consortium to Establish a Registry for AD (CERAD) (35) proposed a diagnostic battery that has now been translated and used in several countries.

The main CERAD battery consists of a relatively brief neurological evaluation designed to help clinicians to make reliable and valid diagnosis of probable AD and a brief neuropsychological battery intended to assess the severity of the overall dementia and the extent to which various cognitive domains are affected. So far the diagnostic accuracy for AD in the early phase is 86%.

The CERAD battery includes the CDR, which relies on subjective assessment by the neurologist. Its administration requires training, and its scoring has been simplified by using the "sum of boxes." The neuropsychological battery, which has a high inter-rater reliability and high re-test reliability, has been augmented by the addition of further measures of delayed verbal recall, Trails A and B, and a simple test of verbal intelligence aimed at estimating the subject's premorbid IQ. One study (36) found that it could distinguish even the mildest cases of AD from nondemented controls. However, in some of the countries that use CERAD, the battery has not yet been extensively validated.

The CERAD 1 includes: Word Fluency (category-animal), the Boston Naming Test, the MMSE, Word List Memory, Constructional Praxis, Word List Delayed Recall, Word List Recognition, plus a behavioral rating scale. A second version of the test, CERAD 2, has been proposed. It includes the Shipley-Hartford Vocabulary, Verbal Paired Associate Learning Test, Recall of Constructional Praxis items, Verbal Paired Associate Recall, Trails A and B, Nelson Adult Reading Test, Word Fluency (letter: "F" and "P"), Clock Drawing, and Finger Tapping.

Alzheimer's Disease Assessment Scale

The Alzheimer's Disease Assessment Scale (ADAS) was designed to measure the severity of the most important symptoms of AD (37). Its subscale ADAS-cog is the most popular cognitive testing instrument used in clinical pharmacological trials for AD. It consists of tasks measuring disturbances of memory, language, praxis, and attention. A review has concluded that in comparison with other rating scales, the ADAS-cog is regarded as more comprehensive, although it is not a substitute for an extensive neuropsychological test study (38). Age and education norms are available for ADAS-cog. It must be remembered that ADAS was not designed for diagnostic use (it assumes that the diagnosis of probable AD has already been reached), and that it does not provide any type of individual or group profile. In addition, it does not take into account psychiatric or behavioral manifestations of AD. Finally, the standardization is limited, which restricts the comparability of results in multicenter international research studies.

Psychometric Assessment of Specific Cognitive Domains

Ideally, a neuropsychological battery should be a collection of reliable, valid tests with known specificity and sensitivity. The tests should be standardized with reference to normal individuals matched for sex, age, education, and also socio-economic characteristics. Notwithstanding the fundamental role of neuro-psychological methods in the diagnosis and in treatment evaluation for dementia, validated psychometric measurements are still not extensively used in dementia assessment. We will briefly describe some of the available tests, subdivided by cognitive area.

Memory

It is commonly accepted that memory is not a unitary cognitive function, but can be fractionated in multiple components with different disease susceptibility. In dementia conditions the evaluation of the different memory processes is mandatory.

Short-term and working memory: Short-term memory (STM) is a system that allows the retention of a limited number of various kinds of information to be retained over short periods of time. This retention process is typically involved in carrying out various types of cognitive tasks, an aspect which is captured by the concept of working memory (39). Baddeley defined working memory "as the system for the temporary maintenance and manipulation of information, necessary for the performance of such complex cognitive activities as comprehension, learning, and reasoning" (40). Working memory is composed of three subsystems: the Phonological Loop, the Visuospatial Sketchpad, and the Central Executive (39). The Phonological Loop enables phonological material in a phonological store to be maintained by a recycling process. The Visuospatial Sketchpad is involved in storing a limited quantity of visuospatial information for a limited time. The Central Executive, which is an attention system, is responsible for the control of the other slave subsystems. It is generally agreed that patients with dementia, in particular AD and FTD, show early in their disease a deficit of executive functions that are underpinned by the Central Executive system (41). In the very earliest stage of the disease, there might be a clear dissociation between the impairment of Central Executive system and the relative preservation of the articulatory loop and the Visuospatial Sketchpad (42). Patients at this stage of the disease, for example, might show great difficulty in performing two different tasks simultaneously and in manipulating information maintained in working memory.

Considering these cognitive aspects, it is not surprising that a number of studies have addressed the assessement of STM in AD and other dementias. The more commonly used measure of STM in AD is the memory span. Two tests are widely used in clinical practice: the digit span and the visuospatial span. In the digit span test, subjects are presented with a series of digits and are required to reproduce immediately the series in the correct order. The number of digits the subject can correctly recall constitutes his digit span. The visuospatial span is usually measured with the Corsi test (43). This consists of nine cubes fastened in a random order to a board. Each time the examiner taps the blocks in a prearranged sequence, the patient must attempt to copy this tapping pattern. In AD patients, memory span is generally reduced for words (44,45), letters (44,46,47), digits (44,46,47), and spatial location (48–50). Although reduced compared to normal old subjects, the memory span in early and in moderate AD is relatively preserved compared to their performance on tasks tapping explicit long term memory. Another approach has been to examine the free-recall accuracy as a function of the serial position of the stimulus after giving the subjects lists of words. Normal adults, both young and old, typically show a *u*-shaped function with a recency (better recall for the first items of the list) and a primacy (better recall for the last items) effect (51). The recency and the primacy effects concern STM and LTM, respectively. In AD patients there is a mild decrease in the recency portion of the curve and a major decrease in the primacy portion. These results suggest that STM is relatively spared in AD compared to LTM (52).

Explicit long-term memory: The evaluation of long-term memory systems is mandatory in dementia. This should include the assessment of episodic memory, i.e., the memory system involved in remembering specific episodes of one's own past (53), whose involvement is often the earliest symptom of AD, and the assessment of semantic memory, i.e., encyclopedic knowledge, and the meaning of words. The presence of episodic memory impairment is actually required for the diagnosis of dementia (1,2). Episodic memory impairment is also a powerful predictor of future dementia in individuals at risk (54–58). The early detection of episodic memory impairment is therefore crucial for the diagnosis of dementia and for the detection of persons that are likely to develop dementia in the future.

There is a general agreement (59,60) that measures of delayed recall are the most effective for the early diagnosis of AD compared to measures of immediate recall. A non-progressive decrease in delay recall is a frequent finding in normal aging, but it is also very common in AD, in such a way to render it unusable for the evaluation of disease progression. The most used tests are learning of a word list and the "story recall test" logical memory (LM), based on the evaluation of the encoding of a written piece immediately after its reading by the examiner and after ten minutes delay with different interferences. The California Verbal Learning Test (CVLT) (61), for the evaluation of short- and long-term memory in dementia using local normative values, is widely applied as part of batteries in multicenter studies (62–64). A deficit in delay recall is typical in the initial phase of dementia. The performances are indeed severely affected in early mild dementia. In the non-verbal domain, the recall of Rey's figure and Corsi's supraspan learning are among the most popular measures.

The theoretical principle of "encoding specificity" underlines the strict dependence between the encoding and retrieval conditions. Indeed, an effective retrieval requires specific encoding, because "what is perceived determines what is stored, and what is stored determines what retrieval cues are effective in providing access to what is stored" (65). It is well known that the encoding specificity effect is lacking or is very weak even in the early stage of AD (54). Most tests currently used for the diagnosis of dementia do not take into account the relationship between encoding and retrieval. One exception is represented by the Free and Cued Selective Reminding Test (FCSRT) (66). The FCSRT shows high sensitivity and specificity for the diagnosis of early dementia (57,67). However, as pointed out by Buschke et al. the FCSRT has two major limitations (54). First, the power of the test is limited by ceiling effects. These ceiling effects make important bias in the comparison of the effect of encoding specificity for aged with dementia and aged without dementia. Buschke and co-workers developed a test, the Double Memory Test (DMT), to remedy the limitations of the FCSRT. The DMT includes two memory tests, one with and one without coordinated acquisition and retrieval. The Category Cued Recall (CCR) memory test optimizes encoding specificity by using the same category cues for acquisition as well as retrieval. Buschke and co-workers compared the DMT with two standard memory tests, Paired Associated (PA) and LM (68), in the diagnosis of early dementia. They found that the CCR had much higher sensitivity (93%) and specificity (99%) than PA (68%, 91%) and LM (48%, 92%). CCR had the greatest advantage in the mildest cases. These results show that tests based on encoding specificity are much more powerful for the diagnosis of early dementia than traditional learning tests. For the screening of dementia, Buschke and co-workers have recently devised a test, the Memory Screen Test, which is a brief, four-item delay free and cued recall memory test (69). This test showed good sensitivity and specificity for the screening of dementia (70), providing efficient, reliable, and valid screening for AD and other dementias.

Attention

Attention is also a non-unitary function. Tests that evaluate vigilance and selective focused attention include the verbal and non-verbal span and letter cancellation tests. Selective divided attention is measured by the Brown-Peterson, Trail B, and Stroop tests. The test most widely used to evaluate selective attention abilities is the "cancellation" test. In this test, of which many variants exist, the subjects are required to detect as quickly as possible a given series of stimuli, for example a letter or a digit, among a great number of distracters. Another widely used test of selective attention is the Stroop test (71). Here the subjects are exposed to ambiguous stimuli, namely names of colors written in an incongruous ink color (for example the word BLUE written in red). In this task, the subjects are required to name as fast as possible the color of the ink in which each word is written and to ignore the word itself.

Executive Functions

The most widely used tests in clinical practice are verbal fluency, Trail Making Test (TMT), and Wisconsin Card Sorting Test (WCST). In the verbal fluency tasks, the subject is required to retrieve as fast as possible words belonging to a specific category (e.g., animals) or beginning with a given letter. Another widely used test of executive functions and mental flexibility is the TMT (72). This test is given in two parts, A and B. The subject must first draw lines to connect consecutively numbered and lettered circles on one work sheet (Part A), and then connect the same number of consecutively numbered and lettered circles on another worksheet by alternating between the two sequences (Part B). The WCST is probably the most widely used test to assess executive functions, in particular "abstract behavior" and "shift of set" (73). In this test, the subject is given a pack of 60 cards on which are printed one to four symbols, triangle, star, cross, or circle, in red, green, yellow, or blue. The patient's task is to place them by one under four-stimulus cards according to a principle that the patient must deduce from the pattern of the examiner responses to the patient's placement of the cards.

Language

Language impairments are a prominent feature of AD (74) and FTD. The mechanisms underlying the language deficits found in persons with AD are often attributed to the direct result of the cognitive deficits, particularly those related to memory. Impaired naming is the major change in language functioning in early AD, and reflects the impairment of semantic memory. Word-finding difficulties tend to be prominent, and their assessment plays a role in the differential diagnosis of the dementias, especially AD (75,76). Naming tests such as the Boston Naming Test (77) are therefore commonly used; as mentioned above it is also part of the CERAD battery. Normative data for normal aging have recently become available (78). Besides naming, other disorders in accessing semantic information or complete loss of semantic knowledge have been described in AD (79). Many studies have also shown impairment in syntactic processing. This deficit has been particularly evident in comprehension of syntactically complex sentences. Again, the poor syntactic processing in the AD population has been ascribed to reduced working memory and difficulty in integrating information (80). Due to its integrative nature, discourse processing, either in production and comprehension, poses great demand in AD. Picture description is used for this aim with a reported decrease in the number of content units and conciseness with increasing severity (81). As the disease progresses, the language impairments become more profound and might resemble fluent aphasia. There are significant auditory and reading comprehension deficits, and language production is fluent and paraphasic. In late stages of dementia, decreasing verbal output often resulting in mutism is the rule. Tests such as the Token Test for the evaluation of language comprehension (82,83) and the Reporter's Test (82) have been used in many studies aimed in particular at differentiating various types of dementia (84). Special tests have also been used to assess repetition (85).

Praxis

Another cognitive deficit encountered in all stages of dementia is apraxia. An evaluation battery proposed by De Renzi and Lucchelli has been used in AD (86). The authors showed that both ideational apraxia and, to a lesser extent, ideomotor apraxia (IMA) are present in AD. Apraxia is a crucial feature of corticobasal degeneration. Spatial orientation and limb praxis are usually spared in FTD (87).

In AD, all aspects of visuoconstruction, including copying, drawing, and construction in 3D, are impaired. The immediate reproduction of Rey's Complex Figure (88) and the Constructional Apraxia test (89) test visuospatial competence as well as planning and perceptual organization. The WAIS-R block design task is impaired in AD (90). Another possible source of constructional difficulties is impaired executive function and global or local attention processes.

Visuospatial Abilities

In AD there are severe impairments of spatial abilities (91). AD patients have difficulties in scanning the visual field in order to locate objects, and may present with a deficit in spatial exploration and Balint's syndrome (gaze apraxia, optic ataxia, and simultagnosia) (92). These impairments lead to deficits in everyday life including problems in writing, drawing, driving, following lines of text when reading, and telling the time from a watch. Some patients, though rarely, may present with spatial hemineglect. There is a disruption of personal and extrapersonal orientation: inability to follow unfamiliar route, but also becoming lost in familiar surroundings. Tests of the ability to undertake the "road map test" in relation to one's own body position showed a prevalence deficit in AD (93).

The two aspects of spatial cognition that are most frequently evaluated in AD are mental rotation and judgement of line orientation. Tests of detection of object rotation or object rotation to solve object matching problems (94,95) show significant impairment. The TMT B (96), described above, is also used to measure the visuomotor planning. Street's test (89) also measures visual and perceptual abilities.

ASSESSMENT OF PSYCHOLOGICAL AND BEHAVIORAL DISTURBANCES

The importance of evaluating non-cognitive aspects of dementia is increasingly appreciated. In particular, the measurement of behavioral disturbances in dementia represents a methodological and clinical challenge (97). Coexistence of cognitive deficits with behavioral changes and psychotic symptoms makes it difficult to obtain a proper characterization of the individual aspects. Several instruments have been developed for the assessment of global, as well as of specific, behavioral symptoms (98). Direct observation is limited to patients in specialized institutions, whereas interview of the caregivers is possible for patients at home. There is a tendency by the caregivers to provide either an above or an under estimation of the deficits, according to the relationship with the patient and the stress level (99).

Neuropsychiatric Inventory

The Neuropsychiatric Inventory (NPI) scale was developed in order to gather data on the presence and nature of psychopathological disorders in patients with cerebral pathologies (100), and addresses particularly patients with AD or other dementias. It is based on caregiver's information obtained by a questionnaire and provides measurements of frequency and severity of behavioral disturbances. The scale relies on the caregiver and evaluates twelve common psychiatric disorders, from delusion, hallucinations, agitation, and depression to anxiety, disinhibition, and apathy. Each single item is correlated to further sub-items that provide more detailed information. Administration time is about 20 minutes. NPI is a valid instrument for behavioral evaluation in AD, VaD, and FTD and may also help in the differential diagnosis of dementia (101).

Clinical Insight Rating Scale

The evaluation of subjective experience is of great value in a patient with dementia, in particular the awareness of the functional, behavioral, and cognitive deficits. There is maintenance of insight, at least in the initial and intermediate phases of disease progression (99). The awareness of disease seems to depend upon the type and severity of dementia, due to the selective involvement of specific brain regions (frontal lobes and right hemisphere, in particular) (102). The Clinical Insight Rating scale represents a standardized approach to achieve this aim for patient examination. It is a semi-structured interview preceded by an interview with the caregiver that should provide information on the reasons for the request for medical examination, the duration of disease, the onset and progression of cognitive symptoms, and their impact on functional and daily activities (103,104).

Assessment of Depression

A particular concern is the evaluation of depression. This is usually achieved with the application of rating scales, such as the Geriatric Depression Scale, but also the Hamilton, Beck, and Cornell scales. The latter properly addresses the evaluation of depressive symptoms in dementia. It is the only scale validated in patient populations, even at moderate-severe stages. It consists of a series of standardized items obtained by patient and caregiver's interviews. It is also based on the patient's own observations and does not require direct answers by the patient to a standardized questionnaire. There are 19 items with graduate scale points from 0 (absence of symptom) to 2 (severe symptom).

FUNCTIONAL SCALES

It should be underlined that all diagnostic criteria require that the cognitive deficits, assessed clinically and quantified by neuropsychological tests, have an impact on the activities of daily living. Several functional scales are used with the aim of evaluating working, social, and relational capacity in patients with dementia (105). These scales present with a series of specific problems, which is mainly concerned with the limited information about their validity and sensitivity. A functional impairment depends also on occupational status and personal attitudes, and it is additionally dependant on the subjective evaluation and clinical interview (1). Nevertheless, standardized examinations are largely used because they can give answers when it is necessary to compare different phases of the disease, thereby measuring disease progression. They are also useful for determining the impact of rehabilitative and pharmacological treatments (106).

More precisely, a functional evaluation is aimed at measuring the individual capacities in concrete activities and in social roles (107).

Living-Instrumental Activities of Daily Living

These rating scales, which have not been developed specifically for dementia, are widely used for functional assessment, and form the basis for more targeted instruments, such as the Activities of Daily Living (ADL) questionnaire (108). ADL consists of instrumental ADL (IADL), which evaluates complex skills, such as managing money, and basic ADL (BADL), which assesses self-maintenance skills. The Barthel Index within the BADL provides valuable measurements of walking, bathing, eating, dressing, and use of toilet. A patient is independent,

dependent or completely dependent when he/she can exert control over all of these functions, needs assistance or is completely dependent on nurse or caregiver help. The ADL are widely used but are influenced by the cognitive status, by the social and frequent usage of the subject, and also by the physical conditions, such as for the BADL (106). A complete autonomy reflects the capacity for the subject to live independently at home. In dementia there is a rapid loss of IADL, and a certain sparing of the BADL, but in the more advanced stages, all the activities are lost. A major problem, however, mainly concerns the limited sensitivity in the early phase of dementia, in particular in individuals with large social and relational interests. To solve this problem the Advanced Activities of Daily Living (AADL) have been introduced. These represent complex and demanding aspects of daily living such as travelling, hobbies, and recreational and social activities (107). The AADL can reveal behavioral modifications that, while not indicative of a specific cognitive impairment, indicate the likelihood of incipient dementia.

A serious problem is the floor effect, since the lowest level of these scales includes individuals with very different degrees of disability. The use of the Bedford Alzheimer Assessment Nursing Scale, for severe disability, allows a precise evaluation of the functional level in each individual, with the possibility of monitoring also the effect of rehabilitative and therapeutic approaches (109).

These indirect functional evaluations, all based on information provided by the patient or very often by the caregiver, have some limits linked to variables that might influence a correct report on the real capacity of the patients. To overcome this problem, there are more direct evaluations based on objective observation of functional capacity of the patient to perform a series of standardized tasks that mimic the basic daily activities. Among these the Physical Performance Test and the Direct Assessment Functional Scale formerly used in the elderly have been applied in the evaluation of patients with dementia (110,111). Finally, it is useful in monitoring of crucial survival abilities, such as walking capacity, equilibrium, and feeding by standardized instruments (Tinetti Scale) (112).

Communicative Abilities of Daily Living

Communicative Abilities of Daily Living (CADL) is a functionally oriented battery which has been proposed to assess aphasic patients in an ecologically valid fashion (113). CADL has been used to investigate functional communication skills in subjects with mild and moderate AD and their performance compared with that of Wernicke's aphasics, normal elderly, and elderly depressed subjects (114). Subjects with mild and moderate AD were impaired on the CADL, and the impairment was more severe in the moderately demented group than in the mildly demented group. Language skills were also impaired in elderly depressed subjects as compared with normal elderly controls; however, the elderly depressed subjects were less impaired than were the mild AD subjects. Finally, although performance of the moderate AD and Wernicke's aphasic subjects did not differ in terms of total CADL score, the performance of these groups' subtests was markedly different.

THE ROLE OF NEUROPSYCHOLOGICAL ASSESSMENT OF DEMENTIA

The pattern of neuropsychological impairment in patients with different forms of dementia reflects the location of brain damage rather than its underlying pathology. Specific pathological conditions are associated with a relatively selective topographical pattern of brain involvement, thus leading to relatively typical neuropsychological pictures. However, there are many exceptions. For example, typical AD is characterized by the early involvement of medial temporal cortex and associative temporoparietal areas; typically, frontal involvement is less severe or delayed. The situation is more complicated in the case of dementias associated with focal lobar involvement in the temporal and frontal lobes. Neuropsychological assessment provides different patient profiles that might help in the differential diagnosis.

The fundamental applications of neuropsychology for the evaluation of dementia are the following:

1. Differential diagnosis between cognitive changes in normal aging and conversion to dementia (early diagnosis)
2. Differential diagnosis among different dementia conditions
3. Quantitative evaluation of disease progression
4. Assessment of severe dementia
5. Monitoring the effect of pharmacological treatments.

Early Diagnosis

It is well accepted that the natural course of dementia from a condition of full health to an established dementia status may last several years. At the beginning the patient might have a deficit limited to memory or to attention (not both), without any disorder of instrumental and daily activities. The cognitive impairment then proceeds to a degree that allows the diagnosis of dementia. In the transitional state between normal aging and mild dementia is fitted the term MCI.

The term MCI is an operational diagnostic term used to describe subjects at risk of developing AD or in the pre-clinical stage of the disease (115). It is reserved for subjects whose impairment is objectively demonstrable but is not pronounced in more than one domain of cognition and does not seriously affect activities of daily living. Neuropsychological assessment in MCI subjects shows impairment in memory tests, especially delayed recall, a possible index of an incipient dementia process, thus supporting the role of cognitive testing in identifying early or pre-clinical AD (116). Identification of pre-clinical AD among MCI subjects might be important for the timely detection of patients to whom currently available treatment options should be offered (117).

Nevertheless, it has been suggested that the proposed criteria for MCI may apply to a heterogeneous population in which memory complaints could be due to somatic diseases, drug-induced states, affective disorders, or other neurological conditions, rather than to an ongoing AD-related process (118). Important aspects in this respect are which kind of memory tests should be used to define impairment (sensitivity and specificity) and if patients with other cognitive non-mnestic deficits should be excluded. The different inclusion and exclusion criteria might account for the reported large variable conversion rate to AD (119). In fact, narrow inclusion criteria might fail to capture the heterogeneity of clinical AD presentations, such as progressive visuospatial or language deficit. The problem is even more complex because the differential diagnosis of these variants might include a greater likelihood of dementia syndromes such as DLB and FTD. MCI has been shown to convert to AD at 10% to 15% a year (115). 20% to 50% of MCI subjects, according to different studies however, may remain stable (115,120). Amnesic MCI usually evolves to AD, whereas MCI with deficits in a single cognitive domain may convert to AD or to FTD, DLB, VaD, primary progressive aphasia, or Parkinson's disease. An MCI in several cognitive domains usually reflects possible AD, VaD, or even normal aging.

The evaluation of memory is the basis for the differential diagnosis between the early onset of dementia, and cognitive changes related to normal aging. The initial phase of AD is marked by a progressive deterioration of episodic memory. When the process advances, the impairment spreads to other cognitive functions, such as semantic memory, language, and visuospatial ability.

A range of cognitive functions other than episodic memory, including semantic memory (knowledge- or fact-based memory), attention, and executive function (high-level control processes), is significantly impaired in the mild stages of AD (118,121,122), and indeed, tests of many different cognitive capacities have been shown to be predictive of future AD diagnosis among memory-impaired subjects (56,59).

An ideal neuropsychological tool for the early detection of dementia should be sensitive enough to differentiate dementia from normal aging and other brain disorders that can mimic dementia, in particular depression. Recent neuropsychological longitudinal research studies have been used in detecting individuals at risk of developing dementia: community-based studies of elderly subjects, studies of MCI with high risk of developing AD, and in presymptomatic individuals with known genetics for autosomal dominant familial AD. These approaches showed that episodic memory deficits might precede the onset of clinical dementia by at least five years (123). Other cognitive domains, such as mental speed, attention, and executive functions can be affected in advance, thus becoming indicators of incipient dementia (59,124). In autosomal dominant AD, subgroups of converters showed low IQ scores and lower verbal memory scores than non-converters (125). In MCI and very early AD, impairment on tests of episodic memory is generally the most predictive measure (57,115), but deficits in semantic memory [semantic knowledge of famous people is also lost in very early AD (126,127)], attention, and mental speed also predict conversion to AD (15,128,129). Longitudinal studies revealed the role of a spatial learning test from the CANTAB computer battery, the PA Learning (PAL) test, which is sensitive in detecting the earliest stage of AD and is also able to distinguish patients with depression (130). In the early phase of AD several extensive cognitive batteries have been designed showing considerable promise (131).

Differential Diagnosis of Dementia

Neuropsychological evaluation should be considered an ancillary tool for the differential diagnosis of dementia within the context of other clinical evidence. It is of secondary role with respect to neuroradiological investigations in the differential diagnosis of AD and cerebro-VaD, and with respect to clinical examination for the differential diagnosis of AD and "subcortical dementia" (such as in the case of Parkinson's disease and Huntington's disease).

Vascular Dementia

VaD is the second most common type of dementia; however, it is increasingly being recognised that VaD is actually a heterogeneous syndrome and that several vascular pathologies can lead to cognitive deterioration (132). In contrast to the striking deficits produced by cortical infarcts, lesions of the subcortical white matter are mainly associated with a non-specific slowing of behavior. Cerebrovascular disease also plays an important role in forms of cognitive decline other than dementia, and as such, it appears to be no less prevalent in old age than AD. In addition, AD and VaD represent the extremes of the clinical spectrum of dementia conditions that includes also various combinations of cerebrovascular and degenerative pathology. It is thus evident how classical diagnostic criteria are often of reduced clinical value (133). The relationship between cerebrovascular lesions, as shown by neuroimaging, and focal neuropsychological signs is difficult to define during clinical follow-up. There is a common belief that the cognitive impairment should be ascribed to mixed vascular and AD types of dementia (134). The prevalence of this kind of dementia is high in the elderly population. A large multi-center study for the treatment of CVD and AD showed a slower rate of progression of cognitive impairment in "pure" VaD in comparison to AD (135) using the ADAS-cog assessment in a two-year follow-up study.

A specific neuropsychological profile, characterized by a prominent impairment of executive and visuospatial functions associated with a relative sparing of episodic memory, has been suggested to be typical of subcortical VaD (136).

Frontotemporal Lobar Degenerations

Frontotemporal lobar degeneration (FTLD/FTD) is characterized by a relatively selective degeneration of frontal and/or temporal cortical areas. According to widely accepted diagnostic criteria (4), three different clinical syndromes are delineated. The frontal variant of FTD is characterized by prevalent behavioral symptoms, with early change in personality and difficulty in modulating behavior, often resulting in inappropriate responses and activities; semantic dementia is associated with prevalent semantic/cognitive impairment; and progressive aphasia is characterized by early non-fluent aphasia (137,138). The differential diagnosis from AD is unreliable on the basis of NINCDS-ADRDA criteria (139). Improved reliability may be achieved by means of clinical features and neuropsychological tests (140). Memory disorder and even dementia are not paramount as early symptoms of FTD, so that at least in the early stages, this syndrome has to be differentiated from psychiatric disorders more than from other types of dementia. Thus, measurements of behavioral impairments are mandatory. A behavioral frontotemporal dysfunction assessment scale validated on patients at the mild stage (MMSE > 18) helps to distinguish between FTD, AD, and VaD (141). The items of this structured interview are classified into four classes: self-monitoring dyscontrol, self-neglect, self-centered behavior, and affective behavior. A score of 1 is given for the class if at least one symptom is present. A total score of 3 or more gives a sensitivity of 100%, a specificity of 93%, and a diagnostic accuracy for FTD of 97%. The assessment of neuropsychiatric symptoms with other standardized scales or inventory is useful in distinguishing dementia patients with FTD and AD (142,143). The Frontal Behavioral Inventory Scale (144) provides a tool to distinguish between the different clinical variants of FTD.

In the frontal variant of FTD it is possible to identify two opposite behavioral profiles (145). Apathy, psychomotor inhibition, lack of emotional reactions, and defective social functioning characterize the more common "apathetic" behavior, whereas impulsiveness, perseverations, disinhibition, and lack of concern for others are associated with the less common "disinhibited" behavior (146).

Diagnostic criteria for FTD are based on the following clinical findings: insidious onset and gradual progression, early decline in social interpersonal conduct, early emotional blunting, and loss of insight. One or more of the following can be associated: oral and manual exploration, hyperphagia, echolalia, impulsive behavior, jocularity, and inappropriate actions or words. A characteristic aspect is the discrepancy between judgment and behavioral alteration that is out of proportion with the memory disorder. Neuropsychology shows significant impairment on frontal lobe tests in the absence of severe amnesia, aphasia, or perceptual disorders. In FTD, an extensive neuropsychological test battery, aimed at assessing the different cognitive domains, including in particular the executive functions, is suggested: the MMSE (147) as a global measure of dementia severity, Tower of London Test, WCST for frontal function, and Raven's Colored Progressive Matrices (148) for abstract reasoning. Also, there are the CVLT (61), Story Recall, and Word Learning (149) tests to assess verbal recall and verbal learning, the recall of Rey's Complex Figure (88) for visual long-term memory, and the Digit Span forward and reverse test (150) to evaluate STM. The pattern of memory decline differs from that of AD: memory performances benefit from cues and from the provision of multiple-choice alternative responses. A deficit of retrieval strategies more than a storage problem has been suggested (84). The TMT A is used to test attention/concentration of the patients, and the TMT B, which also measures visuomotor planning, is used for the assessment of divided attention (96). The immediate reproduction of Rey's Complex Figure (88) and the Constructional Apraxia test for visuospatial competence, as well as planning and perceptual organization and the Street's test (89) for visual and perceptual abilities, are also used. Language ability should be tested not only for the classic naming, repetition, reading, and writing competences, but also for phonological, semantic, and grammatical aspects, as well as language comprehension (e.g., Token Test) (89). With this aim, the BADA Italian standardized aphasia protocol (151) has been used in Italy. In FTD there is an economy of language output, hypophonia, and loss of prosody. Perseveration, echolalia, and stereotypies occur in the course of the disease. Mutism usually ensues in the final stages. Patients have no perceptuospatial difficulty, and skills are preserved even in advanced disease. There is no spatial disorientation, which is an important distinguishing feature from AD. Due to reduced cooperation and concentration deficits, it might be difficult to administer the whole neuropsychological battery to some patients.

Primary progressive aphasia usually presents with insidious and gradual progression of anomia or word-comprehension impairment. Intact premorbid language and absence of a "specific" cause, stroke in particular, are also hallmarks. A non-fluent aphasia is typical. Acalculia and IMA may be present, but there is an absence of significant forgetfulness and apathy for the initial two years. ADL impairment, when present, should be ascribed to language deficits.

Semantic dementia presents with anomia, impairment in word comprehension, and loss of knowledge on semantic tasks (152). A fluent aphasia of the transcortical type is a hallmark. There might be also reading difficulties (surface dyslexia) with inability to read irregularly spelled words, but intact syntactic functions. The Pyramids and Palms test can be used to evaluate the impairment of semantic knowledge (153).

In a series of comparative studies, patients with the clinical diagnosis of probabile AD and FTD showed significantly different neuropsychological profiles. In an object and action naming test, FTD patients were particularly impaired in the latter (154); during word generation on a phonemic cue (f, p, l as initial letters) or a semantic cue (animal, fruit names), FTD patients showed major impairment with the phonemic fluency, whereas AD patients were impaired in semantic fluency.

A brief neuropsychological assessment for the differential diagnosis between FTD and AD has been designed by Siri and coworkers (155). They found considerable overlap between AD and FTD. Four tests (Rey figure recall, phonemic fluency, oral apraxia, and cube analysis) achieved 70% sensitivity and 80% specificity for the correct classification of patients in the FTD or AD group. The conclusion is to include these four tests, as well as other measures sensitive to the frontal impairment, since they can be useful in the differential diagnosis.

Dementia with Lewy Bodies

DLB is diagnosed in vivo on the basis of a series of clinical criteria, which do not include a differential pattern of cognitive impairment in comparison with AD (156). Others instead reported differences in cognitive profiles. Mental status, compared to AD, shows a disproportionately severe attention, fluency, visuoperceptual, as well as visuoconstructive, and visuospatial impairment. Fluctuations are the rule, particularly for attentional aspects. Neuropsychological features are characterized by mild memory deficits, attentional deficits, impaired working memory, and slowed processing speed. The DLB profile was reported to resemble the pattern of dementia found in PD (157). These results are compatible with the view that cognitive dysfunction in DLB reflects combined subcortical and cortical involvement with relative sparing of the medial temporal lobes. A strong predictor of accelerated cognitive decline in DLB is the *APOE* E4 allele.

The clock-face drawing has been used to differentiate DLB and AD type dementia syndromes, with a higher score for Draw than Copy in AD, a pattern not specific for DLB (158).

Alzheimer's Disease and Depression

Neuropsychological deficits such as poor episodic memory are a consistent feature of the early course AD, but they overlap with cognitive impairments in other disorders such as depression, making differential diagnosis difficult. Contributing to this is the fact that some episodic memory tests that are very sensitive to AD, particularly "effortful" tasks such as free recall, are also vulnerable in depression (159,160). It is very important that patients without AD are not falsely "detected" by such a test.

Computerised and traditional tests of memory, attention, and executive function were given to mild AD, questionable dementia, and major depression patients (161). Only a restricted set of neuropsychological measures was sensitive to impairment in questionable dementia compared to the depressed and control group, in particular, tests for episodic and semantic memory and category fluency. A visuospatial associative learning test (the PAL test, see 130) accurately distinguished AD from depressed subjects and revealed a subgroup of questionable dementia patients who performed like AD patients. Elements of contextual and cued recall may account for the task's sensitivity and specificity for AD. The PAL test is thus sensitive and specific for AD, and it may also be sensitive to the specific memory deficits of prodromal AD.

Because of its requirement to combine object-based and contextual information, PAL may be particularly sensitive to the entorhinal/hippocampal damage sustained in AD, and the provision of supportive recall cues may explain its relative insensitivity to strategic, or effortful processes, which may underlie poor memory function in the elderly and in depression. This might be relevant for clinical practise. All the tasks of attention and executive function are of no value in differentiating individuals with questionable dementia and those who are depressed. As a whole, these results suggest that prodromal-early AD differs from depressed and elderly healthy subjects significantly in terms of memory test scores.

Evaluation of Disease Progression

In this field, psychometric instruments should have characteristics that are different with respect to the ones employed in the early diagnosis. First of all, they should not present "floor effects," in particular for episodic memory measurements, nor should they be insufficiently sensitive to impairments in cognitive functions partially spared by the pathological processes (i.e., apraxia, implicit memory). In this respect, visuoperceptive and language tests, in other words, the fundamental assessment of right and left hemispheric cortical function also need appropriate norms and criteria (see "Advanced Tests and Future Research Approaches" section).

Since in the advanced phase of disease all the traditional neuropsychological tests show a "floor effect" and become useless, in the evaluation of severe cognitive impairment, new neuropsychological batteries have been developed (see "Severe Dementia" section).

In a follow-up evaluation, consideration should be given to determining cognitive deficits, functional level in daily activity, and non-cognitive symptoms. According to the severity as assessed by the CDR, the following schema can be followed:

> CDR 0.5: MMSE, extensive psychometric examination, IADL, Barthel Index.
> CDR 1: MMSE, extensive psychometric examination (optional), IADL, Barthel Index.
> CDR 2: MMSE, IADL, Barthel Index, NPI, Tinetti Scale.
> CDR 3: MMSE, Barthel Index, NPI, Tinetti Scale, BANNS Scale.
> CDR 4: Barthel Index, NPI, Tinetti Scale, BANNS Scale.

Severe Dementia

The great increase of the prevalence of age-associated dementias, particularly AD, has become a major health problem. The majority of cases evolve towards a stage of marked severity, which can last many years. Severe dementia is accompanied by loss of autonomy and impairment in activity of daily living ADL, and severe cognitive deficits in several cognitive domains (memory, language, attention, praxis, and visuospatial behavior). This stage of dementia is operationally defined on the basis of scores on global scales such as stage 6–7 on GDS, or 3 or more on CDR. The MMSE threshold for severe dementia is considered below 10. The advanced phases of dementia are very often associated with behavioral and psychiatric symptoms. These aspects, which might appear acutely or sub-acutely in patients who are often old or very old, should always be considered in order to rule out associated pathologies (pneumonia, acute pain, urinary retention, etc.). Aggressiveness is the most frequent disorder (estimated between 30% and 55%) (162). Keene et al. 1999 (163) found that in AD or VaD, aggression is related to more severe dementia and loss of personal care. Sometimes aggressive behavior is associated with conflicts with the family and caregivers. Depression has a prevalence of 17–35% in the literature, the highest percentage for a population of patients with severe dementia (164); it may be also highly correlated with anxiety (165). The best scale for measuring depression in severe dementia is the Cornell Scale (166). Hallucinations, motor disorders, and neurological signs should be considered in the differential diagnosis with AD and other dementias (LBD, FTD, CBD, etc.) (167).

Despite its size, the population of patients with severe dementia has been studied relatively little. In addition, the few studies have dealt almost exclusively with AD, and, as a consequence, little is known about the advanced stages of other dementias. Evaluation tools currently used for dementia are, in most cases, diagnostic instruments designed for patients who are in the early and moderate stages of their disease, and they are therefore generally unsatisfactory for assessing patients with severe dementia (168). For instance, the MMSE often yields a floor effect in cases of advanced dementia so that preserved capacities in these individuals may be overlooked. Researchers investigating advanced dementia have used instruments such as behavioral scales (169) and coma scales (170). The Katz ADL Index is used in the evaluation of functional status and is designed to be used in institutions by a physician or a nurse.

While these scales are based on the observation of behaviors and symptoms, they do not provide a precise evaluation of the cognitive profiles of the patient (171). In recent years, several batteries specifically aimed at testing patients with severe dementia have been proposed. One such scale is the Hierarchic Dementia Scale (172) that includes 20 subtests which cover the entire range of cognitive and motor functions. Other batteries such as the Severe Cognitive Impairment Profile (173) and the Test for Severe Impairment Battery (SIB) are reliable, validated measures of neuropsychological functioning in severely demented patients with AD, though they are not validated outside of the United States. The SIB has been developed keeping into account the specific cognitive and behavioral features of patients with severe dementia (174). This scale is very appropriate for severe dementia since, provided the patients agree to take it, it almost always yields scores that are above 0. Administration time is around 30 minutes and includes evaluation of all cognitive functions plus evaluation of social interaction derived from the CADL. It includes very simple tasks, which are presented with gestual indices. It has the advantage of having been validated not only in its original US version, but also in several languages including French (175,176), Italian (177), and Spanish (178,179).

Monitoring the Effect of Pharmacological Treatments

With regard to monitoring the effects of pharmacological treatments, short neuropsychological batteries, such as ADAS and CAMDEX, are frequently used. They provide quantitative information on the main cognitive areas within a limited time frame, together with information on affective and behavioral disturbances. Clinically, it is more relevant to measure changes in functional impairment than changes in task performances. It is thus necessary to use not only the classic measurements of cognitive deficits but also "ecologic" tasks and functional scales. As for cognitive assessment, the available instruments are limited: Rivermead Behavioral Memory Test (180), and attention and executive function tests for daily living (still to be standardized in many countries). The limits of functional scales have already been discussed.

ADVANCED TESTS AND FUTURE RESEARCH APPROACHES

Neuropsychology is an important asset in the study and treatment of cognitive decline, but must be embedded in a multidisciplinary context. In addition, in order to understand the different symptoms of different diseases in the elderly, one should keep in mind the relevant principles in the neuropsychological assessment of older individuals and the complex relationship between aging and cognition. Neuropsychological assessment aims to identify cognitive impairments in a maximally objective manner. To this end, patients are confronted with standardized tasks, preferably well documented with regard to reliability, validity, and norms. It should be remembered, however, that testing "oldest" elderly people is lacking for many instruments, in particular for normative data. Neuropsychological assessment is a powerful aid in the detection of early dementia, but has certain limitations. Firstly, the test results will be useful only if the subject is fully cooperative. Secondly, individual variation in cognitive performance is—especially in the elderly—considerable, even among people with the same demographic characteristics (age, sex, education); therefore, a wide margin of uncertainty must be allowed before impairment can be inferred. Even so, the impairment may be due to many causes besides brain dysfunction. Finally, a good deal of interpretation may be required in deciding what functional disturbance(s) underlie a deviant test result. For example, the term MCI is reserved for patients whose impairment is objectively demonstrable, but is not pronounced in more than one domain of cognition, and does not seriously affect activities of daily living (181). In MCI, however, while current criteria provide a convenient clinical procedure for identifying people at risk of developing dementia, there are numerous limitations. Firstly, even strict criteria still allow considerable latitude in assessment methods, for instance, in the quality and number of tests used. In connection with this, studies of the prevalence of MCI and its rate of conversion to dementia are poorly comparable and yield highly variable results. It would be very important to reconsider neuropsychological batteries, by implementing new tests, and obtaining normative data in elderly normal individuals with well-defined social, demographic, and educational characteristics. More sensitive instruments for cognitive decline evaluation will be thus available.

Furthermore, different types of dementia may not be equally recognizable by their early symptoms (182). For example, VaD actually consists of a heterogeneous collection of clinical features (132). The combined occurrence of AD and VaD is probably more common than it has been assumed. Lacunar infarcts and white matter lesions in subcortical areas lead to cognitive effects usually quite different from those of AD. Patients with white matter lesions demonstrate a clinical syndrome of subcortical dementia. Their cognitive performance remains largely adequate, though conspicuously slowed. This slowing is accompanied by relatively mild impairments of memory (mostly affecting reproduction) and executive function (mainly reflected by loss of mental flexibility and difficulty in dealing with complex situations). The patients are usually well aware of their limitations. It is thought that subcortical ischaemia contributes substantially to "normal" age-related decline (183,184). On the other hand, multi-infarct dementia, a syndrome caused by large cortical infarcts, leads to multiple functional and cognitive disturbances. An obvious example is the effect of single cortical infarcts, which consist of circumscribed functional disturbances corresponding with the location of the infarct. Assessment of the principal deficit might not be enough, and an extended neuropsychological evaluation is mandatory to define the complete cognitive profile. In addition, unlike AD, cerebrovascular disease is not necessarily progressive. It usually can cause more limited and static cognitive impairment. This requires neuropsychological assessment that is able to define cognitive stability and distinguish a real worsening from fluctuations associated with temporary variables. The problem of evaluation of cognitive fluctuations is crucial in the neuropsychological assessment of DLB. Together with standardized neuropsychological batteries, it can be useful to administer scales for the evaluation of fluctuation in behavioral and cognitive symptoms (185).

Different profiles according to the *disease stages* should be considered in the evaluation of dementia. For example, when an extensive battery of visuospatial perception tests was administered to mild probable AD patients in very early stage, these were not impaired (186). They were impaired only in an object-naming task. After eight months, the performance in the subtests of object perception was unchanged, while there was a significant decline in the total score of the items investigating space perception. A significant worsening was also observed in the Rey's figure copy score and was correlated with the decrease in the spatial perception score. This study confirmed that impairment in visual perceptual tests requiring access to semantic and lexical knowledge is present in the earliest phase of AD, whereas visuospatial and constructional impairments became evident only later. The authors suggest that this pattern of progression may represent the clinical correlate of increasing pathological involvement of posterior associative cortex.

There is also a characteristic cognitive profile and course of dementia in FTD. Nonetheless, cognitive test performance does not clearly distinguish FTD from AD in the early phase. A cross-sectional and longitudinal study was specifically instituted to address the cognitive characteristics of FTD, with the aim of determining which features distinguish FTD from AD. A large series of patients were included, some with a pathologically verified diagnosis of Pick's disease. Information regarding the initial symptoms of dementia were obtained from each patient's caregiver, global dementia severity was estimated by the BDS and the ADL scales, and specific cognitive domains were assessed by administering tests of memory, language, visuospatial, and reasoning abilities and selective attention. Among initial symptoms reported by caregivers, personality change and language impairment were significantly more common in FTD than AD. At initial cognitive testing, deficits in memory were common in both groups, but more prevalent in AD. Patients with FTD had greater impairments on the ADL Scale. During the course of illness, patients with FTD declined significantly faster than those with AD on language tests and on global measures of dementia severity (187). These results in this large co-hort of patients with dementia underline the importance of determining cognitive profiles at the beginning and during the course of the disease, for the differential diagnosis.

The same is supported by another study that suggests a selection of neuropsychological tests are sensitive in the differential diagnosis of AD (155). Neuropsychological performance (including measures of language, semantic memory, visual and spatial perception, and executive functions) was compared in two groups of patients with clinical diagnosis of probable AD or FTD. The aim was to identify a specific cognitive profile for FTD to be used as a sensitive short evaluation for the differential diagnosis with AD. Both groups were severely impaired in most tasks, but interestingly also in "frontal lobe" tests that have been suggested to play an important role in the differential diagnosis. Noteworthy, significant differences were found for a minority of tests that assessed oral praxis, visuospatial perception, and verbal fluency. The authors suggest a shortened testing procedure based on four tests (Rey Complex Figure recall, phonemic fluency, cube analysis, and oral apraxia test), together with other measures sensitive to frontal impairment as a useful tool in the differential diagnosis between AD and FTD.

New research approaches in the neuropsychological evaluation of dementia might derive from neuroimaging studies. Normal subjects executing specific cognitive tasks during functional magnetic resonance imaging (fMRI) or positron emission tomography (PET) acquisitions have shown the activation of complex neural systems. These studies provide evidence for the neural correlates of cognition that go far beyond classical neuropsychological correlates in brain-damaged patients. For example, they suggest that whereas the left temporal neocortex plays a crucial role in all tasks involving lexical-semantic processing, some regions of the left prefrontal convexity are selectively recruited during verb processing. Repetitive transcranial magnetic stimulation (rTMS) also showed different neural correlates for noun and verb processing in the human brain (188). In fact, a shortening of naming latency for actions was observed only after stimulation of left prefrontal cortex. On this basis, noun and verb processing in different dementia types were assessed (154). Object and action naming was tested in probable AD patients with mild to moderate dementia and in a group of FTD patients. AD and FTD patients were impaired in naming compared with control subjects; action naming being more severely impaired. However, the discrepancy between object and action naming was significantly greater in FTD than in AD patients, independent of the severity of dementia or of overall language impairment. The latter finding is compatible with the hypothesis that the frontal lobe plays a crucial role in action naming. The authors suggest a relatively selective impairment in action naming as a characteristic neuropsychological feature of FTD.

New interesting research approaches aimed at identifying specific personality and behavioral profiles in dementia have recently emerged. In FTD, diagnostic criteria agree that alterations in personality and social conduct are a central clinical feature of the disease (4,137). However, quantitative instruments have not been used to systematically measure these changes. Similarly, specific social deficits in the FTD syndrome have not been isolated to either the frontal or temporal variants of the disease. A promising approach is the study of "theory of mind," a key aspect of social cognition related to the prefrontal cortex, which has been reported to be affected in the frontal variant of FTD (189). One source of confusion may be that clinicians and researchers have focused on discrete behavioral changes (138,142,190), since they do not have the tools to observe a patient's social processing on a higher level. Since personality becomes fixed by early adulthood and remains constant throughout old age, significant changes in personality during adulthood typically have a neuropathologic etiology (191). Because the primary brain areas affected in FTD are the frontal lobes, in particular the orbitofrontal and frontal medial cortex, the anterior temporal lobes, the amygdala, and ventral striatum (63), the observed personality changes ostensibly arise from a disruption of these structures. In contrast, early in the disease, social functioning remains preserved in AD, most likely because of the relative sparing of these anterior structures (192,193). It therefore seems important to include investigations of how particular social deficits correlate with neuropsychological functioning and areas of pathology on functional brain scans. It will become possible to further characterize a patient's personality change as a function of the timing of the disease progression. A recent paper suggests the Interpersonal Adjectives Scales, since they were able to differentiate frontal and temporal variants of FTD from patients with AD, who remained within the normal range on all scores, on the basis of both degree and direction of personality change (194,195). On a similar basis, the Frontal Behavioral Inventory Scale is a useful tool for the assessment of behavioral changes in FTD patients.

The identification of clinical subtypes of probable AD, such as the so-called posterior cortical atrophy variant, raises the issue of a more focused neuropsychological assessment. Posterior cortical atrophy presents with prevalent visuospatial deficits, thus evaluation of visuoperceptual abilities and also praxis is necessary. Two batteries have been proposed so far, the Visual Object and Space Perception Battery and the Birmingham Object Recognition Battery. They are both time-demanding, and therefore considering the patient's compliance, a useful evaluation can be achieved by a using a shorter task administration, such as Benton's Line Judgment Orientation and Benton's Face Test.

CONCLUSIONS

Not long ago, cognitive aging was viewed as a general deterioration of cognition (reflected by a decreasing IQ) and dementia as an acceleration of this process. Currently, we know that cognitive decline occurs in various forms, marked by considerable differences in the nature and order of development of behavioral symptoms. This knowledge is an important asset in the early detection, management, and treatment of dementia. The neuropsychological assessment of dementia has a central role and is concerned with all disease stages. The current implicit assumption that all patients with AD tend to evolve and decline in a similar fashion needs to be critically re-examined. Neuropsychological tests allow one to determine various patients' profiles. Future research should determine the possible predictive value of these profiles, which has important implications for therapeutic trials. Clinically, neuropsychological instruments are crucial for the diagnosis, prognosis, and monitoring of pharmacological treatments. In the field of research, its role is even more clear-cut: a correct clinical diagnosis is mandatory in instrumental and pharmacological trials. However, the neuropsychological approach to dementia certainly has limitations and is at its proper place only in a multidisciplinary context. The concerted effort of all branches of neuroscience is required for patient care, as well as research on cognitive decline in aging individuals and in neurological diseases.

REFERENCES

1. American PA. Diagnostic and Statistical Manual of Mental Disorders. 4th ed. Washington DC: American Psychiatric Association,1994.

2. McKhann G, Drachman D, Folstein M, Katzman R, Price D, Stadlan EM. Clinical diagnosis of Alzheimer's disease: report of the NINCDS-ADRDA Work Group under the auspices of Department of Health and Human Services Task Force on Alzheimer's Disease. Neurology 1984; 34:939–944.

3. Roman GC, Tatemichi TK, Erkinjuntti T, et al. Vascular dementia: diagnostic criteria for research studies. Report of the NINDS-AIREN International Workshop. Neurology 1993; 43:250–260.

4. The Lund a, Group, M. Clinical and neuropathological criteria for frontotemporal dementia. The Lund and Manchester Groups. J Neurol Neurosurg Psychiatry 1994; 57:416–418.

5. Folstein MF, Folstein SE, McHugh PR. "Mini-mental state." A practical method for grading the cognitive state of patients for the clinician. J Psychiatr Res 1975; 12:189–198.

6. Grut M, Fratiglioni L, Viitanen M, Winblad B. Accuracy of the Mini-Mental Status Examination as a screening test for dementia in a Swedish elderly population. Acta Neurol Scand 1993; 87:312–317.

7. Strub R, Black F. The mental status examination in neurology. Philadelphia: Davis, 1993.

8. Bisiach E, Cappa S, Vallar G. Guida all'esame neuropsicologico. Milan: Raffaello Cortina, 1983.

9. Hodges J. Cognitive assessment for clinicians. Oxford: Oxford Medical Publications, 1994.

10. Reisberg B, Ferris SH, de Leon MJ, Crook T. The Global Deterioration Scale for assessment of primary degenerative dementia. Am J Psychiatry 1982; 139:1136–1139.

11. Morris JC. Clinical dementia rating: a reliable and valid diagnostic and staging measure for dementia of the Alzheimer type. Int Psychogeriatr 1997; 9:173–176; discussion 177–178.

12. Kalbe E, Salmon E, Perani D, et al. Anosognosia in very mild Alzheimer's disease but not in mild cognitive impairment. Dement Geriatr Cogn Disord 2005; 19:349–356.

13. Weschler D. The measurement of adult intelligence. Baltimore: Williams and Wilkins, 1939.

14. Heaton R, Marcotte T. In: Boller FGJ, Rizzolatti G, eds. Clinical neuropsychological tetsts and assessment techniques. Handbook of Neuropsychology, Amsterdam: Elsevier, 2000; 1:27–52.

15. Devanand DP, Folz M, Gorlyn M, Moeller JR, Stern Y. Questionable dementia: clinical course and predictors of outcome. J Am Geriatr Soc 1997; 45:321–328.

16. Lezak M. Neuropsychological assessment. Oxford: Oxford University Press, 1995.

17. Nakamura H, Nakanishi M, Furukawa TA, Hamanaka T, Tokudome S. Validity of brief intelligence tests for patients with Alzheimer's disease. Psychiatry Clin Neurosci 2000; 54:435–439.

18. Brandt J, Spencer M, McSorley P, Folstein MF. Semantic activation and implicit memory in Alzheimer disease. Alzheimer Dis Assoc Disord 1988; 2:112–119.

19. Mahieux F, Michelet D, Manifacier M-J, Boller F, Fermanian J, Guillard A. Mini-Mental Parkinson: First Validation Study of a new Bedside Test Constructed for Parkinson's disease. Behavioural Neurology 1995; 8:15–22.

20. Tang-Wai DF, Knopman DS, Geda YE, et al. Comparison of the short test of mental status and the mini-mental state examination in mild cognitive impairment. Arch Neurol 2003; 60:1777–1781.

21. Heyman A, Wilkinson WE, Hurwitz BJ, et al. Early-onset Alzheimer's disease: clinical predictors of institutionalization and death. Neurology 1987; 37:980–984.

22. Hughes CP, Berg L, Danziger WL, Coben LA, Martin RL. A new clinical scale for the staging of dementia. Br J Psychiatry 1982; 140:566–572.

23. Marcopulos BA, Gripshover DL, Broshek DK, McLain CA, Brashear HR. Neuropsychological assesment of psychogeriatric patients with limited education. Clin Neuropsychol 1999; 13:147–156.

24. Paul RH, Cohen RA, Moser D, et al. Performance on the Mattis Dementia Rating Scale in patients with vascular dementia: relationships to neuroimaging findings. J Geriatr Psychiatry Neurol 2001; 14:33–36.

25. Suarez SV, Stankoff B, Conquy L, et al. Similar subcortical pattern of cognitive impairment in AIDS patients with and without dementia. Eur J Neurol 2000; 7:151–158.

26. Vitaliano PP, Breen AR, Albert MS, Russo J, Prinz PN. Memory, attention, and functional status in community-residing Alzheimer type dementia patients and optimally healthy aged individuals. J Gerontol 1984; 39:58–64.

27. Tombaugh TN, McIntyre NJ. The mini-mental state examination: a comprehensive review. J Am Geriatr Soc 1992; 40:922–935.

28. Blessed G, Tomlinson BE, Roth M. The association between quantitative measures of dementia and of senile change in the cerebral grey matter of elderly subjects. Br J Psychiatry 1968; 114:797–811.

29. Cosentino S, Jefferson A, Chute DL, Kaplan E, Libon DJ. Clock drawing errors in dementia: neuropsychological and neuroanatomical considerations. Cogn Behav Neurol 2004; 17:74–84.

30. Solomon PR, Hirschoff A, Kelly B, et al. A 7 minute neurocognitive screening battery highly sensitive to Alzheimer's disease. Arch Neurol 1998; 55:349–355.

31. Nasreddine ZS, Phillips NA, Bedirian V, et al. The Montreal Cognitive Assessment. MoCA: a brief screening tool for mild cognitive impairment. J Am Geriatr Soc 2005; 53:695–699.

32. Kalbe E, Kessler J, Calabrese P, et al. DemTect: a new, sensitive cognitive screening test to support the diagnosis of mild cognitive impairment and early dementia. Int J Geriatr Psychiatry 2004; 19:136–143.

33. Roth M, Tym E, Mountjoy CQ, et al. CAMDEX. A standardised instrument for the diagnosis of mental disorder in the elderly with special reference to the early detection of dementia. Br J Psychiatry 1986; 149:698–709.

34. van Hout H, Teunisse S, Derix M, et al. CAMDEX, can it be more efficient? Observational study on the contribution of four screening measures to the diagnosis of dementia by a memory clinic team Int J Geriatr Psychiatry 2001; 16:64–69.

35. Morris JC, Mohs RC, Rogers H, Fillenbaum G, Heyman A. Consortium to establish a registry for Alzheimer's disease (CERAD) clinical and neuropsychological assessment of Alzheimer's disease. Psychopharmacol Bull 1988; 24:641–652.

36. Welsh K, Butters N, Hughes J, Mohs R, Heyman A. Detection of abnormal memory decline in mild cases of Alzheimer's disease using CERAD neuropsychological measures. Arch Neurol 1991; 48:278–281.

37. Rosen WG, Mohs RC, Davis KL. A new rating scale for Alzheimer's disease. Am J Psychiatry 1984; 141:1356–1364.

38. Pena-Casanova J. Alzheimer's Disease Assessment Scale—cognitive in clinical practice. Int Psychogeriatr 1997; 1:105–114.

39. Baddeley A, Hitch G. Working memory The psychology of learning and motivation: advances in research and theory. In: Bower, ed. New York: Academy Press, 1974; 8.

40. Baddeley A. Working memory: the interface between memory and cognition. In: Schacter DLTE, ed. Memory Systems. Cambridge, Ma: The MIT Press, 1994.

41. Baddeley AD, Bressi S, Della Sala S, Logie R, Spinnler H. The decline of working memory in Alzheimer's disease. A longitudinal study. Brain 1991; 114:2521–2542.

42. Spinnler H. Alzheimer's disease: neuropsychological defects according to topographical spreading of neuronal degeneration. In: Denes GPL, ed. Handbook of Clinical and Experimental Neuropsychology. Hove: Psychol. Press, 1999:699–746.

43. Milner B. Interhemispheric differences in the localization of psychological processes in man. Br Med Bull 1971; 27:272–277.

44. Belleville S, Peretz I, Malenfant D. Examination of the working memory components in normal aging and in dementia of the Alzheimer type. Neuropsychologia 1996; 34:195–207.

45. Morris RG. Dementia and the functioning of Articulatory Loop System. Cogn Neuropsychol 1984; 1:143–157.

46. Cherry B, Buckwalter J, Henderson V. Memory span procedures in Alzheimer's disease. Neuropsychology 1996; 10:286–293.

47. Kopelman MD. Rates of forgetting in Alzheimer-type dementia and Korsakoff's syndrome. Neuropsychologia 1985; 23:623–638.

48. Grossi D, Becker JT, Smith C, Trojano L. Memory for visuospatial patterns in Alzheimer's disease. Psychol Med 1993; 23:65–70.

49. Orsini A, Trojano L, Chiacchio L, Grossi D. Immediate memory spans in dementia. Percept Mot Skills 1988; 67:267–272.

50. Spinnler H, Della Sala S, Bandera R, Baddeley A. Dementia, ageing, and the structure of human memory. Cogn Neuropsychol 1988; 5:193–211.

51. Buschke H, Hinrichs J. Controlled rehearsal and recall order in serial list retention. J Exp Psychol 1968; 78:502–509.

52. Wilson RS, Bacon LD, Fox JH, Kaszniak AW. Primary memory and secondary memory in dementia of the Alzheimer type. J Clin Neuropsychol 1983; 5:337–344.

53. Tulving E. Episodic and semantic memory. In: Tulving EDW, ed. Organization of Memory. New York: Academic Press, 1972.

54. Buschke H, Sliwinski MJ, Kuslansky G, Lipton RB. Diagnosis of early dementia by the double memory test: encoding specificity improves diagnostic sensitivity and specificity. Neurology 1997; 48:989–997.

55. Jacobs DM, Sano M, Dooneief G, Marder K, Bell KL, Stern Y. Neuropsychological detection and characterization of preclinical Alzheimer's disease. Neurology 1995; 45:957–962.

56. Masur DM, Sliwinski M, Lipton RB, Blau AD, Crystal HA. Neuropsychological prediction of dementia and the absence of dementia in healthy elderly persons. Neurology 1994; 44:1427–1432.

57. Petersen RC, Smith GE, Ivnik RJ, Kokmen E, Tangalos EG. Memory function in very early Alzheimer's disease. Neurology 1994; 44:867–872.

58. Bondi MW, Monsch AU, Galasko D, Butters N, Salmon DP, Delis DC. Preclinical cognitive markers of dementia of the Alzheimer's type. Neuropsychology 1994; 8:374–384.

59. Linn RT, Wolf PA, Bachman DL, et al. The 'preclinical phase' of probable Alzheimer's disease. A 13-year prospective study of the Framingham cohort. Arch Neurol 1995; 52:485–490.

60. Albert MS. Cognitive and neurobiologic markers of early Alzheimer disease. Proc Natl Acad Sci USA 1996; 93:13547–13551.

61. Banos J, Martin R. California verbal learning test. In: Delis DKJ, Kaplan E, Ober B, San Antonio TX, eds. California Verbal Learning Test. San Antonio, TX: The Psychological Corporation, 2000.

62. Salmon E, Garraux G, Delbeuck X, et al. Predominant ventromedial frontopolar metabolic impairment in frontotemporal dementia. Neuroimage 2003; 20:435–440.

63. Franceschi M, Anchisi D, Pelati O, et al. Glucose metabolism and serotonin receptors in the frontotemporal lobe degeneration. Ann Neurol 2005; 57:216–225.

64. Anchisi D, Borroni B, Franceschi M, et al. Heterogeneity of glucose brain metabolism in Mild Cognitive Impairment predicts clinical progression to Alzheimer's Disease. Heterogeneity of brain glucose metabolism in mild cognitive impairment and clinical progression to Alzheimer disease. Archives of Neurology 2005; 62:1728–1733.

65. Tulving E, Thomson D. Encoding specificity and the retrieval processes in episodic memory. Psychol Rev 1973; 80:352–373.

66. Buschke H. Cued recall in amnesia. J Clin Neuropsychol 1984; 6:433–440.

67. Grober E, Buschke H, Crystal H, Bang S, Dresner R. Screening for dementia by memory testing. Neurology 1988; 38:900–903.

68. Wechsler D. In: Wechsler memory scale-revised manual. ed. The Psychological Corporation, San Antonio TX, 1987.

69. Buschke H, Kuslansky G, Katz M, et al. Screening for dementia with the memory impairment screen. Neurology 1999; 52:231–238.

70. American, Psychiatric, Association. Diagnosticand statistical manual of mental disorders. 3rd ed. Washington, D.C: American Psychiatric Association, 1987.

71. Stroop J. Studies of interference in serial verbal reactions. J Exp Psychol 1935; 18:643–662.

72. Reitan R. Validity of the trail making test as an indication of the organic damage. Percept Mot Skills 1985; 8:271–276.

73. Grant DA, Berg E. The Wisconsin card sort test random layout: directions for administration and scoring. Madison Wisconsin: Wells Printing, 1980.

74. Ramage A, Holland A. In: Boller FGJ, ed. Language in Normal Aging and Age-Related Neurological Disorders. Handbook of Neuropsychology, Amsterdam: Elsevier, 1997; 7.
75. Fuld PA, Katzman R, Davies P, Terry RD. Intrusions as a sign of Alzheimer dementia: chemical and pathological verification. Ann Neurol 1982; 11:155–159.
76. Lukatela K, Malloy P, Jenkins M, Cohen R. The naming deficit in early Alzheimer's and vascular dementia. Neuropsychology 1998; 12:565–572.
77. Kaplan E, Goodglass H, Weintraub S. The Boston Naming Test. Philadelphia: Lea & Febiger, 1983.
78. Saxton J, Ratcliff G, Munro CA, et al. Normative data on the boston naming test and two equivalent 30-item short forms. Clin Neuropsychol 2000; 14:526–534.
79. Nicholas M, Obler LK, Au R, Albert ML. On the nature of naming errors in aging and dementia: a study of semantic relatedness. Brain Lang 1996; 54:184–195.
80. Waters G, Rochon E, Caplan D. Task demands and sentence comprehension in patients with dementia of the Alzheimer's type. Brain Lang 1998; 62:361–397.
81. Tomoeda CK, Bayles KA, Trosset MW, Azuma T, McGeagh A. Cross-sectional analysis of Alzheimer disease effects on oral discourse in a picture description task. Alzheimer Dis Assoc Disord 1996; 10:204–215.
82. De Renzi E, Vignolo L. The token test: a sensitive test to detect receptive disturbances in aphasics. Brain 1962; 85:665–678.
83. Boller F, Vignolo LA. Latent sensory aphasia in hemisphere-damaged patients: an experimental study with the token test. Brain 1966; 89:815–830.
84. Pasquier F, Grymonprez L, Lebert F, Van der Linden M. Memory impairment differs in frontotemporal dementia and Alzheimer's disease. Neurocase 2001; 7:161–171.
85. Holland A, Boller F, Bourgeois M. Repetition in Alzheimer's Disease: A Longitudinal Study. J Neurolinguistics 1986; 2:163–177.
86. De Renzi E, Lucchelli F. Ideational apraxia. Brain 1988; 111:1173–1185.
87. Brun A, Passant U. Frontal lobe degeneration of non-Alzheimer type. Structural characteristics, diagnostic criteria and relation to other frontotemporal dementias. Acta Neurol Scand Suppl 1996; 168:28–30.
88. Rey A. Reattivo della figura complessa. Firenze, Manuale Organizzazioni Speciali 1983.
89. Spinnler H, Tognoni G. Standardizzazione e taratura italiana di test neuropsicologici. Ital J Neurol Sci 1987; 6:5–120.
90. Cahn-Weiner DA, Sullivan EV, Shear PK, et al. Brain structural and cognitive correlates of clock drawing performance in Alzheimer's disease. J Int Neuropsychol Soc 1999; 5:502–509.
91. Stehli Nguyen A, Chubb C, Jacob Huff F. Visual identification and spatial location in Alzheimer's disease. Brain Cogn 2003; 52:155–166.
92. Mendez MF, Turner J, Gilmore GC, Remler B, Tomsak RL. Balint's syndrome in Alzheimer's disease: visuospatial functions. Int J Neurosci 1990; 54:339–346.
93. Armstrong CL, Cloud B. The emergence of spatial rotation deficits in dementia and normal aging. Neuropsychology 1998; 12:208–217.
94. Kaskie B, Storandt M. Visuospatial deficit in dementia of the Alzheimer type. Arch Neurol 1995; 52:422–425.
95. Mendola JD, Cronin-Golomb A, Corkin S, Growdon JH. Prevalence of visual deficits in Alzheimer's disease. Optom Vis Sci 1995; 72:155–167.

96. Giovagnoli AR, Del Pesce M, Mascheroni S, Simoncelli M, Laiacona M, Capitani E. Trail making test: normative values from 287 normal adult controls. Ital J Neurol Sci 1996; 17:305–309.
97. Cummings JL. Behavior as an efficacy outcome. Alzheimer Dis Assoc Disord 1997; 11:v–vi.
98. Cummings JL. Theories behind existing scales for rating behavior in dementia. Int Psychogeriatr 1996; 8:293–300.
99. Zanetti O, Vallotti B, Frisoni GB, et al. Insight in dementia: when does it occur? Evidence for a nonlinear relationship between insight and cognitive status J Gerontol B Psychol Sci Soc Sci 1999; 54:P100–P106.
100. Cummings JL, Mega M, Gray K, Rosenberg-Thompson S, Carusi DA, Gornbein J. The Neuropsychiatric Inventory: comprehensive assessment of psychopathology in dementia. Neurology 1994; 44:2308–2314.
101. Binetti G, Mega MS, Magni E, et al. Behavioral disorders in Alzheimer disease: a transcultural perspective. Arch Neurol 1998; 55:539–544.
102. Bianchetti A, Pezzini A. L'insight nel paziente demente. Dementia Update 1998; 2:45–62.
103. Ott BR, Lafleche G, Whelihan WM, Buongiorno GW, Albert MS, Fogel BS. Impaired awareness of deficits in Alzheimer disease. Alzheimer Dis Assoc Disord 1996; 10:68–76.
104. Vallotti B, Zanetti O, Bianchetti A, Trabucchi M. L'insight del paziente demente: riproducibilita' di due strumenti di valutazione. Giorn Geront 1997; 45:341–345.
105. Corey-Bloom J, Thal LJ, Galasko D, et al. Diagnosis and evaluation of dementia. Neurology 1995; 45:211–218.
106. Reuben D. Use and abuse of assessment instruments. In: Osterwail DRD, Rozzini R, Rubenstein LZ, Trabucchi M, eds. New Frontiers in Geriatric medicine. Kendall: Padova, 1993:17–26.
107. Reuben DB, Solomon DH. Assessment in geriatrics of caveats and names. J Am Geriatr Soc 1989; 37:570–572.
108. Johnson N, Barion A, Rademaker A, Rehkemper G, Weintraub S. The activities of daily living questionnaire: a validation study in patients with dementia. Alzheimer Dis Assoc Disord 2004; 18:223–230.
109. Volicer L, Hurley AC, Lathi DC, Kowall NW. Measurement of severity in advanced Alzheimer's disease. J Gerontol 1994; 49:M223–M226.
110. Loewenstein DA, Amigo E, Duara R, et al. A new scale for the assessment of functional status in Alzheimer's disease and related disorders. J Gerontol 1989; 44:P114–P121.
111. Reuben DB, Siu AL. An objective measure of physical function of elderly outpatients. The physical performance test. J Am Geriatr Soc 1990; 38:1105–1112.
112. Tinetti ME. Performance-oriented assessment of mobility problems in elderly patients. J Am Geriatr Soc 1986; 34:119–126.
113. Holland A. Communicative Abilities in Daily Living. Austin TX: PRO-ED, 1980.
114. Fromm D, Holland A. Functional communication in Alzheimer's disease. J Speech Hear Disord 1989; 54:535–540.
115. Petersen RC, Doody R, Kurz A, et al. Current concepts in mild cognitive impairment. Arch Neurol 2001; 58:1985–1992.

116. Small BJ, Fratiglioni L, Viitanen M, Winblad B, Backman L. The course of cognitive impairment in preclinical Alzheimer disease: three- and 6-year follow-up of a population-based sample. Arch Neurol 2000; 57:839–844.
117. Bozoki A, Giordani B, Heidebrink JL, Berent S, Foster NL. Mild cognitive impairments predict dementia in nondemented elderly patients with memory loss. Arch Neurol 2001; 58:411–416.
118. Ritchie K, Touchon J. Mild cognitive impairment: conceptual basis and current nosological status. Lancet 2000; 355:225–228.
119. Petersen RC, Stevens JC, Ganguli M, Tangalos EG, Cummings JL, DeKosky ST. Practice parameter: early detection of dementia: mild cognitive impairment (an evidence-based review). Report of the quality standards subcommittee of the american academy of neurology. Neurology 2001; 56:1133–1142.
120. Chertkow H, Bergman H, Schipper HM, et al. Assessment of suspected dementia. Can J Neurol Sci 2001; 28:S28–S41.
121. Petersen RC. Mild Cognitive Impairment. New York: Oxford University Press, 2003.
122. Fuld PA, Masur DM, Blau AD, Crystal H, Aronson MK. Object-memory evaluation for prospective detection of dementia in normal functioning elderly: predictive and normative data. J Clin Exp Neuropsychol 1990; 12:520–528.
123. Ritchie K, Artero S, Touchon J. Classification criteria for mild cognitive impairment: a population-based validation study. Neurology 2001; 56:37–42.
124. Chen P, Ratcliff G, Belle SH, Cauley JA, DeKosky ST, Ganguli M. Cognitive tests that best discriminate between presymptomatic AD and those who remain nondemented. Neurology 2000; 55:1847–1853.
125. Fox NC, Warrington EK, Seiffer AL, Agnew SK, Rossor MN. Presymptomatic cognitive deficits in individuals at risk of familial Alzheimer's disease. A longitudinal prospective study. Brain 1998; 121:1631–1639.
126. Thompson SA, Graham KS, Patterson K, Sahakian BJ, Hodges JR. Is knowledge of famous people disproportionately impaired in patients with early and questionable Alzheimer's disease? Neuropsychology 2002; 16:344–358.
127. Estevez-Gonzalez A, Garcia-Sanchez C, Boltes A, et al. Semantic knowledge of famous people in mild cognitive impairment and progression to Alzheimer's disease. Dement Geriatr Cogn Disord 2004; 17:188–195.
128. Tierney MC, Szalai JP, Snow WG, et al. Prediction of probable Alzheimer's disease in memory-impaired patients: a prospective longitudinal study. Neurology 1996; 46:661–665.
129. Albert MS, Moss MB, Tanzi R, Jones K. Preclinical prediction of AD using neuropsychological tests. J Int Neuropsychol Soc 2001; 7:631–639.
130. Blackwell AD, Sahakian BJ, Vesey R, Semple JM, Robbins TW, Hodges JR. Detecting dementia: novel neuropsychological markers of preclinical Alzheimer's disease. Dement Geriatr Cogn Disord 2004; 17:42–48.
131. Darby D, Maruff P, Collie A, McStephen M. Mild cognitive impairment can be detected by multiple assessments in a single day. Neurology 2002; 59:1042–1046.
132. O'Brien JT, Erkinjuntti T, Reisberg B, et al. Vascular cognitive impairment. Lancet Neurol 2003; 2:89–98.
133. Chui HC, Victoroff JI, Margolin D, Jagust W, Shankle R, Katzman R. Criteria for the diagnosis of ischemic vascular dementia proposed by the State of California Alzheimer's disease diagnostic and treatment centers. Neurology 1992; 42:473–480.

134. Roman GC. Defining dementia: clinical criteria for the diagnosis of vascular dementia. Acta Neurol Scand Suppl 2002; 178:6–9.
135. Kurz AF, Erkinjuntti T, Small GW, Lilienfeld S, Damaraju CR. Long-term safety and cognitive effects of galantamine in the treatment of probable vascular dementia or Alzheimer's disease with cerebrovascular disease. Eur J Neurol 2003; 10:633–640.
136. Graham NL, Emery T, Hodges JR. Distinctive cognitive profiles in Alzheimer's disease and subcortical vascular dementia. J Neurol Neurosurg Psychiatry 2004; 75:61–71.
137. Neary D, Snowden JS, Gustafson L, et al. Frontotemporal lobar degeneration: a consensus on clinical diagnostic criteria. Neurology 1998; 51:1546–1554.
138. Edwards-Lee T, Miller BL, Benson DF, et al. The temporal variant of frontotemporal dementia. Brain 1997; 120:1027–1040.
139. Varma AR, Snowden JS, Lloyd JJ, Talbot PR, Mann DM, Neary D. Evaluation of the NINCDS-ADRDA criteria in the differentiation of Alzheimer's disease and frontotemporal dementia. J Neurol Neurosurg Psychiatry 1999; 66:184–188.
140. Rosen HJ, Hartikainen KM, Jagust W, et al. Utility of clinical criteria in differentiating frontotemporal lobar degeneration (FTLD) from AD. Neurology 2002; 58:1608–1615.
141. Lebert F, Pasquier F, Souliez L, Petit H. Frontotemporal behavioral scale. Alzheimer Dis Assoc Disord 1998; 12:335–339.
142. Bozeat S, Gregory CA, Ralph MA, Hodges JR. Which neuropsychiatric and behavioural features distinguish frontal and temporal variants of frontotemporal dementia from Alzheimer's disease? J Neurol Neurosurg Psychiatry 2000; 69:178–186.
143. Kertesz A, Nadkarni N, Davidson W, Thomas AW. The Frontal Behavioral Inventory in the differential diagnosis of frontotemporal dementia. J Int Neuropsychol Soc 2000; 6:460–468.
144. Kertesz A, Davidson W, Fox H. Frontal behavioral inventory: diagnostic criteria for frontal lobe dementia. Can J Neurol Sci 1997; 24:29–36.
145. Perry RJ, Hodges JR. Differentiating frontal and temporal variant frontotemporal dementia from Alzheimer's disease. Neurology 2000; 54:2277–2284.
146. Rosen HJ, Perry RJ, Murphy J, et al. Emotion comprehension in the temporal variant of frontotemporal dementia. Brain 2002; 125:2286–2295.
147. Magni E, Binetti G, Cappa S, Bianchetti A, Trabucchi M. Effect of age and education on performance on the Mini-Mental State Examination in a healthy older population and during the course of Alzheimer's disease. J Am Geriatr Soc 1995; 43:942–943.
148. Basso A, Capitani E, Laiacona M. Raven's coloured progressive matrices: normative values on 305 adult normal controls. Funct Neurol 1987; 2:189–194.
149. Novelli G, Papagno C, Capitani E. Tre test clinici di memoria verbale a lungo termine. Taratura su soggetti normali. Arch Psicol Neurol Psich 1986; 47:278–296.
150. Orsini A, Grossi D, Capitani E, Laiacona M, Papagno C, Vallar G. Verbal and spatial immediate memory span: normative data from 1355 adults and 1112 children. Ital J Neurol Sci 1987; 8:539–548.
151. Miceli G, Laudanna A, Burani C, Capasso R. Batteria per l'Analisi dei Deficit Afasici, BADA. Università Cattolica del Sacro Cuore. Istituto di Psicologia 1994.

152. Hodges JR, Patterson K, Oxbury S, Funnell E. Semantic dementia. Progressive fluent aphasia with temporal lobe atrophy. Brain 1992; 115:1783–1806.

153. Howard D, Patterson K. The pyramids and palm trees test. A Test of Semantic Access From Pictures and Words. Thames Valley: Bury St Edmunds, 1992.

154. Cappa SF, Binetti G, Pezzini A, Padovani A, Rozzini L, Trabucchi M. Object and action naming in Alzheimer's disease and frontotemporal dementia. Neurology 1998; 50:351–355 see comment.

155. Siri S, Benaglio I, Frigerio A, Binetti G, Cappa SF. A brief neuropsychological assessment for the differential diagnosis between frontotemporal dementia and Alzheimer's disease. Eur J Neurol 2001; 8:125–132.

156. McKeith IG, Perry RH, Fairbairn AF, Jabeen S, Perry EK. Operational criteria for senile dementia of Lewy body type (SDLT). Psychol Med 1992; 22:911–922.

157. Walker Z, Allen RL, Shergill S, Katona CL. Neuropsychological performance in Lewy body dementia and Alzheimer's disease. Br J Psychiatry 1997; 170:156–158.

158. Gnanalingham KK, Byrne EJ, Thornton A. Clock-face drawing to differentiate Lewy body and Alzheimer type dementia syndromes. Lancet 1996; 347(9002):696–697.

159. Lichtenberg PA, Ross T, Millis SR, Manning CA. The relationship between depression and cognition in older adults: a cross-validation study. J Gerontol B Psychol Sci Soc Sci 1995; 50:P25–P32.

160. Zakzanis KK, Leach L, Kaplan E. On the nature and pattern of neurocognitive function in major depressive disorder. Neuropsychiatry Neuropsychol Behav Neurol 1998; 11:111–119.

161. Swainson R, Hodges JR, Galton CJ, et al. Early detection and differential diagnosis of Alzheimer's disease and depression with neuropsychological tasks. Dement Geriatr Cogn Disord 2001; 12:265–280.

162. Eastwood R. Adieu to Alzheimer? Can J Psychiatry 1994; 39:251–252.

163. Keene J, Hope T, Fairburn CG, Jacoby R, Gedling K, Ware CJ. Natural history of aggressive behaviour in dementia. Int J Geriatr Psychiatry 1999; 14:541–548.

164. Teri L, Larson EB, Reifler BV. Behavioral disturbance in dementia of the Alzheimer's type. J Am Geriatr Soc 1988; 36:1–6.

165. Teri L, Ferretti LE, Gibbons LE, et al. Anxiety of Alzheimer's disease: prevalence, and comorbidity. J Gerontol A Biol Sci Med Sci 1999; 54:M348–M352.

166. Alexopoulos GS, Abrams RC, Young RC, Shamoian CA. Cornell Scale for Depression in Dementia. Biol Psychiatry 1988; 23:271–284.

167. Leroi I, Voulgari A, Breitner JC, Lyketsos CG. The epidemiology of psychosis in dementia. Am J Geriatr Psychiatry 2003; 11:83–91.

168. Verny M, Hugonot-Diener L, Boller F. Severe dementia and its evaluation: scales for cognition, behavior, and overall functioning. In Handbook of Neuropsychology, 2nd Edition, Edited by Boller F, Cappa S. Amsterdam: Elsevier. Vol. 6. 2001; 463–474.

169. Ritchie K, Ledesert B. The measurement of incapacity in the severely demented elderly: the validation of a behavioural assessment scale. Int J Geriat Psychiatry 1991; 6:217–226.

170. Benesch CG, McDaniel KD, Cox C, Hamill RW. End-stage Alzheimer's disease. Glasgow coma scale and the neurologic examination. Arch Neurol 1993; 50:1309–1315.

171. Panisset M, Saxton J, Boller F. End-stage Alzheimer's disease: Glasgow Coma Scale and the neurologic examination. Arch Neurol 1995; 52:127–128.

172. Cole MG, Dastoor DP. The hierarchic dementia scale: conceptualization. Int Psychogeriatr 1996; 8:205–212.

173. Peavy GM, Salmon DP, Rice VA, et al. Neuropsychological assessment of severely demeted elderly: the severe cognitive impairment profile. Arch Neurol 1996; 53:367–372.

174. Saxton J, Swihart AA. Neuropsychological assessment of the severely impaired elderly patient. Clin Geriatr Med 1989; 5:531–543.

175. Panisset M, Poncet M, Boller F, Simonetto J. Validation de l'échelle CERAD. Premières données françaises., abstract presented at the 2nd French AD symposium. Marseille, 1993.

176. Verny M, Hugonot-Diener L, Saillon A. Evaluation de la Démence Sévère: Echelles Cognitives et Comportementales (Groupe de Travail du Greco). Année Gérontologique 1999; 13:156–168.

177. Pippi M, Mecocci P, Saxton J, et al. Neuropsychological assessment of the severely impaired elderly patient: validation of the Italian short version of the Severe Impairment Battery (SIB). Gruppo di Studio sull'Invecchiamento Cerebrale della Societa Italiana di Gerontologia e Geriatria. Aging (Milano) 1999; 11:221–226.

178. Llinas Regla J, Lozano Gallego M, Lopez O. Validacion de la version española de la severe impairment battery. Neurologia 1995; 10:14–18.

179. Pelissier C, Roudier M, Boller F. Factorial validation of the Severe Impairment Battery for patients with Alzheimer's disease. A pilot study. Dement Geriatr Cogn Disord 2002; 13:95–100.

180. Wilson B, Cockburn J, Baddeley A, Hiorns R. The development and validation of a test battery for detecting and monitoring everyday memory problems. J Clin Exp Neuropsychol 1989; 11:855–870.

181. Petersen RC. Mild cognitive impairment as a diagnostic entity. J Intern Med 2004; 256:183–194.

182. Vicioso BA. Dementia: when is it not Alzheimer disease? Am J Med Sci 2002; 324:84–95.

183. Gunning-Dixon FM, Raz N. The cognitive correlates of white matter abnormalities in normal aging: a quantitative review. Neuropsychology 2000; 14:224–232.

184. Ferro JM, Madureira S. Age-related white matter changes and cognitive impairment. J Neurol Sci 2002; 203–204:221–225.

185. McCusker J, Cole MG, Dendukuri N, Belzile E. The delirium index, a measure of the severity of delirium: new findings on reliability, validity, and responsiveness. J Am Geriatr Soc 2004; 52:1744–1749.

186. Binetti G, Cappa SF, Magni E, Padovani A, Bianchetti A, Trabucchi M. Visual and spatial perception in the early phase of Alzheimer's disease. Neuropsychology 1998; 12:29–33.

187. Binetti G, Locascio JJ, Corkin S, Vonsattel JP, Growdon JH. Differences between Pick disease and Alzheimer disease in clinical appearance and rate of cognitive decline. Arch Neurol 2000; 57:225–232.

188. Cappa SF, Sandrini M, Rossini PM, Sosta K, Miniussi C. The role of the left frontal lobe in action naming: rTMS evidence. Neurology 2002; 59:720–723.

189. Gregory C, Lough S, Stone V, et al. Theory of mind in patients with frontal variant frontotemporal dementia and Alzheimer's disease: theoretical and practical implications. Brain 2002; 125:752–764.
190. Gregory C, Hodges J. Dementia of frontal type and the focal lobar atrophies. Int Rev Psychiatry 1993; 5:397–406.
191. Stuss D, Benson D. The frontal lobes. New York: Raven Press, 1986.
192. Strauss ME, Pasupathi M, Chatterjee A. Concordance between observers in descriptions of personality change in Alzheimer's disease. Psychol Aging 1993; 8:475–480.
193. Siegler IC, Dawson DV, Welsh KA. Caregiver ratings of personality change in Alzheimer's disease patients: a replication. Psychol Aging 1994; 9:464–466.
194. Chatterjee A, Strauss ME, Smyth KA, Whitehouse PJ. Personality changes in Alzheimer's disease. Arch Neurol 1992; 49:486–491.
195. Rankin KP, Kramer JH, Mychack P, Miller BL. Double dissociation of social functioning in frontotemporal dementia. Neurology 2003; 60:266–271.

3

Biomarkers in Blood and Cerebrospinal Fluid

Harald Hampel and Katharina Buerger

Alzheimer Memorial Center and Geriatric Psychiatry Branch, Department of Psychiatry, Ludwig-Maximilian University, Munich, Germany

INTRODUCTION

Alzheimer's disease (AD) is the most common neurodegenerative disorder and afflicts about 10% of the population over 60. Biomarker research in neurodegenerative disorders using blood and cerebrospinal fluid (CSF) is focused on specific targets: early detection, differential diagnosis (classification), tracking of disease progression, and evaluation of therapeutic strategies. With the currently approved antidementia drugs and with the development of novel disease modifying therapeutic strategies (secondary prevention), it is of particular clinical interest to establish early diagnostic and preclinical prognostic biomarkers of AD.

Criteria for a useful biomarker were proposed by an international consensus group on molecular and biochemical markers of AD in 1998 (1). According to these guidelines, a biomarker for AD should detect important aspects of the fundamental neuropathology and be validated in neuropathologically confirmed cases. Its sensitivity for detecting AD should exceed 85% and its specificity in differentiating between AD and other dementias should be at least 75%. Ideally, a biomarker should also be reliable, reproducible, non-invasive, simple to perform, and inexpensive.

Until now, a large number of biomarker studies in AD have been reported (2–4). Relevance for clinical practice and feasibility, however, is questionable for the majority of markers that have been studied so far. Recently, based on accumulating data, the biological markers working group of the NIA neuroimaging in AD initiative suggested a selected set of 13 biomarker candidates as feasible core markers of AD for large-scale multi-center studies (4). Feasibility was determined by the availability of a validated assay for the biological marker in question, with properties that include high precision and reliability of measurement, as well as good description of reagents and standards. Core analytes were those judged by the initiative to have reasonable evidence for association with key mechanisms of pathology implicated in AD. There could be several different reasons to support measuring a biochemical marker, ranging from increasing diagnostic accuracy, enhancing the prediction of progression from mild cognitive impairment (MCI) to clinical AD, or providing insight into a pathway influenced by drug treatment for AD. It is likely that no single marker could serve all these utilities, hence the need for a panel of measures.

In this chapter, currently available data on these 13 putative biomarkers of AD are presented and their potential applicability for clinical use is discussed. Moreover, results on protein 14-3-3 are described briefly, a biomarker that has been established for the diagnosis of primary dementia disorders, such as Creutzfeldt–Jakob disease (CJD). As a perspective for further biomarker research, recent studies on naturally occurring antibodies against beta-amyloid (Aβ) peptide are presented.

β-AMYLOID PEPTIDE 40 AND 42

Extracellular senile plaques consisting of Aβ are one of the histopathological hallmarks of AD (5). Secreted soluble Aβ is found in various body fluids including plasma and CSF (6).

Aβ in Cerebrospinal Fluid

Initial reports on Aβ in CSF as a biomarker for AD were disappointing, with results ranging form a slight decrease in AD, with a large overlap, to no change (7–9). In these studies, total Aβ in CSF was examined. More recent studies have shown two major C-terminal variants of Aβ, with either 40 (Aβ40) or 42 (Aβ42) amino acids. Different ELISA tests have been developed for the measurement of Aβ42 in CSF and plasma (10,11). There are commercially available ELISA-kits for the measurement of Aβ42 and Aβ40 in CSF (e.g., The Genetics, Schlieren, Switzerland; Innogenetics, Gent, Belgium). Several studies reported that Aβ42 concentrations are decreased in CSF of AD patients (12–17). The specificity to distinguish patients with AD from controls has varied from 42% to 88%, and the sensitivity has varied from 72% to 100% in these studies. CSF levels for Aβ42 seem to be unrelated to age. Based on recent data, a cutoff-level of >500 pg/ml has been suggested to discriminate AD from normal aging (18). Further, it has been reported that Aβ42 levels were lower in AD patients with the *APOE* ε4 allele than those without *APOE* ε4 allele (19). The sensitivity of Aβ42 measurement was 83.6% for AD patients carrying an *APOE* ε4 allele, whereas in AD patients without *APOE* ε4 allele it was 54.2%. Decreased CSF Aβ42 levels are not specific for AD since studies showed that half of the patients with vascular dementia (VaD) had decreased CSF Aβ42 (16).

It has been hypothesized that a decrease of Aβ42 in CSF indicates an early stage of AD before clinically overt dementia is detectable. A significant decrease of CSF Aβ42 in MCI subjects compared to controls has been shown, but this study had no follow-up measure (20). In a further study investigating MCI patients, Aβ42 levels did not differ significantly from age-matched normal controls (21). Control subjects in this study, however, were subjects with memory complaints without neuropsychological impairment. Since it has been reported that individuals with memory complaints have a higher risk of dementia (22–24), the control group in this study might represent a subgroup with subclinical AD pathology reflected in altered CSF Aβ42 levels. More recently, it has been shown that Aβ42 protein may be an indicator of early identification of AD in MCI subjects when taking potential confounding factors into account such as age, severity of cognitive decline, time of observation, *APOE* E ε4 (*APOE* ε4) carrier status, and gender (25).

Studies correlating CSF Aβ42 protein concentrations with cognitive performance in AD have been contradictory. Cross-sectionally, the concentration of Aβ42 protein and cognitive measures were either inversely correlated (26–28) or no significant correlation was found (12,15,16,29). In a longitudinal study, a decrease in CSF Aβ42 protein has been found within a three year follow-up (30). A highly significant correlation between low CSF concentrations at baseline and one year serial follow-up was demonstrated. In a separate study, no correlation was found between CSF levels and duration or severity of AD (12). The potential value of Aβ42 during the course of AD progression should be further evaluated.

Several studies have been performed on the potential of CSF Aβ42 to differentiate AD from other neurodegenerative disorders. Compared to control subjects with other neurological conditions, a slight decrease has been described in non-AD dementias (31). Normal or decreased levels of Aβ42 were reported in Parkinson's disease (PD) (11,32). In Lewy body dementia, a disorder also characterized by the presence of senile plaques, low levels of Aβ42 protein have been detected. The range of Aβ42 protein concentrations found in Lewy body dementia overlaps with Aβ42 concentrations found in AD patients (20,33–35). Furthermore, low CSF Aβ42 protein is found in a relatively large percentage of patients with frontotemporal dementia (FTD) and VaD (16,36). In summary, CSF Aβ42 does not seem to significantly support the differential diagnosis of AD.

A satisfying explanation for the decrease of the Aβ42 level in CSF to about 40–50% of control levels in AD (14) is still lacking. One suggested mechanism is that it is caused by the deposition of Aβ42 in plaques, with lower amounts of Aβ being free to diffuse into CSF (11). This explanation is also supported by the finding of a strong correlation between low Aβ42 in ventricular CSF and high numbers of plaques in the neocortex and hippocampus (37). However, subsequent studies also found a marked reduction in CSF Aβ42 in disorders without β-amyloid plaques, such as CJD (38), amyotrophic lateral sclerosis (39), and multiple system atrophy (40). This points to other mechanisms, such as disturbances in Aβ formation and breakdown in AD. Interestingly, one study reported a significant increase of Aβ42 protein in patients with early stage of AD followed by a steady decrease concentration (10). This might be explained by different sets of antibodies and protocols used, as well as by differences in the stage of the disease when the patients were included.

Several CSF studies have shown that concentrations of another amyloid β peptide species, Aβ40, were similar in AD and controls (11,17,41,42). In one study (43), however, a decrease in CSF Aβ40 values was found with significant overlap between the groups. Another study reported that Aβ40 is deposited later in the disease and is prominent in vascular amyloid deposits (44).

In addition to Aβ42 and Aβ40 in CSF alone, the ratio of Aβ42 to Aβ40 has been investigated. The ratio of Aβ42 to Aβ40 is suggested to be superior to the concentration of Aβ42 alone in discriminating patients with AD from normal controls (42). Furthermore, a recent study showed that for the neurochemical diagnosis of AD, the number of correctly classified patients turned out to be slightly higher compared to all groups (non-Alzheimer dementia and control subjects) when the Aβ peptide ratio was used instead of the Aβ42 concentration alone (correct discrimination of AD and controls increases from 86.7% to 94% when Aβ42 is replaced with Aβ peptide ratio); however, this effect failed to reach significance (17).

Aβ in Plasma

Some studies suggest that plasma Aβ40 and Aβ42 levels were two- to threefold higher in patients with familial AD and with presenilin mutations than in subjects with sporadic AD and controls (45). Further, it has been reported that Aβ levels are approximately 100-fold lower in plasma than CSF (45). Some studies demonstrated that plasma Aβ40 and Aβ42 levels are similar in AD and control groups (46,47). However, others have shown that plasma Aβ40 levels are increased in AD patients with *APOE* ε4 allele compared to those without this allele and age-matched controls (46). Because of the potential overlap between the AD patients and controls, measurement of plasma Aβ40 levels is not useful as a diagnostic tool to distinguish patients with sporadic AD from elderly non-demented (ND) controls (46,47). A longitudinal study of unrelated individuals reported that those who subsequently developed AD had higher plasma Aβ42 levels at entry than those who did not develop dementia (48). These results indicate that elevated plasma Aβ42 levels may be detected several years before onset of symptoms, supporting the role of extracellular Aβ42 in the pathogenesis of AD.

However, although blood is easy to obtain, it is still unclear if there are systemic changes specific for AD, and to what extent changes in blood composition reflect pathological changes seen in the brain since plasma Aβ42 levels showed no difference between AD and controls, whereas data with Aβ40 are controversial (with either an increase in AD or no change). One longitudinal study has shown that elevated plasma Aβ42 levels occur before the onset of MCI in some individuals (48).

In summary, Aβ1–42 comes close to fulfilling the criteria for a useful AD diagnostic test as recently summarized by an expert review (49). It is, however, of limited value in differentiating AD from other primary dementias. Further studies will be required to evaluate the whether the ratio of Aβ42 to Aβ40 is superior to the concentration of Aβ42 alone (17).

AMYLOID PROTEIN PRECURSOR

Amyloid β protein is derived through proteolytic processing of a larger membrane bound glycoprotein, the amyloid protein precursor (APP) (50). APP is ubiquitously expressed as an integral membrane protein and is cleaved by proteases called α-, β-, and γ-secretase (51). The sequential cleavage by β- and γ-secretase generate amyloidgenic Aβ peptides and simultaneously soluble β-APP [β-secreted APP (sAPP)]. In contrast, α-secretase cleavage precludes Aβ formation and generates soluble α-sAPP (52).

The total amounts of sAPP, or specifically cleaved forms of APPα and sAPPβ, can be measured and are abundant in CSF. Results of studies measuring the total level of sAPP in AD compared to healthy controls are contradictory, ranging from no significant change (53) to a decrease (7,54). Studies on APP in AD from human brain tissue are also inconsistent. In two studies it was shown that APP levels did not differ between AD and normal human brains (55,56). However, in another study a decline of APP in specific brain areas in AD has been reported (57). In a previous study, the α- and β-secretase cleaved APP was investigated in patients with AD compared to healthy controls and patients with MCI. No significant changes were found for CSF α-sAPP or CSF β-sAPP between patients with AD and healthy controls (52). However, the level of CSFβ-sAPP was significantly increased in patients with MCI compared to healthy controls (52), which might be due to disturbances in APP metabolism. Furthermore, another recent study showed no significant differences in the levels of CSF β-sAPP between AD patients and controls, but the CSF α-sAPP, and total sAPP levels, were significantly lower in AD patients compared to controls (58).

Taken together, β-sAPP in CSF does not currently seem to be an adequate marker for sporadic AD. Nevertheless it is of importance to investigate β-sAPP in larger samples of familial and sporadic AD (58).

TAU PROTEINS

Neurofibrillary tangles are one of the major pathological hallmarks of AD. They consist of paired helical filaments (PHF), derived from abnormally hyper-phosphorylated microtubule-associated protein tau (59). Physiologically, tau is located in the neuronal axons and a component of the cytoskeleton and intracellular transport systems. Due to alternative splicing of tau mRNA, there are six isoforms ranging in size from 352 to 441 amino acids, with molecular weights ranging from 50 to 65 kDa (60), encoded by a single gene consisting of 16 exons on chromosome 17q21. Furthermore, at least 30 phosphorylation sites, either threonine or serine, exist on tau extracted from human brain (61). Due to hyperphosphorylation, tau loses its ability to bind to the microtubules and to stimulate their assembly, and shows an increased tendency to aggregate (62). Total tau (t-tau) and truncated forms of monomeric and phosphorylated tau are released and can be measured in the CSF.

The first promising report on CSF t-tau as a biomarker for AD was published in 1993. An ELISA with a polyclonal reporter antibody was used (63). After this, ELISA methods based on monoclonal antibodies have been developed that detect all isoforms of tau independent of phosphorylation sites (64,65) to measure total and phosphorylated CSF tau protein (66–68).

Total Tau

T-tau, a general marker of neuronal destruction, has been intensively studied in more than 30 studies on 2000 AD patients and 1000 age-matched elderly controls over the last 5–10 years (69). The most consistent finding is a statistically significant increase in CSF t-tau protein in AD. The mean level of CSF t-tau protein concentration is about 300% higher in AD compared to elderly controls. Across the reviewed studies, sensitivity and specificity levels varied due to the different control groups and statistical methods used. Specificity levels were between 65% and 86% and sensitivity between 40% and 86% (14). In several studies, a significant elevation was also found in patients with very early dementia (31,70,71). Overall, in mild dementia, the potential of CSF t-tau protein to discriminate between AD and normal aging is high, with a mean sensitivity of 75% and a specificity of 85% (69). An age-associated increase of t-tau protein has been shown in ND subjects (72). Therefore, the effect of age should be considered when t-tau protein levels are diagnostically employed. Age-dependent reference values for t-tau protein have already been established: for subjects between 21–50 years old at <300 pg/ml, between 51–70 years old at <450 pg/ml, and between 70–93 years old at <500 pg/ml (18).

MCI is a major risk factor for AD. Ten to fifteen percent of patients with MCI have been reported to convert to AD in a year (73). In patients suffering from MCI who converted to AD during follow-up, elevated t-tau levels at baseline were found in a relatively high number of individuals (20,74). Memory impaired subjects who later developed AD could be discriminated by high

CSF t-tau from those who did not progress with 90% sensitivity and 100% specificity (75). Longitudinally, elevated CSF levels of t-tau in MCI subjects were found and still remained elevated after conversion to clinical AD. Another study showed that 88% of patients with MCI had elevated t-tau concentrations and/or low CSF $A\beta_{1-42}$ levels at baseline (13). Thus, elevated CSF t-tau in MCI may have the potential to predict AD, a finding that was supported by a recent study (2). Cross-sectional studies correlating CSF t-tau concentrations with cognitive status in AD have shown a correlation between elevation of t-tau and cognitive decline (26,27,76), though others have found no systematic effect (16,77–80). Longitudinal studies of t-tau in mildly to moderately demented AD patients showed no statistically significant correlation with progression during follow-up (12,81,82). CSF t-tau remained elevated for up to two years in mild to moderate AD. Initial and follow-up levels of t-tau correlated strongly, suggesting a stable rate of neurodegeneration during this time period. It could be hypothesized that CSF t-tau will decrease over time if treatment of AD achieves disease-modification and neuroprotection (83).

An increase of CSF t-tau has also been found in a proportion of cases with other dementia disorders. In VaD, FTD, and dementia with Lewy bodies (DLB), elevated CSF t-tau has been found (20,33,69,74,78,84–88). Other studies, however, found normal levels compared to controls in these disorders (14,16,36,81,89,90). The potential of CSF t-tau, however, is limited in its ability to discriminate AD from other relevant dementia disorders. At a sensitivity level of 81%, CSF t-tau reached a specificity level of only 57% in distinguishing AD from other dementias (16,91). Therefore, t-tau has not been suggested as a marker for the differential diagnosis of AD.

T-tau rather reflects non-specific processes of axonal damage and neuronal degeneration. This notion is further supported by an increase in CSF t-tau in disorders with extensive and/or rapid neuronal degeneration such as CJD (92,93). A highly significant increase of 580% was documented in CJD compared to AD patients. At a cut-off level of 2130 pg/ml, t-tau yielded a sensitivity of 93% and a specificity of 100% between AD and CJD (94). An elevation of CSF t-tau, correlating with clinical severity, has been shown in normal pressure hydrocephalus (95). Moreover, a marked transient increase of CSF t-tau has been demonstrated after acute stroke. The transient increase of CSF t-tau correlated with infarct size measured by cranial computed tomography (96). Elevated levels of CSF t-tau in patients with diffuse axonal damage after traumatic brain injury have been found, thus decreasing with clinical improvement (68).

The differential diagnoses of AD, alcoholic dementia, PD, progressive supranuclear palsy, corticobasal degeneration, and other psychiatric disorders show normal CSF t-tau (20,36,64,97,98), with elevated CSF t-tau concentrations only occasionally being reported (14,36,74,99,100).

In geriatric major depression (MD), an important psychiatric condition in the differential diagnosis of AD, CSF t-tau has also been investigated.

Subgrouping a sample of AD patients, healthy controls, and patients with MD according to age resulted in a correct classification rate of 94.5% in the "young old" subjects (<70 years of age) compared to only 68.4% in the "old old" (70 years of age). This report supports the notion that elevated CSF t-tau particularly in subjects younger than 70 years of age is highly indicative of a neurodegenerative process (72,101).

Phosphorylated Tau

Promising efforts are under way to establish phosphorylated tau (p-tau) in CSF as a putative biological marker for AD. Several ELISA methods have been developed specifically detecting phosphorylation of tau protein at different epitopes, such as threonine 181 and 231 (p-tau$_{181+231}$) (66), threonine 181 (p-tau$_{181}$) (67), threonine 231 and serine 235 (p-tau$_{231+235}$) (102), serine 199 (p-tau$_{199}$) (102), threonine 231 (p-tau$_{231}$) (103), and serine 396 and 404 (p-tau$_{396+404}$) (104).

Although there is no doubt that tau phosphorylation differs in AD, it is hard to speculate why this should be the case. There have been few studies of p-tau$_{199}$ and p-tau$_{181}$ in the human brain. With the exception of one study (105) all that is known about these sites is that they are phosphorylated in advanced AD neuropathological changes (106). Furthermore, it is well established that p-tau$_{231}$ appears early in the pathological development of the disease, even before the formation of PHF in neurons of the hippocampus (105,107). Phosphorylation at both threonine 181 and serine 199 occurs later, and these are only found to any appreciable extent in intracellular tangles (105).

One question, yet to be resolved, is which site of abnormal phosphorylation is most useful for the differentiation between AD and other disease groups. A comparative study examining the different tests (p-tau$_{181}$ vs. p-tau$_{231}$ vs. p-tau$_{199}$) in the same subjects and controls have shown that, applied as single markers, p-tau$_{231}$ and p-tau$_{181}$ reached specificity levels >75% between AD and the combined non-AD group when sensitivity was set at ≥85%. With respect to these data and with respect to the fact that the majority of data on CSF p-tau in AD is available for p-tau$_{181}$ and p-tau$_{231}$, studies on p-tau$_{181}$ and p-tau$_{231}$ will now be described in more detail. Moreover, there is a commercially available assay for p-tau$_{181}$, and a commercial assay for p-tau$_{231}$ will soon become available.

CSF p-tau$_{231}$ distinguished between AD-patients and subjects with other neurological disorders (OND) with a sensitivity of 85% and a specificity of 97% showing elevated CSF p-tau$_{231}$ in AD (103). In this first study describing the assay, a total of 39 CSF samples were prepared and analyzed from individuals with AD, a number of different dementias, other neurological conditions, and controls. The data suggest that the assay can distinguish AD from other dementias (103). In a subsequent study on differential diagnosis of AD using CSF p-tau$_{231}$ in an independent sample, a sensitivity level of 90.2% and a specificity level of 80.0% between AD and non-AD disorders was reported (108). Furthermore, p-tau$_{231}$ significantly improved differential diagnosis compared to t-tau between AD and other non-AD groups, particularly FTD (108). In AD versus FTD, p-tau$_{231}$ correctly allocated 91% of subjects compared to only 66% using t-tau (108). In the differentiation between AD and MD, p-tau$_{231}$ levels were found to be significantly increased in AD patients compared to geriatric MD and healthy controls subjects (109). Results of this study further indicated that p-tau$_{231}$ also has the potential to differentiate between very mild possible AD and MD, even if Mini-Mental State Examination (MMSE) score did not (109).

Recently, the positive and the negative predictive value was calculated for p-tau$_{231}$ in the differential diagnosis of AD (110). A positive predictive value of 77.1% and a negative predictive value of 91.7% were found. The high negative predictive value means that a negative test rules out AD with 90% probability.

Another promising value of p-tau$_{231}$ may be its ability to predict cognitive decline in MCI patients. A longitudinal study showed elevated levels for p-tau$_{231}$ in 77 MCI patients in comparison to healthy controls at baseline (111). High CSF p-tau$_{231}$ levels at baseline significantly correlated with subsequent cognitive decline and conversion to AD. This study suggests that high p-tau$_{231}$ may be a predictor variable for progressive cognitive decline in subjects with MCI. A one-year longitudinal MCI study showed progressive elevation of p-tau$_{231}$ concentrations in MCI subjects compared to healthy controls (112). In a six-year longitudinal serial CSF study, p-tau$_{231}$, but not t-tau, concentrations decreased linearly over time during the clinical progression of AD (113). The decrease of CSF p-tau$_{231}$ with AD progression might reflect the increasing sequestration of p-tau into the tangle, suggesting that p tau becomes more insoluble rather than entering into the CSF, whereas solubility of t-tau remains unaffected.

CSF p-tau$_{181}$ was elevated in AD compared to other dementias and healthy controls and has been proposed as a potential marker for discriminating AD patients from patients suffering from DLB (87). Focussing on the differentiation between AD and DLB, specificity at a given sensitivity level was improved by p-tau$_{181}$ compared to t-tau (34,35). In a study with 101 subjects comparing p-tau$_{181}$ and t-tau in different diagnostic subgroups, p-tau$_{181}$ was increased in patients with probable and possible AD compared with VaD, and dementia in PD (18). Compared with FTD, PD, VaD, and normal aging, both p-tau$_{181}$ and t-tau were increased in probable AD. In possible AD, p-tau$_{181}$ was increased compared to FTD and VaD.

A recent study directly compared the diagnostic performance of p-tau$_{231}$, p-tau$_{181}$, and p-tau$_{199}$ in the same patient cohort, including a large series of patients with AD, DLB, FTD, VaD, and OND (106). The p-tau$_{231}$ and p-tau$_{181}$ assays performed nearly equally well in the discrimination of AD from ND controls, whereas the p-tau$_{199}$ assay showed a weaker discrimination (106). Discrimination between AD and DLB was maximized using p-tau$_{181}$ at a sensitivity of 94% and a specificity of 64%, while p-tau$_{231}$ maximized group separation between AD and FTD with a sensitivity of 88% and a specificity of 92% (106). Thus, differences in the phosphorylation of specific tau epitopes between dementia disorders may be reflected in the CSF level of the corresponding p-tau variant (106).

Interestingly, despite a very marked increase in t-tau in CJD, there is only a slight elevation of p-tau$_{181}$ (114). Furthermore, p-tau$_{181}$ does not change after acute stroke in contrast to t-tau (96). These findings suggest that CSF p-tau is not simply a marker for neuronal damage, like CSF t-tau, but might specifically reflect the phosphorylation state of tau, and thus possibly the formation of tangles in AD.

In summary, p-tau proteins come closest to fulfilling the criteria for a useful biological marker of AD (106). There is a tendency for p-tau proteins to perform differently in the discrimination of AD from other primary dementia disorders.

APOLIPOPROTEIN E

Apolipoprotein E (*APOE*, gene; ApoE, protein) is the major apolipoprotein in the central nervous system where it is involved in the mobilisation and redistribution of cholesterol, necessary for the maintenance of myelin and neuronal membranes during development and following injury (115). However, *APOE* is of special interest in AD research since the presence of the *APOE* ε4 allele has been suggested to be a major risk factor for the development of late-onset AD (116). *APOE* polymorphism influences levels of amyloid deposits in the brain of AD patients and elderly ND controls (117).

Previous studies on CSF *APOE* in AD patients and controls, however, have shown conflicting results. While in some investigations elevated CSF *APOE* levels have been found (118,119), others have reported reduced *APOE* concentrations in CSF (120). Interestingly, in one study *APOE* levels in CSF were reduced in AD patients without the *APOE* ε4 allele, but increased in AD patients and *APOE* ε 4 allele carriers (120). However, another study reported decreased CSF *APOE* concentrations in *APOE* ε 4 allele carriers (118,121); Lindh and colleagues also reported increased levels of *APOE* in CSF in patients with MCI and other dementia disorders than AD compared to healthy controls (118). To investigate whether *APOE* levels in CSF differ with various ages at onset of AD, one study examined *APOE* in early- and late-onset AD, showing significantly lower *APOE* levels in early-onset AD patients and higher in the late-onset group compared to controls (122).

Concerning serum ApoE in AD patients in comparison to controls, studies are still inconclusive. Some studies report decreased serum ApoE levels (123), whereas others have observed similar or elevated serum ApoE levels between AD and controls (119,124).

Taken together, levels of ApoE in CSF and serum seem not to fulfill the criteria for a useful biomarker of AD.

ISOPROSTANES

Several studies have suggested a role for oxidative damage in the pathogenesis of different neurodegenerative diseases, especially AD and amyotrophic lateral sclerosis (ALS) (125–127). Oxidative damage to CNS tissue prominently manifests as lipid peroxidation (LPO).

Isoprostanes are prostaglandin isomers that are producted exclusively from free-radical-catalyzed peroxidation of arachidonic acid (128). Isoprostanes are biochemically stable end-products of LPO that are released by phospholipases, circulate in plasma, and are excreted in urine (129). Therefore, analysis of LPO by measuring isoprostane levels has been performed in brain, CSF, serum, and urine (130–133). Special attention has been focussed on isomers of the F2-isoprostanes (F2α-iPs), especially 8,12-iso-iPF2α-VI. In different studies, it has been reported that 8,12-iso-iPF$_2$-VI levels are elevated in urine, blood, and CSF of AD patients and that these values correlate with memory impairment, CSF tau levels, and the number of *APOE* 4 alleles (130–132,134). The results, however, for blood and urine, in contrast to CSF, have been conflicting since other studies found no elevated F2-isoprostanes levels (135,136). In addition to AD, in early Huntington's disease, meningoencephalitis, and stroke, elevated levels of isoprostanes were also found (137,138), while in ALS, PD, and schizophrenia no increase of isoprostanes has been observed (139,140). Furthermore, CSF F2-isoprostanes concentrations in AD patients are significantly correlated with global indices of brain degeneration such as decreasing brain weight and degree of cerebral cortical atrophy, but not with *APOE* genotype or the tissue density of neuritic plaques or neurofibrillary tangles (140).

In summary, although additional studies are needed to confirm and extend these findings in larger cohorts of MCI and AD patients, F2-isoprostanes seem to be an interesting marker in AD, not only in CSF, but also in serum and urine.

α1-ANTICHYMOTRYPSIN

It has been suggested that a number of molecules associated with inflammation are involved in the pathogenesis of AD. Antichymotrypsin (ACT), one of the serine proteinase inhibitors, plays an important role in inflammation. Interestingly, elevated levels of ACT were found in the brains of patients with AD and were also described as one of the components of senile plaques (141).

ACT has been investigated in CSF and serum in several studies, but the results have been controversial. While in some studies no difference in ACT levels between AD and controls have been found (142), others have described higher levels of ACT in AD than controls (143–145). A recently performed study found that ACT levels correlate with the severity of dementia (146). Further studies are essential to confirm these findings. In addition, investigations on MCI are needed since ACT has not been studied in MCI so far.

In summary, serum and CSF levels of ACT might be independently upregulated in AD. The measurement of ACT in serum could be useful as a screening marker in AD. Further independent studies, however, are still needed.

THE SOLUBLE INTERLEUKIN-6 RECEPTOR COMPLEX

It has been shown that amyloid within senile plaques is associated with activated microglia and astrocytes that express inflammatory proteins and neuroregulatory factors such as interleukin-6 (IL-6). IL-6 has been consistently detected in the frontal, parietal, and occipital cortex and hippocampus of AD patients but not of ND elderly subjects. In further investigations, IL-6 has been demonstrated in diffuse early plaques without neuritic pathology in isocortical (frontal temporal and parietal cortex) and hippocampal brain samples of AD patients. IL-6 immunoreactivity was rare in classical plaques and absent in compact or burned-out plaques. Therefore, it has been suggested that IL-6 expression may appear before neuritic changes rather than follow neuritic degeneration.

Basic studies show that IL-6 exerts its biological actions only by complex interactions with specific soluble or membrane bound receptors, forming the biologically active IL-6 receptor complex (IL-6RC). The component proteins, in addition to the 19.5 kDa cytokine IL-6, are two membrane glycoproteins, an 80 kDa protein referred to as the ligand-binding α-subunit (gp80, IL-6R, or CD126) and a 130 kDa protein referred to as the non-ligand binding, affinity converting, and signal transducing β-receptor (gp130 or CD130). All members of the IL-6 cytokine family [IL-6, IL-11, oncostatin M, leukemia inhibitory factor, ciliary neurotrophic factor, and cardiotrophin-1 (CT-1)] share gp130 as a component critical for signal transduction. In the nervous system, IL-6 can be secreted by microglia, astroglia, neurons, and endothelial cells, the IL-6R by neurons, and gp130 by all cells. Gp130 neuropil immunoreactivity was observed in telencephalic structures including the hippocampus, cerebral cortex, and caudate-putamen. Activation of membrane bound gp130 by IL-6 and the soluble IL-6R was reported to generate a neuronal differentiation signal. Soluble forms of the two receptors ($_s$IL-6R, $_s$gp130) arise by limited proteolysis (shedding) or differential splicing ($_s$IL-6R of 38 kDa and $_s$gp130 of 68kDa). It has been reported that this soluble complex ($_s$IL-6RC) forms a hexameric structure in solution, consisting of the three different proteins with a 2:2:2 stoichiometry. There is a complex regulatory interaction between all $_s$IL-6R components. $_s$IL-6R enhances IL-6 effects by making the ligand accessible to the membrane-bound signal-transducing β-subunit; however, it has also been shown to augment the action of $_s$gp130, which neutralizes IL-6 signals. There are commercially available bioassays (ELISA) to detect the IL-6RC in biological fluids. Using such an assay, significantly decreased CSF concentrations of $_s$IL-6R (101) and $_s$gp130 (147), in the presence of unchanged IL-6 concentrations (148), in AD-patients compared to healthy age-matched controls were reported. In addition, these data indicate that the application of multivariate discriminant analysis using combined CSF t-tau protein and $_s$IL-6RC components may add more certainty to the diagnosis of AD (147). The reported method, however, needs to be extended to an independent group of AD patients, other neurodegenerative conditions, and control subjects to assess the true diagnostic applicability. Interpretation of the relationship between CSF and brain levels of the IL-6RC at present remain speculative and require studies based on simultaneous measurement of corresponding CSF and brain samples.

C-REACTIVE PROTEIN

C-reactive protein (CRP) is a pentraxin acute phase reactant synthesized in the liver. Its plasma level can increase up to 1000-fold during the acute-phase response (149). CRP is not normally found in the brain, but previous studies have demonstrated the presence of CRP in senile plaques and neurofibrillary tangles in the brains of AD patients (150,151). It is up-regulated in AD brains compared to samples from ND individuals (152). In a follow-up study, examining over 1000 cases, it has been observed that men in the upper three quartiles for serum high-sensitivity CRP had a 3-fold, significantly increased risk for all dementias combined, AD, and VaD (153). Remarkably, the serum samples that were investigated had been taken and stored 20–25 years earlier, long before onset of dementia symptoms in any subject. In contrast, another recent study of only 11 AD and 11 ND patients found comparable levels of CRP in AD and ND patients.

In summary, CRP might play a causal role, or merely be a marker of inflammatory processes. Whether the association proves to be direct or indirect, CRP measurements may turn out to be an important adjunct for global risk assessment of dementia (153).

C1Q

C1q, a subcomponent of C1, the first component of the classical complement pathway, is associated with neuritic plaques and with neurons in the hippocampus of AD brain.

There is evidence that C1q, in addition to its normal production in the liver, is also synthesized in the brain by pyramidal neurons and glial cells (154–156). β-pleated, fibrillar Aβ and, more recently, tau-containing neurofibrillary tangles have been found to directly and fully activate the classical complement pathway in vitro in an antibody-independent fashion, (157,158). Of the many different inflammatory mediators that enhance Aβ aggregation, C1q is one of the most potent (159).

In several studies, abundantly elevated C1q levels have been observed in the brains of AD patients compared to unaffected brains (160,161). In CSF, significantly lower levels of C1q have been observed in AD compared to control patients, thus correlating with cognitive deficits (162). In summary, these results support the hypothesis that complement plays a role in the pathogenesis of AD potentially by triggering local inflammation (163).

HOMOCYSTEINE

Homocysteine is a precursor of methionine and cysteine. Folate and vitamin B12 are needed for the conversion of homocysteine to methionine, and vitamin B6 is essential for the conversion of homocysteine to cysteine (164). Deficiencies of folate or vitamin B12, and vitamin B6, result in increased levels of homocysteine. There are a variety of assays to measure homocysteine levels, including immuno-assays and high pressure liquid chromatography (HPLC)-based methods, which have similar performance and high precision (165,166).

Hyperhomocysteinemia is considered a potentially important risk factor for heart disease, carotid atherosclerosis, and stroke (167–170). Atherosclerosis and stroke, in turn, increase the risk for AD (171,172). However, in AD, VaD, and cognitive deterioration, increased levels of homocysteine in serum in combination with decreased vitamin B12 or folic acid are considered as potential risk factors for the development of cognitive impairment (173). A significant increase in total homocysteine levels were demonstrated in a large case control study of 164 patients with AD compared to 108 controls (174). Total homocysteine levels were stable over a three-year follow-up period, and homocysteine levels did not correlate with duration of symptoms. A recent longitudinal study has shown an association between hyperhomocysteinemia and a higher risk of AD (175). In this study, plasma homocysteine levels greater than 14 umol/L almost doubled the risk of AD (175). In another study it has been demonstrated that, independent of low folate levels, higher levels of homocysteine were associated with cognitive decline in a large group of older subjects (176). In contrast, no relation between increased homocysteine concentrations and cognitive decline was observed in a large study with 702 individuals with a mean follow-up duration of 2.7 years (177). A recent MRI study suggested that increased homocysteine was a risk factor for cerebro-vascular disease independent of AD (178). This leads to the question of whether homocysteine is directly linked to mechanisms of AD or indirectly, via cerebrovascular disease.

Besides homocysteinemia, low vitamin B12 and folate levels were also found in AD. Since supplementation with B group vitamins lowers homocysteine levels by up to 30% (174), dietary interventions are now being tried in current studies to explore the benefit on cognitive outcome (4). Furthermore, in the US, fortification of cereal grain products with folic acid was mandated in the late 1990s, and there has already been a decrease in mean values of homocysteine in older individuals. This will make it more difficult to evaluate whether further supplementation has benefits in dementia (4).

Studies of folate supplementation in depression, one of several neuropsy-chiatric diseases also associated with low folate serum levels, have shown benefits even when folate status was not low (179). A potential explanation might be that serum folate concentrations do not reflect concentrations in the CNS or that folate requirements are increased in neuropsychiatric diseases (180).

In summary, elevated homocysteine levels in plasma seem to be a strong, independent risk factor for the development of dementia and AD. Further large-scale studies are currently in progress.

OXYSTEROLS AND CHOLESTEROL METABOLISM

The brain is the most cholesterol-rich organ in the human body. Cholesterol metabolism in the CNS is postulated to be regulated independently and potentially by a unique mechanism because CNS is segregated from the systemic circulation by the blood-brain barrier (181). It is known that cholesterol is synthesised in the brain in situ and that extracerebral cholesterol does not contribute significantly to brain cholesterol content (173,182–184). Converging evidence links cholesterol metabolism and AD (185). It has been hypothesised that increased removal of cholesterol from brain occurs during neurodegenerative processes (173,186). Accumulation of excess cholesterol in hippocampal neurons promotes the cleavage of the APP into amyloidogenic components with consequent acceleration of neuronal degeneration. Conversion of cholesterol to 24S-hydroxycholesterol mediated by cholesterol 24S-hydroxylase is the major pathway for the elimination of brain cholesterol and the maintenance of brain cholesterol homeostasis (173,181,187).

Concentrations of 24S-hydroxycholesterol in plasma and CSF are significantly higher in AD and vascular demented patients at early stages of the disease compared to healthy subjects. Variation in genetic background, time of disease onset, and severity of dementia are potential sources of variance (187–190). In a recent study, an influence of *APOE* ε4 allele on CSF 24S-hydroxycholesterol concentrations, and a gene-dosage effect was observed which might point to the existence of a link between the established AD, risk factor, *APOE* ε4 allele, and CNS cholesterol metabolism. Also, in patients with MCI, increased CSF 24S-hydroxycholesterol levels were found suggesting that high levels of 24S-hydroxycholesterol appear to occur early in the disease process (187).

The relationship between serum cholesterol and lipid levels and the risk of AD is not clear. In one prospective study, high serum cholesterol in midlife appeared to increase the risk of incident AD (189), while another population-based study found no clear relationship between cholesterol levels and AD (191).

Cholesterol-lowering drugs (HMG-CoA reductase inhibitors, or statins) decrease the prevalence of AD (192). Statins reduce the generation of the amyloid precursor protein, the neuronal secretion of beta-amyloid, and de novo cholesterol synthesis (193–196). Recent epidemiological studies indicate that the prevalence of diagnosed AD and VaD is reduced among people taking statins for a longer period of time. High-dose simvastatin treatment (80 mg/day) in patients with hypercholesterolemia leads to a significant decrease in brain-specific serum 24S-hydroxycholesterol concentrations, indicating diminished cholesterol metabolism in the brain (188). As statin treatment not only reduces total and LDL cholesterol levels, but also increases high-density lipoprotein (HDL) levels, statin treatment may help reduce the risk of AD by increasing serum HDL and CSF cholesterol levels. HDL is critical for the maturation of synapses and the maintenance of synaptic plasticity (197,198).

Taken together, although measures of cholesterol metabolism do not appear to be diagnostically useful in AD, they may serve as indices of treatment effects and mechanisms in clinical trials. The mounting evidence implicating cholesterol pathways in AD has led to preliminary studies of statins in patients with AD (183,199). Following treatment with a statin, CSF levels of 24S-hydroxy-cholesterol decreased, but CSF levels of Aβ were not found to be altered.

To study the correlation between cholesterol metabolism and the processing of APP, the effect of statin treatment (simvastatin or atorvastatin) on Aβ in humans was tested (200). Treatment with both statins reduced total plasma cholesterol levels by 56% (p <0.001). No significant change of plasma Aβ40, Aβ42, and total Aβ was found questioning the effect of statins on the processing of APP in humans (200).

3-NITROTYROSINE

In the presence of reactive oxygen species and nitric oxide, 3-nitrotyrosine (3NT) may be formed in constituent proteins in the brain. The predominant pathway appears to involve nitric oxide in the presence of superoxide ion to form peroxynitrite. Peroxynitrite in turn reacts with tyrosine residues in proteins or with free tyrosine to form 3NT (201). 3NT can be found in CSF in specific proteins, e.g., superoxide dismutase (202), or can be found as free 3NT. With normal aging, 3NT concentrations in CSF increase modestly from about 0.75 nM at 40 years to about 2 nM at 80 years (203).

In the brains of patients with AD, regionally specific increases in 3NT have been found in the neocortex and cerebellum (204). In the CSF of patients with AD, the concentration of 3NT is reported (203) to be 11.4 nM, or about sixfold higher than age-matched controls. In this study, concentrations of 3NT in CSF were inversely correlated with MMSE scores, but did not correlate with duration of disease.

Analysis of 3NT is relatively straightforward when done by HDL with electrochemical detection (HPLC/ED) (201). CSF analysis requires only 400 ul, and acid precipitation of proteins is sufficient for the analysis of free 3NT (201,203). The stability of 3NT in plasma proteins, however, is not well established, and thus the significance of 3NT concentrations in this compartment is less clear (201,205). Increased concentrations of 3NT in CSF, along with changes in isoprostanes, and 8OHDG as outlined in this review, are consistent with the suggestion that oxidative stress may play an important role in the pathogenesis of AD. It is not yet clear whether the increase in reactive oxygen species with oxidative stress is proximal or distal in the pathophysiological cascade leading to cell death. As with a number of proposed biomarkers for AD, longitudinal studies are necessary to determine if changes in 3NT in CSF increase monotonically with disease progression, or might have a more complex relationship with disease severity. Even in the absence of a linear relationship with disease severity, measurement of 3NT and other markers of oxidative stress may provide an indirect marker of drug efficacy in subacute clinical trials using putative disease-modifying agents.

14-3-3 PROTEIN IN CREUTZFELDT–JAKOB DISEASE

Several studies have reported an elevation of 14-3-3 protein in CSF of sporadic CJD (206). Levels of this protein are high in 95% of sporadic CJD patients (207). However, although the increase of the 14-3-3 protein in CSF is used as a diagnostic test in CJD, sensitivity and specificity of the 14-3-3 protein test varies between the different subtypes of sporadic CJD, distinguished by electrophoretic mobility of proteinase K-resistant protein (PrP^{sc}) and genotype at codon 129 of the prion protein gene (206,208). The sensitivity of the 14-3-3 test has been shown to be higher in patients with molecular features of classic sporadic CJD rather than in patients with the nonclassic CJD subgroups (94% vs. 77%). The difference appears to be related to the PrP^{sc} type (208).

Furthermore, it should be mentioned that in the differential diagnosis of neurodegenerative disorders, only rare cases other than CJD are positive for 14-3-3. Single cases are reported in AD, stroke, cerebral neoplasia, Hashimoto's encephalopathy, inflammation, and some other rare conditions (206).

In summary, 14-3-3 protein test is a useful CSF test for the clinical diagnosis of CJD, but only in a subgroup of the CJD cases. Disease duration, dependent on the PrP^{sc} genotype, should therefore be taken into consideration (208,209). Concerning discrimination CJD from other forms of dementia, 14-3-3 protein has been proved to be a useful marker (206).

PERSPECTIVE OF BIOMARKER RESEARCH IN AD: β-AMYLOID ANTIBODIES

Naturally occurring antibodies against Aβ have been detected in CSF and blood of patients with AD, neurological diseases, and healthy controls (5,210–212). In a study of Aβ-antibody in CSF by ELISA, Du and colleagues found a statistically significant decrease of antibody levels in patients with AD compared to age-matched healthy control subjects. Brettschneider and colleagues assessed the diagnostic value of serum Aβ42-antibodies for AD. Aβ42-antibody levels were measured using a newly developed immuno-precipitation assay with radiolabelled amyloid β$_{1-42}$ peptide (213). A highly significant decrease of Aβ42-antibody levels in AD patients was found independently of age, cognitive status, and *APOE* ε4 carrier status. Aβ42 antibody levels were correlated with gender only in AD, with a higher level occurring in women. When Aβ42 antibody sensitivity (specificity) was set at $> 80\%$, specificity (sensitivity) was below 50% in correctly allocating patients and healthy controls. These data indicate a potentially pathophysiological decrease of serum Aβ42-antibodies in AD. Aβ42-antibodies in the serum alone, however, appear not to be useful as a diagnostic marker of AD.

So far, very little is known about Aβ-antibodies with respect to their function, induction, specificity, and role in disease processes. However, considering data from recent investigations in transgenic AD mouse models, there is evidence for a therapeutic impact of Aβ-antibodies. A reduction of cerebral plaque load and cognitive impairment was observed after active and passive immunization resulting in increased production or administration of Aβ-antibodies in these animal models (214–220). Unfortunately, the phase II clinical trial of the Aβ vaccination approach had to be withdrawn because of signs consistent with meningo-encephalitis in an increasing number of patients (221). Setbacks in active immunization are shifting the focus to passive administration of antibodies. Dodel and colleagues detected naturally occurring Aβ-antibodies in commercially available immunoglobulin G products. In a clinical approach they investigated patients with different neurological diseases treated with intravenous immunoglobulin (IVIG) preparations. A significant decrease of total Aβ and $Aβ_{1-42}$ in CSF compared to baseline values was observed after treatment. In serum, a significant increase of total Aβ without change in the $Aβ_{1-42}$ level was observed (222). These data are in agreement with observations in transgenic mouse models (220,223). A clinical trial involving the administration of IVIG to five patients with AD with simultaneous measurements of CSF and serum Aβ levels has shown a decrease of total CSF Aβ levels by 30% following IVIG. Total Aβ increased in the serum by 230%. No significant change was found in CSF/ serum Aβ42 levels. ADAS-cog was improved by 3.7 points (± 2.9), though MMSE scores remained essentially unchanged. Although the sample size of this pilot study is too small to draw a clear conclusion, the study provides evidence for a more detailed investigation of IVIG for the treatment of AD (224). Due to the very preliminary nature of the findings, the question of whether soluble Aβ-antibodies in serum and CSF has potential value as a biomarker of biological disease activity or a potential surrogate endpoint for clinical trials cannot be finally answered (225).

DISCUSSION

Results and overall direction of change, respectively, that have been reported so far on the biomarkers as discussed in this chapter are given in Table 1. The majority of studies presented here refer to Aβ42, t-tau, and p-tau in the CSF and yield the most convincing evidence for these core biomarkers to be useful either

Table 1 Results/Directions of Change Reported so far on CSF and Blood Biomarkers as Discussed in this Chapter

Cerebrospinal fluid

Biomarker	Alzheimer's disease	Mild cognitive impairment	VaD	Frontotemporal dementia	DLB	Creutzfeldt–Jakob disease
Aβ42	↓	↓ ↔	↓	↓	↓	↓
Aβ40	↔ ↓	↔	↔	↔	↔	↔
APP	↓ ↔	↑	↔	↔	↔	
t-tau	↑	↑	↑ ↔	↑ ↔	↑ ↔	↑↑↑
p-tau	↑↑	↑	(↑)	↔	(↑)	↔
ApoE	↑ ↓ ↔	↑	↑ ↔	↑ ↔		↑
Isoprostanes	↑				↔	↑
ACT	↑ ↔		↔			
Interleukin-6 receptor complex	↓ ↔					
C1q	↓					
Oxysterols and cholesterol	↑	↑				
3-Nitrotyrosine	↑					
14-3-3 Protein	↑		↑			↑↑↑

Serum

Biomarker	Alzheimer's disease	Mild cognitive impairment	VaD	Frontotemporal dementia	DLB	Creutzfeldt–Jakob disease
Aβ42	↔ ↑	↓ ↑				
Aβ40	↔ ↑	↓ ↑ ↔				
APP						
t-tau						
p-tau						
ApoE	↓ ↔		↔			
Isoprostanes	↔ ↑				↔ ↑	
ACT	↔ ↑					
Interleukin-6 receptor complex	↓					
CRP	↑	↑				
C1q						
Homocysteine	↔ ↑		↔ ↑			
Oxysterols and cholesterol	↓ ↑		↓ ↑	↔		

Overall direction of change of biomarkers in CSF and serum of patients with Alzheimer's disease, mild cognitive impairment, VaD, frontotemporal dementia, LBD, and Creutzfeldt–Jakob disease as far as data are available. Blanks indicate that the issue has not been addressed so far. Please note that the database for this overview, i.e., the number of studies investigating a particular biomarker, varies considerably between markers.

Key: ↑, increased; ↔, not different; ↓, decreased in comparison to non-demented controls, respectively.
Abbreviations: VaD, vascular dementia; DLB, dementia with Lewy bodies.

as diagnostic, classificatory, or prognostic markers of AD. A large number of studies have demonstrated that tests based on CSF t-tau protein and CSF Aβ42 have reasonable specificity and sensitivity when differentiating AD from normal aging. A smaller number of studies show similar accuracy when distinguishing AD from MD. One main criticism of these studies is that few have included postmortem confirmation of diagnosis. Nevertheless, provisional work hints that these tests may also be useful in detecting incipient AD in MCI patients. Unfortunately, the value of these biomarkers to clinicians is limited, as they are not specific enough to accurately separate AD from other common forms of dementia, such as VaD and DLB. The combination of both CSF t-tau protein and CSF Aβ42 does not markedly improve their individual sensitivity.

CSF p-tau, based on different phosphorylation epitopes of tau protein, has now been examined in a number of independent studies. Initial results are extremely promising, showing that different p-tau protein epitopes may substantially contribute to improved diagnostic accuracy of AD compared with healthy aged controls, elderly depressed patients, and those with other types of dementia. Compared with CSF t-tau protein and CSF Aβ42, CSF p-tau is more specific and less influenced by covariables such as age or degree of cognitive decline. This has important implications for the value of CSF p-tau to clinicians. If the marker is abnormal very early in the course of disease relatively independently from the degree of cognitive decline, then the marker may be ideal as a diagnostic test. If, however, the marker is closely linked to current or future cognitive decline, then it may be better suited as a prognostic tool. However, conceptually the two areas may overlap in the case of MCI. Roughly 50% of MCI patients deteriorate to AD over five years, and this group may be considered to have a very early form of AD at baseline. However, about 40% of MCI subjects actually improve over time, suggesting an absence of neurodegenerative pathophysiology. Thus at baseline, it is hoped that an accurate diagnostic test of AD would differentiate between these subgroups, which would also inform prognosis for MCI sufferers as a whole.

Studies of all possible biomarkers to date in AD suggest p-tau comes closest to an ideal diagnostic marker. However, different epitopes of phosphorylated tau may have different strengths and weaknesses. CSF p-tau$_{231}$ may be the most useful in distinguishing AD from FTD, and CSF p-tau$_{181}$ may improve separation between AD and DLB. In addition, CSF p-tau$_{231}$ may be the most useful prognostic marker candidate that predicts cognitive decline to AD in MCI subjects. Further studies are needed to decide whether detection of multiple phospho-epitopes may allow a distinct representation of AD related pathology at different stages of the disease, based on the "evolutionary" model of a sequential phosphorylation pattern of tau protein (105).

In assessing the clinical significance of these findings, several confounding factors have to be taken into account. An important factor is the uncertainty of the clinical diagnostic criteria against which these markers have been tested. Neuropathological studies suggest that high proportions (30–50%) of clinically diagnosed patients with VaD have notable concomitant AD pathology. Similarly, a high proportion of those with clinically diagnosed AD have evidence of vascular pathology (226). For example, in a health maintenance organization dementia registry (90), only 36% of patients had pathologically definite AD and no other findings, while 45% had pathologically definite AD plus coexistent vascular pathological features and 22% had pathological findings of AD plus DLB pathological features. This may be due to the influence of vascular risk factors on the onset and progression of AD, since our clinical criteria may be, at least in part, inadequate, or because the diagnosis of mixed dementia is typically overlooked. Whatever the explanation, in patient samples based on clinical diagnosis, it is difficult to achieve high specificity for CSF biomarkers because the gold standard itself is not completely stable. The only way to resolve this question is to study the markers in neuropathologically verified subjects. There is a related issue with elderly comparison groups. Even if such individuals are asymptomatic and age-matched, it is possible that they harbour presymptomatic AD brain lesions (227). In large samples this will invariably reduce the specificity of even the most accurate AD biomarkers. The true value of a marker to practicing clinicians can only be assessed using representative and heterogeneous populations. Most, if not all, studies to date have been evaluated putative markers in highly selected subgroups, representing relatively pure forms of the disease.

Finally, there are several practical consideration. For example, storage time and freeze-thaw cycles of CSF aliquots may influence results. Equally important, clinicians (neurologists as well as psychiatrists) need to consider a lumbar puncture as a routine investigation. Studies have demonstrated lumbar puncture in geriatric patients as safe and tolerable.

In the near future novel methodological approaches in the characterization and quantification of proteins in biofluids might reveal additional information and potentially new candidate biomarkers. For example, the peptide pattern of a sample can be depicted as a multi-dimensional peptide mass fingerprint with each peptide's position being characterized by its molecular mass and chromatographic behaviour. Such a fingerprint of a CNS sample consists of more than 6000 different signals. First data on this promising new approach to analyse CNS diseases on the peptide level have been recently reported (39).

In conclusion, the newly established immunoassays detecting tau-proteins and Aβ-proteins, as well as the rapidly developing modern structural and functional brain imaging methods (such as MRI, DTI, MRS, fMRI, and PET) open up exciting avenues for early and accurate diagnosis of AD. Beyond diagnosis, it is hoped that markers of prognosis will enable clinicians to monitor whether new treatments of AD are working effectively and inexpensively. The accuracy of any diagnostic test in AD is likely to be increased by the cumulative information from clinical and neuropsychological examination, as well as genetic testing and brain imaging (98). Large international dementia consortia are currently investigating potential AD biomarkers in large-scale multi-center trials.

The reviewed CSF measures may gain a potential clinical utility as biomarkers of disease. However, the preliminary and retrospective nature of the majority of findings, the absence of assay standardization, and the partial lack of comparison patient populations must be addressed in future studies testing the usefulness of these CSF measures, particularly for predictive, diagnostic, or treatment evaluation purposes.

REFERENCES

1. The ronald and nancy reagan research institute of the Alzheimer's association and the national institute on aging working group. Consensus report: molecular and biochemical markers of Alzheimer's disease. Neurobiol Aging 1998; 19:109–116.
2. Hampel H, Mitchell A, Blennow K, Frank RA, Weller L, Moeller H-J. Core biological marker candidates of Alzheimer's disease—perspectives for diagnosis, prediction of outcome and reflection of biological activity. J Neural Transm 2003; 65:1–26.
3. Hampel H, Blennow K. CSF tau and β-amyloid as biomarkers for mild cognitive impairment (MCI). Dialogues Clin Neurosci 2005; 6:373–390.
4. Frank RA, Galasko D, Hampel H, et al. Biological markers for therapeutic trials in Alzheimer's disease. Proceedings of the biological markers working group; NIA initiative on neuroimaging in Alzheimer's disease. National institute on aging biological markers working group. Neurobiol Aging 2003; 24:521–536.
5. Hyman BT, Trojanowski JQ. Consensus recommendations for the postmortem diagnosis of Alzheimer disease from the national institute on aging and the reagan institute working group on diagnostic criteria for the neuropathological assessment of Alzheimer disease. J Neuropathol Exp Neurol 1997; 56:1095–1097.
6. Mehta PD, Kim KS, Wisniewski HM. ELISA as a laboratory test to aid the diagnosis of Alzheimer's disease. Tech Diagn Pathol 1991; 2:99–112.
7. Van Nostrand WE, Wagner SL, Shankle WR, et al. Decreased levels of soluble amyloid beta-protein precursor in cerebrospinal fluid of live Alzheimer disease patients. Proc Natl Acad Sci USA 1992; 89:2551–2555.
8. Farlow M, Ghetti B, Benson MD, Farrow JS, van Nostrand WE, Wagner SL. Low cerebrospinal-fluid concentrations of soluble amyloid beta-protein precursor in hereditary Alzheimer's disease. Lancet 1992; 340:453–454.
9. Van Gool WA, Kuiper MA, Walstra GJ, Wolters EC, Bolhuis PA. Concentrations of amyloid beta protein in cerebrospinal fluid of patients with Alzheimer's disease. Ann Neurol 1995; 37:277–279.
10. Jensen M, Schroeder J, Blomberg M, et al. Cerebrospinal fluid A beta42 is increased early in sporadic Alzheimer's disease and declines with disease progression. Ann Neurol 1999; 45:504–511.
11. Motter R, Vigo-Pelfrey C, Kholodenko D, et al. Reduction of beta-amyloid peptide42 in the cerebrospinal fluid of patients with Alzheimer's disease. Ann Neurol 1995; 38:643–648.
12. Andreasen N, Hesse C, Davidsson P, et al. Cerebrospinal fluid β-Amyloid(1–42) in Alzheimer disease: differences between early- and late-onset Alzheimer disease and stability during the course of disease. Arch Neurol 1999; 56:673–680.

13. Andreasen N, Minthon L, Davidsson P, et al. Evaluation of CSF-tau and CSF-A-beta-42 as diagnostic markers for alzheimer disease in clinical practice. Arch Neurol 2001; 58:373–379.
14. Blennow K, Vanmechelen E, Hampel H. CSF total tau, A-beta42 and phosphorylated tau protein as biomarkers for Alzheimer's disease. Mol Neurobiol 2001; 24:87–97.
15. Galasko D, Chang L, Motter R, et al. High cerebrospinal fluid tau and low amyloid-beta-42 levels in the clinical diagnosis of Alzheimer disease and relation to apolipoprotein E genotype. Arch Neurol 1998; 55:937–945.
16. Hulstaert F, Blennow K, Ivanoiu A, et al. Improved discrimination of AD patients using beta-amyloid (1–42) and tau levels in CSF. Neurology 1999; 52:1555–1562.
17. Lewczuk P, Esselmann H, Otto M, et al. Neurochemical diagnosis of Alzheimer's dementia by CSF Abeta42. Abeta42/Abeta40 ratio and total tau. Neurobiol Aging 2004; 25:273–281.
18. Sjoegren M, Vanderstichele H, Agren H, et al. Tau and Abeta42 in cerebrospinal fluid from healthy adults 21–93 years of age: establishment of reference values. Clin Chem 2001; 47:1776–1781.
19. Tapiola T, Pirttilä T, Mehta PD, Alafuzoff I, Lehtovirta M, Soininen H. Relationship between apoE genotype and CSF beta-amyloid (1–42) and tau in patients with probable and definite Alzheimer's disease. Neurobiol Aging 2000; 21:735–740.
20. Andreasen N, Minthon L, Vanmechelen E, et al. Cerebrospinal fluid tau and A-beta42 as predictors of development of Alzheimner's disease in patients with mild cognitive impairment. Neurosci Lett 1999; 273:5–8.
21. Maruyama M, Arai H, Sugita M, et al. Cerebrospinal fluid amyloid beta(1–42) levels in the mild cognitive impairment stage of Alzheimer's disease. Exp Neurol 2001; 172:433–436.
22. Flicker C, Ferris SH, Reisberg B. A longitudinal study of cognitive function in elderly persons with subjective memory complaints. J Am Geriatr Soc 1993; 41:1029–1032.
23. Clarnette RM, Almeida OP, Forstl H, Paton A, Martins RN. Clinical characteristics of individuals with subjective memory loss in Western Australia: results from a cross-sectional survey. Int J Geriatr Psychiatry 2001; 16:168–174.
24. Schofield PW, Marder K, Dooneief G, Jacobs DM, Sano M, Stern Y. Association of subjective memory complaints with subsequent cognitive decline in community-dwelling elderly individuals with baseline cognitive impairment. Am J Psychiatry 1997; 154:609–615.
25. Hampel H, Teipel SJ, Fuchsberger T, et al. Value of CSF β-Amyloid1–42 and tau as predictors of Alzheimer's disease in patients with mild cognitive impairment. Mol Psychiatry 2004; 9:705–710.
26. Kanai M, Matsubara E, Isoe K, et al. Longitudinal study of cerebrospinal fluid levels of tau, A-beta1–40, and A-beta1–42(43) in Alzheimer's disease: a study in Japan. Ann Neurol 1998; 44:17–26.
27. Nitsch RM, Rebeck GW, Deng M, et al. Cerebrospinal fluid levels of amyloid beta-protein in Alzheimer's disease: inverse correlation with severity of dementia and effect of apolipoprotein E genotype. Ann Neurol 1995; 37:512–518.
28. Samuels SC, Silverman JM, Marin DB, et al. CSF beta-amyloid, cognition, and APOE genotype in Alzheimer's disease. Neurology 1999; 52:547–551.

29. Okamura N, Arai H, Higuchi M, et al. Cerebrospinal fluid levels of amyloid beta-peptide1–42, but not tau have positive correlation with brain glucose metabolism in humans. Neurosci Lett 1999; 273:203–207.

30. Tapiola T, Pirttilä T, Mikkonen M, et al. Three-year follow-up of cerebrospinal fluid tau, beta-amyloid 42, and 40 concentrations in Alzheimer's disease. Neurosci Lett 2000; 280:119–122.

31. Galasko D. Cerebrospinal fluid levels of A beta 42 and tau: potential markers of Alzheimer's disease. J Neural Transm Suppl 1998; 53:209–221.

32. Ida N, Hartmann T, Pantel J, et al. Analysis of heterogeneous A4 peptides in human cerebrospinal fluid and blood by a newly developed sensitive Western blot assay. J Biol Chem 1996; 271:22908–22914.

33. Kanemaru K, Kameda N, Yamanouchi H, Decreased CSF. amyloid beta42 and normal tau levels in dementia with Lewy bodies. Neurology 2000; 54:1875–1876.

34. Parnetti L, Lanari A, Amici S, Gallai V, Vanmechelen E, Hulstaert F. CSF phosphorylated tau is a possible marker for discriminating Alzheimer's disease from dementia with Lewy bodies. Neurol Sci 2001; 22:77–78.

35. Vanmechelen E, Van Kerschaver E, Blennow K, et al. CSF-Phosphotau (181P) as a promising marker for discriminating Alzheimer's disease from dementia with lewy bodies. Neurobiol Aging 2001; 21:272.

36. Sjoegren M, Minthon L, Davidsson P, et al. CSF levels of tau, beta-amyloid(1–42), and GAP-43 in frontotemporal dementia, other types of dementia, and normal aging. J Neural Transm 2000; 107:563–579.

37. Strozyk D, Blennow K, White LR, Launer LJ. CSF A(42) levels correlate with amyloid-neuropathology in a population-based autopsy study. Neurology 2003; 60:652–656.

38. Otto M, Esselmann H, Schulz-Shaeffer W, et al. Decreased beta-amyloid1–42 in cerebrospinal fluid of patients with Creutzfeldt-Jakob disease. Neurology 2000; 54:1099–1102.

39. Sjoegren M, Davidsson P, Wallin A, et al. Decreased CSF β-amyloid42 in Alzheimer's disease and amyotrophic lateral sclerosis may reflect mismetabolism of β-amyloid induced by separate mechanisms. Dement Geriatr Cogn Disord 2002; 13:112–118.

40. Holmberg B, Johnels B, Blennow K, Rosengren L. Cerebrospinal fluid Abeta42 is reduced in multiple system atrophy but normal in Parkinson's disease and progressive supranuclear palsy. Mov Disord 2003; 18:186–190.

41. Wiltfang J, Esselmann H, Cupers P, et al. Elevation of beta-amyloid peptide, 2–42 in sporadic and familial Alzheimer's disease and its generation in PS1 knockout cells. J Biol Chem 2001; 276:42645–42657.

42. Shoji M, Matsubara E, Kanai M, et al. Combination assay of CSF Tau, A-beta1–40, A-beta1–42(43) as a biochemical marker of Alzheimer's disease. J Neurol Sci 1998; 158:134–140.

43. Kahle PJ, Jakowec M, Teipel SJ, et al. Combined assessment of tau and neuronal thread protein in Alzheimer's disease CSF. Neurology 2000; 54:1498–1504.

44. Wisniewski T, Lalowski M, Golabek A, Vogel T, Frangione B. Is Alzheimer's disease an apolipoprotein E amyloidosis? Lancet 1995; 345:956–958.

45. Scheuner D, Eckman C, Jensen M, et al. Secreted amyloid beta-protein similar to that in the senile plaques of Alzheimer's disease is increased in vivo by the

presenilin 1 and 2 and APP mutations linked to familial Alzheimer's disease. Nat Med 1996; 2:864–870.

46. Mehta PD, Pirttilä T, Mehta SP, Sersen EA, Aisen PS, Wisniewski HM. Plasma and cerebrospinal fluid levels of amyloid beta proteins 1–40 and 1–42 in Alzheimer's disease. Arch Neurol 2000; 57:100–105.

47. Tamaoka A, Fukushima T, Sawamura N, et al. Amyloid small beta. Greek protein in plasma from patients with sporadic Alzheimer's disease. J Neurol Sci 1996; 141:65–68.

48. Mayeux R, Tang MX, Jacobs DM, et al. Plasma amyloid beta-peptide 1–42 and incipient Alzheimer's disease. Ann Neurol 1999; 46:412–416.

49. The ronald and nancy reagan research institute of the Alzheimer's association and the national institute on aging working group. Consensus report of the working group molecular and biochemical markers of Alzheimer's disease. Neurobiol Aging 1998; 19:109–116.

50. Kang J, Lemaire HG, Unterbeck A, et al. The precursor of Alzheimer's disease amyloid A4 protein resembles a cell-surface receptor. Nature 1987; 325:733–736.

51. Hooper NM, Karran EH, Turner AJ. Membrane protein secretases. Biochem J 1997; 321:265–279.

52. Olsson A, Höglund K, Sjögren M, et al. Measurement of small alpha. Greek- and small beta, Greek-secretase cleaved amyloid precursor protein in cerebrospinal fluid from Alzheimer patients. Exp Neurol 2003; 183:74–80.

53. Hock C. Early diagnosis and biological markers in Alzheimer's disease (AD) patients. Eur Psychiatry 1998; 13:168.

54. Palmert MR, Cohen ML, Frazzini V, et al. Soluble derivatives of the beta-amyloid protein precursor in cerebrospinal fluid are altered in normal aging and to a greater extent in Alzheimer's disease. Neurobiol Aging 1990; 11:300.

55. Arai H, Lee VM, Messinger ML, Greenberg BD, Lowery DE, Trojanowski JQ. Expression patterns of beta-amyloid precursor protein (beta-APP) in neural and nonneural human tissues from Alzheimer's disease and control subjects. Ann Neurol 1991; 30:686–693.

56. Nordstedt C, Gandy SE, Alafuzoff I, et al. Alzheimer beta/A4 amyloid precursor protein in human brain: aging-associated increases in holoprotein and in a proteolytic fragment. Proc Natl Acad Sci USA 1991; 88:8910–8914.

57. Davidsson P, Bogdanovic N, Lannfelt L, Blennow K. Reduced expression of amyloid precursor protein, presenilin-1 and rab3a in cortical brain regions in Alzheimer's disease. Dement Geriatr Cogn Disord 2001; 12:243–250.

58. Sennvik K, Fastbom J, Blomberg M, Wahlund LO, Winblad B, Benedikz E. Levels of small alpha. Greek- and small beta, Greek-secretase cleaved amyloid precursor protein in the cerebrospinal fluid of Alzheimer's disease patients. Neurosci Lett 2000; 278:169–172.

59. Grundke-Iqbal I, Iqbal K, Tung YC, Quinland M, Wisniewski HM, Binder LI. Abnormal phosphorylation of the microtubule-associated protein τ (tau) in Alzheimer cytoskeletal pathology. Proc Natl Acad Sci USA 1986; 83:4913–4917.

60. Buée L, Bussiere T, Buee-Scherrer V, Delacourte A, Hof PR. Tau protein isoforms, phosphorylation and role in neurodegenerative disorders. Brain Res Brain Res Rev 2000; 33:95–130.

61. Goedert M. Tau protein and the neurofibrillary pathology of Alzheimer's disease. Trends Neurosci 1993; 16:460–465.
62. Iqbal K, Alonso AD, Gondal JA, et al. Mechanism of neurofibrillary degeneration and pharmacologic therapeutic approach. J Neural Transm 2000; 59:213–222.
63. Vandermeeren M, Mercken M, Vanmechelen E, et al. Detection of tau proteins in normal and Alzheimer's disease cerebrospinal fluid with a sensitive sandwich enzyme-linked immunosorbent assay. J Neurochem 1993; 61:1828–1834.
64. Blennow K, Davidsson P, Wallin A, Ekman R. Chromogranin A in cerebrospinal fluid: a biochemical marker for synaptic degeneration in Alzheimer's disease? Dementia 1995; 6:306–311.
65. Vigo-Pelfrey C, Seubert P, Barbour R, et al. Elevation of microtubule-associated protein tau in the cerebrospinal fluid of patients with Alzheimer's disease. Neurology 1995; 45:788–793.
66. Blennow K, Wallin A, Agren H, Spenger C, Siegfried J, Vanmechelen E. Tau protein in cerebrospinal fluid: a biochemical marker for axonal degeneration in Alzheimer disease? Mol Chem Neuropathol 1995; 26:231–245.
67. Vanmechelen E, Vanderstichele H, Davidsson P, et al. Quantification of tau phosphorylated at threonine 181 in human cerebrospinal fluid: a sandwich ELISA with a synthetic phosphopeptide for standardization. Neurosci Lett 2000; 285:49–52.
68. Zemlan FP, Rosenberg WS, Luebbe PA, et al. Quantification of axonal damage in traumatic brain injury: affinity purification and characterization of cerebrospinal fluid tau proteins. J Neurochem 1999; 72:741–750.
69. Blennow K, Hampel H. CSF markers for incipient Alzheimer's disease review. Lancet Neurol 2003; 2:605–613.
70. Kurz A, Riemenschneider M, Buch K, et al. Tau protein in cerebrospinal fluid is significantly increased at the earliest clinical stage of Alzheimer disease. Alzheimer Dis Assoc Disord 1998; 12:372–377.
71. Riemenschneider M, Buch K, Schmolke M, Kurz A, Guder WG. Cerebrospinal protein tau is elevated in early Alzheimer's disease. Neurosci Lett 1996; 212:209–211.
72. Buerger K, Padberg F, Nolde T, et al. CSF tau protein shows a better discrimination in young old (<70 years) than in old patients with Alzheimer's disease, compared with controls. Neurosci Lett 1999; 277:21–24.
73. Petersen RC, Smith GE, Waring SC, Ivnik RJ, Tangalos EG, Kokmen E. Mild cognitive impairment: clinical characterization and outcome. Arch Neurol 1999; 56:303–308.
74. Arai H, Nakagawa T, Kosaka Y, et al. Elevated cerebrospinal fluid tau protein level as a predictor of dementia in memory-impaired individuals. Alzheimer's Res 1997; 3:211–213.
75. Arai H, Morikawa Y, Higuchi M, et al. Cerebrospinal fluid tau levels in neurodegenerative diseases with distinct tau-related pathology. Biochem Biophys Res Commun 1997; 236:261–264.
76. Hock C, Golombowski S, Naser W, Mueller-Spahn F. Increased levels of Tau protein in Cerebrospinal Fluid of Patients with Alzheimer's disease—Correlation with Degree of Cognitive Impairment. Ann Neurol 1995; 37:414–415.
77. Andreasen N, Vanmechelen E, Vanderstichele H, Davidsson P, Blennow K. Cerebrospinal fluid levels of total-tau, phospho-tau and Aβ42 predicts development

of Alzheimer's disease in patients with mild cognitive impairment. Acta Neurol Scand 2003; 107:47–51.

78. Andreasen N, Vanmechelen E, Van de Voorde A, et al. Cerebrospinal fluid tau protein as a biochemical marker for Alzheimer's disease: a community based follow up study. J Neurol Neurosurg Psychiatry 1998; 64:298–305 see comments.

79. Arai H, Terajima M, Miura M, et al. Tau in cerebrospinal fluid: a potential diagnostic marker in Alzheimer's disease. Ann Neurol 1995; 38:649–652.

80. Blomberg M, Jensen M, Basun H, Lannfelt L, Wahlund LO. Increasing cerebrospinal fluid tau levels in a subgroup of Alzheimer patients with apolipoprotein E allele epsilon 4 during 14 months follow-up. Neurosci Lett 1996; 214:163–166.

81. Mecocci P, Cherubini A, Bregnocchi M, et al. Tau protein in cerebrospinal fluid: a new diagnostic and prognostic marker in Alzheimer disease? Alzheimer Dis Assoc Disord 1998; 12:211–214.

82. Sunderland T, Wolozin B, Galasko D, et al. Longitudinal stability of CSF tau levels in Alzheimer patients. Biol Psychiatry 1999; 46:750–755.

83. Galasko D. Lewy bodies and dementia. Curr Neurol Neurosci Rep 2001; 1:435–441.

84. Fabre SF, Forsell C, Viitanen M, et al. Clinic-based cases with frontotemporal dementia show increased cerebrospinal fluid tau and high apolipoprotein E epsilon4 frequency, but no tau gene mutations. Exp Neurol 2001; 168:413–418.

85. Green AJ, Harvey RJ, Thompson EJ, Rossor MN. Increased tau in the cerebrospinal fluid of patients with frontotemporal dementia and Alzheimer's disease. Neurosci Lett 1999; 259:133–135.

86. Higuchi M, Tashiro M, Arai H, et al. Glucose hypometabolism and neuropathological correlates in brains of dementia with Lewy bodies. Exp Neurol 2000; 162:247–256.

87. Sjoegren M, Davidsson P, Tullberg M, et al. Both total and phosphorylated tau are increased in Alzheimer's disease. J Neurol Neurosurg Psychiatry 2001; 70:624–630.

88. Vanmechelen E, Vanderstichele H, Davidsson P, et al. CSF-phospho-tau as a promising marker for discriminating Alzheimer disease from Lewy Body dementia. Neurosci Lett 2000; 285:49–52.

89. Arai H, Satoh-Nakagawa T, Higuchi M, et al. No increase in cerebrospinal fluid tau protein levels in patients with vascular dementia. Neurosci Lett 1998; 256:174–176.

90. Itoh N, Arai H, Urakami K, et al. Large-scale, multicenter study of cerebrospinal fluid tau protein phosphorylated at serine 199 for the antemortem diagnosis of Alzheimer's disease. Ann Neurol 2001; 50:150–156.

91. Parnetti L, Reboldi GP, Gallai V. Cerebrospinal fluid pyruvate levels in Alzheimer's disease and vascular dementia. Neurology 2000; 54:735–737.

92. Otto M, Wiltfang J, Cepek L, et al. Tau protein and 14-3-3 protein in the differential diagnosis of Creutzfeldt-Jakob disease. Neurology 2002; 58:192–197.

93. Otto M, Wiltfang J, Tumani H, et al. Elevated levels of tau-protein in cerebrospinal fluid of patients with Creutzfeldt-Jakob disease. Neurosci Lett 1997; 225:210–212.

94. Kapaki E, Kilidireas K, Paraskevas GP, Michalopoulou M, Patsouris E. Highly increased CSF tau protein and decreased beta-amyloid (1–42) in sporadic CJD: a discrimination from Alzheimer's disease? J Neurol Neurosurg Psychiatry 2001; 71:401–403.

95. Kudo T, Mima T, Hashimoto R, et al. Tau protein is a potential biological
     marker for normal pressure hydrocephalus. Psychiatry Clin Neurosci 2000; 54:
     199–202.
96. Hesse C, Rosengren L, Andreasen N, et al. Transient increase in total but not
     phospho-tau in human cerebrospinal fluid after acute stroke. Neurosci Lett 2001;
     297:187–190.
97. Morikawa Y, Arai H, Matsushita S, et al. Cerebrospinal fluid tau protein levels in
     demented an nondemented alcoholics. Alcohol Clin Exp Res 1999; 23:575–577.
98. Shoji M, Matsubara E, Murakami T, et al. Cerebrospinal fluid tau in dementia
     disorders: a large scale multicenter study by a Japanese study group. Neurobiol
     Aging 2002; 23:363–367.
99. Mitani K, Furiya Y, Uchihara T, et al. Increased CSF tau protein in corticobasal
     degeneration. J Neurol 1998; 245:44–46.
100. Urakami K, Mori M, Wada K, et al. A comparison of tau protein in cerebrospinal
     fluid between corticobasal degeneration and progressive supranuclear palsy.
     Neurosci Lett 1999; 259:127–129.
101. Hampel H, Goernitz A, Buerger K. Advances in the development of biomarkers for
     Alzheimer's disease: from CSF total tau and Abeta(1–42) proteins to phosphory-
     lated tau protein. Rev Brain Res Bull 2003; 61:243–253.
102. Ishiguro K, Ohno H, Arai H, et al. Phosphorylated tau in human cerebrospinal
     fluid is a diagnostic marker for Alzheimer's disease. Neurosci Lett 1999;
     270:91–94.
103. Kohnken R, Buerger K, Zinkowski R, et al. Detection of tau phosphorylated at
     threonine 231 in cerebrospinal fluid of Alzheimer's disease patients. Neurosci Lett
     2000; 287:187–190.
104. Hu YY, He SS, Wang X, et al. Levels of nonphosphorylated and phosphorylated tau
     in cerebrospinal fluid of Alzheimer's disease patients: an ultrasensitive bienzyme-
     substrate-recycle enzyme-linked immunosorbent assay. Am J Pathol 2002;
     160:1269–1278.
105. Augustinack JC, Schneider A, Mandelkow EM, Hyman BT. Specific tau
     phosphorylation sites correlate with severity of neuronal cytopathology in
     Alzheimer's disease. Acta Neuropathol 2002; 103:26–35.
106. Hampel H, Buerger K, Zinkowski R, et al. Measurement of phosphorylated tau
     epitopes in the differential diagnosis of Alzheimer disease: a comparative
     cerebrospinal fluid study. Arch Gen Psychiatry 2004; 61:95–102.
107. Vincent I, Zheng JH, Dickson DW, Kress Y, Davies P. Mitotic phosphoepitopes
     precede paired helical filaments in Alzheimer's disease. Neurobiol Aging 1998;
     19:287–296.
108. Buerger K, Zinkowski R, Teipel SJ, et al. Differential diagnosis of Alzheimer's
     disease with CSF tau protein phosphorylated at threonine 231. Arch Neurol 2002;
     59:1267–1272.
109. Buerger K, Zinkowski R, Teipel SJ, et al. Differentiation of geriatric major
     depression from Alzheimer's disease with CSF Tau protein phosphorylated at
     threonine 231. Am J Psychiatry 2003; 160:376–379.
110. Mitchell A, Brindle N. CSF phosphorylated tau—does it constitute an
     accurate biological test for Alzheimer's disease? Int J Geriatr Psychiatry 2003;
     18:407–411.

111. Buerger K, Teipel SJ, Zinkowski R, et al. CSF tau protein phosphorylated at threonine 231 correlates with cognitive decline in MCI subjects. Neurology 2002; 59:627–629.

112. de Leon MJ, Segal S, Tarshish CY, et al. Longitudinal cerebrospinal fluid tau load increases in mild cognitive impairment. Neurosci Lett 2002; 333:183–186.

113. Hampel H, Buerger K, Kohnken R, et al. Tracking of Alzheimer's disease progression with CSF tau protein phosphorylated at threonine 231. Ann Neurol 2001; 49:545–546.

114. Riemenschneider M, Wagenpfeil S, Vanderstichele H, et al. Phospho-tau/total tau ratio in cerebrospinal fluid discriminates Creutzfeldt-Jakob disease from other dementias. Mol Psychiatry 2003; 8:343–347.

115. Ignatius MJ, Gebicke-Harter PJ, Skene JH, et al. Expression of apolipoprotein E during nerve degeneration and regeneration. Proc Natl Acad Sci USA 1986; 83:1125–1129.

116. Saunders AM, Schmader K, Breitner JCS, et al. Apolipoprotein E Epsilon4 allele distributions in late-onset Alzheimer's disease and in other amyloid-forming diseases. Lancet 1993; 342:710–711.

117. Schmechel DE, Saunders AM, Strittmatter WJ, et al. Increased amyloid beta-peptide deposition in cerebral cortex as a consequence of apolipoprotein E genotype in late-onset Alzheimer disease. Proc Natl Acad Sci USA 1993; 90:9649–9653.

118. Lindh M, Blomberg M, Jensen M, et al. Cerebrospinal fluid apolipoprotein E (apoE) levels in Alzheimer's disease patients are increased at follow up and show a correlation with levels of tau protein. Neurosci Lett 1997; 229:85–88.

119. Taddei K, Clarnette R, Gandy SE, Martins RN. Increased plasma apolipoprotein E (apoE) levels in Alzheimer's disease. Neurosci Lett 1997; 113:29–32.

120. Hesse C, Larsson H, Fredman P, et al. Measurement of apolipoprotein E (apoE) in cerebrospinal fluid. Neurochem Res 2000; 25:511–517.

121. Pirttila T, Koivisto K, Mehta PD, et al. Longitudinal study of cerebrospinal fluid amyloid proteins and apolipoprotein E in patients with probable Alzheimer's disease. Neurosci Lett 1998; 249:21–24.

122. Song H, Saito K, Seishimaa M, Nomaa A, Urakamib K, Nakashimab K. Cerebrospinal fluid apo E and apo A-I concentrations in early- and late-onset Alzheimer's disease. Neurosci Lett 1997; 231:175–178.

123. Siest G, Bertrand P, Herbeth B, et al. Apolipoprotein E polymorphisms and concentration in chronic diseases and drug responses. Clin Chem Lab Med 2000; 38:841–852.

124. Slooter AJ, de Knijff P, Hofman A, et al. Serum apolipoprotein E level is not increased in Alzheimer's disease: the Rotterdam study. Neurosci Lett 1998; 248:21–24.

125. Beal MF. Aging, energy, and oxidative stress in neurodegenerative diseases. Ann Neurol 1995; 38:357–366.

126. Markesbery WR. The role of oxidative stress in Alzheimer disease. Arch Neurol 1999; 56:1449–1452.

127. Tu PH, Gurney ME, Julien JP, Lee VM, Trojanowski JQ. Oxidative stress, mutant SOD1, and neurofilament pathology in transgenic mouse models of human motor neuron disease. Lab Invest 1997; 76:441–456.

128. Morrow JD, Roberts LJ. The isoprostanes: unique bioactive products of lipid peroxidation. Prog Lipid Res 1997; 36:1–21.

129. Morrow JD, Awad JA, Boss HJ, Blair IA, Roberts LJ, II. Non-cyclooxygenase-derived prostanoids (F2-isoprostanes) are formed in situ on phospholipids. Proc Natl Acad Sci USA 1992; 89:10721–10725.
130. Pratico D, Clark CM, Liun F, Rokach J, Lee VY, Trojanowski JQ. Increase of brain oxidative stress in mild cognitive impairment: a possible predictor of Alzheimer disease. Arch Neurol 2002; 59:1475.
131. Pratico D, Clark CM, Lee VM, Trojanowski JQ, Rokach J, FitzGerald GA. Increased 8,12-iso-iPF2alpha-VI in Alzheimer's disease: correlation of a noninvasive index of lipid peroxidation with disease severity. Ann Neurol 2000; 48:809–812.
132. Pratico D. Alzheimer's disease and oxygen radicals: new insights. Biochem Pharmacol 2002; 63:563–567.
133. Pratico D, Uryu K, Leight S, Trojanoswki JQ, Lee VM. Increased lipid peroxidation precedes amyloid plaque formation in an animal model of Alzheimer amyloidosis. J Neurosci 2001; 21:4183–4187.
134. Montine KS, Bassett CN, Ou JJ, Markesbery WR, Swift LL, Montine TJ. Apolipoprotein E allelic influence on human cerebrospinal fluid apolipoproteins. J Lipid Res 1998; 39:2443–2451.
135. Montine TJ, Shinobu L, Montine KS, et al. No difference in plasma or urinary F2-isoprostanes among patients with Huntington's disease or Alzheimer's disease and controls. Ann Neurol 2000; 48:950.
136. Montine TJ, Milatovic D, Gupta RC, Valyi-Nagy T, Morrow JD, Breyer RM. Neuronal oxidative damage from activated innate immunity is EP2 receptor-dependent. J Neurochem 2002; 83:463–470.
137. Montine KS, Quinn JF, Zhang J, et al. Isoprostanes and related products of lipid peroxidation in neurodegenerative diseases. Chem Phys Lipids 2004; 128:117–124.
138. Montine TJ, Beal MF, Robertson D, et al. Cerebrospinal fluid F2-isoprostanes are elevated in Huntington's disease. Neurology 1999; 52:1104–1105.
139. Pratico D, Lee MYV, Trojanowski JQ, Rokach J, Fitzgerald GA. Increased F2-isoprostanes in Alzheimer's disease: evidence for enhanced lipid peroxidation in vivo. FASEB J 1998; 12:1777–1783.
140. Montine TJ, Markesbery WR, Zackert W, Sanchez SC, Roberts LJ, II, Morrow JD. The magnitude of brain lipid peroxidation correlates with the extent of degeneration but not with density of neuritic plaques or neurofibrillary tangles or with APOE genotype in Alzheimer's disease patients. Am J Pathol 1999; 155:863–868.
141. Abraham CR, Selkoe DJ, Potter H. Immunochemical identification of the serine protease inhibitor alpha 1-antichymotrypsin in the brain amyloid deposits of Alzheimer's disease. Cell 1988; 52:487–501.
142. Pirttila T, Mehta PD, Frey H, Wisniewski HM. Alpha 1-antichymotrypsin and IL-1 beta are not increased in CSF or serum in Alzheimer's disease. Neurobiol Aging 1994; 15:313–317.
143. Matsubara E, Hirai S, Amari M, et al. Alpha 1-antichymotrypsin as a possible biochemical marker for Alzheimer-type dementia. Ann Neurol 1990; 28:561–567.
144. Licastro F, Morini MC, Polazzi E, Davis LJ. Increased serum alpha 1-antichymotrypsin in patients with probable Alzheimer's disease: an acute phase reactant without the peripheral acute phase response. J Neuroimmunol 1995; 57:71–75.

145. Harigaya Y, Shoji M, Nakamura T, Matsubara E, Hosoda K, Hirai S. Alpha 1-antichymotrypsin level in cerebrospinal fluid is closely associated with late onset Alzheimer's disease. Intern Med 1995; 34:481–484.
146. Licastro F, Masliah E, Pedrini S, Thal LJ. Blood levels of alpha-1-antichymotrypsin and risk factors for Alzheimer's disease: effects of gender and apolipoprotein E genotype. Dement Geriatr Cogn Disord 2000; 11:25–28.
147. Han X, Holtzman DM, McKeel DW, Jr., Kelley J, Morris JC. Substantial sulfatide deficiency and ceramide elevation in very early Alzheimer's disease: potential role in disease pathogenesis. J Neurochem 2002; 82:809–818.
148. Hampel H, Sunderland T, Kötter HU, et al. Moeller H-J: Decreased soluble interleukin-6 receptor in cerebrospinal fluid of patients with Alzheimer's disease. Brain Res 1998; 780:356–359.
149. Pepys MB, Baltz ML. Acute phase proteins with special reference to C-reactive protein and related proteins (pentaxins) and serum amyloid A protein. Adv Immunol 1983; 34:141–212.
150. Iwamoto T, Okada T, Ogawa K, Yanagawa K, Uno M, Takasaki M. Brain MRI findings in patients with initial cerebral thrombosis and the relationship between incidental findings, aging, and dementia. Nippon Ronen Igakkai Zasshi 1994; 31:879–888.
151. Duong T, Nikolaeva M, Acton PJ. C-reactive protein-like immunoreactivity in the neurofibrillary tangles of Alzheimer's disease. Brain Res 1997; 749:152–156.
152. McGeer PL, Akiyama H, Itagaki S, McGeer EG. Immune system response in Alzheimer's disease. Can J Neurol Sci 1989; 16:516–527.
153. Schmidt R, Schmidt H, Curb JD, Masaki K, White LR, Launer LJ. Early inflammation and dementia: a 25-year follow-up of the Honolulu-Asia aging study. Ann Neurol 2002; 52:168–174.
154. Shen Y, Li R, McGeer RG, McGeer PL. Neuronal expression of mRNAs for complement proteins of the classical pathway in Alzheimernext term brain. Brain Res 1997; 769:391–395.
155. Terai K, Walker DG, McGeer EG, McGeer PL. Neurons express proteins of the classical complement pathway in Alzheimer disease. Brain Res 1997; 769:385–390.
156. Fischer B, Schmoll H, Riederer P, Bauer J, Platt D, Popa-Wagner A. Complement C1q and C3 mRNA expression in the frontal cortex of Alzheimer's patients. J Mol Med 1995; 73:465–471.
157. Rogers J, Cooper NR, Websters S, et al. Complement activation by beta-amyloid in Alzheimer's disease. Proc Natl Acad Sci USA 1992; 89:10016–10020.
158. Eikelenboom P, Stam FC. Immunoglobulins and complement factors in senile plaques. An immunoperoxidase study. Acta Neuropathol 1982; 57:239–242.
159. Webster S, Rogers J. Relative efficacies of amyloid beta peptide (A beta) binding proteins in A beta aggregation. J Neurosci Res 1996; 46:58–66.
160. Akiyama H, Barger S, Barnum S, et al. Inflammation and Alzheimer's disease. Neurobiol Aging 2000; 21:383–421.
161. Brachova L, Lue LF, Schultz J, el Rashidy T, Rogers J. Association cortex, cerebellum, and serum concentrations of C1q and factor B in Alzheimer's disease. Brain Res Mol Brain Res 1993; 18:329–334.
162. Smyth MD, Cribbs DH, Tenner AJ, et al. Decreased levels of C1q in cerebrospinal fluid of living Alzheimer patients correlate with disease state. Neurobiol Aging 1994; 15:609–614.

163. Afagh A, Cummings BJ, Cribbs DH, Cotman CW, Tenner AJ. Localization and cell association of C1q in Alzheimer's disease brain. Exp Neurol 1996; 138:22–32.

164. LeBoeuf R. Homocysteine and Alzheimer's disease. J Am Diet Assoc 2003; 103:304–307.

165. Moller J, Ahola L, Abrahamsson L. Evaluation of the DPC IMMULITE 2000 assay for total homocysteine in plasma. Scand J Clin Lab Invest 2002; 62:369–373.

166. Zighetti ML, Chantarangkul V, Tripodi A, Mannucci PM, Cattaneo M. Determination of total homocysteine in plasma: comparison of the Abbott IMx immunoassay with high performance liquid chromatography. Haematologica 2002; 87:89–94.

167. Perry IJ, Refsum H, Morris RW, Ebrahim SB, Ueland PM, Shaper AG. Prospective study of serum total homocysteine concentration and risk of stroke in middle-aged British men. Lancet 1995; 346:1395–1398.

168. Bostom AG. Homocysteine: "expensive creatinine" or important modifiable risk factor for arteriosclerotic outcomes in renal transplant recipients? J Am Soc Nephrol 1999; 11:149–151.

169. Vasan RS, Beiser A, D'Agostino RB, et al. Plasma homocysteine and risk for congestive heart failure in adults without prior myocardial infarction. JAMA 2003; 289:1251–1257.

170. Tanne D, Sela BA. Neurological implications of hyperhomocysteinemia in patients with atherothrombotic disease. Ital Heart J 2003; 4:577–579.

171. Hofman A, Ott A, Breteler MM, et al. Atherosclerosis, apolipoprotein, E and prevalence of dementia and Alzheimer's disease in the Rotterdam study. Lancet 1997; 349:151–154.

172. Snowdon DA, Greiner LH, Mortimer JA, Riley KP, Greiner PA, Markesbery WR. Brain infarction and the clinical expression of Alzheimer disease. The nun study. J Am Med Assoc JAMA 1997; 277:813–817.

173. Teunissen CE, de Vente J, Steinbusch HW, De Bruijn C. Biochemical markers related to Alzheimer's dementia in serum and cerebrospinal fluid. Neurobiol Aging 2002; 23:485–508.

174. Clarke R, Smith AD, Jobst KA, Refsum H, Sutton L, Ueland PM. Folate, vitamin B12, and serum total homocysteine levels in confirmed Alzheimer disease. Arch Neurol 1998; 55:1449–1455.

175. Seshadri S, Beiser A, Selhub J, et al. Plasma homocysteine as a risk factor for dementia and Alzheimer's disease. N Engl J Med 2002; 346:476–483.

176. Morris MS, Bostom AG, Jacques PF, Selhub J, Rosenberg IH. Hyperhomocysteinemia and hypercholesterolemia associated with hypothyroidism in the third US National Health and Nutrition Examination Survey. Arteriosclerosis 2001; 155:195–200.

177. Kalmijn S, Launer LJ, Lindemans J, Bots ML, Hofman A, Breteler MM. Total homocysteine and cognitive decline in a community-based sample of elderly subjects: the Rotterdam study. Am J Epidemiol 1999; 150:283–289.

178. Miller JW, Green R, Mungas DM, Reed BR, Jagust WJ. Homocysteine, vitamin B6, and vascular disease in AD patients. Neurology 2002; 58:1471–1475.

179. Passeri M, Cucinotta D, Abate G, et al. Oral 5″-methyltetrahydrofolic acid in senile organic mental disorders with depression: results of a double-blind multicenter study. Aging (Milano) 1993; 5:63–71.

180. Shea TB, Rogers E. Homocysteine and dementia. N Engl J Med 2002; 346:2007–2008.
181. Michikawa M. The role of cholesterol in pathogenesis of Alzheimer's disease: dual metabolic interaction between amyloid beta-protein and cholesterol. Mol Neurobiol 2003; 27:1–12.
182. Fagan AM, Holtzman DM. Astrocyte lipoproteins, effects of apoE on neuronal function, and role of apoE in amyloid-beta deposition in vivo. Microsc Res Tech 2000; 50:297–304.
183. Fassbender K, Stroick M, Bertsch T, et al. Effects of statins on human cerebral cholesterol metabolism and secretion of Alzheimer amyloid peptide. Neurology 2002; 59:1257–1258.
184. Jurevics H, Morell P. Cholesterol for synthesis of myelin is made locally, not imported into brain. J Neurochem 1995; 64:895–901.
185. Hartmann T. Cholesterol, A-beta, and Alzheimer's disease. Trends Neurosci 2001; 24:45–48.
186. Bjorkhem I, Lutjohann D, Diczfalusy U, Stahle L, Ahlborg G, Wahren J. Cholesterol homeostasis in human brain: turnover of 24S-hydroxycholesterol and evidence for a cerebral origin of most of this oxysterol in the circulation. J Lipid Res 1998; 39:1594–1600.
187. Papassotiropoulos A, Lutjohann D, Bagli M, et al. 24S-hydroxycholesterol in cerebrospinal fluid is elevated in early stages of dementia. J Psychiatr Res 2002; 36:27–32.
188. Lutjohann D, von Bergmann K. 24S-hydroxycholesterol: a marker of brain cholesterol metabolism. Pharmacopsychiatry 2003; 36:102–106.
189. Notkola IL, Sulkava R, Pekkanen J, et al. Serum total cholesterol, apolipoprotein E epsilon 4 allele, and Alzheimer's disease. Neuroepidemiology 1998; 17:14–20.
190. Kivipelto M, Helkala EL, Laakso MP, et al. Midlife vascular risk factors and Alzheimer's disease in later life: longitudinal, population based study. BMJ 2001; 322:1447–1451.
191. Romas SN, Tang MX, Berglund L, Mayeux R. APOE genotype, plasma lipids, lipoproteins, and AD in community elderly. Neurology 1999; 53:517–521.
192. Wolozin B, Kellman W, Ruosseau P, Celesia GG, Siegel G. Decreased prevalence of Alzheimer disease associated with 3-hydroxy-3-methyglutaryl coenzyme A reductase inhibitors. Arch Neurol 2000; 57:1439–1443.
193. Fassbender K, Simons M, Bergmann C, et al. Simvastatin strongly reduces levels of Alzheimer's disease beta -amyloid peptides Abeta 42 and Abeta 40 in vitro and in vivo. Proc Natl Acad Sci USA 2001; 98:5856–5861.
194. Refolo LM, Pappolla MA, LaFrancois J, et al. A cholesterol-lowering drug reduces beta-amyloid pathology in a transgenic mouse model of Alzheimer's disease. Neurobiol Dis 2001; 8:890–899.
195. Puglielli L, Konopka G, Pack-Chung E, et al. Acyl-coenzyme: a cholesterol acyltransferase modulates the generation of the amyloid beta-peptide. Nat Cell Biol 2001; 3:905–912.
196. Sparks DL, Kuo YM, Roher A, Martin T, Lukas RJ. Alterations of Alzheimer's disease in the cholesterol-fed rabbit, including vascular inflammation. Preliminary observations. Ann N Y Acad Sci 2000; 903:335–344.

197. Koudinov AR, Berezov TT, Koudinova NV. The levels of soluble amyloid beta in different high density lipoprotein subfractions distinguish Alzheimer's and normal aging cerebrospinal fluid: implication for brain cholesterol pathology? Neurosci Lett 2001; 314:115–118.

198. Mauch DH, Nagler K, Schumacher S, et al. CNS synaptogenesis promoted by glia-derived cholesterol. Science 2001; 294:1354–1357.

199. Simons M, Schwarzler F, Lutjohann D, et al. Treatment with simvastatin in normocholesterolemic patients with Alzheimer's disease: A 26-week randomized, placebo-controlled, double-blind trial. Ann Neurol 2002; 52:346–350.

200. Hoglund K, Wiklund O, Vanderstichele H, Eikenberg O, Vanmechelen E, Blennow K. Plasma levels of beta-amyloid(1–40), beta-amyloid(1–42), and total beta-amyloid remain unaffected in adult patients with hypercholesterolemia after treatment with statins. Arch Neurol 2004; 61:333–337.

201. Holtzman DM, Fagan AM, Han X. CSF sulfatide levels: a possible biomarker for Alzheimer's disease at the earliest clinical stages. Neurology 2002; 58:A361.

202. Aoyama K, Matsubara K, Fujikawa Y, et al. Nitration of manganese superoxide dismutase in cerebrospinal fluids is a marker for peroxynitrite-mediated oxidative stress in neurodegenerative diseases. Ann Neurol 2000; 47:524–527.

203. Trojanowski JQ, Lee VM. Brain degeneration linked to "fatal attractions" of proteins in Alzheimer's disease and related disorders. J Alzheimer's Dis 2001; 3:117–119.

204. Hensley K, Maidt ML, Yu Z, Sang H, Markesbery WR, Floyd RA. Electrochemical analysis of protein nitrotyrosine and dityrosine in the Alzheimer brain indicates region-specific accumulation. J Neurosci 1998; 18:8123–8132.

205. Tierney MC, Fisher RH, Lewis AJ, et al. The NINCDS-ADRDA work group criteria for the clinical diagnosis of probable Alzheimer's disease: a clinicopathologic study of 57 cases. Neurology 1988; 38:359–364.

206. Zerr I, Poser S. Clinical diagnosis and differential diagnosis of CJD and vCJD. With special emphasis on laboratory tests. Acta Pathologica, Microbiologica, Et Immunologica Scandinavica APMIS 2002; 110:88–98.

207. Zerr I, Schulz-Schaeffer WJ, Giese A, et al. Current clinical diagnosis in Creutzfeldt-Jakob disease: identification of uncommon variants. Ann Neurol 2000; 48:323–329.

208. Castellani RJ, Colucci M, Xie Z, et al. Sensitivity of 14-3-3 protein test varies in subtypes of sporadic Creutzfeldt-Jakob disease. Neurology 2004; 63:436–440.

209. Van Everbroeck B, Quoilin S, Boons J, Martin JJ, Cras P. A prospective study of CSF markers in 250 patients with possible Creutzfeldt-Jakob disease. J Neurol Neurosurg Psychiatry 2003; 74:1210–1214.

210. Gaskin F, Finley J, Fang Q, Xu S, Fu SM. Human antibodies reactive with beta-amyloid protein in Alzheimer's disease. J Exp Med 1993; 177:1181–1886.

211. Xu S, Gaskin F. Increased incidence of anti-beta-amyloid autoantibodies secreted by Ebstein-Barr virus transformed B cell lines from patients with Alzheimer's disease. Mech Ageing Dev 1997; 94:213–222.

212. Du Y, Dodel RC, Hampel H, et al. Reduced CSF levels of amyloid-beta peptide antibody in Alzheimer's disease. Neurology 2001; 57:801–805.

213. Brettschneider S, Morgenthaler NG, Teipel SJ, et al, Decreased serum amyloid-β1–42-autoantibody levels in Alzheimer's disease using a newly developed

immunoprecipitation assay with radiolabelled amyloid β1–42 peptide. Biological Psychiatry submitted.

214. Schenk D, Barbour R, Dunn W, et al. Immunization with amyloid-beta attenuates Alzheimer-disease-like pathology in the PDAPP mouse. Nature 1999; 400:173–177.
215. Bard F, Cannon C, Barbour R, et al. Peripherally administered antibodies against amyloid beta-peptide enter the central nervous system and reduce pathology in a mouse model of Alzheimer disease. Nat Med 2000; 6:916–919.
216. Chen KS, Knox J. A learning deficit related to age and beta-amyloid plaques in a mouse model of Alzheime's disease. Nature 2000; 408:975–979.
217. Janus CPJ, McLaurin J. A-beta peptide immunization reduces behavioural impairment and plaques in a model of Alzheimer's disease. Nature 2000; 408:979–982.
218. Morgan DDD, Gottschall PE. A-beta peptide vaccination prevents meory loss in an animal model of Alzheimer's disease. Nature 2000; 408:982–985.
219. Weiner HL, Lemere CA, Maron R, et al. Nasal administration of amyloid-beta peptide decreases cerebral amyloid burden in a mouse model of Alzheimer's disease. Ann Neurol 2000; 48:567–579.
220. DeMattos RB, Parsadanian M. Plaque-associated disruption of CSF and plasma amyloid-beta equilibrium in a mouse model of Alzheimer's disease. J Neurochem 2002; 81:229–236.
221. Senior K. Dosing in phase II trial of Alzheimer's vaccine suspended. Lancet Neurol 2002; 1:3.
222. Dodel R, Hampel H, Depboylu C, et al. Human antibodies against amyloid beta-peptide: A potential treatment for Alzheimer disease. Ann Neurol 2002; 52:253–256.
223. DeMattos RB, Cummings DJ, Dodart JC, Paul SM. Peripheral anti A-beta antibody alters CNS and A-beta clearance and decreases brain A-beta burden in a mouse model of Alzheimer's disease. Proc Natl Acad Sci USA 2001; 98:8850–8855.
224. Dodel RC, Du Y, Depboylu C, et al. Intravenous immunoglobulins containing antibodies against beta-amyloid for the treatment of Alzheimer's disease. J Neurol Neurosurg Psychiatry 2004; 75:1472–1474.
225. Dodel RC, Hampel H, Du Y. Immunotherapy for Alzheimer's disease. Lancet Neurol 2003; 2:215–220.
226. de la Torre JC. Alzheimer disease as a vascular disorder: nosological evidence. Stroke 2002; 33:1152–1162.
227. Rosler N, Wichart I, Jellinger KA. CSF Abeta40 and Abeta42: Natural course and clinical usefulness. J Alzheimer's Dis 2001; 3:599–600.

4

Genetics: Facts and Perspectives

Sandro Sorbi, Paolo Forleo, Francesca Massaro,
and Andrea Ginestroni

Department of Neurological and Psychiatric Sciences, University
of Florence, Florence, Italy

INTRODUCTION

There has been a major expansion in recent years on research into the genetic causes of dementia, and a simple search on the PubMed database including the terms "Dementia" and "Genetics" in March 2005 identified more than 13,000 references from 1964. Following the description of Alzheimer's first case, the first suggestion that genetic factors may play a role in Alzheimer's disease (AD) were reported in a paper of Lua (1920) and subsequently in a case report by Flugel (1922), both speculating a possible genetic inheritance of the disease. Since then, from 1930 to 1990, more than 50 pedigrees with a familial form of AD have been described, suggesting that familial aggregation is a common feature of AD. This observation has been successively confirmed by several epidemiological studies (1,2). The analysis of these collected families and the possible genotype-phenotype correlations, together with the outstanding progress of molecular biological techniques, have made the field of dementia genetics in the past 15 years an area of intense research and fruitful discoveries. This information assembled in the past few years has led to the principal finding that analysis of the genetic mechanisms underlying familial clustering of the disease is likely to be directly relevant to the pathogenesis of the common and apparently sporadic forms of AD. In addition, today's knowledge of genetic factors is currently evolving and leading to the progressive definition of a putative cascade of biochemical events that, applied to early diagnosis, therapeutic trials, treatment, and preventive approaches, could provide fundamental advances to prevent and cure AD and other dementias.

Alzheimer's Disease

AD is a genetically complex and heterogeneous neurodegenerative disorder characterized by memory loss that leads to progressive and irreversible cognitive decline until death.

The neuropathology of AD is characterized by widespread neuronal degeneration, the abundant presence of neuritic plaques, containing beta-amyloid, and neurofibrillary tangles, mainly composed of tau aggregates, dystrophic cortical neurites, and amyloid microangiopathy. Senile plaques are located in the extracellular space of the brain and are mainly formed by a highly hydrophobic peptide that contains a 42 amino acid residues (A beta 1–42), produced from its precursor amyloid precursor protein (APP) through proteolytic processing (see Chapter 11).

Since 1991, the results of genetic studies have led to the identification of gene mutations and polymorphisms that can either cause AD or substantially increase the risk of developing the disease. Mutations in three genes (Table 1), *APP*, located on chromosome 21, and presenilin-1 (*PSEN1*) and presenilin-2 (*PSEN2*), located on chromosomes 14 and 1 respectively, result in familial AD (FAD). The FAD cases account for approximately 5% to 10% of all early onset AD cases, and mutations in *PSEN1* are the most frequent. Although more than 140 different *PSEN1* mutations are described in more than 200 families with different ethnic origins, only 10 different mutations among 13 families have been reported for the *PSEN2* gene, and only about 20 families with *APP* mutations are known (3,49).

Amyloid Precursor Protein

Following the identification of β-amyloid (Aβ) and APP, there was considerable speculation as to the causation of AD as being genetic. In the next few years, several different missense mutations were found in exons 16 and 17 of *APP* in families with early onset AD. All mutations are missense mutations lying within or close to the domain encoding beta-amyloid peptide.

Table 1 Genes Involved in Alzheimer's Disease

Gene name	Chromosomal location	Identified genetic mutations	Effect of mutation on Alzheimer's disease pathogenesis
APP	21q21	18	↑ Aβ production and aggregation
PSEN1	14q24	142	↑ Aβ 42/40 ratio
PSEN2	1q42	10	↑ Aβ 42/40 ratio

The *APP* mutations account for a very small proportion (2–3%) of all published cases of FAD and 5–7% of reported cases of early onset FAD. The pathogenicity of these mutations has been strongly supported by the fact that they are virtually 100% penetrant in FAD kindreds where they occur in affected or at-risk individuals, but are absent in age-matched controls. Swedish and Flemish mutations at codon 670/671 and at codon 692 are rare; mutations at codon 717 have been described in about 20 families worldwide from different ethnic origins, including Anglo-Saxon, Italian, and Japanese subjects (4–6). Mutations in APP have been shown to affect the release of Aβ in transfected cells and patient fibroblasts. Transgenic mice expressing the APP V717F mutation produce numerous Aβ deposits in the form of classical senile plaques, and the brains of these animals exhibit other neuropathological features of AD including neuronal and synaptic loss and gliosis (6,7).While the APP codon 717 mutations are associated with overproduction of $A\beta_{1-42}$, the Swedish double missense mutant leads to an increase in total Aβ secretion. The Swedish mutant involves the substitution of the two N-terminal amino acids of the Aβ domain, presumably rendering APP more susceptible to β-secretase activity. Therefore, FAD mutations in *APP* appear to affect both Aβ release and the intracellular trafficking of APP.

Presenilins

Mutations in *PSEN1* (8) and in the related *PSEN2* (9,10) are found to be causative in about 50% of kindreds with FAD. The coding region of *PSEN1* is derived from 10 exons (numbered 3–12). So far, mutations have been found in six of the 10 coding exons, with exons 5 and 8 accounting for 65% of the mutations. As some mutations result in a later onset age, it cannot yet be excluded that mutations in *PSEN1* may also result in late onset forms (>65 years) of the disease.

The FAD mutations in *PSEN1* are missense mutations causing single amino acid changes or, rarely, exonic deletions and appear to be 100% penetrant and are best classified as autosomal dominant "causative" gene defects. In contrast, only ten *PSEN2* mutations have been identified, suggesting that mutations on *PSEN2* gene are a rare but possible cause of disease and that FAD mutations are considerably more frequent in *PSEN1* than in *PSEN2*.

In 1995 a large Italian AD kindred was identified with a mutation in *PSEN2* consisting of a methionine to valine substitution at residue 239 (9).This mutation is characterized by some peculiarities of the clinical and neuropathologic phenotype compared to sporadic AD. In the autopsy analysis (11) of two probands, in addition to neurofibrillary changes and Aβ deposits, ectopic neurons in the subcortical white matter containing neurofibrillary tangles were observed. Furthermore, an unusually high number of ghost tangles in the cerebral cortex were found. The major peculiarity of this family was the clinical onset with epileptic seizures before the dementia (Fig. 1).

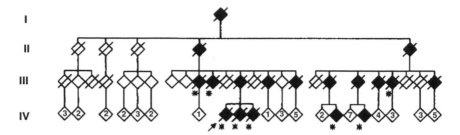

Figure 1 An example of familial Alzheimer's disease pedigree of a large Italian family carrying PSEN2 Met239Val mutation. * Indicates the affected members bearing the mutation. *Source*: From Ref. 11.

The combination of molecular and biochemical studies in the familial forms of Alzheimer's dementia supported the "amyloid hypothesis" as the main mechanism involved in the pathogenesis.

Mutations in the APP and presenilin genes invariably increase production of Aβ42 leading to enhanced deposition of this toxic fragment in the brain parenchyma (12–14) and consequently neuronal death. Abnormal accumulation of Aβ peptide could be considered a possible trigger of the disease and, together with neurofibrillary tangle formation and neuronal dysfunction, lead to the classical clinical picture of severe memory decline and loss of higher cortical functions. The mechanism by which $A\beta_{1-42}$ accumulates in the brain has been partially clarified in the last few years.

Formation of Aβ42 requires proteolytic processing of APP. APP is a type I transmembrane protein with a largely undefined function that undergoes a primary glycosylation step in the Golgi apparatus and endoplasmic reticulum, which is then transported to the plasma membrane where it is partly internalized via endocytosis through a clathrin-dependent pathway. During these metabolic steps, one of two proteolytic processes occurs. In the major metabolic pathway the APP molecule is cleaved by alpha-secretase into two fragments, a large N-terminal soluble form of APP (APPs alpha), which is eventually released into the extracellular fluid, and a C-terminal fragment (CTF) termed C83 bound to the membrane. An alternative minor pathway involves cleavage of APP at position -1 of the Aβ portion of APP by beta-secretase leading to the formation again of a large soluble protein (APPs beta) and a CTF termed C99 (Fig. 2).

Cleavage by an enzyme, gamma-secretase, of C83 leads to the formation of p3 (amino acids 16–42 of Aβ), precluding the formation of intact Aβ. Metabolism of C99 by gamma-secretase releases peptides $A\beta_{1-40}$ and pathogenic $A\beta_{1-42}$.

Alpha-secretase processing of APP does not result in the formation of amyloidogenic fragments and is therefore not implicated in the formation of Aβ or in the development of AD. Several different enzymes appear to account for

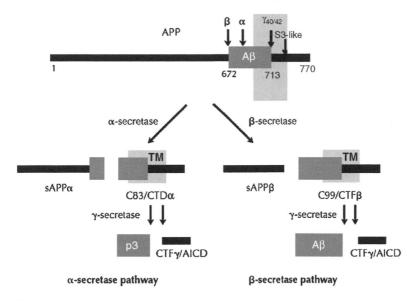

Figure 2 Amyloid precursor protein (APP) cleavage and α- and β-secretase pathways and production of β-amyloid peptide. *Abbreviations*: AICD, APP intracellular domain; CTF, C-terminal fragment; sAPP, soluble APP; TM, transmembrane. *Source*: From Ref. 15.

Alpha-secretase activity including enzymes of the disintegrin and metalloprotease class [ADAM 10 and ADAM 17 or tumor necrosis factor-α converting enzyme (TACE)], with these enzymes showing alpha-secretase activity regulated by proteolytic processing and phosphorylation (16).

β-secretase is involved in the first step of Aβ generation, and inhibition of this protease provides a possible target for drugs against AD (17). Several lines of research have identified the transmembrane aspartyl protease beta-site APP cleaving enzyme (BACE1) as the putative beta-secretase. BACE1 is a type I transmembrane protein, primarily expressed in neurons and localized in intracellular endosomes and in the trans-Golgi network where the interaction occurs. Experimental enhancement of BACE1 expression (18) leads to the generation of C99, C89, and APPs beta, and a decrease in the levels of alpha-secretase cleavage products. This phenomenon has recently been demonstrated also in sporadic AD (19), but the role in the pathogenesis of the sporadic form of the disease is still to be elucidated. In contrast, antisense inhibition of BACE1 decreases β-secretase activity and Aβ production. A homologue of BACE1, BACE2, has been identified by genetic database comparison and mapped to chromosome 21 (20). The speculation of a possible involvement of BACE2 in the processing of APP and ultimately in the generation of Aβ, given its proximity to the obligate Down syndrome region, has though failed to be confirmed, since major expression of BACE2 is localized outside of the brain and inhibition studies using antisense tools or protease overexpression does not lead to variation in Aβ production.

Gamma-secretase catalyzes the intramembrane proteolysis of APP, and this process is closely linked to the development of $A\beta_{1-42}$ peptide. This protease cleaves APP to produce C83 and C99 and releases the APP intracellular domain (AICD) into the cytoplasm, which can bind to cytoplasmic adaptor proteins and translocate to the nucleus where it may regulate gene expression. The gamma-secretase activity has several substrates in addition to APP, perhaps the most important of which is Notch, a family of cell-surface receptors which are essential for correct embryonic development. Recent findings suggest that gamma-secretase is a complex of at least four integral membrane proteins: presenilin, nicastrin, Aph-1, and Pen-2 (21), with the presenilins being the active site of gamma-secretase.

Sequence analysis of presenilins demonstrates two intramembrane aspartate residues, closely associated with the hydrophobic region that undergoes endoproteolysis leading to the formation of the two active presenilin heterodimers. Mutation of the two aspartate residues results in the blockade of gamma-secretase cleavage of the C99 peptide, leading to a reduction of Abeta production with simultaneous accumulation of C83 and C99 fragments and simultaneous abolition of presenilin endoproteolytic processing (22). In addition there is a close intracellular relationship between APP and PSEN1, which coprecipitate together in small amounts to form complexes and are located in the same intracellular vesicle compartments.

The evidence presented above supports the notion that a complex flow of events, known as "amyloid cascade theory," triggered by as yet unknown stimuli or promoted by a single genetic defect, increases Aβ42 production. A chronic imbalance between the production and clearance of fibrillogenic Aβ peptide with a tendency to misfold and aggregate progressively reduces the efficacy of synaptic transmission, promotes a microglial and astrocytic activation, and disrupts neuronal membrane homeostasis and potentiates oxidative stress to the cell. Recent findings suggest that the toxicity of Aβ does not lie in the insoluble fibrils that accumulate but rather in the soluble oligomeric intermediates (23). Soluble Aβ oligomers are found in human AD cerebrospinal fluid, and their total amount correlates with the severity of the disease better than senile plaques (24). Evidence suggests that the soluble oligomers can directly compromise synaptic function and that senile plaques may function as reservoirs of fibrous polymers that are in equilibrium with the diffusible species (25).

Because APP is axonally transported and processed in presynaptic terminals, synapses are sites where oligomers of Aβ may accumulate in high amounts. Soluble oligomers of Aβ42 inhibit long term potentiation in the hippocampus of rodents, which may suggest that these oligomers are responsible for memory impairment in AD patients. In transgenic mouse models of AD, synaptic dysfunction and memory impairment can occur in the absence of any evidence of Aβ deposition or neuronal degeneration (26). Evidence for frank cellular apoptosis in AD is controversial, but there is a growing recognition that apoptotic mechanisms may play a role in disease pathogenesis. Experimental studies suggest that Aβ can activate caspase through the extrinsic pathway, implicating binding of extracellular Aβ to cell receptors, while other studies suggest that the intrinsic pathway may be more relevant. Accumulation of Aβ in the endoplasmic reticulum or endosomes may activate apoptotic mechanisms through the unfolded protein response or endoplasmic reticulum stress; alternatively, intracellular Aβ may bind to alcohol dehydrogenase within mitochondria and activate apoptosis through mitochondrial stress. One of the consequences of caspase activation is cleavage of tau protein. Fragments of tau, particularly those that contain the microtubule binding domain which is critical for self interaction, more readily aggregate into fibrils than full length tau, but the precise way in which Aβ accumulation induces a cascade of neuronal metabolic changes that includes the hyperphosphorylation of wild type tau molecules in AD is the subject of active study, and several kinases have been proposed as possible candidates (Fig. 3).

Genetic Analysis in Alzheimer's Disease

With the identification of mutations in *APP, PSEN1*, and *PSEN2* as causes of AD, there is the possibility of using genetic testing to give a positive diagnosis of AD in individuals with AD dementia and also the potential for predictive testing in at-risk individuals. The majority of cases of dementia associated with mutations in *APP, PSEN1*, and *PSEN2* are early onset (generally age at onset of less than 65 years), and almost without exception where a family history is known, carriers will develop disease, though there are cases where *PSEN1* mutations are not fully penetrant (28). These cases of FAD are, however, rare (29), and not necessarily seen except in large specialist centers, and therefore the possibility of genetic testing is only applicable to a very small minority of dementia cases. Identification of a genetic basis for early onset dementia has, though, similar implications to that found for Huntington's disease, and therefore almost identical procedures will apply.

When presented with an individual with *early onset* dementia, patients and families are naturally anxious to know what the diagnosis is, and also if there is any likelihood that the disorder may be inherited. Frequently, evidence is brought forward by families of dementia in a previous generation or of dementia in a sibling. It should be stressed here that a positive family history of dementia is often apparent in a great many cases of AD, and some studies show up to 40% of AD cases with an affected relative (30). These cases are often though, of late onset, and not necessarily suitable for any genetic testing. In such circumstances, taking a brief family history is warranted, with particular attention being paid to the age at onset of symptoms in affected family members, as within families with early onset autosomal dominant dementia, age at onset is frequently very similar

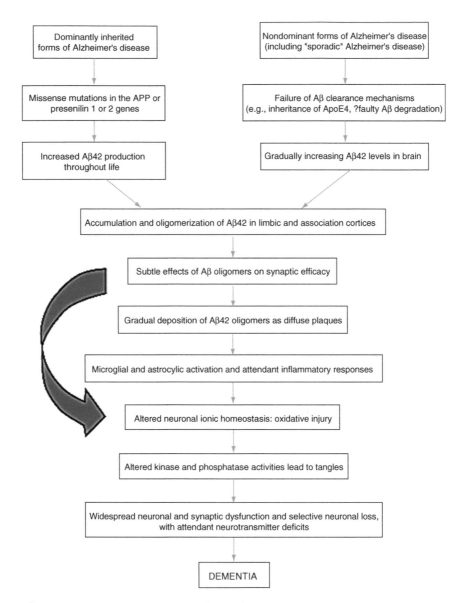

Figure 3 A hypothetical sequence of the pathogenetic steps of Alzheimer's disease based on currently available evidence. *Source*: From Ref. 27.

and may be one indication that a mutation in a particular gene may be present and require further investigation (29,31–35). A patient's and family's knowledge of a family history of dementia, however, brings with it certain anxieties, and appropriate specialist counselling measures should be instituted prior to, and during, any investigations (36,37). If an individual is, however, presented with early onset dementia suggesting AD, genetic analysis can be instituted if access to facilities and appropriate technical support is present. In the first instance, only the proband should be tested for the most likely mutations which will entail sequencing the *PSEN1* gene, followed by exons 16 and 17 of *APP*, and then, if available, all coding exons of *PSEN2*, since such mutations of the latter are rare. Given the fact that in many families with suspected AD, there is no evidence of mutations in *APP, PSEN1*, and *PSEN2* (29), it should be noted that families may face a degree of uncertainty over the findings of any testing, and therefore following testing, appropriate support should be made readily available (37).

If mutations in *APP, PSEN1*, or *PSEN2* are identified, then confirmation of diagnosis can be made, appropriate care and treatment of the patient provided, support and counselling given to the family (36,38), and the possibility of predictive testing undertaken. Predictive testing, however, has certain issues associated with it (38) and should not be undertaken lightly due to the impact upon life choices for the individual, and should only be undertaken in those families where a mutation has been identified in an affected individual. Once again, extensive counselling and support should be provided. In those found to be at risk of developing AD because of the presence of a defined mutation, additional support could be given in the form of longitudinal neuropsychiatric assessment to determine if there are signs of cognitive impairment. Longitudinal magnetic resonance imaging (MRI) studies (39,40) and possibly positron emission tomography (PET) scanning may predict cognitive changes and give the possibility of disease slowing treatments including cholinesterase inhibitors (41) or vaccination against $A\beta$, if it is possible given the side effects (42), then further supportive measures can be undertaken.

Apolipoprotein E and Other Genes Potentially Associated with Alzheimer's Disease

The current knowledge, mainly derived from studies on familial AD, points out that a single genetic defect occurring in these pathways could lead to dementia. Despite the increasing number of *APP, PSEN1*, and *PSEN2* mutations detected so far, research on novel candidate genes or molecules implicated in the sporadic form of AD has not reached a sufficient power or level of evidence compared to the only recognized risk factor to date, Apolipoprotein E.

Since 1993, over 150 association studies have replicated and confirmed the early findings (43) reporting an increased frequency of the Apolipoprotein E E4 allele in AD and the association of this allele with late onset AD (LOAD) and sporadic forms of AD. Apolipoprotein E (ApoE, protein; *APOE*, gene) is a 37 KDa protein involved in cholesterol transport in the brain and periphery. The three major isoforms of human ApoE (ApoE E2, ApoE E3, ApoE E4) are coded by the E2, E3, and E4 alleles, ApoE E3 being the most frequent isoform. ApoE E4 differs from ApoE E3 in a Cys/Arg change at position 112. It is now widely accepted that *APOE* E4 allele confers, in terms of relative risk, an increased risk of AD, whereas the E2 allele appears to have a protective effect. The risk for AD conferred by *APOE* E4 allele increases in a dose-dependent fashion, being eight times more likely for carriers of a double dose of E4 allele compared to *APOE* E3 carriers. Further epidemiological studies and genotype-phenotype correlations have suggested that E3/E4 and E4/E4 genotypes are more frequent in female patients with AD, with a compelling dose effect, and also that particular ethnic populations (i.e., African Americans) show a higher frequency of the *APOE* E4 allele, and therefore have an increased risk of developing AD. In addition, several studies, although controversial, have shown a role for ApoE in the mechanistic processes that lead to brain injury and ultimately to dementia. ApoE may contribute to amyloid and tau deposition in AD, binding to amyloid in a isoform specific manner enhancing aggregation, and in a similar way, interfering with tau binding to microtubules. *APOE* E4 is strongly associated with increased neuritic plaques, and the presence of this allele increases the odds ratio for cerebral amyloid angiopathy. In addition, *APOE* E4 carriers have shown reduced glucose metabolism and choline acetyltransferase activity in selected brain regions, demonstrate an accelerated cognitive decline, and are poor responders to memory-enhancing drugs prescribed for AD.

Several studies have shown that the E4 allele is also overrepresented in mild cognitive impairment (MCI), and an increased frequency of the allele is a strong predictor of clinical progression from MCI to AD. Although the E4 allele alone does not imply conversion to AD in MCI, the combination of genetic assessment with functional brain imaging is now seen as a promising preclinical AD detection strategy (see Chapter 8). Recent PET studies have demonstrated an association between the E4 allele and an abnormal reduction of glucose metabolism in normal individuals carrying the E4 genotype in the same brain regions as found in AD patients. It remains unknown if this is a predictor of future cognitive decline. In addition, there is evidence that the E4 allele leads to greater longitudinal metabolic decline in healthy elderly persons converting to MCI. Nonetheless, no study has been carried out to assess the impact of the E4 allele on brain physiology in the conversion from MCI to AD (44).

Several studies have addressed the utility of *APOE* genotyping in the diagnosis of AD, and the suggestion has been made that the presence of the E4 allele is indicative of AD in a patient presenting with dementia (45). The presence of an *APOE* E4 allele is, however, neither sufficient or specific to support a clinical diagnosis of AD on the basis of genetic testing alone (46), and currently it offers little significant gain over currently used diagnostic tools. For prediction of dementia development, there is almost universal agreement that *APOE* genotyping should not be offered or used (47,48), and therefore it remains a tool for academic use only.

APOE E4 allele frequency has also been associated with a number of neurological diseases, mainly degenerative, in which the major pathogenic step is represented by proteinaceous aggregates in the brain. This has suggested a putative role of ApoE in the clearance and internalization of small peptides that tend to accumulate in the brain. An increased E4 frequency was shown in patients with traumatic brain injury with a poor neurologic recovery, possibly due to enhanced β-amyloid deposition. The role of ApoE has also been suggested in increasing oxidative stress and in altering inflammation-related astrocyte and glial activation, and given the fact that ApoE is the major component of very-low density lipoproteins, a function in determining intracellular cholesterol distribution and homeostasis has been proposed.

However, despite all the evidence presented above, *APOE* remains a genetic risk factor that is neither sufficient nor necessary to cause AD, and only increases the risk of devloping disease.

Since mutations in *APP, PSEN1*, and *PSEN2* genes account for less than 10% of early onset FAD cases, and the presence of the *APOE* E4 allele is not a causative determinant for AD, several other genetic factors predisposing or causing the disease must exist.

Other Genetic Loci for Alzheimer's Disease

The current strategies to identify novel candidate genes (Table 2) or loci that could be related to sporadic AD or other dementias are today principally based on linkage analysis studies that provide new chromosomal regions to investigate, and on genetic association studies (family based or case-control designed), applied to detect genetic variants (polymorphisms) in molecules implicated in the disease-specific pathways or in biologically disease-related genes.

In comparison with early-onset forms of AD, the genetic basis of LOAD appears much more complex. Most LOAD cases are sporadic, with no family history of the disease. Genetic susceptibility at multiple genes and interaction between them and/or environmental factors are likely to be responsible for the aetiology of LOAD. Linkage analysis narrows down a chromosomal candidate region which may harbour dozens of genes (positional candidate genes) and consequently hundreds or thousands of single nucleotide polymorphisms. Some of these genes may be functional candidates with respect to pathogenic mechanisms of interest. Besides the chromosome 19 region harbouring *APOE*, multiple genome scans and linkage analyses have identified important chromosomal regions that potentially harbour additional LOAD genes on chromosomes 1, 5, 9, 10, 12, and 21 (containing *APP*), in addition to several loci with possible linkage (50). Although there are disagreements among linkage reports on the locations of putative AD genes on these chromosomes, given the overwhelming linkage evidence, it now seems logical to subject the relevant linkage regions to an exhaustive gene hunt. The application of refined methods that account for disease phenotype heterogeneity and the inclusion of informative covariates accounting for locus heterogeneity (age at onset, gender, *APOE* genotype, etc.) would be useful in either reducing or eliminating the background noise, allowing the identification of genes related to a defined stratum of LOAD. Replicating linkage for complex diseases represents a challenging prospect, and usually requires a sample far larger than the original to see a similar signal.

Table 2 Susceptibility Genes for Alzheimer's Disease

Gene	Chromosomal location	Association with Alzheimer's disease
APOE	19q32.2	+
ACE	17q23	+/−
ACT	14q32.1	+/−
BACE 1	11q23	+/−
BChE	3q26.1–q26.2	+/−
BH	17q11.1–q11.2	+/−
CATD	11p15.5	+/−
CST3	20p11.2	+/−
CTNNA3	10q21	+/−
5-HTT	17q11.1–q12	+/−
IDE	10q23–q25	+/−
LRP 1	12q13.1–13.3	+/−
NCSTN	1q23	+/−
NOS3	7q35	+/−
PEN2	19q13	+/−
PLAU	10q22	+/−
PS1 promoter	14q24	+/−
TGF-β1	19q13.1–q13.3	+/−
UBQLN1	9q21.2–q21.3	+/−
VLDL-R	9pter–p23	+/−
α2M	12p13.3–12.3	+/−

+/− indicates the positive and negative association studies. For specific indications on association studies of a specific gene, visit the "Alzgene" database (http://www.alzforum.org/res/com/gen/alzgene/default.asp).
Source: From Ref. 3.

The collection of additional families for linkage studies may be useful in addressing the issue of power. However, there is no guarantee that this would provide more meaningful information about the linkage regions than we already have from the existing linkage data. In addition, possible candidate genes should be confirmed with case-control association analyses, although often giving inconsistent results on populations with different ethnic background and if limited to a relatively small number of cases and controls. Carefully designed high-resolution large linkage genome scans together with association studies on relatively large case-control cohorts may provide useful additional and/or confirmatory information on the locations of putative AD genes.

In addition, genome-wide linkage or association studies can only identify potentially important chromosomal regions that may harbour functional genes, but the next steps must be focused to investigate these regions with fine or linkage mapping and to perform functional tests on these plausible biological and positional candidate genes.

A recent full genome scan indicated two major regions of interest on chromosome 19q13 and on chromosome 11q25 related to early onset FAD (51). These regions contain, apart from *APOE*, two interesting candidates, namely the *PEN2* gene, encoding a protein relevant to gamma-secretase activity, and the *BACE1* gene. To date, association studies on small populations with newly discovered polymorphisms in nicastrin and BACE1 have yielded contrasting or negative results (52).

Numerous proteins, enzymes, and proteases involved in the mechanism of degradation, clearance, and toxicity of Aβ have been investigated as possible candidate genes of susceptibility for developing AD. In particular, recent studies suggest new susceptibility loci on chromosome 10q. Over 240 genes in this region are thought to be strong positional and biological candidates able to interfere with AD-related biochemical pathways such as the urokinase-plasminogen activator (PLAU) gene and the insulin degrading enzyme (IDE).

PLAU is a serine protease (chromosome 10q22.2) that converts the inactive zymogen plasminogen into its active form plasmin. Although the plasmin proteolytic cascade is traditionally involved in fibrinolysis and cell migration, the plasmin system seems to be relevant to Aβ clearance. Ledesma and colleagues (53) report that plasminogen and its proteolytic fragment plasmin are present on the membrane of cultured mature hippocampal neurons where plasmin could cleave APP at the alpha site precluding the formation of APP, and could promote Aβ degradation. Recently a positive association with a single C/T nucleotide polymorphism of *PLAU* (P141L) and LOAD has suggested a possible effect on the risk of developing AD, but these results have been not replicated by other studies (54–57).

IDE gene (located on chromosome 10q24) encodes for an enzyme able to degrade Aβ monomers, thereby modulating cerebral Aβ levels. Indeed loss of IDE function in knockout mice and a rat mutant model leads to increased cerebral Aβ levels. Moreover, IDE appears to degrade the AICD. Despite initial reports of significant linkage of *IDE* in a family-based sample, negative data have been found in successive case-control studies (58–61).

Other known Aβ degrading enzymes such as neprilysin and endothelin converting enzyme-2 (*ECE2*) encoded by genes on chromosome 3, and plasminogen and the tissue-type plasminogen activator encoded by genes on chromosome 6, despite their potential and clinically relevant roles on AD neuropathogenesis, have not been positively associated with AD in case control or family based studies. Finally, Bertram, and Hiltunen have recently suggested an association with the ubiquilin 1 (*UBQLN1*) gene (located on chromosome 9q22) because of its potential role in the proteasomal degradation of proteins and its interaction with PS1 and PS2 (62). These data have, however, not been replicated yet.

Regarding the Aβ clearance, increasing evidence suggests that the low-density lipoprotein receptor-related protein (LRP) mediates the efflux of Aβ from the brain to the periphery. LRP is a scavenger receptor that can bind a variety of ligands, including ApoE, APP, and alpha2 macroglobulin. Aβ can form a complex with ApoE or alpha-2-macroglobulin and, after binding to LRP, is internalized to endosomes for degradation or directly exported into the plasma. Several studies have tested alpha 2 macroglobulin and LRP1 genes in patients with AD with contrasting results (63–66). In summary, the alpha-2-macroglobulin gene might be considered a risk factor only in LOAD cases with a family history (67), while study of the LRP1 gene performed to date does not support any association with disease.

The exact mechanism of Aβ toxicity is unclear. One hypothesis appears to involve the induction of apoptosis, but to date there is no evidence for an association with specific apoptosis candidate genes. Another hypothesis is based on the role of inflammation in AD: although inflammation and the up-regulation of inflammatory mediators is observed in the AD brain around senile plaques, none of the various members of cytokine family (such as interleukin 1-alpha, interleukin 1-beta, interleukin-6) have been reported to be associated with disease with additional evidence of genetic linkage. However, interesting data based on a number of full-genome screens in AD have shown positive genetic linkage and association with the TNF alpha gene (50).

Perspectives

The knowledge of genes involved in the amyloid cascade has moved towards the development of specific targets for possible therapeutic approach. There is a great interest in identifying small molecular inhibitors of the beta and gamma secretases, although problems have arisen with these strategies because these proteases also process other critical substrates (e.g., gamma secretase processes Notch). Possible selective inhibitors for APP include nonsteroidal anti-inflammatory drugs and cholesterol-lowering drugs (20).

An alternative approach is to prevent aggregation of the Aβ peptide and/or promote its clearance. In this field, early work in APP transgenic mice demonstrates that immunization with Aβ significantly attenuates AD-like pathology and ameliorates memory deficits (68,69). Although the mechanism by which brain Aβ is reduced following vaccination remains controversial, recent preliminary reports indicate that Aβ immunization may lower senile plaque load and stabilize behavioral decline in humans with AD (70,71). However, the findings of an adverse effect involving meningoencephalitis in approximately 6% of active Aβ-vaccinated patients in early clinical trials conducted in 300 patients (42) raise questions about the safety of this approach. The development of efficacious and safe immunogens with careful antigen and antibody selection, as well as of new vaccination techniques for immuntherapy of AD, can be expected in the future to maximize efficacy and minimize serious adverse events. An alternative active approach that may carry a lower risk of adverse events is mucosal (nasal or oral) vaccination. This method has been tested in APP transgenic mice and has led to significant decreases in plaque burden, Aβ levels, neuritic dystrophy, and gliosis (72).

For the identification of AD genes it would be useful to combine the genetic map information with gene expression profiling data, which in itself provides a powerful instrument to rapidly identify a set of genes differently expressed between normal and diseased tissues (73). Only the integration of the information from genetic maps (location of genes) and genomic maps based on gene expression and indicating specific genes may lead to the rapid identification of causal genes. The combination of these two strategies may prove to be useful for AD, and this is already evidenced by preliminary studies (74).

Another important aspect that should be considered in order to gain an understanding of the genetic basis of complex disorders is gene–gene interaction. With the exception of *APOE*, which is universally recognized to have a high risk associated with AD, the general understanding is that several genes, each with a moderate effect, are involved in the aetiology of a complex disease such as AD. Therefore it has been hypothesized that other possible candidate genes, having a small effect on the risk of AD, may not be detectable in all association studies due to power or sample heterogeneity issues, but that they may show a considerable effect in conjunction with other candidate genes. Much larger case-control samples are required for gene–gene interaction studies as stratification of the data reduces the power considerably, and this represents a limitation. With the exception of a few published cases-controls studies that have utilized more than 1000 subjects, most genetic studies use a smaller sample, raising questions about the meaningfulness of the association data rather than providing promising future aims. Only significant results from appropriately powered studies could be considered for replication in other samples from different populations.

Frontotemporal Dementias

Frontotemporal dementias (FTD) are complex clinical entities, characterized neuropathologically by glial and neuronal tau deposition with widespread neuronal loss and gliosis (see Chapter 11), with a marked clinical and genetic heterogeneity. The nosological classification is still under debate, even though Consensus Criteria have been published (75). Common clinical features include presenile age of onset (35 to 75 years age range) and psychotic symptoms at onset with late memory impairment. Often extrapyramidal signs or motor neuron involvement is present.

The disorder is quite rare, with a prevalence of 10–15 per 100,000 individuals aged less than 65 years, and representing about 15–20% of all the presenile dementing syndromes. At least three clinical syndromes have been described in the past: a frontal variant of FTD, with pronounced changes in behavior and personality, semantic dementia, and primary progressive (nonfluent) aphasia. These latter forms of the disease are purely sporadic, but approximately 40% of all FTD cases are familial, with a large clinical variability between and within kinships with FTD.

Linkage analysis studies, trying to homogenize different families with diverse clinical patterns, have led, more or less simultaneously worldwide, to the identification of a significant locus on chromosome 17, in the same region as the tau protein gene (*TAU*). Initial sequencing of *TAU* in chromosome 17-linked families showed negative results. An early report of an intronic mutation in 1998 led to the subsequent identification of *TAU* defects as the cause of FTD in some families. The reason for this initial delay could be related to the structure of *TAU*, which is composed of 15 exons, of which 11 are expressed in the adult brain. Exons 2, 3, and 10 are subject to alternative splicing, producing six different isoforms of the protein. These six isoforms are characterized by the presence of two diverse functional domains, the first being composed of variable NH2-terminal inserts that interact with plasma membranes and the second by three or four COOH-terminal microtubule binding repeats that ensure binding with tubulin and promote microtubule assembly (Fig. 4).

The first molecular variation found in *TAU* was an intronic mutation (77). Further identification of novel mutations clustering in exon 10 and nearby in intron 10, where the mutations affects tau splicing resulting in an altered 3/4 repeat ratio, provided direct evidence that intronic mutations could alter gene structure with loss of protein function. In fact, alterations in splice regulation caused by these mutations may disrupt a putative stem-loop structure or impair the binding of regulatory proteins to the repeat region (78). Such a different conformation of mutated tau could promote excessive deposition of the protein (also in absence of hyperphosphorylation) due to microtubule malfunction, and slowing intraneuronal transport of substrates. Thus, precipitation of tau aggregates and subsequent NFT formation could be interpreted as the consequence of this process.

To date more than 100 families with FTD have been identified with over 30 different mutations in *TAU* (78). Nucleotide changes include missense mutations, deletions, and splice site mutations. A direct correlation between the site of mutation and a specific cellular pathology has been predicted by early studies, suggesting that, for example, tau aggregates predominantly composed by filaments with four repeats were more common in patients with exon or intron 10 mutations. Today, with the discovery of novel pathogenic mutations, this is no longer confirmed, since mutations not clustering in the exon-intron 10 region could not necessarily lead to a specific neuronal or glial pathology or lead to a selective deposition of a particular isoform, (i.e., aberrant insoluble tau filaments lacking isoforms with a specific number of NH2-terminal inserts).

Most missense mutations in the microtubule-binding region reduce the ability of tau to interact with microtubules interfering with correct microtubule assembly. The primary effect of these mutations may be equivalent to a partial loss of function, with resultant microtubule destabilisation and deleterious effects on cellular processes, such as rapid axonal transport.

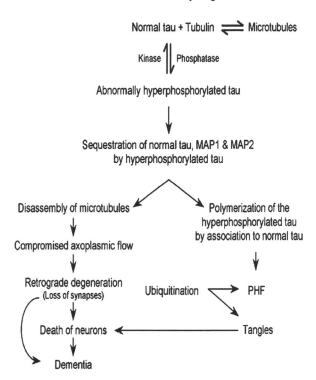

Figure 4 Mechanism of neurofibrillary degeneration. Tau is a major microtubule-associated protein of a normal mature neuron where it stimulates assembly and establishes microtubules. In a normal brain, tau contains 2–3 mol phosphate/mol of the protein for its optimal activity. Hyperphosphorylation of tau depresses this normal biological activity. In Alzheimer's disease and other tauopathies, tau becomes abnormally hyperphosphorylated. The tangles are ubiquitinated for degradation by the non-lysosomal ubiquitin pathway, but apparently this degradation, if any, is minimal. *Source*: From Ref. 76.

The intronic mutations and most coding region mutations in exon 10 increase the splicing of exon 10, thus changing the ratio between three- and four-repeat isoform and resulting in the overproduction of four-repeat tau. The possible existence of different binding sites on microtubules for three-repeat and four-repeat tau could explain the cytoplasmic accumulation of the overproduced isoform with the effect of a "gain of toxic function" mechanism that leads to neurodegeneration (79,80).

The heterogeneity of pathological manifestation of tau mutations is also reflected in clinical phenotypes in mutated families. As far as is known, there are no clear relationship between the clinical presentation and the position of the mutation, although early reports speculated on a more close association between particular clinical features and mutation location. Additional clinical features of *TAU* mutation families described so far include seizures at onset, pure AD phenotype or late onset dementia, progressive supranuclear palsy, and predominant motor neurone involvement with acute respiratory failure. Moreover different phenotypes can be expressed in a single family such as a pathological diagnosis of FTD in the father, and corticobasal degeneration in the offspring. These findings support the notion that additional genetic or environmental factors may account for this marked phenotypic heterogeneity.

There are, however, families with an FTD-like presentation that do not show mutation in *TAU*, and in a recent study the relevance of *TAU* mutations in FTD and related dementias was addressed (81). Mutations in *TAU* gene were only identified in just over 6% of familial or sporadic cases, with 25% of cases with a positive family history of FTD showing mutations. Even cases with FTD showing linkage to chromosome 17 often do not show mutation in *TAU*, suggesting that other genes may cause FTD (82). In apparently sporadic individuals only 4–5% of cases show mutation of *TAU*, again suggesting that these are rare causes of FTD.

Other rare forms of FTD occur with specific additional phenotypes, and these may provide indications in the early differential diagnosis of FTD coupled with genetic testing. A large Danish pedigree has been described which initially showed the pathology of DLDH (OMIM 600795) though subsequently showed tau-positive inclusions in neurones and glia (83). This family demonstrates linkage to a small region on the short arm of chromosome 3p11, and the causative gene is suggested to be *CHMP2B* (84). Other forms of FTD with linkage to chromosome 9q21–22 and a clinical and pathological feature of ALS (Hosler et al. 2000:OMIM 105550) occur, and in these the feature of ALS would suggest a differential diagnosis, but again the causative gene is unknown. Early onset FTD in the thirties with the additional features of inclusion body myopathy and Paget's disease shows linkage to chromosome 9p13 (OMIM#167320), and Watts and colleagues have identified mutations in the Valosin-containing protein gene (*VCP*) to be the cause of this disorder (85). In these cases, frontal cortical and cerebellar atrophy with ubiquitin and VCP-positive inclusions in neurons are a particular neuropathological feature.The clinical features of a progressive myopathy linked with Paget's disease in approximately half of cases and FTD in about one-third would suggest a diagnosis of this disorder and would warrant referral for genetic testing. Although tauopathies have been considered to result from genetic defects, screening for tau gene mutations in sporadic cases, FTD3, FTD/ALS9, FTD/CBD9, and familial PSP is not likely to identify pathogenic mutations (86).

Dementia with Lewy Bodies

Dementia with Lewy bodies (DLB), which neuropathologically is diagnosed by an abnormal aggregation of alpha-synuclein, is not now thought to be a rare cause of familial neurodegenerative disease. Alpha-synucleinopathies are a group of neurodegenerative disorders typically characterized by the loss of selective neuronal populations associated with the accumulation of pathological aggregates of alpha-synuclein, a normal synaptic protein that has been implicated in neurotransmission or in the organization and regulation of synaptic vesicles. This heterogenous group also includes also Parkinson's disease, dementia that occurs during the course of Parkinson's disease, and primary autonomic failure.

In 1996 consensus guidelines were proposed for the clinical and neuropathological diagnosis of DLB (87). The core clinical features for a diagnosis of probable and possible DLB are: fluctuating cognitive impairment, recurrent visual hallucinations, and parkinsonism. The consensus criteria arbitrarily suggest that if dementia occurs within 12 months of the onset of extrapyramidal motor symptoms, the patient should be diagnosed with possible DLB, while if the clinical history of parkinsonism is longer than 12 months, the diagnosis of Parkinson's disease dementia should be more appropriate. Lewy bodies (LB) are relatively large spherical eosinophilic cytoplasmic intraneuronal inclusion bodies that range from approximately 4 to 30 μ in diameter, first described by Frederich Lewy in 1912 in the substantia innominata and the dorsal motor nucleus of the vagus in a case of Parkinson's disease. These proteinaceous inclusions are a defining hallmark of Parkinson's disease and dementia with LB, but there are as yet no definite pathological criteria that separate the different alpha-synucleopathies either from each other or from AD and vascular pathology. Consensus criteria for DLB include ubiquitin immunohistochemistry for LB identification, although the recently developed alpha-synuclein immunochemistry is a better marker for visualizing LB and also shows previously under-recognised neuritic pathology, termed Lewy neurites (88). Pathological alpha-synuclein aggregates can constitute the fibrils of typical classical LB in the pigmented nuclei of the brainstem, in neocortex and amygdala, or Lewy neurites in the Ammon's horn.

Alpha synuclein is a dynamic molecule: it adopts an unfolded random coil structure in aqueous solution, shows an alpha helical structure upon binding to acid phospholipid vesicles, and is able to form insoluble fibrils with a high beta-sheet content resembling the filaments found in LB. Although mutations in alpha synuclein facilitate the transformation to a beta sheet structure, wild type alpha synuclein can adopt a beta sheet conformation possibly due to saturation effects, unknown protein-protein interaction, or environmental or genetic factors. Indeed, several studies suggest that the age-related increase in oxidative damage to membranes promotes the aggregation of alpha synuclein (Fig. 5). APP, chromogranin A, synphilin 1, and synaptophysin are axonally transported proteins that have been reported in LB (see Chapter 11). Even neurofilament and tubulin seem to be implicated in LB formation as immunohistochemical analysis shows their presence. It is possible that the presence of Lewy neurites and neurotransmitter deficits are more likely to be directly associated with clinical symptoms than density of cortical LB.

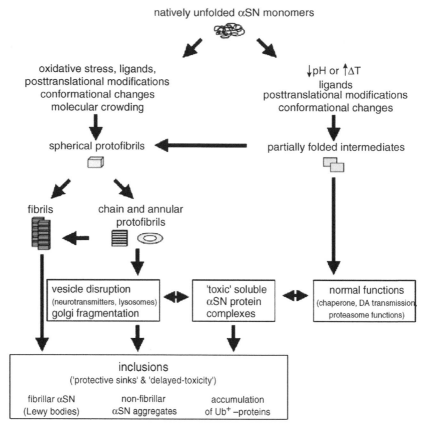

Figure 5 (*See color insert.*) Molecular pathophysiology of α-synuclein (αSN) monomers converting into partially folded, toxic, and/or aggregated forms. Putative toxic forms of αSN include fibrillar aggregates (Lewy bodies, Lewy neurites, cytoplasmic glial inclusions); amorphous aggregates; oligomers; protofibrils; soluble forms including partially folded intermediates, Ser-129-phosphorylated αSN, nitrosylated, and ubiquitylated. *Source*: From Ref. 89.

Currently, the mechanisms responsible for the abnormal aggregation of alpha-synuclein in insoluble and toxic forms remain to be explained. One possibility is that there is a pathological upregulation of normal, wild-type alpha-synuclein due to mRNA hyperexpression. Another is that alpha-synuclein could become insoluble or more able to aggregate. Alternatively, an inefficient proteasome system could process toxic protofibrils of the alpha-synuclein proteins, which are then sequestered into LB (90). The last mechanism could represent an effort by neurons to counteract biological stress inside the cell.

Sporadic and familial cases of DLB have been reported. Genetic investigation of familial DLB has been very limited and in most cases negative.

Recently a novel genetic mutation, E46K, has been found in the alpha synuclein gene (*SNCA*) in a Basque family with autosomal dominant parkinsonism and the typical pathological hallmarks of DLB (91), suggesting that genetic causes of DLB share common mechanisms with genetic forms of PD (92,93). In the recently described family with triplication of *SNCA* (94), some family members presented with a clinical picture that could be considered to fulfil criteria for DLB. However multiplication of *SCNA* has been investigated in pathologically confirmed patients with DLB, without positive results (95). Beta synuclein is a member of the synuclein family, and is highly homologous to alpha synuclein, both being involved in synaptic function. In a recent report, Ohtake and Limprasert suggest that mutations in beta-synuclein gene may predispose to DLB (96). The recent identification of the dardarin gene (*LRRK2*) in families with parkinsonism, frequently with dementia or a DLB presentation (97,98), suggests the possibility that this gene may be important in some DLB/PD cases.

Understanding the pathophysiology of DLB appears important for developing novel therapeutic strategies. Neuroprotection appears interesting since there is evidence in DLB of significant neuronal dysfunction but no striking cortical neuronal degeneration (see Chapter 11). Therefore, the consistent evidence that DLB is more treatable than other neurodegenerative disorders with available pharmacological management, make important the accurate identification of patients with DLB and their differentiation from other common types of dementia.

SUMMARY

An understanding of the genetics of dementia and AD has provided vital clues to the underlying biology that leads to this disorder with the identification of *APP, PSEN1,* and *PSEN2.* Genetic analysis, whilst useful in certain circumstances, cannot currently be used for the majority of cases, as the *APOE* gene, the only robustly identified gene for LOAD, is neither necessary nor sufficient for the development of this disorder.

REFERENCES

1. Rocca WA, Amaducci L. The familial aggregation of Alzheimer's disease: an epidemiological review. Psychiatr Dev 1988; 6:23–36.
2. Breitner JC, Silverman JM, Mohos RC, et al. Familial aggregation in Alzheimer's disease: comparison of risk among relatives of early-and late-onset cases, and among male and female relatives in successive generations. Neurology 1988; 38:207–212.
3. Available at: http://www.alzforum.org/res/com/mut/default.asp.
4. Mullan M, Houlden H, Windelspecht M, et al. A locus for familial early-onset Alzheimer's disease on the long arm of chromosome 14, proximal to the alpha 1-antichymotrypsin gene. Nat Genet 1992; 2:340–342.

5. Hendriks L, van Duijn CM, Cras P, et al. Presenile dementia and cerebral haemorrhage linked to a mutation at codon 692 of the beta-amyloid precursor protein gene. Nat Genet 1992; 1:218–221.

6. Goate A, Chartier-Harlin MC, Mullan M, et al. Segregation of a missense mutation in the amyloid precursor protein gene with familial Alzheimer's disease. Nature 1991; 349:704–706.

7. Games D, Adams D, Alessandrini R, et al. Alzheimer-type neuropathology in transgenic mice overexpressing V717F beta-amyloid precursor protein. Nature 1995; 373:523–527.

8. Sherrington R, Rogaev EI, Liang Y, et al. Cloning of a gene bearing missense mutations in early-onset familial Alzheimer's disease. Nature 1995; 375:754–760.

9. Levy-Lahad E, Wasco W, Poorkaj P, et al. Candidate gene for the chromosome 1 familial Alzheimer's disease locus. Science 1995; 269:973–977.

10. Rogaev EI, Sherrington R, Rogaeva EA, et al. Familial Alzheimer's disease in kindreds with missense mutations in a gene on chromosome 1 related to the Alzheimer's disease type 3 gene. Nature 1995; 376:775–778.

11. Marcon G, Giaccone G, Cupidi C, et al. Neuropathological and clinical phenotype of an Italian Alzheimer family with M239V mutation of presenilin 2 gene. J Neuropathol Exp Neurol 2004; 63:199–209.

12. Citron M, Westaway D, Xia W, et al. Mutant presenilins of Alzheimer's disease increase production of 42-residue amyloid beta-protein in both transfected cells and transgenic mice. Nat Med 1977; 3:67–72.

13. Scheuner D, Eckman C, Jensen M, et al. Secreted amyloid beta-protein similar to that in the senile plaques of Alzheimer's disease is increased in vivo by the presenilin 1 and 2 and APP mutations linked to familial Alzheimer's disease. Nat Med 1996; 2:864–870.

14. Gibson GE, Vestling M, Zhang H, et al. Abnormalities in Alzheimer's disease fibroblasts bearing the APP670/671 mutation. Neurobiol Aging 1997; 18:573–580.

15. Pastor P, Goate AM. Molecular genetics of Alzheimer's disease. Curr Psychiatry Rep 2004; 6:125–133.

16. Buxbaum JD, Liu KN, Luo Y, et al. Evidence that tumor necrosis factor alpha converting enzyme is involved in regulated alpha-secretase cleavage of the Alzheimer amyloid protein precursor. J Biol Chem 1998; 273:27765–27767.

17. Vassar R. Beta-secretase (BACE) as a drug target for Alzheimer's disease. Adv Drug Deliv Rev 2002; 54:1589–1602.

18. Vassar R, Bennett BD, Babu-Khan S, et al. Beta-secretase cleavage of Alzheimer's amyloid precursor protein by the transmembrane aspartic protease BACE. Science 1999; 286:735–741.

19. Yang LB, Lindholm K, Yan R, et al. Elevated beta-secretase expression and enzymatic activity detected in sporadic Alzheimer disease. Nat Med 2003; 9:3–4.

20. Tanzi RE, Bertram L. Twenty years of the Alzheimer's disease amyloid hypothesis: a genetic perspective. Cell 2005; 120:545–555.

21. De Strooper B, Saftig P, Craessaerts K, et al. Deficiency of presenilin-1 inhibits the normal cleavage of amyloid precursor protein. Nature 1998; 391:387–390.

22. Wolfe MS, Xia W, Ostaszewski BL, et al. Two transmembrane aspartates in presenilin-1 required for presenilin endoproteolysis and gamma-secretase activity. Nature 1999; 398:513–517.

23. Hardy J, Selkoe DJ. The amyloid hypothesis of Alzheimer's disease: progress and problems on the road to therapeutics. Science 2002; 297:353–356.

24. Lue LF, Kuo YM, Roher AE, et al. Soluble amyloid beta peptide concentration as a predictor of synaptic change in Alzheimer's disease. Am J Pathol 1999; 155:853–862.

25. Selkoe DJ. Cell biology of protein misfolding: the examples of Alzheimer's and Parkinson's diseases. Nat Cell Biol 2004; 6:1054–1061.

26. Oddo S, Caccamo A, Shepherd JD, et al. Triple-transgenic model of Alzheimer's disease with plaques and tangles: intracellular Abeta and synaptic dysfunction. Neuron 2003; 39:409–421.

27. Selkoe DJ. American college of physicians; American physiological society. "Alzheimer disease: mechanistic understanding predicts novel therapies." Ann Intern Med 2004; 140:627–638.

28. Rossor MN, Fox NC, Beck J, et al. Incomplete penetrance of familial Alzheimer's disease in a pedigree with a novel presenilin-1 gene mutation. Lancet 1996; 347:1560.

29. Janssen JC, Beck JA, Campbell TA, et al. Early onset familial Alzheimer's disease: mutation frequency in 31 families. Neurology 2003; 60:235–239.

30. Lautenschlager NT, Cupples LA, Rao VS, et al. Risk of dementia among relatives of Alzheimer's disease patients in the MIRAGE study: what is in store for the oldest old? Neurology 1996; 46:641–650.

31. Fox NC, Kennedy AM, Harvey RJ, et al. Clinicopathological features of familial Alzheimer's disease associated with the M139V mutation in the presenilin 1 gene. Pedigree but not mutation specific age at onset provides evidence for a further genetic factor. Brain 1997; 120:491–501.

32. Harvey RJ, Ellison D, Hardy J, et al. Chromosome 14 familial Alzheimer's disease: the clinical and neuropathological characteristics of a family with a leucine—> serine (L250S) substitution at codon 250 of the presenilin 1 gene. J Neurol Neurosurg Psychiatry 1998; 64:44–49.

33. Janssen JC, Hall M, Fox NC, et al. Alzheimer's disease due to an intronic presenilin-1 (PSEN1 intron 4) mutation: a clinicopathological study. Brain 2000; 123:894–907.

34. Palmer MS, Beck JA, Campbell TA, et al. Pathogenic presenilin 1 mutations (P436S & I143F) in early-onset Alzheimer's disease in the U.K. Mutations in brief no. 223. Online. Hum Mutat 1999; 13:256.

35. Rossor MN, Newman S, Frackowiac RS, et al. Alzheimer's disease families with amyloid precursor protein mutations. Ann NY Acad Sci 1993; 695:198–202.

36. Coon DW, Davies H, McKibben C, et al. The psychological impact of genetic testing for Alzheimer disease. Genet Test 1999; 3:121–131.

37. McConnell LM, Koenig BA, Greely HT, et al. Genetic testing and Alzheimer disease: recommendations of the stanford program in genomics, ethics, and society. Genet Test 1999; 3:3–12.

38. Fogarty M. Genetic testing, Alzheimer disease, and long-term care insurance. Genet Test 1999; 3:133–137.

39. Fox NC, Warrington EK, Stevens JM, et al. Atrophy of the hippocampal formation in early familial Alzheimer's disease. A longitudinal MRI study of at-risk members of a family with an amyloid precursor protein 717Val-Gly mutation. Ann NY Acad Sci 1996; 777:226–232.

40. Schott JM, Fox NC, Frost C, et al. Assessing the onset of structural change in familial Alzheimer's disease. Ann Neurol 2003; 53:181–188.

41. Hashimoto M, Kazui H, Matsumoto K, et al. Does donepezil treatment slow the progression of hippocampal atrophy in patients with Alzheimer's disease? Am J Psychiatry 2005; 162:676–682.

42. Orgogozo JM, Gilman S, Dartigues JF, et al. Subacute meningoencephalitis in a subset of patients with AD after Abeta42 immunization. Neurology 2003; 61:46–54.

43. Corder EH, Saunders AM, Strittmatter WJ, et al. Gene dose of apolipoprotein E type 4 allele and the risk of Alzheimer's disease in late onset families. Science 1993; 261:921–923.

44. Mosconi L, Perani D, Sorbi S, et al. MCI conversion to dementia and the APOE genotype: a prediction study with FDG-PET. Neurology 2004; 63:2332–2340.

45. Roses AD, Saunders AM. Apolipoprotein E genotyping as a diagnostic adjunct for Alzheimer's disease. Int Psychogeriatr 1997; 9:277–288; discussion 317-21.

46. Relkin MR, Kwon YJ, Tsai J, et al. The National Institute on Aging/Alzheimer's Association recommendations on the application of apolipoprotein E genotyping to Alzheimer's disease. Ann NY Acad Sci 1996; 802:149–176.

47. Brodaty H, Conneally M, Gauthier S, et al. Consensus statement on predictive testing for Alzheimer disease. Alzheimer Dis Assoc Disord 1995; 9:182–187.

48. Lovestone S. Early diagnosis and the clinical genetics of Alzheimer's disease. J Neurol 1999; 246:69–72.

49. Available at: http://www.molgen.ua.ac.be/ADMutations/default.cfm.

50. Bertram L, Tanzi RE. Alzheimer's disease: one disorder, too many genes? Hum Mol Genet 2004; 13:R135–R141.

51. Blacker D, Bertram L, Saunders AJ, et al. Results of a high-resolution genome screen of 437 Alzheimer's disease families. Hum Mol Genet 2003; 12:23–32.

52. Cruts M, Dermaut B, Rademakers R, et al. Amyloid beta secretase gene (BACE) is neither mutated in nor associated with early-onset Alzheimer's disease. Neurosci Lett 2001; 313:105–107.

53. Ledesma MD, Dotti CG. The conflicting role of brain cholesterol in Alzheimer's disease: lessons from the brain plasminogen system. Biochem Soc Symp 2005;129–138.

54. Finckh U, van Hadeln K, Muller-Thomsen T, et al. Association of late-onset Alzheimer disease with a genotype of PLAU, the gene encoding urokinase-type plasminogen activator on chromosome 10q22.2. Neurogenetics 2003; 4:213–217.

55. Myers AJ, Marshall H, Holmans P, et al. Variation in the urokinase-plasminogen activator gene does not explain the chromosome 10 linkage signal for late onset AD. Am J Med Genet B Neuropsychiatr Genet 2004; 124:29–37.

56. Ertekin-Taner N, Allen M, Fadale D, et al. Genetic variants in a haplotype block spanning IDE are significantly associated with plasma Abeta42 levels and risk for Alzheimer disease. Hum Mutat 2004; 23:334–342.

57. Papassotiropoulos A, Tsolaki M, Wollmer MA, et al. No association of a non-synonymous PLAU polymorphism with Alzheimer's disease and disease-related traits. Am J Med Genet B Neuropsychiatr Genet 2005; 132:21–23.

58. Prince JA, Feuk L, Gu HF, et al. Genetic variation in a haplotype block spanning IDE influences Alzheimer disease. Hum Mutat 2003; 22:363–371.

59. Boussaha M, Hannequin D, Verpillat P, et al. Polymorphisms of insulin degrading enzyme gene are not associated with Alzheimer's disease. Neurosci Lett 2002; 329:121–123.

60. Abraham R, Myers A, Wavrant-DeVrieze F, et al. Substantial linkage disequilibrium across the insulin-degrading enzyme locus but no association with late-onset Alzheimer's disease. Hum Genet 2001; 109:646–652.

61. Nowotny P, Hinrichs AL, Smemo S, et al. Association studies between risk for late-onset Alzheimer's disease and variants in insulin degrading enzyme. Am J Med Genet B Neuropsychiatr Genet 2005; 136:62–68.

62. Bertram L, Hiltunen M, Parkinson M, et al. Family-based association between Alzheimer's disease and variants in UBQLN1. N Engl J Med 2005; 352:884–894.

63. Pritchard A, Harris J, Pritchard CW, et al. Association study and meta-analysis of low-density lipoprotein receptor related protein in Alzheimer's disease. Neurosci Lett 2005; 382:221–226.

64. Goto JJ, Tanzi RE. The role of the low-density lipoprotein receptor-related protein (LRP1) in Alzheimer's A beta generation: development of a cell-based model system. J Mol Neurosci 2002; 19:37–41.

65. Van Leuven F, Thiry E, Lambrechts M, et al. Sequencing of the coding exons of the LRP1 and LDLR genes on individual DNA samples reveals novel mutations in both genes. Atherosclerosis 2001; 154:567–577.

66. Scott WK, Yamaoka LH, Bass MP, et al. No genetic association between the LRP receptor and sporadic or late-onset familial Alzheimer disease. Neurogenetics 1998; 1:179–183.

67. Blacker D, Wilcox MA, Laird NM, et al. Alpha-2 macroglobulin is genetically associated with Alzheimer disease. Nat Genet 1998; 19:357–360.

68. Schenk D, Hagen M, Seubert P. Current progress in beta-amyloid immunotherapy. Curr Opin Immunol 2004; 16:599–606.

69. Gandy S, Walker L. Toward modeling hemorrhagic and encephalitic complications of Alzheimer amyloid-beta vaccination in nonhuman primates. Curr Opin Immunol 2004; 16:607–615.

70. Nicoll JA, Wilkinson D, Holmes C, et al. Neuropathology of human Alzheimer disease after immunization with amyloid-beta peptide: a case report. Nat Med 2003; 9:448–452.

71. Ferrer I, Boada Rovira M, Sanchez Guerra ML, et al. Neuropathology and pathogenesis of encephalitis following amyloid-beta immunization in Alzheimer's disease. Brain Pathol 2004; 14:11–20.

72. Selkoe DJ. Defining molecular targets to prevent Alzheimer disease. Arch Neurol 2005; 62:192–195.

73. Kamboh MI. Molecular genetics of late-onset Alzheimer's disease. Ann Hum Genet 2004; 68:381–404.

74. Li YJ, Oliveira SA, Xu P, et al. Glutathione S-transferase omega-1 modifies age-at-onset of Alzheimer disease and Parkinson disease. Hum Mol Genet 2003; 12:3259–3267.

75. The Lund and Manchester Groups. Clinical and neuropathological criteria for frontotemporal dementia. J Neurol Neurosurg Psychiatry 1994; 57:416–418.
76. Iqbal K, Alonso Adel C, Chen S, et al. Tau pathology in Alzheimer disease and other taupathies. Biochim Biophys Acta. 2005; 1739:198–210.
77. Hutton M, Lendon CL, Rizzu P, et al. Association of missense and 5′-splice-site mutations in tau with the inherited dementia FTDP-17. Nature 1998; 393:702–705.
78. Hutton M. Missense and splice site mutations in tau associated with FTDP-17: multiple pathogenic mechanisms. Neurology 2001; 56:S21–S25.
79. Goedert M, Jakes R. Mutations causing neurodegenerative taupathies. Biochim Biophys Acta 2005; 1739:240–250.
80. Yancopoulou D, Spillantini MG. Tau protein in familial and sporadic diseases. Neuromolecular Med 2003; 4:37–48.
81. Stanford PM, Brooks WS, Teber ET, et al. Frequency of tau mutations in familial and sporadic frontotemporal dementia and other tauopathies. J Neurol 2004; 251:1098–1104.
82. van Swieten JC, Rosso SM, van Herpen E, et al. Phenotypic variation in frontotemporal dementia and parkinsonism linked to chromosome 17. Dement Geriatr Cogn Disord 2004; 17:261–264.
83. Yancopoulou D, Crowther RA, Chakrabarti L, et al. Tau protein in frontotemporal dementia linked to chromosome 3 (FTD-3). J Neuropathol Exp Neurol 2003; 62:878–882.
84. Skibinski G, Parkinson NJ, Brown JM, et al. Mutations in the endosomal ESCRTIII-complex subunit CHMP2B in frontotemporal dementia. Nat Genet 2005; 37:806–808.
85. Watts GD, Wymer J, Kovach MJ, et al. Inclusion body myopathy associated with paget disease of bone and frontotemporal dementia is caused by mutant valosin-containing protein. Nat Genet 2004; 36:377–381.
86. Morris HR, Katzenschlager R, Janssen JC, et al. Sequence analysis of tau in familial and sporadic progressive supranuclear palsy. J Neurol Neurosurg Psychiatry 2002; 72:388–390.
87. McKeith IG, Galasko D, Kosaka K, et al. Consensus guidelines for the clinical and pathologic diagnosis of dementia with lewy bodies (DLB): report of the consortium on DLB international workshop. Neurology 1996; 47:1113–1124.
88. Spillantini MG, Schmidt ML, Lee VM, et al. Alpha-synuclein in lewy bodies. Nature 1997; 388:839–840.
89. Dev KK, Hofele K, Barbieri S, et al. Part II: Alpha-synuclein and its molecular pathophysiological role in neurodegenerative disease. Neuropharmacology 2003; 45:14–44.
90. McKeith I, Mintzer J, Aarsland D, et al. Dementia with lewy bodies. Lancet Neurol 2004; 3:19–28.
91. Zarranz JJ, Alegre J, Gomez-Esteban JC, et al. The new mutation, E46K, of alpha-synuclein causes Parkinson and lewy body dementia. Ann Neurol 2004; 55:164–173.
92. Polymeropoulos MH, Lavedan C, Leroy E, et al. Mutation in the alpha-synuclein gene identified in families with Parkinson's disease. Science 1997; 276:2045–2047.
93. Hardy J, Cookson MR, Singleton A. Genes and parkinsonism. Lancet Neurol 2003; 2:221–228.

94. Singleton AB, Farrer M, Johnson J, et al. Alpha-synuclein locus triplication causes Parkinson's disease. Science 2003; 302:841.
95. Johnson J, Hague SM, Hanson M, et al. SNCA multiplication is not a common cause of Parkinson disease or dementia with lewy bodies. Neurology 2004; 63:554–556.
96. Ohtake H, Limprasert P, Fan Y, et al. Beta-synuclein gene alterations in dementia with lewy bodies. Neurology 2004; 63:805–811.
97. Paisan-Ruiz C, Jain S, Evans EW, et al. Cloning of the gene containing mutations that cause PARK8-linked Parkinson's disease. Neuron 2004; 44:595–600.
98. Zimprich A, Biskup S, Leitner P, et al. Mutations in LRRK2 cause autosomal-dominant parkinsonism with pleomorphic pathology. Neuron 2004; 44:601–607.

5

Approaches to the Identification of Novel Diagnostic and Therapeutic Targets in Dementia

Kate E. Wilson

Institute for Ageing and Health, University of Newcastle, Newcastle General Hospital, Newcastle upon Tyne, Tyne and Wear, U.K.

Chris Morris

Wolfson Unit of Clinical Pharmacology, Chemical Hazards and Poisons Division–Newcastle, Health Protection Agency, and School of Neurology, Neurobiology, and Psychiatry, The Medical School, University of Newcastle upon Tyne, Newcastle upon Tyne, Tyne and Wear, U.K.

INTRODUCTION

With the increasing prevalence of dementia in the elderly and the recognition that the syndrome itself is a heterogeneous disorder, there is a pressing need to identify not only effective treatments, but also diagnostic aids that will selectively and specifically define the different forms of dementia. Population-based studies backed by neuropathological assessment are few; however, they show that Alzheimer's disease (AD), while still the major form of dementia, accounts for about 60% of cases, with vascular dementia, dementia with Lewy bodies, frontal lobe syndromes, and mixed pathology disorders also contributing to the overall problem (1). Combining diagnostics and therapeutics will provide the most significant benefits for patients, but with different syndromes making up the total picture, it is vital to ensure that the diagnosis is correct. A major problem with dementia diagnosis currently is the fact that gold standard diagnosis can only come postmortem (see Chapter 11). Clinical diagnosis, while highly accurate in many tertiary referral centers, comes only after extensive examination over a period of months, during which time specific treatments need to be applied. The ability to provide a rapid and accurate diagnosis could therefore lead to significant improvements in dementia treatment.

But how, particularly when the underlying basis for many aspects of dementia is unknown, is it possible to identify new diagnostic targets, or new targets for therapy? Can a technique also be applied early enough to provide presymptomatic diagnosis? Various systems which are currently in use or are in development allow potential novel diagnostic targets to be identified. These methods, collectively termed functional genomics, permit the rapid and often wholesale analysis of cells or tissues in a disease state or the effects of pharmacological treatment, making the identification of changes possible in a short space of time.

FUNCTIONAL GENOMICS

The various genome projects that have set out to define the molecular basis for many major organisms, including man, and have provided the foundation for the global analysis of cell and tissue function using functional genomics (2). By cataloguing all the possible genes in an organism, the genome projects have allowed the production of reagents capable of detecting all the expressed genes, or a reference with which to identify gene products by. The former is exemplified by the production of whole genome microarrays, now the method of choice for determining gene expression, and the latter by the bioinformatics tools which, when coupled to various mass spectrometry (MS) methods, can be used for high throughput protein and peptide identification. For the identification of diagnostic targets in dementia, the application of these methods allows the production of a catalogue from which to choose suitable candidates for further testing.

MICROARRAY-BASED GENE EXPRESSION PROFILING

Several methods exist which allow the analysis of all the expressed genes within a tissue or cell type, such as those based on subtractive cDNA methodology (3), differential display-based methods (4,5), or serial analysis of gene expression (6). Many of these methods can be used by standard laboratories with the minimum of molecular biology equipment, though a problem with their use is in the relatively labor-intensive nature of the methods. The advent of gene expression microarrays has, however, largely superseded these technologies since it allows the rapid and comprehensive analysis of gene expression, or a focused approach to the analysis of a specific set of genes. Microarrays are high densities of specific DNA sequences either as single stranded chemically synthesised oligonucleotides or as cDNAs (often produced by PCR from defined clones), present as a highly ordered array on a solid support of usually glass or plastic (7). Several thousand individual sequences can be spotted or synthesised on an array, with each single spot, often only a few microns across, representing a single mRNA species. Microarrays are probed using a reverse hybridization procedure where the RNA sample is labeled, normally with a fluorescent reporter molecule, and then hybridized to the DNA sequences on the array. Since hybridization is roughly proportional to the amount of an mRNA species present in the sample, the presence of this highly ordered array allows each individual gene sequence to be analyzed for the amount of mRNA present in the sample.

For any given tissue or cell, there will be a specific set of genes that are expressed and which defines the nature of that tissue or cell. Of the 35,000–40,000 genes in the human genome, normally in any cell only a limited fraction of these genes will be expressed, perhaps only 20–30% of the genome for any given cell type (2). The complexities of the brain, with multiple neuronal types, vasculature, and supporting glia, mean that the gene expression profile of any one brain area can be extensive, and it has been suggested that perhaps half of the genome is represented by genes specific to the brain (2). Microarrays have been designed which are sufficient size that they represent most if not all of the possible genes in the human genome. For the definition of brain function in health and in disease, such arrays have the capacity to rapidly assess and identify those genes that are expressed within a specific tissue. By extracting RNA from brain tissue and applying it to a microarray, it is therefore possible to determine which genes are being expressed by that tissue and also the relative amount of the particular transcript present. Comparing healthy tissue with diseased therefore permits the identification of which genes are present or absent and also to what extent any particular gene is being expressed.

One potential problem of brain tissue is its highly complex nature stemming from the numerous cell types and connections. In the various forms of dementia, pathology is often restricted to specific anatomical locations, but also key lesions are restricted to certain cell types (see Chapter 11). For example, neurofibrillary tangle formation in AD may be restricted to large pyramidal neurons, sparing interneurons (8–10). Even in areas associated with pathology, only a limited subset of the vulnerable neurons may be affected, leaving some free of pathology. Because of this cellular heterogeneity, it can be difficult to detect gene expression changes in a single cell type due to dilution effects or the effects of pathology. Using laser capture microdissection, it is, however, possible using a focused laser beam to cut through a thin tissue section and isolate single cells of a given type, or small areas of tissue (11). Using this methodology, specific cell groups such as neurons can be profiled independently of any other surrounding cells, allowing a diseased neuron to be compared with its unaffected neighbor (12). While there may be only a few picograms of RNA in a single neuron, this is insufficient to use on a microarray as normally an array requires microgram amounts of RNA. It is, however, possible to use linear amplification methods to amplify endogenous RNA in a reliable and unbiased manner from nanogram amounts of RNA for microarray analysis (13,14). By combining methods such as laser capture microdissection with linear amplification of RNA and microarray-based gene expression profiling, it is possible to determine gene expression profiles in isolated neurons or glia in health and disease (15). This has been achieved to some extent in dementia with expression profiling having been reported in AD in particular. Perhaps of significance is the report by Blalock and colleagues who studied AD cases and also individuals with mild cognitive impairment (MCI) in order to identify genes expressed at the earliest stages of dementia (16). This study analysing hippocampal gene expression identified mRNA up-regulation in several pathways involved with oligodendrocyte differentiation and lipid metabolism, though a down-regulation of energy metabolism pathways was evident (16). Similarly, analysis of hippocampal CA1 gene expression in AD has been used to show that there is up-regulation of some of the inflammatory signalling pathways in AD, possibly associated with reactive gliosis (17). This latter study also showed decreased neurotrophin and apoptotic signalling, possibly being associated with the loss of pyramidal neurones and neurofibrillary tangle formation (17).

The primary results of a microarray experiment represent only the beginning of a particular gene expression study. Standard levels of analysis identify significantly altered levels of gene expression using relatively conservative changes, often ± 2 standard deviations from mean of control expression levels, making subtle changes in gene expression difficult to detect. Using bioinformatics approaches, however, allows the detection of specific pathways that are affected, frequently using clustering algorithms that place differentially expressed genes into families and pathways based on gene ontology terms. Since the results of a microarray analysis are at best semi-quantitative, all microarray experiments require further validation, normally by semi-quantitative real time PCR (Q-RT-PCR). It is therefore possible to accurately determine the levels of gene expression for a specific gene identified using the microarray, by comparison with an appropriate housekeeping gene. Q-RT-PCR systems now exist which make it possible to determine the levels of expression for either a few specific genes in several samples, or to determine expression levels of a hundred or more genes in a single sample. By this route it is a relatively straightforward task to validate the primary targets from a microarray analysis, but also to analyze additional components of the pathway identified as being potentially changed on the basis of bioinformatics analysis. Microarray analysis and Q-RT-PCR therefore can determine differential gene expression in highly selected tissue samples.

But what of the tissue to be used in the identification of specific markers for dementia diagnosis? One approach will be the use of suitable animal models, most notably transgenic models showing the pathological changes associated with dementia, which allows considerable control over agonal and pre- and post-mortem effects. The use of transgenic models offers the opportunity to look not just at end stage disease as is often the case with human postmortem material, but to look at early stage pathology and even animals before the development of pathology. One caveat of such an approach would be the complexity of the pathology in dementia involving amyloid deposition, tangle formation, gliosis, vascular changes, and white matter pathology, which is difficult to accurately reproduce in an animal model. The use of human material is therefore perhaps preferable, though not without difficulties in analysis. Methods for the isolation of high-quality intact RNA from postmortem brain for gene expression profiling are well established (18,19). A major problem with postmortem material is, however, the uncertainties over what happens to the expression of particular genes as a result of premortem and postmortem changes which may impact upon the interpretation of results. It has been known for several years that RNA quality and the expression of certain genes is heavily affected by how an individual dies (20). Recently this has been extended by comparing gene expression in normal individuals who died suddenly with an absence of any premortem phase, with individuals who had various lengths of premortem illness (21). The presence of any significant premortem coma (often seen as a reduction in the pH of tissue) is reflected in an increase in transcripts for certain stress response genes and in the levels of transcription factors involved in the mediation of these processes, and a decrease in the levels of mRNAs for energy metabolism transcripts and those involved in proteolytic events (21). Previous studies on AD where a down-regulation of energy metabolism genes was seen may be an example of this (16,17). Considerable care is therefore required in not only obtaining high-quality RNA, but also in ensuring that case and control material is carefully matched for short postmortem delay and good agonal state. This, and particularly the latter, can be difficult to achieve particularly with dementia cases that often die in terminal coma due to bronchopneumonia, though with access to large tissue banks, it is possible to obtain well-matched samples.

One possibility that may avoid the problems associated with postmortem tissue or animal models may be to use peripheral tissues, and in this instance, lymphocytes or fibroblasts may provide the most accessible source. Given that there is a considerable genetic influence on the development of neuro-degenerative diseases and particularly AD (see Chapter 4), it can be argued that the underlying genetic changes that occur in the brain will also be evident in the periphery if that gene is expressed in a similar manner. It is also apparent that changes in the brain impact upon the periphery as there are anatomical connections between the central nervous system (CNS) and the periphery, and soluble factors (cytokines, trophic molecules) can egress from the brain and have an effect. This can be seen in changes in gene expression in lymphocytes in response to various forms of CNS insult (22). It should therefore be possible to investigate, for example, gene expression in lymphocytes from patients with vascular dementia to determine if there are differential gene expression changes compared to, for example, elderly normal individuals.

The application of microarray-based gene expression profiling to disease tissue or animal models has the potential therefore to identify the changes that uniquely define dementia, and moreover, different forms of dementia. These markers, alone or in combination, provide the basis for the development of tests to identify dementia in its earliest stages, and to provide a specific diagnosis.

Cases with MCI may be one particularly fruitful source of information since, if the individuals die early in the disease course without developing dementia, these cases may provide information relating to the gene expression changes associated with the primary cause of disease allowing such therapies and markers to be developed. By using proteomic methods to identify the protein products of these gene changes in cerebrospinal fluid (CSF), plasma, etc., or by gene expression profiling of lymphocytes, it may be possible to develop novel tests for rapid diagnosis. If gene expression changes are confined to the CNS, then the development of neuroimaging ligands utilizing these targets would be one route to improving diagnosis. Altered gene expression also provides the foundation for potential new therapeutic strategies based on specific biochemical pathways affected in disease, and may afford opportunities for more rational disease-based treatment.

PROTEOMICS

Proteomics, the analysis of the protein complement of a cell or tissue, represents the natural extension to functional genomic studies where mRNA expression is mapped. While the sequencing of the human genome has revealed 35,000–40,000 genes, the proteome is much larger and also more dynamic in nature presenting a unique challenge. Alternative splicing of genes results in different isoforms of a protein while post-translational modifications also lead to multiple gene products from a single gene. Furthermore, proteins also differ physically due to amino acid composition, for example, strongly basic, acidic, or hydrophobic, as well as differences in protein folding that have an effect along with protein-protein interactions. Given the complexity of the brain, and also where comparisons between healthy and diseased tissue are involved, the data sets generated by proteomic techniques can be extremely large. While microarray-based gene expression profiling can provide a rapid means to identify potential candidates for further analysis, it can be argued that changes in gene expression are not necessarily reflected by changes in the respective protein (23). High-throughput proteomic techniques are therefore ideal for the direct identification of biomarkers of disease, not only in postmortem or biopsy tissue, but also in serum, plasma, and CSF, making the discovery of novel diagnostics and treatment markers more effective.

Currently, no single method in a single pass is capable of accurately identifying all proteins expressed by a cell or tissue due to the enormous variation in the physical and chemical properties of proteins. A standard approach in proteomic methodologies, particularly for tissue samples, is therefore to use fractionation methods to reduce complex samples and simplify analysis. Standard methods include centrifugation in order to separate a cell or tissue sample into, for example, cytoplasmic and mitochondrial fractions. Alternatively, the use of various detergents, high pH, and chaotropes can be applied to samples to extract insoluble proteins such as membrane proteins followed by chromatographic separation, which can in itself be used directly on samples. With comparative proteomic methods, removal of certain proteins is often practiced, and this is frequently the case when analyzing body fluids, where, for example, the plasma may have 10,000 different proteins and peptides with concentrations ranging from fg/ml to mg/ml. Methods to remove the most abundant proteins in a fraction which are not thought to contribute to proteome variation are often practiced, such as removal of albumin or immunoglobulin from plasma or serum samples. By a combination of these techniques, it is possible to generate a series of fractions which are sufficiently refined to allow accurate analysis. This combination of analytical techniques, applied to even a single sample, results in generation of very large data sets, which now means that automation and development of high-throughput methods is becoming increasingly important in proteomic studies, as well as tools such as protein databases for rapid data analysis. Since an ideal biomarker of disease will reflect the underlying mechanism or pathology of a disease, the use of automated methods is becoming common to detect these changes, particularly where proteomic methods are being used to identify diagnostic targets.

2D Gel Electrophoresis

Two-dimensional polyacrylamide gel electrophoresis (2D-PAGE) is the most commonly used technique in proteomics since it is a highly effective method for simultaneously separating complex protein mixtures (24,25). It is the only technique currently available which allows thousands of proteins to be resolved with one format in a single experiment and remains unchallenged as such. Proteins are firstly separated by charge [isoelectric point (pI)] using isoelectric focusing, followed by separation by mass in the second-dimension gel, recent advances allowing up to 10,000 individual spots to be distinguished on a single large format gel (26).

First-dimension isoelectric focusing separates proteins according to their pI (the pH at which a protein has no net charge) using immobilized pH gradients composed of thin gel strips into which ampholytes (charged carrier molecules) are incorporated. In an electric field, proteins migrate through the gel due to the pH gradient effect created by the ampholytes and stop migrating once their charge is net neutral. These strips are available in a variety of formats, from wide pH ranges covering many pH units to narrow ranges which cover just one or two pH units. While broad range strips are ideal for initial experiments, for example, large scale sample screening, narrow range strips have the advantage of allowing much greater resolution. A series of gels can be overlapped to provide greater visualization of proteins within the same range as a broad range strip yet with much greater resolution, improving image analysis and protein identification (24,26). Despite the advances in technology, 2D-PAGE remains unsuitable for highly acidic or basic proteins since a lack of good ampholytes means that focusing below pH3 and above pH11 is poor. This tends to result in reduced separation of membrane-associated proteins, which are often very acidic, due to reduced solubility in the absence of detergents, the presence of which would interfere with the focusing step. Additional pre-separation methods are therefore needed to solubilize membrane proteins prior to analysis.

Following first-dimension separation by pI, proteins are separated by molecular weight in polyacrylamide gels containing SDS, an anionic detergent which denatures proteins, converting them into essentially linear molecules and imparting a net negative charge. When combined with a reducing agent such as DTT, proteins are therefore separated exclusively by mass. The resulting protein spot map can be visualized using a variety of stains. Silver and Coomassie are relatively simple staining techniques requiring little specialist equipment and are therefore the most frequently used methods. Silver staining has a higher sensitivity than traditional radiolabeling or Coomassie Brilliant Blue staining, capable of detecting 100 pg of protein per spot (27). Recently fluorescent dyes such as SYPRO and CyDyes have been developed with sensitivity similar to silver stains. A major advantage of these stains is their compatibility with MS since more traditional methods often require destaining before proteins can be identified by MS (28–30). Traditionally one of the biggest disadvantages of 2D-PAGE was the poor reproducibility; however, the advent of fluorescent techniques has greatly improved this, though silver and Coomassie stains are still routinely used in many labs and provide a simple method for building proteome databases and reference maps for various organisms or tissues (see http://ca.expasy.org/ch2d).

A new development in 2D-PAGE ideally suited to the identification of protein biomarkers is fluorescence difference gel electrophoresis (DIGE). This uses different fluorescent cyanine dyes (e.g., Cy2, Cy3, Cy5) to pre-label protein samples prior to 2D electrophoresis. Each dye, since it fluoresces at a different wavelength, can be visualized by scanning the 2D gel at dye-specific wavelengths, and the images overlaid to give a combined image which can be analyzed using various software packages (31,32). This technique allows direct comparison between samples to show either the presence or absence of a particular protein in test compared to control sample or differences in protein abundance, thereby reducing the effect of gel-to-gel variation and therefore improving reproducibility (33). Since multiple samples can be separated on a single gel, an internal standard can be incorporated into all gels within an experiment. Using this approach, studies have demonstrated that there is little variation between multiple operators, and differentially expressed spots can be easily identified and analyzed (33,34). Two labeling techniques are available for DIGE studies, minimal and saturation labeling, which in both cases have minimal effect on the charge of the protein and add approximately 600 Da to the mass. These CyDyes have a greater sensitivity, being capable of detecting 0.1 ng albumin, and over a greater dynamic range, around 10^3–10^4 (35). This makes the use of the dye labeling technique ideal for applications in which there is a limited sample, for example, where analysis of a single cell type is required and so can be coupled to sample acquisition methods such as laser capture microdissection (36,37).

Several approaches in neuroscience have used traditional 2D gel-based approaches, and in the majority of instances have utilized prefractionation of samples prior to analysis. For example, drug treatment has been analyzed by 2D-PAGE to identify the effects of anti-depressive drugs on the brain proteome (38). Proteins involved in neurogenesis, such as IGF-1 and HCNP, and synaptic plasticity, such as Rab4a and HSP10, were induced by venlafaxine or fluoxetine, defining pathways by which these compounds can effect long-term changes in brain structure by treatment. The pathological effects of drug-induced seizures on brain protein expression indicate changes in heat shock and antioxidant proteins along with synaptic proteins (39,40), which complements work using microarray gene expression profiling on the action of anti-epileptic drugs (41). In dementia, 2D studies using silver staining of AD and control brains have visualized over 1500 proteins (42), though this is considerably less than can be achieved with fluorescence-based detection methods. Analysis of the normal human CSF proteome has produced a list of over 480 proteins using silver-stained 2D gels in several studies, but again these represent the most abundant proteins (43,44). Variations in Apolipoprotein E in the CSF have, however, been identified between patients with sporadic or variant CJD (45), and between Alzheimer's and schizophrenia patients (46). Several proteins have been identified as significantly different in the CSF between AD and control, including a number of glycoproteins, again including Apolipoprotein E, but also Apolipoproteins J and A1, raising the possibility that these protein changes simply represent the presence of neurodegeneration. Here liquid phase IEF was used as a pre-fractionation step prior to 2D-PAGE (47). The identification of these possible markers for AD has not, though, been validated in any large cohorts, and therefore additional studies are required. The use of 2D-PAGE, however, provides a basis for other proteomic methods to build on in dementia biomarker identification.

Isotope-Coded Affinity Tagging

While 2D-PAGE is limited in its capacity to analyze membrane proteins, isotope coded affinity tagging (ICAT) is a new methodology in comparative proteomic analysis that is particularly suited to membrane protein analysis as the system is compatible with strong detergents, making it the ideal complement to DIGE (48,49). With ICAT, samples are labeled with either an isotopically light or heavy thiol reactive reagent which also contains a biotin affinity tag. Both samples are then mixed together and subjected to proteolytic digestion, typically by trypsin, and the resulting peptide mixture is then fractionated by avidin affinity chromatography which isolates only the ICAT labelled peptides. These are then identified by liquid chromatography (LC) and tandem MS (48–50). The eight-dalton difference between the light and heavy reagents (containing eight hydrogen or eight deuterium atoms respectively) is detected by MS, allowing direct comparison between test and control sample. The first generation ICAT reagents have recently been improved by incorporating an acid-cleavable linker, allowing removal of the biotin affinity tag prior to MS but leaving the peptide isotopically labeled. This simplifies the analysis so that greater numbers of peptides can be identified and quantified (51). ICAT labeling has been employed to study protein changes induced in cultures of cortical neurons by the chemotherapeutic agent campothecin and analyzed by LC/MS, demonstrating changes in proteins involved in transcriptional regulation, protein synthesis, and signal transduction (52). This method is suited to the study of relatively insoluble proteins such as membrane proteins since these can be extracted using strong ionic detergent prior to the labeling and digestion steps, creating peptides which are also more soluble than whole proteins (48). Given that many ligands for positron emission tomography (PET) and single photon emission computed tomography (SPECT) are membrane receptors, the use of methods such as ICAT have the potential to isolate novel targets for the development of new neuroimaging ligands in dementia.

Multidimensional Protein Identification Technology

Since the proteome of even a single cell is highly complex, for example, a typical human cell contains many thousand different proteins and protein isoforms, direct analysis is virtually impossible, and further complicated since several times this number of peptides is produced by trypsin digestion prior to MS. No single separation technique can separate all proteins and so multidimensional techniques are often required for proteome studies. Multidimensional protein identification technology (MudPIT) is an automated technique combining LC and MS. This is similar to ICAT, though MudPIT tends to use online separation techniques whereby samples flow between the different components of the system automatically (53). Various LC techniques in sequence (affinity, size exclusion, reversed phase) allow separation of complex samples. The flowthrough from these columns is directly fed into an electrospray ionization (ESI) MS in which the microcapillary tube used for injection has a diameter as small as 1–2 μm allowing flow rates as low as 5 nl/min (53,54), greatly reducing the amount of sample required for analysis. MudPIT is particularly useful for membrane-associated proteins, kinases, and transcription factors which are difficult to detect using 2D-PAGE due to their low abundance (55). A similar method has been used to characterize the serum proteome following digestion with trypsin and fractionation using strong cation exchange and reversed phase HPLC, with identification using ion-trap MS (56). Nearly 500 proteins were directly identified, demonstrating the use of MudPIT methods in identifying proteomic changes with minimal sample handling but maximal throughput. Using first-dimension anion exchange followed by reverse phase separation, tryptic peptides from a post-synaptic density preparation were injected directly by electrospray into a quadrupole time of flight mass spectrometer, identifying 492 proteins associated with signal transduction, the synaptic scaffold, adaptor proteins, and cell-cell adhesion molecules (57). While some of the proteins were associated with other cell types such as glial fibrillary acidic protein (57), the use of affinity purification may enhance the ability to accurately define only those proteins specifically associated with certain cell or organelle fractions (58).

Perhaps of direct relevance to dementia is the identification of markers which indicate changes within the CNS and which are amenable to analysis by, for instance, neuroimaging. Combining methods such as comparative 2D-PAGE, ICAT, and MuDPIT has the potential to identify either novel pathways indicating disease mechanisms, or biomarkers that may be present in CSF. As with methods analysing RNA, analysis of proteins is not, however, without its difficulties. For human postmortem material, while there is some suggestion that it is possible to identify phosphoproteins (59), analysis of animal material postmortem suggests that primary signalling pathways, many which rely on specific phosphorylation events, may rapidly alter postmortem (60). This may be particularly relevant to human studies, as similar changes appear to happen, with rapid down-regulation of signaling pathways postmortem (Wilson, unpublished). Many of these methods though have the potential to be used in comparative approaches and several are now being used to provide a preliminary analysis of dementia.

FLUID ANALYSIS

One major goal in the diagnosis of any particular form of dementia would be the availability of a simple screening tool based on key feature of the biology of the disease. CSF and plasma testing provides an obvious route to disease marker identification that could be applied in a routine setting (see Chapter 3). For AD, markers such as Aβ determination in plasma have shown negative results, and in CSF have yielded conflicting results (61). Identification of elevations in hyperphosphorylated tau in CSF in AD has improved specificity (62,63), though the paucity of any studies with neuropathological assessment and the wide variation of Aβ and tau levels with any individual patient perhaps makes the interpretation of these findings premature (61,64–66). Newer markers (47) have also not been validated and therefore new markers are required. While peripheral markers have been suggested to occur in many neurodegenerative diseases, none have so far proved robust (61). This has been due to the commonly held view that while there is CNS disease, there is little impact upon the periphery due to presence of the blood-brain barrier and the very specific cell groups affected in diseases such as AD (67). This view has recently been challenged, with the finding that there are marked changes in lymphocyte gene expression following CNS damage (22). Furthermore, in many psychiatric diseases, there is expression of CNS proteins on lymphocytes, and their expression mirrors that found in the CNS (68,69). It is therefore possible that in diseases such as AD there are changes associated with

CNS disease in the peripheral circulation which are particularly amenable to proteomic and also genomic investigation, and especially by certain MS methods.

Mass Spectrometry

MS is the preferred method for the identification of proteins by providing structural information such as peptide mass and amino acid sequence, as well as information on protein modifications. The data obtained can then be used to identify a protein by searching various databases. MS measures the mass-to-charge ratio (m/z) of gaseous ions produced by accelerating an ionized particle, in this case the protein or peptide, through a rarefied atmosphere to a detector. Often peptide mass fingerprint analysis is used where the isolated protein to be analyzed is digested enzymatically, to cleave the protein at specific bonds giving a reproducible pattern of digestion. MS is then performed on the peptide mixture, giving masses with high accuracy the mass fingerprint of the protein. This fingerprint is then compared to databases containing theoretical protein cleavage data producing a list of the closest matching proteins (70). Much of this has been achieved by matrix-assisted laser desorption/ionization (MALDI) MS which can be used not only to identify isolated proteins, but also to directly identify peptides from tissue samples (71). Ultra high resolution methods such as FT-NMR-MS are now being used which may allow the detection and characterization of low-abundance peptides in body fluids (72).

Matrix-Assisted Laser Desorption/Ionization

Body fluids are extremely complex, and it has been estimated that human plasma may contain well over 10,000 analytes, spanning a concentration range of 10 orders of magnitude (73). Methods are required that can not only detect these numerous different analytes at the various concentrations, but can also distinguish these different analytes. One method that has received wide use in this respect is surface-enhanced laser desorption/ionization (SELDI) where, like MALDI, a laser beam is used to desorb analyte ions from a solid into the gaseous phase for analysis by MS (74,75). While a sample such as plasma or CSF would contain many thousands of potential peptides and would generate an extremely complex series/smear of peaks with MALDI, SELDI utilizes a solid phase chromatographic surface on the MALDI target plate in order to reduce the number of peptide peaks analyzed at any one time (76). For example, the plasma sample is applied to a target which has a cationic affinity support which binds only peptides with high affinity for that particular support. By use of a mild ionization procedure, SELDI produces a limited series of mass peaks for each affinity support, and by using targets with different affinity supports, it is therefore possible to analyze different subsets of proteins to build up a picture of the proteins present. Using this approach it is possible to analyze a given tissue, and by comparing the peak profiles of the tissue, to identify peptides which differ between, for instance, case and control.

One major drawback, however, is the use of a relatively mild ionization procedure which limits the eventual mass resolution of the system. Furthermore, this also provides only a mass/charge ratio for any peak which could potentially correspond to several, if not hundreds, of possible peptide sequences. Peptide identification is therefore difficult unless the peptide is identified in several different runs, and frequently the specific peptide peak has to be isolated and identified by more traditional methods such as chromatography. Direct separation using LC (2D LC) and fractionation of samples (77) along with high-throughput liquid-handling robotics are now though being coupled directly to MALDI and ESI-MS to produce more powerful systems. Here it is possible to directly analyze the individual protein peaks in the peptide profile using TOF/TOF MS and MS^n, and the identity of the peptide can be determined rapidly. There is therefore the prospect that proteins and peptides identified in a complex mass spectrum as being differentially expressed between cases and controls can be directly identified. For example, Aβ has been identified in the lens of Alzheimer's patients suggesting that the pathological features of the disease overlap between brain and lens (78). The identification of ovarian and prostate cancer-associated biomarkers have also demonstrated the usefulness of direct MS-based analysis of biological fluids for rapid discovery of markers which have extremely high specificity and sensitivity in a clinical setting (79,80).

Protein Microarrays

Protein microarrays are gaining in popularity as miniature ligand-binding assays which can be used for complex protein samples since they allow detection and also quantitation of proteins. With protein arrays, a frequent approach is where antibodies are immobilized at a high density on a solid support such as a treated glass microscope slide. When exposed, each individual antibody captures its target protein from the sample. By arraying hundreds or thousands of antibodies on a single slide, this method allows large-scale and high-throughput analysis using small sample volumes and relatively low protein concentrations (81,82). Like gene arrays, protein arrays are probed by direct labeling of the protein sample with fluorescent dyes (e.g., Cy3 or Cy5) and the abundance of a protein being related to the fluorescent intensity of the particular spot on the array (82). One problem with this approach is low sensitivity, though new approaches include multiplexed sandwich immunoassays with ultra-high femtomolar sensitivity (83). A major problem with this approach is the relatively limited availability of antibodies, and in particular monoclonal antibodies, which allow arrays to be reproduced particularly on the large scale required in proteomics. While antibody arrays are an obvious choice for protein detection microarrays, an alternative is the use of recombinant antibody fragments or immunoglobulin fragments expressed on the surface of bacteriophage which provides a rapid means of producing reagents (84). The generation of large-scale protein microarrays based on antibody fragments is now being explored and it may soon be possible to use this high-throughput approach and with the reproducibility that derives from recombinant techniques (85,86).

Antibody microarrays, since they are perhaps more suited to analysis of fluid samples, are now being used in focused clinical analysis. In neurology, these arrays have been used to analyze cord serum of children with cerebral palsy using an antibody array capable of detecting 78 cytokines, chemokines, and growth factors. In this instance, 12 analytes were found to be higher in cases compared to matched controls (87). These techniques have uses as tools in differential diagnosis of disease, both clinically and in the research setting; for example, panels of antibodies or peptides known to be differentially expressed in various disorders can be used to identify specific patterns of changes in CSF, plasma, or serum, providing a rapid and easy diagnostic test, often with very high sensitivity (83). Alternatively, with a wide enough panel of antibodies coupled to the array or by using liquid-based multianalyte analysis (88), it may be possible to directly analyze fluids in order to detect differential protein expression for diagnostic purposes.

CONCLUSIONS

The diagnosis of dementia can only be achieved by the skilled clinician using various clinical tools and personal judgement to assess the individual patient. Currently the *definitive* diagnosis of dementia, particularly in the early stages, is not possible, and reagents and tools are required which will assist the clinician in achieving this. Using a combination of methods should, however, allow determination of the gene and protein expression patterns of key brain regions in health and disease which can define not only the presence of dementia, but of a specific form of dementia such as AD. Techniques such as those described here are already becoming routine in the search for biomarkers that can be used to predict and diagnose disease, and to produce highly specific diagnostic tests. This will be particularly useful in dementia diagnosis where, for example, symptoms tend to overlap in the various different common forms, and yet accurate diagnosis is required if the most effective treatments are to be used. However, if biomarkers are to be used as diagnostic tools, techniques are required which are not only sensitive and reliable but also reproducible allowing for multi-center use. Ultimately, the technologies described here will help to unravel both the genetic and environmental factors that predispose and precipitate the development of dementia. These global technologies should therefore be seen, not simply as a rapid means of identifying biological changes associated with dementia, but as a route to more traditional methods of cell biological analysis for establishing how dementia develops, and how new diagnostic tools can be produced.

ACKNOWLEDGMENTS

Supported by grants from the Alzheimer's Research Trust, Alzheimer's Scotland, Alzheimer's Society, Commission of the European Communities, GE Healthcare, Medical Research Council, and The Health Protection Agency.

REFERENCES

1. Neuropathology Group of the Medical Research Council Cognitive Function and Ageing Study (MRC CFAS). Ince: pathological correlates of late-onset dementia in a multicentre, community-based population in England and Wales. Lancet 2001; 357:169–175.
2. Bishop JR, Ellingrod VL. Neuropsychiatric pharmacogenetics: moving toward a comprehensive understanding of predicting risks and response. Pharmacogenomics 2004; 5:463–477.
3. Hara E, Kato T, Nakada S, Sekiya S, Oda K. Subtractive cDNA cloning using oligo(dT)30-latex and PCR: isolation of cDNA clones specific to undifferentiated human embryonal carcinoma cells. Nucleic Acids Res 1991; 19:7097–7104.
4. Liang P, Pardee AB. Differential display of eukaryotic messenger RNA by means of the polymerase chain reaction. Science 1992; 257:967–971.
5. Mahadeva H, Starkey MP, Sheikh FN, Mundy CR, Samani NJ. A simple and efficient method for the isolation of differentially expressed genes. J Mol Biol 1998; 284:1391–1398.
6. Velculescu VE, Zhang L, Vogelstein B, Kinzler KW. Serial analysis of gene expression. Science 1995; 270:484–487.
7. Xiang CC, Brownstein MJ. Fabrication of cDNA microarrays. Methods Mol Biol 2003; 224:1–7.
8. Hof PR, Nimchinsky EA, Celio MR, Bouras C, Morrison JH. Calretinin-immunoreactive neocortical interneurons are unaffected in Alzheimer's disease. Neurosci Lett 1993; 152:145–148.
9. Hof PR, Cox K, Young WG, Celio MR, Rogers J, Morrison JH. Parvalbumin-immunoreactive neurons in the neocortex are resistant to degeneration in Alzheimer's disease. J Neuropathol Exp Neurol 1991; 50:451–462.
10. Hof PR, Morrison JH. Neocortical neuronal subpopulations labeled by a monoclonal antibody to calbindin exhibit differential vulnerability in Alzheimer's disease. Exp Neurol 1991; 111:293–301.
11. Emmert-Buck MR, Bonner RF, Smith PD, et al. Laser capture microdissection. Science 1996; 274:998–1001.
12. Mikulowska-Mennis A, Taylor TB, Vishnu P, et al. High-quality RNA from cells isolated by laser capture microdissection. Biotechniques 2002; 33:176–179.
13. Xiang CC, Chen M, Kozhich OA, et al. Probe generation directly from small numbers of cells for DNA microarray studies. Biotechniques 2003; 34:386–393.
14. Van Gelder RN, von Zastrow ME, Yool A, Dement WC, Barchas JD, Eberwine JH. Amplified RNA synthesized from limited quantities of heterogeneous cDNA. Proc Natl Acad Sci USA 1990; 87:1663–1667.

15. Kamme F, Salunga R, Yu J, et al. Single-cell microarray analysis in hippocampus CA1: demonstration and validation of cellular heterogeneity. J Neurosci 2003; 23:3607–3615.

16. Blalock EM, Geddes JW, Chen KC, Porter NM, Markesbery WR, Landfield PW. Incipient Alzheimer's disease: microarray correlation analyzes reveal major transcriptional and tumor suppressor responses. Proc Natl Acad Sci USA 2004; 101:2173–2178.

17. Colangelo V, Schurr J, Ball MJ, Pelaez RP, Bazan NG, Lukiw WJ. Gene expression profiling of 12,633 genes in Alzheimer hippocampal CA1: transcription and neurotrophic factor down-regulation and up-regulation of apoptotic and pro-inflammatory signaling. J Neurosci Res 2002; 70:462–473.

18. Bahn S, Augood SJ, Ryan M, Standaert DG, Starkey M, Emson PC. Gene expression profiling in the post-mortem human brain—no cause for dismay. J Chem Neuroanat 2001; 22:79–94.

19. Harrison PJ, Heath PR, Eastwood SL, Burnet PW, McDonald B, Pearson RC. The relative importance of premortem acidosis and postmortem interval for human brain gene expression studies: selective mRNA vulnerability and comparison with their encoded proteins. Neurosci Lett 1995; 200:151–154.

20. Hardy JA, Wester P, Winblad B, Gezelius C, Bring G, Eriksson A. The patients dying after long terminal phase have acidotic brains; implications for biochemical measurements on autopsy tissue. J Neural Transm 1985; 61:253–264.

21. Li JZ, Vawter MP, Walsh DM, et al. Systematic changes in gene expression in postmortem human brains associated with tissue pH and terminal medical conditions. Hum Mol Genet 2004; 13:609–616.

22. Tang Y, Nee AC, Lu A, Ran R, Sharp FR. Blood genomic expression profile for neuronal injury. J Cereb Blood Flow Metab 2003; 23:310–319.

23. Anderson L, Seilhamer J. A comparison of selected mRNA and protein abundances in human liver. Electrophoresis 1997; 18:533–537.

24. Klose J. Protein mapping by combined isoelectric focusing and electrophoresis of mouse tissues. A novel approach to testing for induced point mutations in mammals. Humangenetik 1975; 26:231–243.

25. O'Farrell PH. High resolution two-dimensional electrophoresis of proteins. J Biol Chem 1975; 250:4007–4021.

26. Klose J, Kobalz U. Two-dimensional electrophoresis of proteins: an updated protocol and implications for a functional analysis of the genome. Electrophoresis 1995; 16:1034–1059.

27. Lauber WM, Carroll JA, Dufield DR, Kiesel JR, Radabaugh MR, Malone JP. Mass spectrometry compatability of two-dimensional gel protein stains. Electrophoresis 2001; 22:906–918.

28. Berggren K, Chernokalskaya E, Steinberg TH, et al. Background-free, high sensitivity staining of proteins in one- and two-dimensional sodium dodecyl sulfate-polyacrylamide gels using a luminescent ruthenium complex. Electrophoresis 2000; 21:2509–2521.

29. Berggren KN, Chernokalskaya E, Lopez MF, Beechem JM, Patton WF. Comparison of three different fluorescent visualization strategies for detecting Escherichia coli ATP synthase subunits after sodium dodecyl sulfate-polyacrylamide gel electrophoresis. Proteomics 2001; 1:54–65.

30. Berggren KN, Schulenberg B, Lopez MF, et al. An improved formulation of SYPRO ruby protein gel stain: comparison with the original formulation and with a ruthenium II tris (bathophenanthroline disulfonate) formulation. Proteomics 2002; 2:486–498.

31. Leimgruber RM, Malone JP, Radabaugh MR, LaPorte ML, Violand BN, Monahan JB. Development of improved cell lysis, solubilization and imaging approaches for proteomic analyzes. Proteomics 2002; 2:135–144.

32. Witzman FA, Li J. Cutting-edge technology II. Proteomics: core technologies and applications in physiology. Am J Physiol Gastrointest Liver Physiol 2002; 282:G735–G741.

33. Tonge R, Shaw J, Middleton B, et al. Validation and development of fluorescence two-dimensional gel electrophoresis proteomics technology. Proteomics 2001; 1:377–396.

34. Yan JX, Devenish AT, Wait R, Stone T, Lewis S, Fowler S. Fluorescence two-dimensional difference gel electrophoresis and mass spectrometry based proteomic analysis of Escherichia coli. Proteomics 2002; 2:1682–1698.

35. Shaw J, Rowlinson R, Nickson J, et al. Evaluation of saturation labelling two-dimensional gel electrophoresis fluorescent dyes. Proteomics 2003; 3:1181–1195.

36. Banks RE, Dunn MJ, Forbes MA, et al. The potential use of laser capture microdissection to selectively obtain distinct populations of cells for proteomic analysis—preliminary findings. Electrophoresis 1999; 20:689–700.

37. Mouledous L, Hunt S, Harcourt R, Harry JL, Williams KL, Gutstein HB. Proteomic analysis of immunostained, laser-capture microdissected brain samples. Electrophoresis 2003; 24:296–302.

38. Khawaja X, Xu J, Liang JJ, Barrett JE. Proteomic analysis of protein changes developing in rat hippocampus after chronic antidepressant treatment: implications for depressive disorders and future therapies. J Neurosci Res 2004; 75:451–460.

39. Krapfenbauer K, Berger M, Lubec G, Fountoulakis M. Changes in the brain protein levels following administration of kainic acid. Electrophoresis 2001; 22:2086–2091.

40. Krapfenbauer K, Berger M, Friedlein A, Lubec G, Fountoulakis M. Changes in the levels of low-abundance brain proteins induced by kainic acid. Eur J Biochem 2001; 268:3532–3537.

41. Gu J, Lynch BA, Anderson D, et al. The antiepileptic drug levetiracetam selectively modifies kindling-induced alterations in gene expression in the temporal lobe of rats. Eur J Neurosci 2004; 19:334–345.

42. Tsuji T, Shiozaki A, Kohno R, Yoshizato K, Shimohama S. Proteomic profiling and neurodegeneration in Alzheimer's disease. Neurochem Res 2002; 27:1245–1253.

43. Sickmann A, Dormeyer W, Wortelkamp S, Woitalla D, Kuhn W, Meyer HE. Towards a high resolution separation of human cerebrospinal fluid. J Chromatogr B Analyt Technol Biomed Life Sci 2002; 771:167–196.

44. Davidsson P, Folkesson S, Christiansson M, et al. Identification of proteins in human cerebrospinal fluid using liquid-phase isoelectric focusing as a prefractionation step followed by two-dimensional gel electrophoresis and matrix-assisted laser desorption/ionisation mass spectrometry. Rapid Commun Mass Spectrom 2002; 16:2083–2088.

45. Choe LH, Green A, Knight RS, Thompson EJ, Lee KH. Apolipoprotein E and other cerebrospinal fluid proteins differentiate ante mortem variant Creutzfeldt-Jakob disease from ante mortem sporadic Creutzfeldt-Jakob disease. Electrophoresis 2002; 23:2242–2246.

46. Johnson G, Brane D, Block W, et al. Cerebrospinal fluid protein variations in common to Alzheimer's disease and schizophrenia. Appl Theor Electrophor 1992; 3:47–53.

47. Puchades M, Hansson SF, Nilsson CL, Andreasen N, Blennow K, Davidsson P. Proteomic studies of potential cerebrospinal fluid protein markers for Alzheimer's disease. Mol Brain Res 2003; 118:140–146.

48. Moseley MA. Current trends in differential expression proteomics: isotopically coded tags. Trends Biotechnol 2001; 19:S10–S16.

49. Gygi SP, Rist B, Gerber SA, Turecek F, Gelb MH, Aebersold R. Quantitative analysis of complex protein mixtures using isotope-coded affinity tags. Nat Biotechnol 1999; 17:994–999.

50. Patton WF. Detection technologies in proteome analysis. J Chromatogr B 2002; 771:3–31.

51. Sechi S, Oda Y. Quantitative proteomics using mass spectrometry. Curr Opin Chem Biol 2003; 7:70–77.

52. Yu LR, Johnson MD, Conrads TP, Smith RD, Morrison RS, Veenstra TD. Proteome analysis of camptothecin-treated cortical neurons using isotope-coded affinity tags. Electrophoresis 2002; 23:1591–1598.

53. Wolters DA, Washburn MP, Yates JR, III. An automated multidimensional protein identification technology for shotgun proteomics. Anal Chem 2001; 73:5683–5690.

54. Graves PR, Haystead TA. Molecular biologist's guide to proteomics. Microbiol Mol Biol Rev 2002; 66:39–63 table of contents.

55. Washburn MP, Ulaszek R, Deciu C, Schieltz DM, Yates JR, III. Analysis of quantitative proteomic data generated via multidimensional protein identification technology. Anal Chem 2002; 74:1650–1657.

56. Adkins JN, Varnum SM, Auberry KJ, et al. Toward a human blood serum proteome: analysis by multidimensional separation coupled with mass spectrometry. Mol Cell Proteomics 2002; 1:947–955.

57. Yoshimura Y, Yamauchi Y, Shinkawa T, et al. Molecular constituents of the postsynaptic density fraction revealed by proteomic analysis using multidimensional liquid chromatography-tandem mass spectrometry. J Neurochem 2004; 88:759–768.

58. Vinade L, Chang M, Schlief ML, et al. Affinity purification of PSD-95-containing postsynaptic complexes. J Neurochem 2003; 87:1255–1261.

59. Swatton JE, Prabakaran S, Karp NA, Lilley KS, Bahn S. Protein profiling of human postmortem brain using 2-dimensional fluorescence difference gel electrophoresis (2-D DIGE). Mol Psychiatry 2004; 9:128–143.

60. Li J, Gould TD, Yuan P, Manji HK, Chen G. Post-mortem interval effects on the phosphorylation of signaling proteins. Neuropsychopharmacology 2003; 28:1017–1025.

61. Green AJ. Cerebrospinal fluid brain-derived proteins in the diagnosis of Alzheimer's disease and Creutzfeldt-Jakob disease. Neuropathol Appl Neurobiol 2002; 28:427–440.

62. Shoji M, Matsubara E, Murakami T, et al. Cerebrospinal fluid tau in dementia disorders: a large scale multicenter study by a Japanese study group. Neurobiol Aging 2002; 23:363–370.
63. Blennow K, Vanmechelen E, Hampel H. CSF total tau, Abeta42 and phosphorylated tau protein as biomarkers for Alzheimer's disease. Mol Neurobiol 2001; 24:87–97.
64. Sunderland T, Linker G, Mirza N, et al. Decreased beta-amyloid1–42 and increased tau levels in cerebrospinal fluid of patients with Alzheimer disease. JAMA 2003; 289:2094–2103.
65. Clark CM, Xie S, Chittams J, et al. Cerebrospinal fluid tau and beta-amyloid: how well do these biomarkers reflect autopsy-confirmed dementia diagnoses? Arch Neurol 2003; 60:1696–1702.
66. Teunissen CE, Lutjohann D, von Bergmann K, et al. Combination of serum markers related to several mechanisms in Alzheimer's disease. Neurobiol Aging 2003; 24:893–902.
67. Heinonen O, Soininen H, Syrjanen S, et al. beta-Amyloid protein immunoreactivity in skin is not a reliable marker of Alzheimer's disease. An autopsy-controlled study. Arch Neurol 1994; 51:799–804.
68. Yoon IS, Li PP, Siu KP, et al. Altered TRPC7 gene expression in bipolar-I disorder. Biol Psychiatry 2001; 50:620–626.
69. Ilani T, Ben-Shachar D, Strous RD, et al. A peripheral marker for schizophrenia: increased levels of D3 dopamine receptor mRNA in blood lymphocytes. Proc Natl Acad Sci USA 2001; 98:625–628.
70. Dunn MJ. Studying heart disease using the proteomic approach. Drug Discov Today 2000; 5:76–84.
71. Jespersen S, Chaurand P, van Strien FJ, Spengler B, van der Greef J. Direct sequencing of neuropeptides in biological tissue by MALDI-PSD mass spectrometry. Anal Chem 1999; 71:660–666.
72. Liu T, Qian WJ, Strittmatter EF, et al. High-throughput comparative proteome analysis using a quantitative cysteinyl-peptide enrichment technology. Anal Chem 2004; 76:5345–5353.
73. Anderson NL, Anderson NG. The human plasma proteome: history, character, and diagnostic prospects. Mol Cell Proteomics 2002; 1:845–867.
74. Hutchens TW, Yip TT. New desoprtion strategies for the mass-spectrometric analysis of macromolecules. Rapid Commun Mass Spectrom 1993; 7:576–580.
75. Merchant M, Weinberger SJ. Recent developments in surface-enhanced laser desorption/ionisation-time of flight-mass spectrometry. Electrophoresis 2000; 21:1164–1167.
76. Issaq HJ, Veenstra TD, Conrads TP, Felschow D. The SELDI-TOF MS approach to proteomics: protein profiling and biomarker identification. Biochem Biophys Res Commun 2002; 292:587–592.
77. Heine G, Zucht HD, Schuhmann MU, et al. High-resolution peptide mapping of cerebrospinal fluid: a novel concept for diagnosis and research in central nervous system diseases. J Chromatogr B Analyt Technol Biomed Life Sci 2002; 782:353–361.
78. Goldstein LE, Muffat JA, Cherny RA, et al. Cytosolic beta-amyloid deposition and supranuclear cataracts in lenses from people with Alzheimer's disease. Lancet 2003; 361:1258–1265.

79. Petricoin EF, Ardekani AM, Hitt BA, et al. Use of proteomic patterns in serum to identify ovarian cancer. Lancet 2002; 359:572–577.
80. Wright GLJ, Cazares LH, Leung SM, et al. Proteinchip(R) surface enhanced laser desorption/ionization (SELDI) mass spectrometry: a novel protein biochip technology for detection of prostate cancer biomarkers in complex protein mixtures. Prostate Cancer Prostatic Dis 1999; 2:264–276.
81. Templin MF, Stoll D, Schrenk M, Traub PC, Vohringer CF, Joos TO. Protein microarray technology. Drug Discov Today 2002; 7:815–822.
82. Haab BB, Dunham MJ, Brown PO. Protein microarrays for highly parallel detection and quantitation of specific proteins and antibodies in complex solutions. Genome Biol 2001; 2. RESEARCH0004.
83. Schweitzer B, Roberts S, Grimwade B, et al. Multiplexed protein profiling on microarrays by rolling-circle amplification. Nat Biotechnol 2002; 20:359–365.
84. Lopez MF, Pluskal MG. Protein micro- and macroarrays: digitizing the proteome. J Chromatogr B 2003; 787:19–27.
85. Eickhoff H, Konthur Z, Lueking A, et al. Protein array technology: the tool to bridge genomics and proteomics. Adv Biochem Eng Biotechnol 2002; 77:103–112.
86. Angenendt P, Nyarsik L, Szaflarski W, et al. Cell-free protein expression and functional assay in nanowell chip format. Anal Chem 2004; 76:1844–1849.
87. Kaukola T, Satyaraj E, Patel DD, et al. Cerebral palsy is characterized by protein mediators in cord serum. Ann Neurol 2004; 55:186–194.
88. Swartzman EE, Miraglia SJ, Mellentin-Michelotti J, Evangelista L, Yuan PM. A homogeneous and multiplexed immunoassay for high-throughput screening using fluorometric microvolume assay technology. Anal Biochem 1999; 271:143–151.

6

Quantitative and Functional Magnetic Resonance Imaging Techniques

Giovanni B. Frisoni and Nicola Filippini

*Laboratory of Epidemiology Neuroimaging and Telemedicine (LENITEM),
IRCCS San Giovanni di Dio FBF—The National Center for Research
and Care of Alzheimer's Disease, Brescia, Italy*

IMAGE ACQUISITION: TECHNICAL FEATURES

Structural Magnetic Resonance Imaging

Hydrogen atoms are at the core of the physics of magnetic resonance imaging (MRI) used for clinical purposes: hydrogen nuclei are made by single protons with spinning properties that give the ability to interact with surrounding inhomogeneous magnetic fields. Each hydrogen nucleus produces its own magnetic field whose strength and direction can be represented by a vector known as magnetic dipole moment (MDM). The 1.5 Tesla scanner magnet commonly used for MRI generates a magnetic field 30,000 times greater than earth's that both orients the spin of hydrogen nuclei in the direction of the main magnetic field, and at the same time leads off the "precession" phase, that is, all hydrogen nuclei precess at the same frequency, although not at the same phase. The scanner includes a radio wave emitter that excites hydrogen nuclei by deflecting their spin along the x-y plane. The radio frequency pulse applied enables hydrogen nuclei to precess at the same phase. Hydrogen nuclei revert back to their original spin once the radio wave emission is interrupted, and give back the absorbed energy as radio waves that are picked up by an antenna. The emitted radio wave signal is then analyzed and processed.

The signal characteristics denote some of the properties of the emitting atoms. Clinical MRI makes use of the signal emitted by hydrogen atoms, which are largely represented by water molecules (99.9%) and also have a strong resonant frequency (42.577 MHz). The MRI signal gives information about proton density, i.e., water density, and two more peculiar features are used: T1 and T2 relaxation times. T1, also known as "spin-lattice," denotes the time hydrogen atoms required to revert to their initial magnetic equilibrium state before magnetization. T2, or "spin-spin," denotes the time hydrogen atoms required to revert to their original orientation (dephase). T1 and T2 amplitudes denote the difference between the MDMs of different tissue in the z-axis and in the x-y plane, respectively, and the energy exchange of hydrogen atoms with the surrounding molecules. In the water molecule, energy exchange is low and T1 and T2 are long, while in fatty tissue and in protein rich tissue the opposite is true. Relaxation times of some tissues are reported in Table 1.

Repetition and echo times (TR and TE) can be modified by the scanner operator in order to obtain greater tissue contrast based on T1 and T2: a short TR enhances T1 differences, while a long TE enhances T2 differences.

Brain imaging acquisition time is relatively slow, ranging between 10 and 30 minutes. The bone signal is weak—black—due to low proton mobility, while water—having long T1 and T2—will show black in T1-weighted and white in T2-weighted images. A number of CNS (central nervous system) diseases feature increased brain tissue water content and show as T1-hypointense and T2-hyperintense images. Gray and white matter can be sharply differentiated on T1-weighted sequences. Due to its higher water and lower lipid content, the gray matter is hypointense in T1 and hyperintense in T2 images relative to the white matter.

MRI sequences that are usually applied in clinical practice are: T1 (anatomic sequence), where the cerebrospinal fluid (CSF) is black, the gray matter is dark gray, and the white matter is light gray; T2 (so-called "myelographic" or "pathological" sequence), where the CSF is white, the gray matter is light gray, and the white matter is dark gray; fluid-attenuated inversion

Table 1   T1 and T2 Values at 1.5 T

	T1 (msec)	T2 (msec)
Heart	870	57
Liver	250	44
Kidney	560	58
Fat	260	84
Gray matter	920	101
White matter	790	92

Source: From Ref. 1.

recovery (FLAIR), similar to T2 images, but where the CSF is suppressed and set to black, to allow better lesion contrast in proximity to CSF spaces; and proton density (PD), where intensity is proportional to water content. Figure 1 shows the above sequences of a 40- and a 70-year-old healthy person.

Functional Magnetic Resonance Imaging

Functional magnetic resonance imaging (fMRI) is a tool that, by exploiting the principles of traditional MRI, allows mapping and study of brain function, i.e., "looking at the brain while it works." Effects of blood oxygen on signal decaying rate (T2*) were first reported in MRI images by Seiji Ogawa and colleagues in 1990 (2) who noted that cortical blood vessels became more visible as blood oxygen was lowered. They understood this to be due to the creation of local magnetic field inhomogeneities, and thus signal losses, from deoxyhemoglobin and termed it the Blood Oxygenation Level-Dependent (BOLD) method. Robert Turner, at the NIH, demonstrated that with ultra-fast echo-planar imaging, he was able to observe the time course of these oxygenation changes while an animal breathed an oxygen-deprived nitrogen atmosphere. Shortly thereafter, Kenneth Kwong and colleagues (3) reported seeing similar changes in humans during breath-holding. The use for fMRI of the BOLD signal is based on the assumption that cortical activation produces physiological and MRI parameter changes: increased blood flow, increased oxygen consumption, increased oxyhemoglobin, and decreased deoxyhemoglobin level, all leading to T2* changes and MRI signal detection.

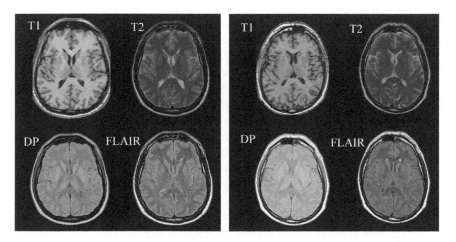

Figure 1 Axial magnetic resonance images of a 40- (*left*) and 70-year-old healthy person (*right*). The images do not show any abnormal findings. The only minimal enlargement of subarachnoid and frontal ventricular spaces of the older person should be appreciated. *Abbreviations*: FLAIR, fluid-attenuated inversion recovery; DP, proton density.

In active areas, blood flow can rise by 30–50%, while oxygen extraction increases by only 5%. This leads to both a local increase of oxyhemoglobin concentration, which has diamagnetic properties, and a reduction of deoxyhemoglobin, which has paramagnetic properties. Changes of the oxy/deoxyhemoglobin ratio in brain tissue is considered the physical-chemical basis of fMRI. Indeed Pauling and Coryell showed that the presence of paramagnetic substances in the blood could act as vascular markers acting as a natural endogenous contrast agent (4). As such, the BOLD signal is an indirect marker of brain activity as it does not evaluate brain activity but hemodynamic changes. Some believe that BOLD signal changes are generated more by synaptic than neuronal body activity (5); this implies that the region(s) apparently active during fMRI experiments can be remote from the true site of neuronal activation. Moreover, as synaptic activity can be either excitatory or inhibitory, the interpretation of fMRI results may be much less straightforward than is currently believed (6). Recently Logothetis and colleagues have analyzed the relationship between BOLD signal and local neural activity by simultaneously acquiring electrophysiological and fMRI data from monkeys (7–9), finding that the BOLD signal does reflect a local increase of neural activity (10) due to both excitatory and inhibitory interneurons (11).

Presently fMRI, based on oxygen consumption, and PET, based on glucose consumption, are the main functional techniques used to evaluate brain activity. Although positron emission tomography (PET) and fMRI have a high spatial resolution, the temporal resolution is limited due to the slower hemodynamic changes related to neuronal depolarization. This is the reason for the combined approach of PET/fMRI (high spatial resolution) with EEG/MEG (high temporal resolution). Comparative studies between fMRI and PET have shown good agreement, although important differences have also been highlighted (12–14).

Combined measurements of BOLD signal, CBF, cerebral metabolic rate of oxygen ($CMRO_2$), and oxygen extraction ratio (OER) have been performed. Feng and colleagues have shown that CBF, $CMRO_2$, and OER changes reached their maximum approximately one second earlier than the BOLD signal change (15). Non-invasive methods have been developed to improve the specificity of fMRI data; one of the most interesting approaches is the so-called arterial spin labeling (ASL) method, which allows simultaneous measurements of BOLD and CBF responses providing a direct measurement of perfusion. Disadvantages of ASL are lower signal-to-noise ratio than BOLD contrast and longer TR (16). With the ASL method, Obata and colleagues have shown discrepancies between BOLD and flow dynamics in primary and supplementary motor areas (17), while Uludag and colleagues have suggested that ASL measurements of CBF change may be a more reliable marker of neural activity than BOLD (18).

The BOLD signal is divided into three stages (Fig. 2). The "initial negative dip" (20) appears about one second after neuronal activation and consists of a mild signal intensity decrease under baseline. It is believed to be due to the sudden deoxyhaemoglobin increase, subsequent to a stimulus-driven increase in oxygen consumption, that immediately follows neuronal activation, temporarily

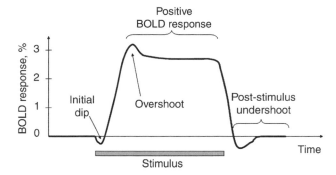

Figure 2 Schematic representation of the common features of the fMRI BOLD response to neuronal stimulation. *Source*: From Ref. 19.

uncoupled with the circulatory response. The "positive BOLD response" that follows is a marked increase of signal intensity due to increased blood flow and decreased oxy-/deoxyhemoglobin ratio. In this phase, the signal peak is reached. At the very beginning of the positive bold response a sudden increase of the BOLD signal can often be appreciated ("overshoot"), presumably due to a slow cerebral blood volume adjustment in the face of a swift increase in cerebral blood flow (21). The same principle applies to the start of the third stage ("undershoot"), where the end of the task is followed by an abrupt below threshold decrease of cerebral blood flow and a persistently high cerebral blood volume which takes longer to return back to baseline values.

In this section two experimental designs typically used in fMRI research will be briefly considered: block design and event related design. The former lasts between 20 and 30 seconds, where between six and nine seconds are needed to reach the activity peak, and between eight and 20 seconds to return to the baseline level; the latter is variable. A BOLD response based on a typical "block design" is divided into a "stimulation period" alternated with a "control period" (or "resting period").

The fMRI signal believed to be proportional to neuronal activation is the difference between signal in the active and that in the control condition. Activation maps are obtained through subtraction of the rest from the active image. Well-defined functions such as motor and sensory tasks give relatively sharp fMRI signals (22), while emotions, for example, due to slow and variable beginning and impossibility to die off quickly, are more problematic. Despite such methodological problems, some researchers have been able to successfully study complex functions such as bereavement and empathy (23,24) using a different technique that is the "event-related design." In fact, it is difficult to measure some cognitive states, like emotions, or some tasks not well temporally defined, such as those analyzed in a typical "oddball paradigm," with a block design technique (25). The event-related design is a technique to detect hemodynamic responses to brief stimuli or events (26). Individual, single trial

Table 2 Levels of Increasing Technological Sophistication of Tools to Rate Structural and Functional Imaging Findings in Patients with Cognitive Impairment

Medium	Technical requirements	Regional atrophy		Subcortical cerebrovascular disease	
		Measure	Expertise	Measure	Expertise
Visual rating	Routine acquisition	Visual rating scales: Scheltens' MTL atrophy score (14)	1–3 days	Visual rating scales: ARWMC scale (15)	1–2 weeks
		Linear measures: width of the temporal horn (16)	1–3 days		
Volumetry	3D T1 acquisition manual or semiautomatic post-processing	Volumetric measures: hippocampal and entorhinal cortex volumes (17,18)	2–4 weeks	Volumetric measures: thresholding of WMHs (19)	1 day
Computational neuroanatomy	3D T1 acquisition software for computerized post-processing serial scans	Prospective whole brain assessment: brain boundary shift integral (20)	–	None	–

Expertise denotes the training time needed to obtain accurate measurements.

Abbreviations: ARWMC scale, Age-Related White Matter Changes scale; MTL, medial temporal lobe; WMHs, white matter hyperintensities.

Source: From Ref. 28.

events are measured rather than a temporally integrated signal (27), as happens for the block design. The main advantage of the event-related design is that accidents such as habituation, anticipation, and strategy effects are greatly limited, thus enhancing the possibility to draw powerful inferences.

QUANTITATIVE MAGNETIC RESONANCE IMAGING TOOLS TO RATE REGIONAL ATROPHY AND CEREBROVASCULAR DISEASE

A number of tools of varying technological sophistication have been developed to rate the structural changes taking place in the brains of patients with cognitive impairment, ranging from simple subjective rating scales to sophisticated computerized algorithms. Which tool should be used in the clinical practice is not obvious. The aim of this section is to review those tools that the clinical neurologist might use in his/her routine clinical practice. Part of its contents have been published in a consensus document of the Neuroimaging Working Group of the European Alzheimer's Disease Consortium (EADC) (28). The EADC is an EU-funded association of 43 centers of excellence for the research and care of Alzheimer's disease and related disorders of 13 European countries (29). The tools have been categorized based on increasing levels of technological intensity and practical usability. The features assessed by the reviewed tools are the two main morphostructural issues of relevance in the clinical diagnosis of cognitive disorders, i.e., regional atrophy and subcortical cerebrovascular disease (Table 2).

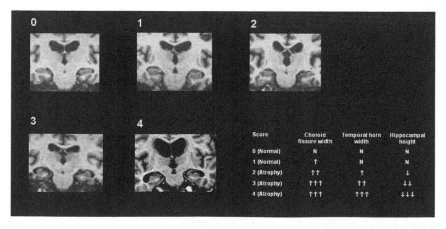

Score	Choroid fissure width	Temporal horn width	Hippocampal height
0 (Normal)	N	N	N
1 (Normal)	↑	N	N
2 (Atrophy)	↑↑	↑	↓
3 (Atrophy)	↑↑↑	↑↑	↓↓
4 (Atrophy)	↑↑↑	↑↑↑	↓↓↓

Figure 3 Magnetic resonance–based visual rating of medial temporal lobe atrophy. Score: 0 (absent), 1 (minimal), 2 (mild), 3 (moderate), and 4 (severe). The small table in the lower right corner of the figure reports the criteria for score assignment.

Visual Rating

Regional Atrophy: Visual Rating Scales

MRI can directly visualise the hippocampus and other critical medial temporal lobe (MTL) structures in substantial cytoarchitectonic detail. Scheltens and colleagues (30) have developed a subjective visual rating scale to assess MTL atrophy on plain MRI films (the subjective MTL atrophy score). T1 weighted sequences are used and six coronal slices (slice thickness of 5 mm) parallel to the brainstem axis are acquired from a midsagittal scout image, the first image being acquired directly adjacent to the brainstem. The score is assigned based on visual rating of the width of the choroid fissure, width of the temporal horn, and height of the hippocampal formation (Fig. 3). In 41 patients with AD and 66 non-demented controls, the subjective MTL atrophy score showed a correct classification of 96%, comparing favourably with volumetry (93%) (31). In a prospective study of 31 patients with minor cognitive impairment, the subjective MTL atrophy score improved the predictive accuracy of age and delayed recall score for AD at follow-up (32).

Subcortical Cerebrovascular Disease: Visual Rating Scales

The European Task Force on Age-Related White Matter Changes (33) has developed the Age-Related White Matter Changes (ARWMC) scale (34). This is a 4-point scale which rates white matter changes separately in five areas: frontal, parieto-occipital, temporal, infratentorial/cerebellum, and "basal ganglia" (striatum, globus pallidus, thalamus, internal/external capsule, and insula). The first three areas are scored as (0) no lesions (including symmetrical, well-defined caps or bands), (1) focal lesions, (2) beginning confluence of lesions, or (3) diffuse involvement of the entire region, with or without involvement of U fibers.

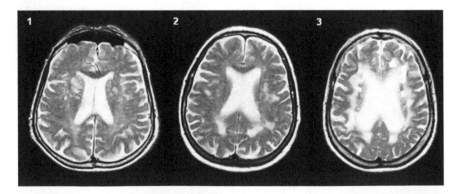

Figure 4   Visual rating scales for subcortical cerebrovascular disease: the Age-Related White Matter Changes (ARWMC) scale. Grade 1, focal lesions; grade 2, early beginning confluent lesions; and grade 3, confluent lesions with diffuse involvement of a lobe. *Source*: From Ref. 34.

The infratentorial/cerebellum and basal ganglia are scored as (0) no lesions, (1) only one focal lesion (>5 mm), (2) more than one focal lesion, or (3) confluent lesions. The final result of the rating are five separate scores to grade subcortical cerebrovascular disease in the different brain regions in each hemisphere (Fig. 4). The interrater reliability was found to be moderate (k=0.48). Figure 4 provides instances of three patients of increasing severity.

One should not forget to detect lacunes, which can be recognized on MRI scans as round areas with regular contours, usually larger than 5 mm, located more often in the basal ganglia, and featuring hyperintensity in T2 and protonic density and hypointensity in T1 sequences.

Volumetry

Regional Atrophy: Volumetric Measures

A T1-weighted 3D-technique is employed for MRI image acquisition magnetization prepared rapid acquisition gradient recalled echo or spoiled gradient (MP-RAGE or SPGR). After acquisition, the digital images need to be reconstructed on coronal, 1–2 mm-thick slices. The hippocampus is then manually traced on all the contiguous slices where it can be appreciated (Fig. 5). In expert hands, the reliability is high, intraclass correlation coefficients for hippocampal measurements being 0.95 for intrarater and 0.90 for interrater variability (35).

Subcortical Cerebrovascular Disease: Thresholding of White Matter Hyperintensities

Quantification of the volume of white matter hyperintensities (WMHs) based on MRI can provide an objective measure of the severity of subcortical

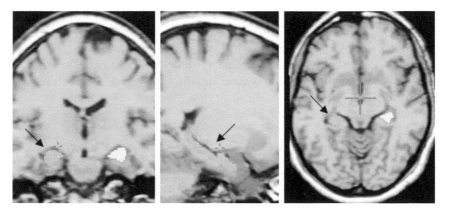

Figure 5 Regional atrophy assessment: hippocampal volumetry. Instance of manual tracing of the right hippocampus (*black arrow*) with simultaneous view of the traced region of interest in the coronal, sagittal, and axial planes.

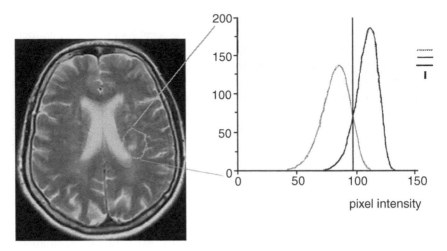

Figure 6 Volumetry through thresholding of white matter hyperintensities as marker of subcortical cerebrovascular disease. Automatic segmentation comprises histogram representation of the pixel intensity distribution, Gaussian modeling of the pixel distribution separately for normal and hyperintense white matter, and identification of the optimal intensity cutoff to separate normal from hyperintense white matter pixels.

cerebrovascular disease. A number of semi-automated methods have been developed, most based on the notion that pixels of normal white matter can be accurately separated from those of hyperintense white matter. A conventional spin-echo, double-echo T2, or FLAIR sequence in the axial orientation is used for MRI acquisition. Digital information is generally transferred for processing and analysis to a separate workstation. Measuring involves manual tracing followed by automatic thresholding. Manual tracing is carried out of a crudely defined region of interest (ROI) within the white matter that completely includes all the hyperintense white matter (Fig. 6).

Intrarater and interrater reliabilities of this method are good (36). WMH volume has been found to be correlated with other features believed to be indicative of subcortical cerebrovascular disease (parkinsonism and depression) and predictive of cognitive impairment in a group of 369 cognitively intact community-dwelling older men (37).

Computational Neuroanatomy

Recently, advances in neuroscience and neuroimaging have led to an increasing recognition that certain neuroanatomical structures may be affected preferentially by particular diseases. Neurodegenerative brain diseases mark the brain with a morphological "signature"; detecting this may be useful to enhance diagnosis, particularly in diseases lacking in other diagnostic tools. Moreover, structural changes provide markers to track the biological progression of disease. In 1993, despite a lack of support from clinical variables, interferon beta was approved by the Food and Drug Administration based on data from MRI (38).

Recent developments in computer science may help detect early sensitive and specific disease signatures. The new approaches are automated, avoiding error-prone and labour-intensive manual measurements. Second, such algorithms can offer unprecedented precision as some can detect brain volume differences of 0.5% between images from the same subject (39).

The effort to develop such algorithms has been referred to as computational neuroanatomy (40).

The individual algorithms can be categorized into two broad classes: algorithms devised to detect group differences at one point in time and algorithms devised to detect prospective changes over time. The first category may be useful to define disease-specific signatures. The second can be applied to one or more individuals to track natural disease progression or as modified by treatment. While most tools have been developed to compare groups, some are being adapted to analyze individual cases, an issue of the greatest interest for the practicing physician.

Computational anatomy algorithms generally involve some or all of the following steps: (1) brain extraction (brain is separated from non-brain voxels), (2) tissue segmentation (voxels representing gray and white matter and cerebro-spinal fluid are separated based on intensity values), (3) spatial normalization (also called registration; the voxels of interest are matched to a template or an earlier scan from the same individual), and (4) statistical comparison of different subject groups or points in time. The pivotal step of all methods is registration. Here, cross-sectional methods match images of interest to a reference stereotactic template (a typical brain or a typical hippocampus, etc.) or vice versa, while prospective methods match sequential images of the same patients taken at different times.

Registration strategies differ in scope (i.e., analysis of the whole brain or preselected regions-of-interest) and mathematical approach (accounting for global or local variability of the brain's size and shape). Some cross-sectional methods that account for global variability are completely automated (such as voxel-based morphometry based on statistical parametric mapping by Ashburner and Friston; see Chapter 7) (41), while those that account for local variability often require manually positioned landmarks to precisely match the image to the template (such as cortical pattern matching) (42). Longitudinal methods use the complexity of each individual's brain structure to align accurately an individual's serial images [such as the brain-boundary shift integral (BBSI) algorithm] (43).

To perform well, all methods need high spatial resolution and clear differentiation between tissue types. Usually, 3D high-resolution T1-weighted MR images [spoiled gradient (SPGR) or magnetization prepared rapid acquisition gradient recalled echo (MP-RAGE)] acquired with conventional 1.5T MR scanners and 1 mm^3 voxels (ideally isotropic) across the cranium provide sufficient detail and contrast.

Cross-Sectional Atrophy Assessment

Voxel-based morphometry: Ashburner & Friston's method (41) requires that registered gray matter images are smoothed with an 8–12 mm filter. This leads to normally distributed data and allows the use of statistical parametric tools. The statistical approach of the A&F method (SPM) is based on the general linear model, and identifies regions of tissue with increased or decreased density or concentration that are significantly related to the effects under study. Ideally, the threshold for significance should be set at $p < 0.05$ corrected for multiple comparisons, but when there is a prior hypothesis of the expected effect a more liberal threshold of $p < 0.001$ uncorrected has also been applied. However, like every statistical test, the larger the effect size and group size, the higher the sensitivity of the method for identifying differences.

A protocol to carry out voxel-based morphometry based on SPM in patients with neurodegenerative disorders has been developed ("optimized VBM") which requires images to be registered onto a "customized template," i.e., an average image of the cases under study (44). The optimized protocol includes (1) generation of customized template, (2) generation of customized prior probability maps, and (3) main VBM steps: normalization of the original MRI images, segmentation of normalized images, cleaning of gray matter images, modulation of gray matter images, and smoothing of modulated images. Customized prior probability maps are computed by generating a customized gray matter template through segmenting the original images into gray matter, white matter, and cerebrospinal fluid, cleaning the GM, normalizing the cleaned GM images to the

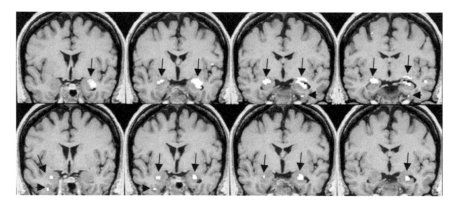

Figure 7 Gray matter changes in Alzheimer's disease assessed with Ashburner and Friston's voxel-based morphometry. Black arrows indicate voxels of decreased gray matter density ($p < .0001$ uncorrected for multiple comparisons) in the amygdalar/hippocampal complex and temporal cortex in 29 mild to moderate (*upper row*, mean MMSE 21 G4) and three very mild (*lower row*, MMSE 26 and 27) AD subjects compared with 26 nondemented controls. *Source*: From Ref. 45.

customized GM template to determine the normalization parameters, smoothing the cleaned images, applying the normalization parameters to the smoothed images, and averaging.

With voxel-based morphometry, hippocampal atrophy has been visualized in Alzheimer's disease (Fig. 7) as well as reduced volume in the posterior cingulate gyrus and adjacent precuneus, and the temporoparietal association cortex (45). In a small group of three very mild AD patients with Mini Mental State Examination (MMSE) scores of 26 and 27, atrophy has been shown to affect the amygdalar/hippocampal complex bilaterally, indicating that the technique is sensitive also in small groups and in the earliest stages of the disease (Fig. 7).

Cortical pattern matching: This is a sensitive approach that measures the topologic variability of the cortex (46–49). The approach consists of cortical flattening and sulcal matching that aims to obtain an average cortical model for a group of subjects. All MRI scans are first aligned to a standardized 3D coordinate space. From each individual's MRI scan, a 3D cortical surface model is extracted, consisting of a network of discrete triangular tiles, and some sulcal/gyral landmarks are identified on the cortical model, which is then flattened. Then, sulcal features are co-registered to a template of sulcal curves, derived from a large group of normal subjects, with a warping technique. The warped images are averaged, and measures of gray matter density can be analyzed with statistical tools similar to those used by A&F's voxel-based morphometry. This technique can be executed on high-end desktop machines such as the Macintosh G4, as well as Silicon Graphics Interface or Sun workstations running UNIX. These algorithms are often used in client-server mode, connecting to a supercomputer for very large-scale analyzes (50).

Cortical pattern matching allows mapping of changes in cortical gray matter density or thickness with great accuracy. Figure 8 shows the atrophic changes found in a group of 26 mild to moderate AD patients (51).

Prospective Atrophy Assessment: Whole Brain Assessment with the Brain Boundary Shift Integral

Serial scans within the same subject have the advantage that the wide inter-individual variability of brain morphology is not an issue, and comparing pre-post images of the same subject(s) carries much less error than comparing a case to controls. Information on prospective global changes can be obtained by rigidly matching serial scans and subtracting the superimposed images. The difference reflects the volume of brain tissue lost or gained [e.g., BBSI (43)]. The rate of atrophy in a group of 18 AD patients was significantly greater than in 31 controls (Fig. 8: 2.78% vs. 0.24% per year with no overlap between the groups) (39). Moreover, the rate of global cerebral volume loss was strongly correlated with rate of cognitive change measured with the MMSE in 29 AD patients (52).

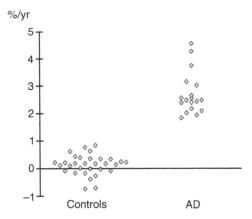

Figure 8 Rate of global brain atrophy computed with the BBSI method in 18 Alzheimer's disease patients and 31 controls. Tissue loss was 2.78% in patients and 0.24% per year in controls. Note the lack of overlap between the groups. *Source*: From Ref. 39.

Information on local changes can be obtained by using non-linear registration, which permits compression or expansion of each voxel to obtain a precise registration (voxel compression method). The resulting deformation fields provide a map [voxel compression map (VCM)] of the amount of compression or expansion applied at each voxel. This reflects the amount of brain tissue or CSF lost or gained over time in the interval between scans. Typical patterns of change in different conditions (for example, normal aging vs. Alzheimer's disease) can be tapped by registering and averaging individual VCMs and comparing the resulting averages. The method allowed the detection of loss of brain tissue in asymptomatic individuals carrying an autosomal dominant mutation known to cause AD more than two years before the appearance of symptoms (53,54).

The BBSI technique might be particularly useful in detecting disease in asymptomatic subjects at high risk of developing AD. Prospective measurements of brain atrophy have become a very relevant issue with the advent of drugs that might alter the natural history of AD by slowing its progression. Rates of brain atrophy measured from serial registered MRI are being used as a surrogate outcome of drug effectiveness in clinical trials.

QUANTITATIVE MAGNETIC RESONANCE IMAGING FOR THE CLINICAL DIAGNOSIS

The traditional approach for imaging in the diagnostic pathway of dementia holds that structural imaging [computed tomography (CT) or MRI] is useful to exclude potentially treatable intracranial causes of cognitive deterioration (the so called pseudodementias). While the increasing expertise of professionals has led to a decrease in the prevalence of pseudodementias—such that reversible causes of cognitive impairment are recognized before the "dementia" label is attached to the patient (55)—current guidelines still advise at least one structural imaging exam during the course of any dementing disorder (56). The justification of this approach is that no clinical rule can identify 100% of cases with potentially treatable intracranial causes (57).

The enhanced anatomical detail allowed by recent MRI scanners has permitted the delineation of atrophic patterns for different forms of dementia. This has led to a shift from the use of imaging as an exclusion exam to an inclusionary approach (58). Such an approach is informative in a much larger proportion of cases than the negative approach. However, it should be highlighted that in the diagnostic workup of patients with dementia, imaging exams fall in a path where they have been preceded by history taking, physical, and neurological examination, neuropsychological screening, laboratory exams, and often detailed neuropsychological testing, such that at the time when imaging is acquired the physician has already collected information that may have provided more or less strong diagnostic clues. Thus, the clinically pregnant question is: what is the diagnostic added value of imaging?

Scheltens and colleagues (58) have computed that the weighted (corrected for number of people in the study) sensitivity and specificity for detection of mild to moderate Alzheimer's disease using visual assessment of medial temporal lobe

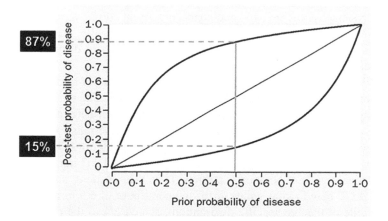

Figure 9 Post-test probability of Alzheimer's disease with visual assessment of medial temporal atrophy (sensitivity 85% and specificity 88%) for any given pre-test probability. The upper curve shows the incremental diagnostic gain from a positive result (i.e., presence of atrophy) and the lower curve shows that from a negative result (i.e., absence of atrophy). In the case of a pre-test probability of Alzheimer's disease of 0.50 (the same as tossing a coin), a positive result adds 0.27 to give a post-test probability of 0.87 and a negative result lowers the post-test probability to 0.15. *Source*: From Ref. 58.

atrophy compared with controls can be calculated as 85% and 88%. The practical implications of the results are given in Fig. 9, showing the incremental diagnostic gain of a positive and negative visual assessment of medial temporal lobe atrophy at any given pre-test chance (before taking MRI). For instance, in the case of a pre-test probability of Alzheimer's disease in a clinical setting of 0.50 (the same as tossing a coin), a positive result adds 0.27 to give a post-test probability of 0.87 and a negative result lowers the post-test probability to 0.15.

Obviously, the higher the pre-test probability of Alzheimer's disease, the smaller the incremental gain obtained through neuroimaging exams. It should be noted that to date naturalistic studies assessing the incremental value of imaging exams—as well as studies assessing the incremental diagnostic value of any other test used for the differential diagnosis of the dementias—are lacking. Thus, strictly speaking, the inclusionary approach of imaging is poorly supported by evidence. However, this fate is unfortunately shared by most radiologic and non-radiologic diagnostic exams currently used in clinical medicine (59).

The Dementias

Alzheimer's Disease

The preceding sections have already clearly outlined what structural MRI can show in patients with Alzheimer's disease, i.e., atrophy of medial temporal structures (hippocampus, entorhinal cortex, and amygdala), of the parietotemporal region, and posterior cingulate. With ordinary analysis tools, i.e., the MRI film and the physician's own eyeballs and connected visual cortex, atrophy can more easily be appreciated in medial temporal structures, while that in the parietotemporal and posterior cingulate cortex is more difficult to discriminate from age-associated changes.

Figure 10 shows how regional atrophy can be studied in a patient with AD using assessment tools of increasing technological complexity. The anatomy of the medial temporal lobe is such that hippocampal atrophy can be appreciated even with CT. A CT-based marker of hippocampal atrophy (the radial width of the temporal horn) has been shown to be sensitive and specific to AD in both clinical and pathological series (60,61). Values greater than 5.3 mm denote clinically significant medial temporal atrophy (45). The patient shown in Figure 10 had a CT-based radial width of the temporal horn of 6.9 mm (above the 99th percentile of the age-specific distribution), scored 2/4 to the right and 3/4 to the left on the MRI-based visual rating scale for medial temporal atrophy (normal values 0 and 1), had the smallest (between right and left) hippocampal volume of 91.5 (below the 2nd percentile of the age-specific distribution), and a single-case analysis with voxel-based morphometry (age-adjusted at $p < .05$ uncorrected vs. 173 nondemented controls between 40 and 80 years of age) showed regional gray matter loss bilaterally in the medial temporal and posterior cingulate-precuneus regions.

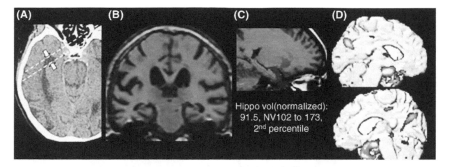

Hippo vol(normalized):
91.5, NV102 to 173,
2nd percentile

Figure 10 Regional atrophy in a 74-year-old patient with mild Alzheimer's disease (MMSE = 23/30) studied using assessment tools of increasing technological complexity. (**A**) Computed tomography (CT)–based radial width of the temporal horn: 6.9 mm, above the 99th percentile of the age-specific distribution; (**B**) conventional magnetic resonance imaging (MRI)–based visual rating scale for medial temporal atrophy: 3/4 to the right and left, normal values 0 and 1; (**C**) digital MRI–based hippocampal volumetry: smallest (between right and left) normalized hippocampal volume of 91.5 (below the 2nd percentile of the age-specific distribution); (**D**) digital MRI-based single-case voxel-based morphometry: regional gray matter loss bilaterally in the medial temporal and posterior cingulate-precuneus regions.

In a relatively large series of 55 AD patients and 42 controls, hippocampal volumetry has shown a classification sensitivity and specificity of 94% and 90%, respectively (62). Small hippocampal volume has been found to be predictive of subsequent conversion to AD in 80 patients with amnestic mild cognitive impairment (MCI) independently of neuropsychological tests, Apolipoprotein E genotype, and cerebrovascular comorbidity (63). Of the 13 MCI patients with hippocampal volume 2.5 SDs below the age-specific mean, six (46%) converted to AD within the following six years, while of the 54 with hippocampal volume between 2.5 SDs and the age-specific mean, converters were 19 (35%), and of the 13 with hippocampal volume above the mean, only two (15%) converted (63).

Frontotemporal Lobar Degeneration

This is a syndrome including—according to recent clinical criteria (64)—frontal dementia, progressive aphasia, and semantic dementia. The frontal variant of frontotemporal lobar degeneration (FTLD) is mainly characterized by marked alterations of behavior and personality and by attention and executive function impairment (65), while semantic dementia is characterized by progressive deterioration of semantic memory with relative sparing of other cognitive functions (66), and progressive aphasia is a slowly progressive impairment of speech production (67). The most frequent etiology is nonspecific cortical degeneration, i.e., neuronal loss associated with gliosis of the superficial cortical layers in the frontal and temporal lobes ["dementia lacking distinctive histology" described by

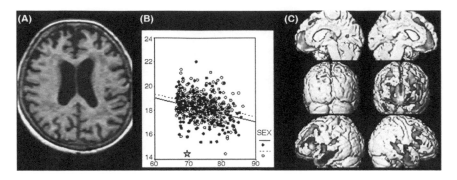

Figure 11 Frontal atrophy in a 69-year-old patient with frontotemporal lobar degeneration—frontal dementia type of mild severity (MMSE 21/30, clinical dementia rating 1) studied using assessment tools of increasing technological sophistication. (**A**) Conventional magnetic resonance imaging (MRI)–based visual assessment: mild to moderate enlargement of cortical sulci in the anterior frontal and temporal regions; (**B**) digital MRI-based lobar volumetry: normalized frontal gray matter volumes of 142 (below the 99th percentile of the age- and gender-specific distribution—open and filled dots denote women and men); (**C**) digital MRI-based single-case voxel-based morphometry: regional gray matter loss in anterior frontal and temporal regions (anterior cingulate, orbitomesial, dorsolateral frontal, and temporopolar areas).

Knopman and colleagues (68)]. Visual assessment of traditional structural imaging allows the rater to appreciate mild to moderate enlargement of cortical sulci in the anterior frontal and temporal regions (Fig. 11). This can be substantiated with a digital analysis of frontal lobar gray matter volumes, showing marked tissue loss on both sides, more marked to the left (Fig. 11). FDG PET also showed typical and distinctive patterns of glucose metabolism in FTD (69,70).

Recently Miller and colleagues have suggested a different pattern of brain atrophy to distinguish the FTLD variants (frontal dementia, progressive aphasia, and semantic dementia) based on voxel-based morphometry analysis. Frontal and semantic dementias seemed to be mainly characterized by common regions of atrophy located in the ventromedial frontal cortex, the posterior orbital frontal regions bilaterally, the insula, and the left anterior cingulate cortex. Specific regions of atrophy in frontal but not semantic dementia affected the right dorsolateral frontal cortex and the left premotor cortex, while semantic dementia patients showed atrophy in the anterior temporal cortex and the amygdala/anterior hippocampal region bilaterally (71). In the progressive aphasia group voxel-based morphometry showed a predominance of frontal atrophy (67), and reduced gray matter in the left superior temporal and inferior parietal regions (71).

Dementia with Lewy Bodies

The Newcastle group has investigated the accuracy of visual assessment of medial temporal lobe atrophy in the differential diagnosis between dementia with Lewy bodies and AD (72). Barber and colleagues (72) have shown that clinically significant atrophy affected 100% of AD, 62% of Lewy body dementia patients, and 4% of controls. Thus, the absence of medial temporal atrophy had 100% specificity for dementia with Lewy bodies versus AD, while the presence of atrophy had a sensitivity of only 38% versus controls. These data indicate that in patients where the differential diagnosis lies between dementia with Lewy bodies and AD, the absence of atrophy is strongly suggestive of the former. Unfortunately, this happens in a minority (less than half) of Lewy body dementia patients.

Structural and functional imaging has allowed the elucidation of the pathophysiology of visual hallucinations in dementia with Lewy bodies. Burton and colleagues (73) have shown that hallucinations in dementia with Lewy bodies are not due to occipital atrophy: unexpectedly, the occipital lobe volume of Lewy body dementia patients with hallucinations is greater than that of patients without hallucinations, and this holds true also in AD. Notably, despite structural integrity, functional imaging techniques (see Chapters 7 and 8) have shown marked occipital hypofunction in Lewy body dementia patients (74).

Other Forms of Dementia with Parkinsonism

The sections on AD, frontotemporal degeneration, and dementia with Lewy bodies have suggested that profiles of atrophy in multiple cerebral regions can be used to differentiate the degenerative dementias and that atrophy in a single region is generally poorly informative.

Atrophy in a single region is poorly informative in the case of dementia in Parkinson's disease, (75–77) where hippocampal atrophy has been shown to be of a degree similar to that found in AD and is therefore of no use in discriminating between the two conditions (35).

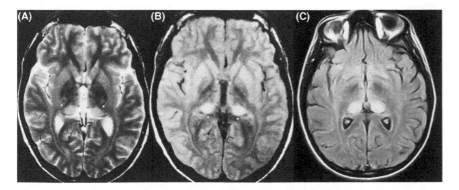

Figure 12 The "pulvinar sign" in a patient with the new variant of Creutzfeldt–Jakob disease. (**A**) T2-weighted, (**B**) proton density-weighted, and (**C**) FLAIR magnetic resonance scans. *Source*: From Refs. 80, 82.

Creutzfeldt–Jakob Disease

About 7 in 10 patients with sporadic Creutzfeldt–Jakob disease show hyperintense lesions in the caudate and putamen and mild thalamic hyperintensities on T2-weighted images (78,79). The low sensitivity and specificity of these findings make them of little use in differential diagnosis. However, the new variant of Creutzfeldt–Jakob disease (due to bovine transmission) shows mild caudate and putaminal findings and marked thalamic hyperintensities. These are located at the level of the pulvinar nucleus ("pulvinar sign") and represent a moderately sensitive (80%) but highly specific (100%) marker (Fig. 12) (80,81). The sign can be appreciated particularly well with FLAIR sequences (82). The pulvinar sign has been included in a suggestion for clinical criteria for the diagnosis of the disease (81) and appears to be the diagnostically most useful instrumental sign in that the EEG is often nonspecific and 14-3-3 protein CSF levels have low sensitivity (81).

Vascular Dementia

The clinical diagnosis of vascular dementia is a thorny issue for the lack of a pathological standard. Consequently, although structural imaging is key to directly appreciate the vascular lesions, its role and usefulness are still hotly debated.

NINDS-AIREN criteria (83) allow four forms of vascular dementia: (1) multiple infarcts due to embolism or large vessel disease, (2) strategic infarcts (due to embolism, large or small vessel disease), (3) multiple lacunes in the basal

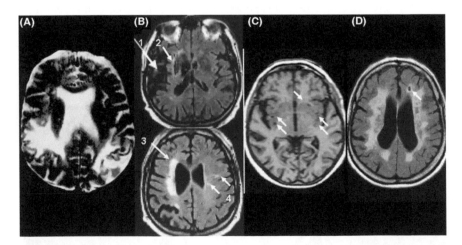

Figure 13 Vascular dementia due to (**A**) multiple infarcts due to large vessel disease but no small vessel disease; (**B**) multiple infarcts (1: temporal, 2: striatal) associated with small vessel disease (3: watershed, 4: white matter lesions of the periventricular and deep subcortical white matter); (**C**) multiple lacunes in the basal ganglia; and (**D**) extensive lesions of the periventricular white matter associated with one deep frontal lacune in the white matter.

ganglia and white matter (generally due to small vessel disease), and (4) extensive lesions of the periventricular white matter (due to small vessel disease). Figure 13 shows cases of vascular dementia with multiple infarcts due to large vessel disease but no small vessel disease, multiple infarcts associated with small vessel disease, and extensive lesions of the periventricular white matter.

While the number, volume, and site necessary for multiple infarcts to give vascular dementia is undetermined, strategic infarcts associated with dementia (or—better—cognitive impairment in multiple domains) have been described in the left angular gyrus, mono- or bilaterally in the thalamus, and bilaterally in the globus pallidus (Fig. 14).

The diagnosis of vascular dementia due to extensive lesions of the periventricular white matter and its differentiation from AD is particularly difficult, although it is clinically relevant due to the poorer prognosis of the former (85). Specific diagnostic criteria for subcortical vascular dementia have been developed where imaging plays a major role, but these await validation (86). Fazekas and colleagues (87,88) have shown that small punctate lesions of the white matter (<5 mm, round, and with regular margins), when not associated with confluent lesions, may not be due to vascular changes (87) and do not progress over time (88). On the contrary, larger (>5 mm) lesions with irregular margins (so called "confluent" as they appear to originate from the confluence of smaller lesions) are due to vascular changes and progress over time (Fig. 15) (88).

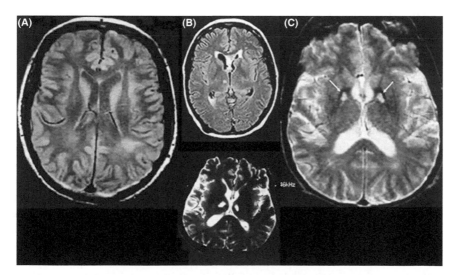

Figure 14 Vascular dementia following strategic lesion. (**A**) Subcortical lesion in the left angular gyrus (proton density-weighted image). (**B**) Unilateral (*upper*, FLAIR image) and bilateral (*lower*, T2-weighted image) lesions following occlusion of the thalamic paramedian artery. (**C**) Bilateral infarcts in the *globus pallidus* (T2 weighted image). *Source*: From Ref. 84.

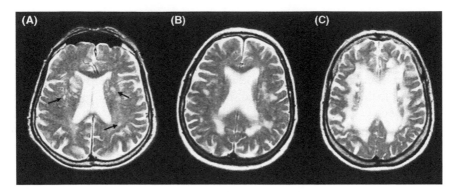

Figure 15 Increasing severity of white matter hyperintensities on T2-weighted magnetic resonance images. (A) Small punctate lesions of the white matter (<5 mm, round, and with regular margins—*arrows*) when not associated with confluent lesions may not be due to vascular changes and do not progress over time. On the contrary, larger (>5 mm) lesions with irregular margins (early and late confluent—**B** and **C**) are due to vascular changes and progress over time. *Source*: From Ref. 88.

Structural Imaging in Mild Cognitive Impairment

The concept of MCI is aimed at detecting patients in the transition from normality to Alzheimer's dementia. The contribution of structural imaging to the diagnosis of MCI should be placed into the more general context of the search for the signature of AD with instrumental exams.

MCI patients have a higher incidence of dementia than cognitively intact persons of similar age (between 6% and 25% vs. 0.2–2.3% per year) (89). Pathological and epidemiological evidence indicate that the vast majority of MCI patients developing dementia have AD, but a relevant proportion of MCI patients (as high as 60%) (90) remain stable and never go on to develop dementia (91). The practical consequence of these observations is that the diagnosis of MCI is clinically unhelpful in certain circumstances, as many MCI patients have Alzheimer's disease but many do not. Pathological and clinical data indicate that some biological indicators of Alzheimer's disease (the neurobiological "signature" or "fingerprint," including imaging indicators) might be used to distinguish those MCI patients who will progress (i.e., those who already have Alzheimer's) from those who will not (i.e., those who do not have Alzheimer's). Biological indicators are hippocampal atrophy (due to early plaque and tangle deposition in the medial temporal lobe), high concentrations of tau protein in the CSF (due to neuronal/axonal damage following neurofibrillary tangle deposition), and functional defects in the temporoparietal and posterior cingulate cortex (due to deafferentation from medial temporal damage) (see Chapter 8). Indeed, when compared to non-progressors, MCI patients who will progress to dementia feature lower hippocampal volume measured through high-resolution structural

MRI, (63,92) high levels of tau protein in the CSF, and perfusion and metabolic defects [PET and single photon emission computed tomography (SPECT)] (93–96).

Jack et al. have tested the hypothesis that MRI-based measurements of hippocampal volume are related to the risk of future conversion to Alzheimer's disease in older patients with MCI (63). Eighty consecutive patients who met criteria for the diagnosis of MCI were recruited from the Mayo Clinic Alzheimer's Disease Center/Alzheimer's Disease Patient Registry. At entry enrolled subjects underwent an MRI examination, in order to obtain volumes of both hippocampi, and for a period of time were also followed longitudinally, on average 32.6 months, with approximately annual clinical/cognitive assessments. During the period of observation 27 of the 80 MCI patients became demented, and hippocampal atrophy at baseline was associated with crossover from MCI to AD. The conclusions of Jack and colleagues were that MCI patients who will progress to dementia feature lower hippocampal volume as measured through high-resolution structural MRI.

Whether imaging or non-imaging markers are more promising for future use in a routine clinical setting is still unknown. The accuracy of single markers varies between 40% and 100%, (63,92–94,97,98) but studies are poorly comparable for the doubtful reliability of current criteria when used in different memory clinics, the heterogeneity of MCI patients enrolled, and the small study groups.

Voxel-based morphometry analysis in MCI has shown a significant agreement in showing that patients had highly significant gray matter loss predominantly affecting the medial temporal lobe, the hippocampal regions, the thalamus, the cingulate gyrus, and extending also into the temporal neocortex (99–102).

A few studies have tried to include use of more than one Alzheimer's disease biomarker to discriminate MCI progressors from non-progressors. Okamura and colleagues (103) studied 30 MCI patients, 22 of whom did and eight who did not progress to cognitive impairment in the following three years, and found that a high ratio between tau in the CSF and posterior cingulate perfusion on SPECT could identify progressors with sensitivity of 89% and specificity of 90%. El Fakhri and colleagues (104) studied 17 healthy controls, 56 non-demented patients with memory problems who did not develop AD during three to five years of follow-up, and 27 nondemented patients with memory problems who developed AD during follow-up. Combining information coming from SPECT and structural MRI at baseline allowed the correct classification of 94% of patients. If these early findings can be replicated in larger and methodologically rigorous studies, the possibility to diagnose Alzheimer's disease before dementia has developed might become a reality using functional and structural tools.

MICROSTRUCTURAL IMAGING: DIFFUSION AND MAGNETIZATION TRANSFER IMAGING

In AD, the detection of gray matter loss in T1-weighted images has allowed a better understanding of the biological basis of the clinical signs and symptoms, an ability to monitor disease progression, and an assessment of the effect of the disease-modifying drugs presently under study. However, gray matter loss on T1-weighted images has limited ability to capture the whole range of morphostructural changes associated with the neurodegeneration of AD. First, tissue shrinkage on T1-weighted images cannot discriminate neuronal from glial and axonal loss as well as neuronal loss from age-associated shrinkage of healthy neurons. Second, T1-weighted images cannot appreciate the white matter damage that might arise in AD from neurofilament tau pathology. Techniques to probe into the finer structure of the brain have recently been developed such as diffusion tensor and magnetization transfer imaging that are providing increasingly valuable information in elucidating the pathophysiology of AD.

Diffusion tensor imaging is based on the physical properties of moving water protons. Motion is higher where protons have no constraints (e.g., in the CSF) and lower where protons are confined within organized tissues such as the intracellular matrix or the axonal cytoplasm. MRI can detect and quantify such motion through the apparent diffusion coefficient (ADC) (Table 3). In the white matter, not only is the ADC lower than in the CSF, but proton motion is highly oriented in the direction of the axonal fiber (i.e., anisotropic), and the direction of the motion can be quantified through the fractional anisotropy index (FA). Axonal loss and demyelination due to Wallerian degeneration are picked up as increased ADC and decreased FA. Gliosis of the white matter, by disrupting the

Table 3 Techniques to Probe into the Brain Microstructure with Magnetic Resonance Imaging

	Physical phenomenon	Measure	Indicative of	Affected by
Diffusion	Mean diffusivity of water	Apparent diffusion coefficient	Axonal density	Cell and axonal density, glial reaction, water content, neurofilament pathology
Diffusion tensor	Mean diffusivity of water in the 3 planes	Fractional anisotropy	Axonal density and coherence in a given plane	Same as above
Magnetization transfer	Transfer of magnetization between large macromolecules and water protons	Magnetization transfer ratio	Integrity of protein matrices and cell membranes	Density of macromolecules

Source: From Ref. 28.

normal axonal structure, also gives rise to decreased FA, but the ADC is normal or decreased due to the boundaries to proton motion represented by glial cell membranes (Table 3). Neurofilament and tau pathology is associated with normal ADC and FA, cell membranes being intact.

Magnetization transfer imaging is based on the exchange of magnetization between free and macromolecule bound protons and allows one to indirectly observe semisolids, such as protein matrices and cell membranes (Table 3). Changes in tissue structural integrity such as gliosis lead to decreased bound and increased free protons which show as decreased magnetization transfer ratio (Table 3).

There are grounds to believe that microstructural pathology exceeding the macrostructural changes can be appreciated through T1-weighted images present in AD, and this is strongly correlated with cognitive performance. Of the two pathological hallmarks of the disease, senile plaques and neurofibrillary tangles, the latter involves the cytoskeleton and neurobiological studies have shown that it affects axonal transport (105). Moreover, pathological studies have shown that neurofibrillary tangle density is more closely related to cognitive performance than senile plaques (106). Structural T1-weighted MRI studies have shown that the correlation between regional atrophy and global cognitive impairment is relatively weak (107).

When structural changes are assessed with magnetization transfer and diffusion imaging, a stronger correlation emerges (107). Bozzali and colleagues have studied 18 AD patients with MMSE between 5 and 25 and 16 elderly controls and found that the Pearson's r correlations with the MMSE were 0.21 for global brain volume, 0.31 for global diffusivity of the gray matter, and 0.58 for a magnetization transfer index of the gray matter. A composite score compounding information on atrophy and magnetization transfer reached $r = 0.65$, indicating that 42% of the MMSE variance was accounted for by these two markers (108). Hanyu and colleagues have studied 35 AD patients with MMSE between 9 and 25 and found that the MMSE was highly correlated with the magnetization transfer ratio in the gray matter of the hippocampus ($r = 0.70$, corresponding to 49% of the explained variance). The same group had previously shown in a group of 23 AD patients with similar range of severity (four had MMSE < 10, 13 had MMSE 11–20, and six had MMSE > 21) that the MMSE had a strong correlation with both anisotropy ($r = 0.65$) and magnetization transfer ratio ($r = 0.64$) (109). However, the correlation with the total callosal area, a proxy of white matter atrophy, was significantly higher, reaching $r = 0.74$ (56% of explained variance). Yoshiura and colleagues have studied 34 AD patients with MMSE between 3 and 28 and found that the mean diffusivity of the white matter in the posterior cingulate gyrus was significantly correlated with the MMSE ($r = 0.53$, 28% explained variance) (110). Twenty-five patients with MCI have so far been studied with MT in two studies. Not unexpectedly, both have found that MT measures of MCI patients are intermediate between those of normal controls and AD patients (111,112).

Other studies have reported high correlations between global cognitive performance and measures of diffusion of the white matter (113) and of T of the gray and white matter (111), but have included controls in the correlation. This design can be criticized in that it inflates group variance through the unlikely assumption that the amount of variance of cognitive performance in healthy subjects that can be accounted for by MR measures of brain structural integrity is similar to that in Alzheimer's patients, and that the biological underpinnings are also similar.

Taken together, these studies suggest that microstructural pathology of the gray and white matter might be a strong correlate of cognitive impairment in AD. However, although one study corrected diffusion and MT measures for brain volume, thus at least partly accounting for the effect of atrophy (111), all the others have so far failed to partial out the effect of global or regional atrophy from that of diffusion and MT measures. Thus, it still remains to be determined whether microstructural change has an effect on cognitive impairment independently of the effect of macrostructural pathology.

Individual imaging modalities have variable relationships with cognitive impairment in AD patients. Future studies will need to combine imaging modalities in order to obtain a multispectral image of a brain where the variance inter-modality and among different areas of the same modality might outline a specific disease pattern. A pioneering study (114) has obtained information on diffusion, MT, and proton spectroscopy in a single MRI exam in order to define profiles of microstructural and biochemical changes in individual patients with a range of neurological diseases (MS, subcortical vascular encephalopathy, major stroke, AD, Alexander's disease, and haemangioma), but the specificity of the profiles still needs to be assessed. Prospective studies will need to assess the progression of microstructural involvement with cognitive deterioration and compare this correlation with that of other markers used to monitor the biological progression of the disease and as surrogate outcome measure in clinical trials (40).

FUNCTIONAL MAGNETIC RESONANCE IMAGING IN DEMENTIAS AND MILD COGNITIVE IMPAIRMENT

fMRI studies are providing unprecedented insight into the physiological mechanisms of the brain in a variety of conditions, from traditional neuro-psychological task to emotional perceptions to ethical choices. In the normal brain, fMRI allows mapping of the regions that are activated during a task with spatial resolution presently around 1 mm at 3.0 Tesla and below 1 mm at 4–7 Tesla. Given the known functional specificity of gray matter structures, the pattern of activation allows investigators to determine the basic functions exploited to carry out a given task.

Neurodegenerative disorders affect the normal activation pattern in a number of ways. As expected, in AD patients functional activation is decreased in the areas most affected by AD pathology. Some studies of verb processing, verbal and non-verbal learning, and working memory have found a reduced activation of the areas activated in healthy persons to carry out the same task (115–120)

(Table 4). Interestingly, medial temporal activation patterns in MCI patients during a memory task have been found to be as much reduced as in AD patients, possibly suggesting that the functional damage of AD neuropathology in the medial temporal lobe is very early (116).

Some studies have provided evidence that in AD and frontotemporal dementia reduced activation of normally active areas is accompanied by cortical reorganization. An enlarged area of activation has been found in the medial temporal lobe and other cortical areas with verbal and non-verbal learning, working memory, semantic, and visuospatial tasks (Table 4) (117–119,121–123,125,126,129,130). This finding is consistent with the recruitment of wider networks in an attempt to preserve cognitive function. It is conceivable that such compensatory mechanism may be functional in the relatively early stages of the disease, while in later stages activation decreases. Again, functional reorganization occurs in the early stages of the disease (121).

One of the most interesting findings obtained through the use of fMRI in the study of dementing disturbances relates to the involvement of the default network in AD (123). In young adults, a specific set of regions consistently shows deactivation that generalizes across a wide range of tasks and stimulus modalities, and has been detected by using both positron emission tomography and fMRI (131–134). These commonly deactivated regions include large sections of the lateral parietal cortex, the medial parietal cortex (including posterior cingulate and precuneus), and the medial frontal cortex. The function of the default network is monitoring the environment, monitoring one's internal state and emotions, and various forms of undirected thought. Engaging in goal-directed, active tasks may redirect processing resources from default activities to task-specific processes and regions. Lustig and colleagues have studied the magnitude and dynamic temporal properties of typically deactivated regions by using fMRI in 32 young adults, 27 older adults without dementia, and 23 older adults with mild AD. These were imaged while performing an active semantic classification and a passive fixation baseline task. Deactivation in lateral parietal regions was equivalent across groups; in medial frontal regions, it was reduced by aging but was not reduced further by AD. Of greatest interest, the posterior cingulate region showed differences between young adults and older adults without dementia and an even more marked difference with AD (Fig. 16). The region was initially activated by all three groups, but the response in young adults quickly reversed, whereas AD individuals maintained activation throughout the task.

These results can be interpreted as being related to damage of the entorhinal/perirhinal cortex—a major source of projections to the posterior cingulate cortex. It could be hypothesized that the deactivation of the default network might disengage monitoring of environment, internal states and emotions, and undirected thought, and allow the selective allocation of specific cognitive resources to a given task. AD patients might be unable to do so, and the

(*Text continues on page 187.*)

Table 4 Functional MRI Studies with Relevance to Dementia and Alzheimer's Disease

Reference	Aim	Results	Test performance
Dickerson et al., 2004 (121)	Study functional activation pattern of MCI during a visual encoding task	Enlarged hippo and parahippo activation with greater clinical impairment and subsequent memory decline Enlarged hippo and parahippo activation was correlated with better memory performance at baseline	
Grossman et al., 2003 (115)	Neural basis for verb processing in AD	Reduced activation in AD of normally activated cortical regions (post-lat temp and inf fr regions)	Poorer in AD
Lipton et al., 2003 (122)	Study working memory in 2 monozygotic twins discordant for AD	Enlarged parietal and reduced prefrontal cortex activation	Poorer in the AD twin
Lustig et al., 2003 (123)	Study activation-deactivation pattern in a semantic classification task	No deactivation in AD of the normally deactivated medial post par cortex Enlargement in normal aging and AD of normally activated regions (dorsal front cortex)	Poorer in normal aging and AD
Machulda et al., 2003 (116)	Study activation patterns of AD and MCI patients and normals during a visual encoding task	Reduced activation in AD and MCI of normally activated regions (medial temp lobe) Association between activation and performance on recognition and recall	Poorer in AD and MCI
Rombouts et al., 2003 (117)	Study working memory in frontotemporal dementia	Reduced activation in frontotemporal dementia of regions activated in AD (fr and par cortex) Greater cerebellar activation in frontotemporal dementia	Similar in frontotemporal dementia and AD
Sperling et al., 2003 (118)	Study the effect of aging and AD on activation patterns during a learning task	Reduced activation with aging of the dorsolat prefr cortex and enlarged activation of par cortex	

Li et al., 2002 (124)	Search for a functional MRI marker of early AD	Reduced activation in AD of medial temp and increased of medial par and post cing regions Functional synchrony of the hippocampus separates AD from controls with sens and spec of 80% and 90%	Poorer in AD
Prvulovic et al., 2002 (125)	Study visuospatial processing in AD	Enlargement in AD of normally activated cortical regions (sup temp lobule and occ-temp cortex) Atrophy partly accounts for differences between AD and controls	
Kato et al., 2001 (119)	Study nonverbal learning in AD	Reduced activation in AD of normally activated regions (medial temp lobe and prefr temp and par association cortices) and enlarged activation of visual associative cortex	Poorer in AD
Bookheimer et al., 2000 (126)	Study activation pattern of apoE4+ normal persons during encoding task and the predictive power of activation patterns on subsequent memory decline	Greater magnitude and enlargement in e4+ of normally activated cortical regions (hippoc, par, and prefr regions). Greater activation predicted memory decline after 2 years	Similar in e4+ and e4−
Johnson et al., 2000 (127)	Study the relationship between functional MRI activation and cerebral atrophy with a semantic classification task in AD	Marked effect in AD of regional cortical atrophy on activation of the left inf fr but not of the left sup temp gyri No effect of atrophy in controls	Poorer in AD
Pihlajamaki et al., 2000 (128)	Study verbal fluency in normal persons	Verbal fluency activates the medial temp lobe	
Rombouts et al., 2000 (120)	Study nonverbal learning in AD	Reduced activation in AD of normally activated regions (hippoc and parahippoc gyri)	Poorer in AD

(Continued)

Table 4 Functional MRI Studies with Relevance to Dementia and Alzheimer's Disease (*Continued*)

Reference	Aim	Results	Test performance
Thulborn et al., 2000 (129)	Study visuospatial attention in AD	Activation in AD of silent areas (bilat dorsolat prefr cortex) Reversal of the normal right > left activation in the intraparietal sulcus	Poorer in AD
Saykin et al., 1999 (130)	Anatomic substrate of semantic memory impairment in AD	Enlargement in AD of normally activated cortical regions (inf and middle fr gyrus)	Poorer in AD

Abbreviations: MCI, mild cognitive impairment; AD, Alzheimer's disease; MRI, magnetic resonance imaging.

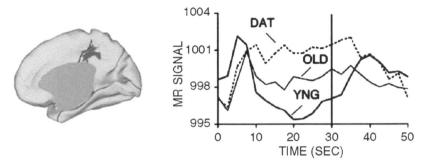

Figure 16 Effects of age and dementia on activation of the posterior cingulate area of the default network during a semantic classification task: the region is initially activated in all three groups, but the response in young adults quickly reverses, whereas DAT individuals maintain activation throughout the task. (*Left*) Medial parietal posterior cingulate cortex. (*Right*) Mean time courses of blood oxygenation level–dependent signal across active task and passive fixation baseline conditions. *Source*: From Ref. 123.

activation of the default monitoring system might interfere with the activation of task-specific regions, leading to poor performance in cognitive tasks. Better understanding of the impairment of the default network in AD and other dementias might help to understand the cognitive processes of patients while in the resting state rather than performance in a challenged state—which has largely been investigated in the last 30 years—as well as alertness and attention to outer and inner stimuli. The neural basis of insight and awareness of own cognitive deficits and of the surrounding environment, the development of agitation following minor environmental stimulation in some AD patients, and the context-dependent performance in activities of daily living might also be elucidated.

Some issues should always be kept in mind when interpreting fMRI results in neurodegenerative conditions. First, fMRI does not allow differentiating systems that can exert either activation or inhibition. This is a major hindrance for tracking the cortical remodelling that likely takes place in AD and other neurodegenerative disorders, whether excited or inhibited. Second, in normal persons the same task gives rise to greater activation based on subjective difficulty (cognitive tasks give more activation in persons with lower IQ, the so-called "neural efficiency" hypothesis) (135,136). As disease specific tasks are more difficult for patients with neurodegenerative disorders than normal persons, this might tend to give greater activation. Unfortunately, the specific contribution of subjective task difficulty cannot be assessed with current experimental designs. Thus, the fMRI signal of patients with neurodegenerative conditions is the summation of three trends: (1) lower activation due to neuronal or synaptic damage, (2) greater activation due to compensatory recruitment, and (3) greater activation due to subjective task difficulty. Their contribution to brain activation remains to be investigated.

ACKNOWLEDGMENTS

Samantha Galluzzi and Lorena Bresciani helped edit the manuscript.

REFERENCES

1. Lai CM, Lauterbur PC. True three-dimensional image reconstruction by nuclear magnetic resonance zeugmatography. Phys Med Biol 1981; 26:851–856.
2. Ogawa S, Lee TM. Magnetic resonance imaging of blood vessels at high fields: in vivo and in vitro measurements and image simulation. Magn Reson Med 1990; 16:9–18.
3. Kwong K, Belliveau J, Chesler D, et al. Real time imaging of perfusion change and blood oxygenation change with EPI. Society of magnetic resonance in medicine eleventh annual meeting. 1992:301. Abstract.
4. Pauling L, Coryell C. The magnetic properties and structure of hemoglobin, oxyhemoglobin, and carbon monoxyemoglobin. Proc Natl Acad Sci USA 1936; 22:210–216.
5. Arthurs OJ, Boniface S. How well do we understand the neural origins of the fMRI BOLD signal? Trends Neurosci 2002; 25:27–31.
6. Lassen NA, Kanno I. The metabolic and hemodynamic events secondary to functional activation—notes from a workshop held in Akita. Japan Magn Reson Med 1997; 38:521–523.
7. Logothetis NK, Guggenberger H, Peled S, Pauls J. Functional imaging of the monkey brain. Nat Neurosci 1999; 2:555–562.
8. Logothetis NK. The neural basis of the blood-oxygen-level-dependent functional magnetic resonance imaging signal. Philos Trans R Soc Lond B Biol Sci 2002; 357:1003–1037. Review.
9. Logothetis NK, Pauls J, Augath M, Trinath T, Oeltermann A. Neurophysiological investigation of the basis of the fMRI signal. Nature 2001; 412:150–157.
10. Logothetis NK, Wandell BA. Interpreting the BOLD signal. Annu Rev Physiol 2004; 66:735–769. Review.
11. Logothetis NK, Pfeuffer J. On the nature of the BOLD fMRI contrast mechanism. Magn Reson Imaging 2004; 22:1517–1531.
12. Mottaghy FM, Krause BJ, Schmidt D, et al. [Comparison of PET and fMRI activation patterns during declarative memory processes]. Nuklearmedizin 2000; 39:196–203.
13. Veltman DJ, Friston KJ, Sanders G, Price CJ. Regionally specific sensitivity differences in fMRI and PET: where do they come from? Neuroimage 2000; 11:575–588.
14. Devlin JT, Russell RP, Davis MH, et al. Susceptibility-induced loss of signal: comparing PET and fMRI on a semantic task. Neuroimage 2000; 11:589–600.
15. Feng CM, Liu HL, Fox PT, Gao JH. Dynamic changes in the cerebral metabolic rate of O2 and oxygen extraction ratio in event-related functional MRI. Neuroimage 2003; 18:257–262.
16. Bandettini P. Selective of the optimal pulse sequence for functional MRI. In: Jezzard P, Matthews PM, Smith SM, eds. Functional MRI: An Introduction to Methods. New York: Oxford University Press, 2001:177–195.

17. Obata T, Liu TT, Miller KL, et al. Discrepancies between BOLD and flow dynamics in primary and supplementary motor areas: application of the balloon model to the interpretation of BOLD transients. Neuroimage 2004; 21:144–153.
18. Uludag K, Dubowitz DJ, Yoder EJ, Restom K, Liu TT, Buxton RB. Coupling of cerebral blood flow and oxygen consumption during physiological activation and deactivation measured with fMRI. Neuroimage 2004; 23:148–155.
19. Jezzard P, Matthews PM, Smith SM. Funcitional MRI: An Introduction to Methods. New York: Oxford University Press, 2003:160.
20. Menon RS, Ogawa S, Tank DW, Ugurbil K. Tesla gradient recalled echo characteristics of photic stimulation-induced signal changes in the human primary visual cortex. Magn Reson Med 1993; 30:380–386.
21. Mandeville JB, Marota JJ, Ayata C, Moskowitz MA, Weisskoff RM, Rosen BR. MRI measurement of the temporal evolution of relative CMRO(2) during rat forepaw stimulation. Magn Reson Med 1999; 42:944–951.
22. David A, Blamire A, Breiter H. Functional magnetic resonance imaging. A new technique with implications for psychology and psychiatry. Br J Psychiatry 1994; 164:2–7.
23. Gundel H, O'Connor MF, Littrell L, Fort C, Lane RD. Functional neuroanatomy of grief: an FMRI study. Am J Psychiatry 2003; 160:1946–1953.
24. Singer T, Seymour B, O'Doherty J, Kaube H, Dolan RJ, Frith CD. Empathy for pain involves the affective but not sensory components of pain. Science 2004; 303:1157–1162.
25. Matthews PM, Jezzard P. Functional magnetic resonance imaging. J Neurol Neurosurg Psychiatry 2004; 75:6–12. Review.
26. Josephs O, Henson RN. Event-related functional magnetic resonance imaging: modelling, inference and optimization. Philos Trans R Soc Lond B Biol Sci 1999; 354:1215–1228. Review.
27. Donaldson DL, Buckner RL. Effective paradigm design. In: Jezzard P, Matthews PM, Smith SM, eds. Functional MRI: An Introduction to Methods. New York: Oxford University Press, 2001:177–195.
28. Frisoni GB, Scheltens P, Galluzzi S, et al. Neuroimaging tools to rate regional atrophy, subcortical cerebrovascular disease, and regional cerebral blood flow and metabolism: consensus paper of the EADC. J Neurol Neurosurg Psychiatry 2003; 74:1371–1381.
29. www.alzheimer-europe.org/EADC.
30. Scheltens P, Leys D, Barkhof F, et al. Atrophy of medial temporal lobes on MRI in "probable" Alzheimer's disease and normal ageing: diagnostic value and neuropsychological correlates. J Neurol Neurosurg Psychiatry 1992; 55:967–972.
31. Wahlund LO, Julin P, Johansson SE, Scheltens P. Visual rating and volumetry of the medial temporal lobe on magnetic resonance imaging in dementia: a comparative study. J Neurol Neurosurg Psychiatry 2000; 69:630–635.
32. Visser PJ, Verhey FR, Hofman PA, Scheltens P, Jolles J. Medial temporal lobe atrophy predicts Alzheimer's disease in patients with minor cognitive impairment. J Neurol Neurosurg Psychiatry 2002; 72:491–497.
33. Scheltens P, Erkinjunti T, Leys D, et al. White matter changes on CT and MRI: an overview of visual rating scales. European task force on age-related white matter changes. Eur Neurol 1998; 39:80–89.

34. Wahlund LO, Barkhof F, Fazekas F, et al. European task force on age-related white matter changes. A new rating scale for age-related white matter changes applicable to MRI and CT. Stroke 2001; 32:1318–1322.

35. Laakso MP, Partanen K, Riekkinen P, et al. Hippocampal volumes in Alzheimer's disease, Parkinson's disease with and without dementia, and in vascular dementia: An MRI study. Neurology 1996; 46:678–681.

36. DeCarli C, Maisog J, Murphy DG, Teichberg D, Rapoport SI, Horwitz B. Method for quantification of brain, ventricular, and subarachnoid CSF volumes from MR images. J Comput Assist Tomogr 1992; 16:274–284.

37. DeCarli C, Miller BL, Swan GE, Reed T, Wolf PA, Carmelli D. Cerebrovascular and brain morphologic correlates of mild cognitive impairment in the national heart, lung, and blood institute twin study. Arch Neurol 2001; 58:643–647.

38. Paty DW, Li DK. Interferon beta-1b is effective in relapsing-remitting multiple sclerosis. II. MRI analysis results of a multicenter, randomized, double-blind, placebo-controlled trial. UBC MS/MRI study group and the IFNB multiple sclerosis study group. Neurology 1993; 43:662–667.

39. Fox NC, Freeborough PA. Brain atrophy progression measured from registered serial MRI: validation and application to Alzheimer's disease. J Magn Reson Imaging 1997; 7:1069–1075.

40. Ashburner J, Csernansky JG, Davatzikos C, Fox NC, Frisoni GB, Thompson PM. Computer-assisted imaging to assess brain structure in healthy and diseased brains. Lancet Neurol 2003; 2:79–88.

41. Ashburner J, Friston KJ. Voxel-based morphometry—the methods. Neuroimage 2000; 14:805–821.

42. Thompson PM, Mega MS, Toga AW. Disease-specific brain atlases. In: Toga AW, Mazziotta JC, eds. Brain Mapping: The Disorders. New York: Academic Press, 2000:131–177.

43. Freeborough PA, Fox NC, Kitney RI. Interactive algorithms for the segmentation and quantitation of 3-D MRI brain scans. Comput Methods Programs Biomed 1997; 53:15–25.

44. Good CD, Johnsrude IS, Ashburner J, Henson RN, Friston KJ, Frackowiak RS. A voxel-based morphometric study of ageing in 465 normal adult human brains. Neuroimage 2001; 14:21–36.

45. Frisoni GB, Testa C, Zorzan A, et al. Detection of gray matter loss in mild Alzheimer's disease with voxel based morphometry. J Neurol Neurosurg Psychiatry 2002; 73:657–664.

46. Nichols TE, Holmes AP. Nonparametric permutation tests for functional neuroimaging: a primer with examples. Hum Brain Mapp 2002; 15:1–25.

47. Thompson PM, Toga AW. A surface-based technique for warping 3-dimensional images of the brain. IEEE Trans Med Imaging 1996; 15:1–16.

48. Thompson PM, Cannon TD, Narr KL, et al. Genetic influences on brain structure. Nat Neurosci 2001; 4:1253–1258.

49. Davatzikos C. Spatial normalization of 3D brain images using deformable models. J Comput Assist Tomogr 1996; 20:656–665.

50. Thompson PM, Hayashi KM, de Zubicaray G, et al. Detecting dynamic and genetic effects on brain structure using high-dimensional cortical pattern matching. Proc Int Symp Biomed Imaging 2002;7–10.

51. Thompson PM, Mega MS, Woods RP, et al. Cortical change in Alzheimer's disease detected with a disease-specific population-based brain atlas. Cereb Cortex 2001; 11:1–16.
52. Smith SM, De Stefano N, Jenkinson M, Matthews PM. Normalised accurate measurement of longitudinal brain change. J Comput Assist Tomogr 2001; 25:466–475.
53. Resnick SM, Goldszal AF, Davatzikos C, et al. One-year age changes in MRI brain volumes in older adults. Cereb Cortex 2000; 10:464–472.
54. Davatzikos C, Resnick SM. Sex differences in anatomic measures of interhemispheric connectivity: correlations with cognition in women but not in men. Cereb Cortex 1998; 8:635–640.
55. Clarfield AM. The decreasing prevalence of reversible dementias: an updated meta-analysis. Arch Intern Med 2003; 163:2219–2229.
56. Knopman DS, DeKosky ST, Cummings JL, et al. Practice parameter: diagnosis of dementia (an evidence-based review). Report of the quality standards subcommittee of the American academy of neurology. Neurology 2001; 56:1143–1153.
57. Gifford DR, Holloway RG, Vickrey BG. Systematic review of clinical prediction rules for neuroimaging in the evaluation of dementia. Arch Intern Med 2000; 160:2855–2862.
58. Scheltens P, Fox N, Barkhof F, De Carli C. Structural magnetic resonance imaging in the practical assessment of dementia: beyond exclusion. Lancet Neurol 2002; 1:13–21.
59. Sackett DL, Haynes RB. The architecture of diagnostic research. BMJ 2002; 324:539–541.
60. Frisoni GB, Geroldi C, Beltramello A, et al. Radial width of the temporal horn: a sensitive measure in Alzheimer disease. AJNR Am J Neuroradiol 2002; 23:35–47.
61. Rossi A, Catala M, Biancheri R, Di Comite R, Tortori-Donati P. MR imaging of brain-stem hypoplasia in horizontal gaze palsy with progressive scoliosis. AJNR Am J Neuroradiol 2004; 25:1046–1048.
62. Laakso MP, Soininen H, Partanen K, et al. MRI of the hippocampus in Alzheimer's disease: sensitivity, specificity, and analysis of the incorrectly classified subjects. Neurobiol Aging 1998; 19:23–31.
63. Jack CR, Jr., Petersen RC, Xu YC, et al. Prediction of AD with MRI-based hippocampal volume in mild cognitive impairment. Neurology 1999; 52:1397–1403.
64. Neary D, Snowden JS, Gustafson L, et al. Frontotemporal lobar degeneration: a consensus on clinical diagnostic criteria. Neurology 1998; 51:1546–1554.
65. Perry RJ, Hodges JR. Differentiating frontal and temporal variant frontotemporal dementia from Alzheimer's disease. Neurology 2000; 54:2277–2284.
66. Gorno-Tempini ML, Rankin KP, Woolley JD, Rosen HJ, Phengrasamy L, Miller BL. Cognitive and behavioral profile in a case of right anterior temporal lobe neurodegeneration. Cortex 2004; 40:631–644.
67. Rosen HJ, Kramer JH, Gorno-Tempini ML, Schuff N, Weiner M, Miller BL. Patterns of cerebral atrophy in primary progressive aphasia. Am J Geriatr Psychiatry 2002; 10:89–97.
68. Knopman DS, Mastri AR, Frey WH, II, Sung JH, Rustan T. Dementia lacking distinctive histologic features: a common non-Alzheimer degenerative dementia. Neurology 1990; 40:251–256.

69. Salmon E, Garraux G, Delbeuck X, et al. Predominant ventromedial frontopolar metabolic impairment in frontotemporal dementia. Neuroimage 2003; 20:435–440.
70. Franceschi M, Anchisi D, Pelati O, et al. Cerebral glucose metabolism and 5-HT2A receptor distribution in the frontal variant of frontotemporal lobe degeneration. Ann Neurol 2004; 56:216–225.
71. Rosen HJ, Gorno-Tempini ML, Goldman WP, et al. Patterns of brain atrophy in frontotemporal dementia and semantic dementia. Neurology 2002; 58:198–208.
72. Barber R, Ballard C, McKeith IG, Gholkar A, O'Brien JT. MRI volumetric study of dementia with Lewy bodies: a comparison with AD and vascular dementia. Neurology 2000; 54:1304–1309.
73. Burton EJ, Karas G, Paling SM, et al. Patterns of cerebral atrophy in dementia with Lewy bodies using voxel-based morphometry. Neuroimage 2002; 17:618–630.
74. Lobotesis K, Fenwick JD, Phipps A, et al. Occipital hypoperfusion on SPECT in dementia with lewy bodies but not AD. Neurology 2001; 56:643–649.
75. Woods SP, Troster AI. Prodromal frontal/executive dysfunction predicts incident dementia in Parkinson's disease. J Int Neuropsychol Soc 2003; 9:17–24.
76. Ivory SJ, Knight RG, Longmore BE, Caradoc-Davies T. Verbal memory in non-demented patients with idiopathic Parkinson's disease. Neuropsychologia 1999; 37:817–828.
77. Vingerhoets G, Verleden S, Santens P, Miatton M, De Reuck J. Predictors of cognitive impairment in advanced Parkinson's disease. J Neurol Neurosurg Psychiatry 2003; 74:793–796.
78. Schroter A, Zerr I, Henkel K, Tschampa HJ, Finkenstaedt M, Poser S. Magnetic resonance imaging in the clinical diagnosis of Creutzfeldt-Jakob disease. Arch Neurol 2000; 57:1751–1757.
79. Zerr I, Schulz-Schaeffer WJ, Giese A, et al. Current clinical diagnosis in Creutzfeldt-Jakob disease: identification of uncommon variants. Ann Neurol 2000; 48:323–329.
80. Zeidler M, Sellar RJ, Collie DA, et al. The pulvinar sign on magnetic resonance imaging in variant Creutzfeldt-Jakob disease. Lancet 2000; 355:1412–1418.
81. Will RG, Zeidler M, Stewart GE, et al. Diagnosis of new variant Creutzfeldt-Jakob disease. Ann Neurol 2000; 47:575–582.
82. Collie DA, Summers DM, Sellar RJ, et al. Diagnosing variant Creutzfeldt-Jakob disease with the pulvinar sign: MR imaging findings in 86 neuropathologically confirmed cases. AJNR Am J Neuroradiol 2003; 24:1560–1569.
83. Roman GC, Tatemichi TK, Erkinjuntti T, et al. Vascular dementia: diagnostic criteria for research studies. Report of the NINDS-AIREN International Workshop. Neurology 1993; 43:250–260.
84. Miao J, Galluzzi S, Beltramello A, Giubbini R, Zanetti O, Frisoni GB. Bilateral pallidal lesions following major haemorrhage: description of a case. J Neurol 2001; 248:806–808.
85. Rockwood K, Wentzel C, Hachinski V, Hogan DB, MacKnight C, McDowell I. Prevalence and outcomes of vascular cognitive impairment. Vascular cognitive impairment investigators of the Canadian study of health and aging. Neurology 2000; 54:447–451.
86. Erkinjuntti T, Inzitari D, Pantoni L, et al. Research criteria for subcortical vascular dementia in clinical trials. J Neural Transm Suppl 2000; 59:23–30.

87. Fazekas F, Kleinert R, Offenbacher H, et al. Pathologic correlates of incidental MRI white matter signal hyperintensities. Neurology 1993; 43:1683–1689.

88. Schmidt R, Enzinger C, Ropele S, Schmidt H, Fazekas F. Austrian stroke prevention study. Progression of cerebral white matter lesions: 6-year results of the Austrian stroke prevention study. Lancet 2003; 361:2046–2048.

89. Petersen RC, Doody R, Kurz A, et al. Current concepts in mild cognitive impairment. Arch Neurol 2001; 58:1985–1992.

90. Bennett DA, Wilson RS, Schneider JA, et al. Natural history of mild cognitive impairment in older persons. Neurology 2002; 59:198–205.

91. Frisoni GB, Padovani A, Wahlund LO. The predementia diagnosis of Alzheimer disease. Alzheimer Dis Assoc Disord 2004; 18:51–53.

92. Bosscher L, Scheltens, Ph. MRI of the medial temporal lobe for the diagnosis of Alzheimers' disease. In: Qizilbash N, Schneider LS, Chui H et al., eds. Evidence-Based Dementia Practice. Oxford (U.K.): Blackwell, 2002:154–161.

93. Arnaiz E, Jelic V, Almkvist O, et al. Impaired cerebral glucose metabolism and cognitive functioning predict deterioration in mild cognitive impairment. Neuroreport 2001; 12:851–855.

94. Chetelat G, Desgranges B, De La Sayette V, Viader F, Eustache F, Baron JC. Mild cognitive impairment: Can FDG-PET predict who is to rapidly convert to Alzheimer's disease? Neurology 2003; 60:1374–1377.

95. Anchisi D, Borroni B, Franceschi M, et al. Heterogeneity of glucose brain metabolism in mild cognitive impairment predicts clinical progression to Alzheimer's Disease. Arch Neurol 2005; 62:1–6.

96. Borroni B, Anchisi D, Paghera B, et al. Combined 99mTc-ECD SPECT and neuropsychological studies in MCI for the assessment of conversion to AD. Neurobiol Aging 2006; 27:24–31.

97. Buerger K, Teipel SJ, Zinkowski R, et al. CSF tau protein phosphorylated at threonine 231 correlates with cognitive decline in MCI subjects. Neurology 2002; 59:627–629.

98. Riemenschneider M, Lautenschlager N, Wagenpfeil S, Diehl J, Drzezga A, Kurz A. Cerebrospinal fluid tau and beta-amyloid 42 proteins identify Alzheimer disease in subjects with mild cognitive impairment. Arch Neurol 2002; 59:1729–1734.

99. Chetelat G, Desgranges B, De La Sayette V, Viader F, Eustache F, Baron JC. Mapping gray matter loss with voxel-based morphometry in mild cognitive impairment. Neuroreport 2002; 13:1939–1943.

100. Karas GB, Scheltens P, Rombouts SA, et al. Global and local gray matter loss in mild cognitive impairment and Alzheimer's disease. Neuroimage 2004; 23:708–716.

101. Pennanen C, Testa C, Laakso MP, et al. A voxel based morphometry study on mild cognitive impairment. J Neurol Neurosurg Psychiatry 2005; 76:11–14.

102. Hirata Y, Matsuda H, Nemoto K, et al. Voxel-based morphometry to discriminate early Alzheimer's disease from controls. Neurosci Lett 2005; 382:269–274. Epub 2005.

103. Okamura N, Arai H, Maruyama M, et al. Combined analysis of CSF tau levels and [(123)I]Iodoamphetamine SPECT in mild cognitive impairment: implications for a novel predictor of Alzheimer's disease. Am J Psychiatry 2002; 159:474–476.

104. El Fakhri G, Kijewski MF, Johnson KA, et al. MRI-guided SPECT perfusion measures and volumetric MRI in prodromal Alzheimer disease. Arch Neurol 2003; 60:1066–1072.

105. Terwel D, Dewachter L, Van Leuven F. Axonal transport, tau protein, and neurodegeneration in Alzheimer's disease. Neuromol Med 2002; 2:151–165.

106. Berg L, McKeel DW, Jr., Miller JP, Baty J, Morris JC. Neuropathological indexes of Alzheimer's disease in demented and nondemented persons aged 80 years and older. Arch Neurol 1993; 50:349–358.

107. Bozzali M, Falini A, Franceschi M, et al. White matter damage in Alzheimer's disease assessed in vivo using diffusion tensor magnetic resonance imaging. J Neurol Neurosurg Psychiatry 2002; 72:742–746.

108. Hanyu H, Asano T, Iwamoto T, Takasaki M, Shindo H, Abe K. Magnetization transfer measurements of the hippocampus in patients with Alzheimer's disease, vascular dementia, and other types of dementia. AJNR Am J Neuroradiol 2000; 21:1235–1242.

109. Hanyu H, Asano T, Sakurai H, et al. Diffusion-weighted and magnetization transfer imaging of the corpus callosum in Alzheimer's disease. J Neurol Sci 1999; 167:37–44.

110. Yoshiura T, Mihara F, Ogomori K, Tanaka A, Kaneko K, Masuda K. Diffusion tensor in posterior cingulate gyrus: correlation with cognitive decline in Alzheimer's disease. Neuroreport 2002; 13:2299–2302.

111. Van Der Flier WM, Van Den Heuvel DM, Weverling-Rijnsburger AW, et al. Cognitive decline in AD and mild cognitive impairment is associated with global brain damage. Neurology 2002; 59:874–879.

112. Kabani NJ, Sled JG, Shuper A, Chertkow H. Regional magnetization transfer ratio changes in mild cognitive impairment. Magn Reson Med 2002; 47:143–148.

113. Rose SE, Chen F, Chalk JB, et al. Loss of connectivity in Alzheimer's disease: an evaluation of white matter tract integrity with colour coded MR diffusion tensor imaging. J Neurol Neurosurg Psychiatry 2000; 69:528–530.

114. Back T, Mockel R, Hirsch JG, et al. Combined MR measurements of magnetization transfer, tissue diffusion and proton spectroscopy. A feasibility study with neurological cases. Neurol Res 2003; 25:292–300.

115. Grossman M, Koenig P, DeVita C, et al. Neural basis for verb processing in Alzheimer's disease: an fMRI study. Neuropsychology 2003; 17:658–674.

116. Machulda MM, Ward HA, Borowski B, et al. Comparison of memory fMRI response among normal, MCI, and Alzheimer's patients. Neurology 2003; 61:500–506.

117. Rombouts SA, van Swieten JC, Pijnenburg YA, Goekoop R, Barkhof F, Scheltens P. Loss of frontal fMRI activation in early frontotemporal dementia compared to early AD. Neurology 2003; 60:1904–1908.

118. Sperling RA, Bates JF, Chua EF, et al. fMRI studies of associative encoding in young and elderly controls and mild Alzheimer's disease. J Neurol Neurosurg Psychiatry 2003; 74:44–50.

119. Kato T, Knopman D, Liu H. Dissociation of regional activation in mild AD during visual encoding: a functional MRI study. Neurology 2001; 57:812–816.

120. Rombouts SA, Barkhof F, Veltman DJ, et al. Functional MR imaging in Alzheimer's disease during memory encoding. AJNR Am J Neuroradiol 2000; 21:1869–1875.

121. Dickerson BC, Salat DH, Bates JF, et al. Medial temporal lobe function and structure in mild cognitive impairment. Ann Neurol 2004; 56:27–35.

122. Lipton RB, Dodick D, Sadovsky R, et al. ID migraine validation study. A self-administered screener for migraine in primary care: the ID migraine validation study. Neurology 2003; 61:375–382.

123. Lustig C, Snyder AZ, Bhakta M, et al. Functional deactivations: change with age and dementia of the Alzheimer type. Proc Natl Acad Sci USA 2003; 100:14504–14509.

124. Li SJ, Li Z, Wu G, Zhang MJ, Franczak M, Antuono PG. Alzheimer Disease: evaluation of a functional MR imaging index as a marker. Radiology 2002; 225:253–259.

125. Prvulovic D, Hubl D, Sack AT, et al. Functional imaging of visuospatial processing in Alzheimer's disease. Neuroimage 2002; 17:1403–1414.

126. Bookheimer SY, Strojwas MH, Cohen MS, et al. Patterns of brain activation in people at risk for Alzheimer's disease. N Engl J Med 2000; 343:450–456.

127. Johnson SC, Saykin AJ, Baxter LC, et al. The relationship between fMRI activation and cerebral atrophy: comparison of normal aging and alzheimer disease. Neuroimage 2000; 11:179–187.

128. Pihlajamaki M, Tanila H, Hanninen T, et al. Verbal fluency activates the left medial temporal lobe: a functional magnetic resonance imaging study. Ann Neurol 2000; 47:470–476.

129. Thulborn KR, Martin C, Voyvodic JT. MR Functional imaging using a visually guided saccade paradigm for comparing activation patterns in patients with probable Alzheimer's disease and in cognitively able elderly volunteers. AJNR Am J Neuroradiol 2000; 21:524–531.

130. Saykin AJ, Flashman LA, Frutiger SA, et al. Neuroanatomic substrates of semantic memory impairment in Alzheimer's disease: patterns of functional MRI activation. J Int Neuropsychol Soc 1999; 5:377–392.

131. Cabeza R. Hemispheric asymmetry reduction in older adults: the HAROLD model. Psychol Aging 2002; 17:85–100.

132. Gusnard DA, Raichle ME, Raichle ME. Searching for a baseline: functional imaging and the resting human brain. Nat Rev Neurosci 2001; 2:685–694.

133. Mazoyer B, Zago L, Mellet E, et al. Cortical networks for working memory and executive functions sustain the conscious resting state in man. Brain Res Bull 2001; 54:287–298.

134. McKiernan KA, Kaufman JN, Kucera-Thompson J, Binder JR. A parametric manipulation of factors affecting task-induced deactivation in functional neuroimaging. J Cogn Neurosci 2003; 15:394–408.

135. Haier RJ, Jung RE, Yeo RA, Head K, Alkire MT. Structural brain variation and general intelligence. Neuroimage 2004; 23:425–433.

136. Gray JR, Thompson PM. Neurobiology of intelligence: science and ethics. Nat Rev Neurosci 2004; 5:471–482.

7

Perfusion Imaging with Single Photon Emission Computed Tomography

Nadine J. Dougall and Klaus P. Ebmeier

*Division of Psychiatry, Gordon Small Center for Research in Old Age
Psychiatry, University of Edinburgh, Edinburgh, U.K.*

SINGLE PHOTON EMISSION COMPUTED TOMOGRAPHY

As its name suggests, single photon emission computed tomography (SPECT) relies on the three-dimensional reconstruction of gamma emitter distributions in the brain. Without the advantage of the special geometry of positron annihilation into two photons travelling in opposite directions, SPECT has to use collimators to limit the field of view of the photon detectors. This implies that a significant amount of the radiation is absorbed by the collimator walls and does not contribute to the reconstructed image. Consequently, the sensitivity of SPECT is reduced compared with PET. Other differences between PET and SPECT derive from the different radioactive half-life of the gamma and positron emitters: short half-lives of positron-emitters make several repeat examinations within a short period possible, while longer half-lives of gamma-emitters allow for the examination of metabolic or pharmacological processes that require longer periods to establish. Further, the replacement of carbon atoms of the ligand with the positron emitter ^{11}C can generate radio-ligands with identical pharmacological properties, whereas substitution with the gamma-emitters ^{123}Iodine or ^{99m}Technetium is likely to change the ligand's chemical properties. Consequently, the generation of new SPECT ligands has proceeded at a disappointingly slow rate, partially because of the need to establish their pharmacological properties after synthesis.

BLOOD FLOW TRACERS

Four SPECT tracers are now available for "cerebral blood-flow" studies. ^{133}Xe is an inert gas that is inhaled, equilibrates with body tissues, and, after supply is stopped, its initial washout rate from tissue is proportional to regional cerebral blood flow (rCBF). Its advantage is that it can be calibrated against absolute CBF, but unfortunately, its gamma radiation is too soft (81 keV) to yield high quality images beyond the surface of the cortex. Iodinated compounds rely on the availability of ^{123}I (radioactive half-life 13.2 hours; 159 keV) and a radio-chemist, who can synthesize the radiotracer to a high standard of purity within a reasonable time to injection. The radio-tracer N-isopropyl-[^{123}I] beta-iodoam-phetamine [(^{123}I) IMP] was the first such SPECT ligand available, but currently it is almost exclusively used in Japan. In Europe and North America, ^{99m}Tc-substituted ligands have taken over from [^{123}I] IMP. ^{99m}Tc has a half-life of 6 hours and generates gamma radiation of 141 keV energy, which allows for resolutions down to 5 mm. Two ligands are commercially available, hexamethyl-propylene amine oxime (HMPAO, Exametazime, Ceretec®) and N′-1, 2-ethylenediy (bis-L-cysteine) diethyl ester (ECD, bicisate, Neurolite®). The cerebral distribution of all three tracers differs slightly, suggesting that their first pass uptake into brain cells is due to and modified by different mechanisms. For example, in a case control study of 90 volunteers, tracer uptake in large areas of the parietal, occipital, and superior temporal cortices was lower in a group imaged with ^{99m}Tc-HMPAO compared to the ^{99m}Tc-ECD group. Increases, on the other hand, were seen in the subcortical nuclei, parts of the brain stem, hippocampus, and small areas of the cerebellum (1). In another confirmatory comparative study, HMPAO-SPECT images showed relatively high radioactivity in the basal ganglia and cerebellum, whereas in the ECD-SPECT images, high levels were observed in the medial aspect of the occipital lobe. These regions with high radioactivity were not apparent in the rCBF-PET images (2). Because uptake in medial temporal lobe differs between ^{99m}Tc-HMPAO and ^{99m}Tc-ECD, specific and separate diagnostic criteria for temporal lobe pathology, such as in dementia and temporal lobe epilepsy, are necessary (3). Moreover, different effects of the diagnostic confounder age on perfusion can be observed, depending on whether HMPAO or ECD is used (4).

There is some controversy about which is the best diagnostic agent, and this will have to be decided on empirical grounds for each diagnosis separately (see below). Here, we want to make some general points about the differences between the first pass uptake perfusion markers ^{123}I-IMP, ^{99m}Tc-HMPAO, and ^{99m}Tc-ECD. ^{99M}Tc-HMPAO is less stable after reconstitution, so that images show more background facial uptake and retention when compared with ^{99m}Tc-ECD images (5). Stabilization of HMPAO with methylene blue or cobalt chloride improves image quality and reduces background activity in comparison to that of unstabilized ^{99m}Tc-HMPAO, without reaching the quality obtained with ^{99m}Tc-ECD (6). On the other hand, a comparison between early and delayed images using both HMPAO and ECD showed that HMPAO is more stable in the brain with no washout over time (7).

Both HMPAO and ECD underestimate perfusion in high flow areas, a phenomenon that can be demonstrated with acetazolamide, which causes greater increases in uptake with IMP than with the other two tracers (8,9).

Uptake of ECD depends on esterase activity, both cytosolic and membrane bound (10), whereas HMPAO retention depends on the presence of glutathione (11). This may, most of the time, ensure that variations in perfusion determine the variability of tracer uptake, but it has to be understood that such variability may also be due to factors specifically interfering with the tracer's retention mechanism. This will be of particular importance in pathological tissue. It appears that HMPAO uptake in ischemic brain behaves like a rCBF tracer, i.e., is increased in areas of luxury perfusion, while ECD and IMP do not show increased uptake, just like regional oxygen consumption, or may even be reduced, as a marker of discrete tissue damage (12–14). Similarly, ictal, inflammatory, and some neoplastic hyperperfusion is more obvious with HMPAO than with ECD SPECT (15–20). However, relative lack of stability after reconstitution of HMPAO make ECD a logistically more useful and effective tracer for ictal and peri-ictal studies (21,22).

Vascular lesions and hypo-perfusion in dementia appear to be detected more easily with IMP or ECD than with HMPAO (23,24), although this may have little impact on actual diagnostic accuracy (25). The situation may be reversed in AIDS encephalopathy, with greater diagnostic accuracy for HMPAO than IMP (26).

ALZHEIMER'S DEMENTIA

The characteristic pattern of AD perfusion deficits in parietal and temporal lobes is generally accepted and has been acknowledged in clinical guidelines (Figs. 1 and 2) (27). SPECT can provide rich information for the differential diagnosis of dementia, but routine use is still controversial. Research studies have increasingly documented modulating effects of age and gender on the typical perfusion pattern of AD. Although confirmation of these effects is still required, the discussion here will hopefully facilitate image interpretation and improve the usefulness of the diagnostic changes observed with SPECT.

Effect of Age

Although presenile onset AD is recognized for its faster clinical decline and greater symptom severity, the wider effect of age on SPECT AD diagnosis across the whole aging spectrum has yet to be fully explored. One of the first studies by Burns et al. (28) found age of onset correlated positively with parietal deficits and negatively with medial temporal lobe perfusion. Jagust et al. (29) then reported relative left frontal hypoperfusion in presenile AD compared with senile-onset AD, and Caffarra et al. (30) tried to replicate this finding with patients matched by illness severity, concluding that presenile AD was not associated with greater SPECT changes than senile AD. O'Brien et al. (31) confirmed that the right

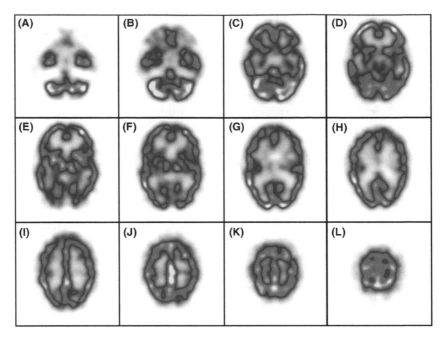

Figure 1 (*See color insert.*) Tc99m HMPAO SPECT scan of a healthy volunteer (MMSE=30); note that the parietal and temporal lobes are well perfused.

occipital hypoperfusion observed in their presenile patients did not distinguish them from senile onset patients after controlling for severity and duration of illness. However, Habert et al. (32) found a reduction in the early onset group in bi-parietal and left temporo-occipital areas. Many possible reasons exist for the lack of consensus of these early results, including confounding variables of age, age of onset, illness severity, and image analysis method.

Recently, and with the benefit of enhanced imaging system resolution and sophisticated data processing, the question of age has been revisited. A study by Hanyu et al. (33) using 3D stereotactic surface projection (3DSSP) found that younger AD had perfusion deficits in parietal lobe and posterior cingulate compared with younger controls, and older AD subjects had reduced perfusion in medial temporal and medial frontal areas, compared with older controls. Comparing young with old AD patients directly, the younger patients had more severe decreases in parieto-temporal and medial parietal lobes and the older group had decreases in medial temporal, medial, and orbital frontal and medial occipital lobes. Because posterior cingulate reductions were more severe in younger patients, the authors conclude that the sensitivity of SPECT is reduced for diagnosing AD in elderly cases.

Kemp et al. (34) found that 79% of a late onset AD group had medial temporal reductions compared with posterior association cortex, and conversely,

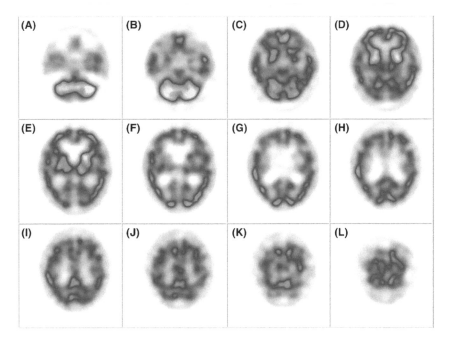

Figure 2 (*See color insert.*) Tc99m HMPAO SPECT scan of Alzheimer's disease (MMSE = 22), a characteristic pattern of perfusion deficits in parietal and temporal lobes.

85% of the early onset AD group had reductions in posterior association cortices compared with medial temporal lobe. In contrast, Nitrini et al. (35) observed bilateral parieto-temporal perfusion deficits in 23% of an early onset group and 71% of the late onset group—by combining parietal and temporal regions, perhaps the subtle differences detected by Kemp and Hanyu were lost.

Dougall et al. (36), in a multi-center study comparing young and old AD patients with age-matched mixed groups of healthy volunteers and depressed subjects, found that an increase in diagnostic accuracy was achieved for younger AD but not for the older AD group by using statistical parametric mapping (SPM) maps in conjunction with SPECT images. Kaneko et al. (37), using 3D-SSP and posterior cingulate reductions as a marker against other dementias, found that the frequency of posterior cingulate hypoperfusion was greater in presenile AD than in senile onset AD patients, thus providing further evidence of the heterogeneity of AD across age groups.

Summary

Clinicians should be alert to possible age-related changes in the interpretation of SPECT. Later onset AD appears to involve more medial temporal deficits and increased image heterogeneity, and is therefore more challenging to diagnose. On the other hand, younger onset AD has been associated with parietal and posterior cingulate reductions. SPM and 3D-SSP appear to be more helpful in early than late onset AD.

Effect of Gender

In a retrospective study of 104 SPECT scans of probable AD patients (NINCDS-ADRDA), Nitrini et al. (35) found that disease severity, age of onset, and being male was associated with bilateral parieto-temporal hypoperfusion. Thirty-nine percent of females and 59% of males had this perfusion pattern. In a separate study by Swartz et al. (38) of 63 probable and possible AD patients, both lower MMSE scores and male gender significantly predicted reduced temporal and parietal perfusion.

In a study by Ott et al. (39), left-right symmetric perfusion occurred more frequently in male than female demented patients with probable AD (NINCDS-ADRDA). Unilateral perfusion deficits in female probable AD patients were found to be almost always on the left side; female gender and shorter disease duration were independent predictors of unilateral left hemisphere CBF reduction.

TECHNIQUES TO IMPROVE DIAGNOSTIC ACCURACY

In the investigation of diagnostic differences, early SPECT studies used subjective visual inspection or quantitative region-of-interest (ROI) analysis which is less subjective but still observer dependent. Substantial progress has been made since then to develop objective quantitative techniques free of observer bias and with increased sensitivity to diagnose subtle changes associated with early dementia. Multivariate statistical techniques such as SPM, 3D-SSP, 3D fractal analysis (3D-FA), discriminant function analysis (DFA), or neural nets (NN) have crossed over from research to clinical practice with some success.

Statistical Parametric Mapping

SPM normalizes SPECT images to standard stereotactic space, allowing for direct statistical voxel-based comparison of scans between diagnostic groups. For example, in a comparison with a normal comparison group, Lee et al. (40) found reductions in left temporo-parietal cortex for mild AD and reductions in bilateral posterior parieto-temporal cortex, contiguous parts of anterior occipital lobes, and posterior cingulate gyri for moderate AD. A further study by Bonte et al. (41) comparing AD with FTD found an absence of reduced perfusion in posterior cingulate cortex to differentially diagnose FTD.

Few studies have directly compared SPM with visual assessment or ROI analysis. In a multi-center study comparing AD patients with depressed and healthy volunteers, Ebmeier et al. (42) reported that with SPM, between-rater variability was reduced, with greatest improvement in diagnostic accuracy for less experienced raters, and furthermore, normalizing to cerebellum was found to increase the spatial extent of reductions observed on SPMs compared with global normalization (43). In the same multi-center study, Dougall et al. (36) found that SPM used together with visual assessment increased specificity but not sensitivity.

3D Stereotactic Surface Projection

A multi-observer ECD-SPECT study by Honda et al. (44) directly compared visual SPECT assessment with SPECT alongside 3D-SSP of patients with AD, memory problems and healthy volunteers. Accuracy measured by area under the ROC curve (AUC) was enhanced for SPECT with 3D-SSP. Accuracy was further improved with an automated algorithm using bilateral posterior cingulate gyri in a 3D-SSP template. Adding 3D-SSP to SPECT increased specificity, but not sensitivity.

3D Fractal Analysis

3D fractal analysis (3D-FA) objectively measures spatial perfusion differences by calculating an index of heterogeneity called a fractal dimension. Yoshikawa et al. (45) used both 3D-SSP and 3D-FA to compare VaD patients with healthy volunteers. With 3D-SSP, reduced perfusion in VaD could be divided into two abnormal patterns: global reduction and a decrease in frontal regions only. 3D-FA demonstrated a difference between VaD and controls and a complete discrimination from patients with moderate and severe VaD. A correlation was found in VaD patients between the fractal dimension of image heterogeneity and cognitive impairment measured with the MMSE (46).

Using 3D-FA, Nagao et al. (47) found differences between AD subjects and controls, and since then Nagao et al. (48) have found differences in heterogeneity between FTD and AD subjects.

Neural Networks

Neural networks (NN) are used to model complex nonlinear datasets where relationships exist between SPECT perfusion patterns and diagnosis. They are trained to recognize patterns for disease simply by presentation of a scan training set, so that new cases can then be classified by likely diagnosis. Using this method, Chan et al. (49) found high diagnostic accuracy measured by AUC. Dawson et al. (50) reported a sensitivity for AD of 75% against a specificity against controls of 69%. Page et al. (51) found NN classified diagnosis more accurately than alternative statistical techniques and visual assessment ratings. The largest and most recent study by Warkentin et al. (52) using NN with ^{133}Xe SPECT obtained a high diagnostic accuracy measured by AUC, with 86% sensitivity for AD and 90% specificity against controls.

Discriminant Function Analysis

DFA derives combinations of variables that best discriminate between diagnostic groups, and can be used to predict group membership of new cases. For example, O'Mahony et al. (53) used DFA in a comparison of probable AD with normal controls, determining an optimal cut-off with a sensitivity of 87% and a specificity of 100%, then correctly categorized 93% of 15 subsequent new cases. In another study by O'Brien and colleagues (54), optimal separation was achieved between AD and controls with a sensitivity of 77% and specificity of 82%. Both studies were similar for MMSE score, age, and subject follow-up.

Partial Volume Correction

The lower spatial resolution of SPECT can cause partial volume effects—rCBF in smaller brain structures is poorly estimated—further exacerbated with age-related atrophy. An ECD study by Kanetaka et al. (55) of early AD and controls using SPM analysis found that partial volume correction increased diagnostic accuracy; using posterior cingulate hypoactivity, the area under the ROC curve was much increased with both global and cerebellar mean normalization.

COHORT STUDIES

Cohort studies of consecutive patients are particularly relevant as they mimic clinical imaging practice. To date, published cohort studies are very heterogeneous in their diagnostic composition. For instance, cohort studies have recruited consecutive outpatients from a memory clinic (56–59), while other studies have recruited consecutive patients with memory problems from a nuclear medicine department (60), a neuropsychiatry unit including neurological disorders (61), and from neuropsychology (62) (summarized in Table 1).

VASCULAR DEMENTIA

Several studies have attempted to discriminate AD from vascular dementia (VaD) with varying success—typically using AD criteria of temporo-parietal or posterior deficits and diffuse multi-focal abnormalities for VaD.

Early Onset AD vs. VaD

Early studies reported promising results in spite of imaging systems with limited resolution. Smith et al. (63) obtained a sensitivity for AD versus VaD of 73% against a specificity of 88%, Battistin et al. (64) a sensitivity for probable AD of 90% and a specificity against VaD of 80%, and Launes et al. (57), comparing AD with VaD, found a sensitivity of 64% against a specificity of 85%.

(*Text continues on page 209.*)

Table 1 SPECT Cohort Studies Are Heterogeneous in Diagnostic Mix and Not Generalizable to the General Population

First author (year)	Diagnosis confirmed by follow-up	No. of AD in cohort	Clinical definition of AD patient group	Age average (years)	MMSE mean score	No. non AD in cohort	Clinical definition of control group	Age average	MMSE mean score	Sensi-tivity (%)	Speci-ficity (%)
Herming-haus (1998)	No	6	Probable AD	NR	NR	27	Non-AD consecutive cohort of MC out-patients—other dementia, pseudode-mentia, or no dementia	NR	NR	71.0	96.0
Launes (1991)	No	36	Assumed probable AD	65	NR	62	Non-AD cohort of out-patients from MC (non-demented)	NR	NR	63.9	83.9

(Continued)

Table 1 SPECT Cohort Studies Are Heterogeneous in Diagnostic Mix and Not Generalizable to the General Population (*Continued*)

First author (year)	Diagnosis confirmed by follow-up	No. of AD in cohort	Clinical definition of AD patient group	Age average (years)	MMSE mean score	No. non AD in cohort	Clinical definition of control group	Age average	MMSE mean score	Sensitivity (%)	Specificity (%)
Lee (2001)	Yes, mean 11.1 months	58	Probable AD	NR	NR	57	Non-AD consecutive cohort of patients from Nuclear Medicine Dept with memory impairment—PD with dementia (12), Picks (3), systemic lupus (3), VaD (30), head trauma (4), Behcet's disease (3)	NR	NR	87.9	70.2

Masterman (1997)	Yes, at 1 month	51	Probable AD	76	17.0	31	Unlikely AD patients from MC who had a SPECT scan—VaD (19), PD (2), FTD (2), CJD (1), age, associated memory impairment (3), others (4)	73	22	74.5	54.8
Pasquier (1997)	No	127	Probable AD	73	17.2	115	Non-AD cohort of consecutive patients from MC—FTD (47), VaD (21), DLB (12), anxiety/depression (14), others (21)	68	22	61.4	71.3
Velakoulis (1998)	No	9	AD (clinical criteria NR)	63	NR	47	Non-AD consecutive cohort of neuropsychiatry unit patients with cognitive impairment—FTD (9), VaD (4), other dementia (9), neurological diagnosis (7), head injury (4), PD (2), others (12)	NR	NR	88.9	78.7

(Continued)

Table 1 SPECT Cohort Studies Are Heterogeneous in Diagnostic Mix and Not Generalizable to the General Population (*Continued*)

First author (year)	Diagnosis confirmed by follow-up	No. of AD in cohort	Clinical definition of AD patient group	Age average (years)	MMSE mean score	No. non AD in cohort	Clinical definition of control group	Age average	MMSE mean score	MMSE Sensitivity (%)	Specificity (%)
Villa (1995)	No	23	Probable AD	68	17.9	40	Non AD cohort of patients from neuropsychology with cognitive impairment—VaD (12) PSP (7) focal ventricular lesion (12) circumscribed cortical degeneration (9)	68.4	NR	91.3	72.5

Abbreviations: AD, Alzheimer's disease; CJD, creutzfeldt–jakob disease; DLB, dementia with lewy bodies; FTD, frontotemporal dementia; MC, memory clinic; MMSE, mini mental state examination; NR, not reported; PD, parkinson's disease; PSP, progressive supranuclear palsy; SPECT, single photon emission computed tomography; VaD, vascular dementia.

Later Onset AD vs. VaD

Weinstein et al. (65) did not find differences between older groups of AD and VaD, concluding SPECT was not ready for routine use. In a comparison of SPECT with MRI, Butler et al. (66) investigated late onset severe AD versus VaD and found that SPECT correctly classified 77% of patients compared with 50% by MRI. Late onset dementia was also examined by McKeith et al. (67), who reported perfusion deficits for AD compared with VaD in right and left frontal, right and left anterior, and posterior parietal areas. DeFigueiredo et al. (68) found that using left parietal and left and right temporal areas to train a neural network, AD was discriminated from VaD with a sensitivity of 80.0% against specificity of 86.4%; however, the AD group had lower MMSE scores than the VaD group.

AD vs. VaD—Detecting Early Dementia

Considering the differential diagnosis of early dementia, hippocampal perfusion deficits have been reported in AD compared with VaD by Villa et al. (62), with a sensitivity of 91.0% against a specificity of 75.0%. In a consecutive SPECT study by Starkstein et al. (69), VaD patients had lower perfusion in frontal, superior, and basal ganglia areas compared with AD patients (mean MMSE 19.0 and 19.9, respectively).

AD vs. VaD with Follow-Up Confirmation of Diagnosis

A number of studies have followed up patients to confirm original diagnosis. Bergman et al. (70) recruited patients with possible or probable AD and VaD, followed-up at 12 months, and found a relatively poor sensitivity for AD of 55% and a specificity of 71% against VaD. Masterman et al. (56) compared probable AD with VaD, followed-up for 1 month, and achieved a sensitivity of 74.5% with a relatively poor specificity of 57.9%; Pasquier et al. (59) obtained a sensitivity of 61% for probable AD against a poor specificity of 48% for VaD.

In more recent follow-up studies, Varma et al. (71) recruited consecutive early onset probable AD and VD, finding a sensitivity of 77% for AD and a specificity against VaD of 67%; Lee et al. (60), with a mean follow-up of 11 months in a study of consecutive patients with probable AD versus VaD and using bilateral or unilateral temporo-parietal deficits as diagnostic criterion, found a high sensitivity for AD 87.9%, compared with a specificity against VaD of 76.7%.

Heterogeneity of Perfusion in AD and VaD

Using 3D-FA, Yoshikawa et al. (72) found higher heterogeneity of perfusion in AD and VaD patients than in matched controls, AD heterogeneity was posterior dominant, and VaD was anterior dominant—the anterior/ posterior ratio derived by 3D-FA may thus be diagnostic of AD if < 1 and of VaD if > 1.

Systematic Review of AD vs. VaD

All extractable HMPAO-SPECT data published up to December 2002 were combined in a systematic review and meta-analysis by Dougall et al. (73): 13 studies with total numbers of 527 AD and 266 VaD (Table 2) gave a pooled weighted sensitivity for AD of 71.3% (95%CI 67.5–75.2) against a pooled weighted specificity against VaD of 75.9% (95% CI 70.8–81.1). Only two of the thirteen studies used quantitative analysis to classify subjects; increased use of objective multivariate statistical methods utilising whole SPECT datasets will possibly improve the discriminative ability of SPECT.

Summary

Younger onset severely demented AD and VaD patients can be differentiated; results for later onset dementia are not as conclusive. Early AD may have reduced hippocampal perfusion, whereas early VaD may have reduced perfusion in frontal and possibly basal ganglia areas.

FRONTOTEMPORAL DEMENTIA

SPECT perfusion deficits in anterior areas of the brain (frontal and anterior temporal cortex) are associated with a frontal lobe dementing process.

Earlier FTD vs. AD

There is some evidence that FTD patients have reduced frontal, temporal, and basal ganglia perfusion compared with controls; compared with AD they had reduced perfusion in orbito-frontal, frontal dorso-lateral, anterior temporal, and basal ganglia regions (74). Read et al. (75) found bilateral frontal reductions of SPECT images in 88% of FTD compared with none of the AD, after pathological verification of the diagnoses; unilateral left frontal hypoperfusion has also been reported by Frisoni et al. (76).

Pasquier et al. (59) found frontal decreases in 68% of FTD patients, but these were also present in 50% of probable AD patients; conversely, temporo-parietal reductions were observed in 61% of patients with probable AD as opposed to 17% in FTD. Pickut et al. (77) used discriminant function analysis (DFA) to separate FTD from AD on the basis of frontal reductions and achieved a sensitivity of 74% for FTD with a specificity of 81% against AD. Charpentier et al. (78), in a more sophisticated DFA with 5 predictor ROIs and MMSE, derived a decision rule, which correctly categorized 100% of FTD and 90% of ATD scans.

Velakoulis et al. (61) used as criterion bilateral parieto-temporal deficits and found a sensitivity of 89% for AD and a specificity against FTD of 67%; conversely, using frontal hypo-perfusion, the sensitivity for AD was 56% with a specificity against FTD of 100%. In a study by Talbot et al. (79) explicitly addressing the odds of a specific dementia diagnosis from perfusion patterns, bilateral anterior perfusion reductions increased the odds of a patient having FTD

Table 2 HMPAO-SPECT Studies Comparing Alzheimer's Disease and Vascular Dementia (1985–2002 Inclusive)

First author	Year	Diagnosis con-firmed by clini-cal follow-up	Num-ber	AD group	Age average (years)	MMSE mean score	Number	VaD group	Age average	MMSE mean score	MMSE Sensi-tivity (%)	Specificity (%)
Battistin	1990	No	19	Probable AD	67.7	9.0	15	VaD	71.5	16.9	89.5	80.0
Bergman	1997	Yes by 12 months; then every 6–12 months	58	Mixed prob & poss AD	75.5	21.6	17	VaD	72.9	22.4	55.0	70.6
Butler	1995	No	11	Probable AD	80.2	14.0	11	VaD	79.0	10.6	81.8	81.8
deFigueir-edo	1995	No	20	Probable AD	72.3	14.5	22	VaD	77.0	20.8	80.0	86.4
Launes	1991	No	36	Assumed prob AD	64.9	NR	33	VaD	68.0	NR	63.9	84.8
Lee	2002	Yes average 11.1 months	58	Probable AD	NR	NR	30	VaD	NR	NR	87.9	76.7

(Continued)

Table 2 HMPAO-SPECT Studies Comparing Alzheimer's Disease and Vascular Dementia (1985–2002 Inclusive) (*Continued*)

First author	Year	Diagnosis confirmed by clinical follow-up	Number	AD group	Age average (years)	MMSE mean score	Number	VaD group	Age average	MMSE mean score	Sensitivity (%)	Specificity (%)
Masterman	1997	Yes at 1 month	51	Probable AD	76.0	17.0	19	VaD	NR	NR	74.5	57.9
Pasquier	1997	No	127	Probable AD	72.8	17.2	21	VaD	71.9	21.6	61.4	47.6
Pavics	1999	No	33	Probable AD	67.0	19.0	18	VaD	68.0	23.0	70.0	66.7
Sloan	1995	No	43	AD (DSM-III-R)	70.1	18.8	25	VaD	76.0	20.2	74.4	92.0
Smith	1988	No	26	AD(DSM-III-R)	64.6	NR	25	VaD	67.8	NR	73.0	88.0
Varma	2002	Yes, 6 monthly for 1–3years	22	Probable AD	62.8	18.0	18	VaD	66.4	21.0	77.3	66.6
Villa	1995	No	23	Probable AD	67.9	17.9	12	VaD	68.9	NR	91.0	75.0

Abbreviations: AD, Alzheimer's disease; MMSE, mini mental state examination; NR, not reported; SPECT, single photon emission computed tomography; VaD, vascular dementia.

as opposed to AD (likelihood ratio = 15.9) and decreased the odds of a patient having AD as opposed to FTD (likelihood ratio = 0.1).

Recent FTD Studies

Pagani et al. (80) compared FTD, AD, and normal controls in a 3D standardized volume of interest analysis. They found fronto-temporal, anterior cingulate, and caudate nucleus reductions for FTD compared with normal controls. Pagani et al. (81) expanded this study using cluster analysis; a joint feature vector for the separation of scans by diagnosis yielded correct classification of 98% of FTD against controls and 94% of AD against FTD.

With an anterior-posterior perfusion ratio, Sjogren et al. (82) achieved a sensitivity of 86% for FTD and specificity against early onset AD of 96% and late onset AD of 80%. Nagao et al. (48) used DFA-derived anterior and anterior-posterior fractal dimensions that separated FTD from AD and controls with a sensitivity of 86% and specificity of 84%.

While hypoperfusion in the posterior cingulate has been found to be specific to AD, Bonte et al. (41) found that the absence of impaired perfusion favors FTD.

Varrone et al. (83) used SPM and found that relatively lower perfusion was observed in right medial frontal, anterior cingulate, and temporal areas as well as orbitofrontal and ventrolateral prefrontal cortex in FTD compared with AD. Comparing AD with FTD, a perfusion decrease in bilateral superior parietal cortex was observed, more extensive on the left than the right with involvement of superior occipital and temporo-occipital regions.

Systematic Review of AD vs. FTD

A meta-analysis of AD from FTD up to December 2002 and, using temporo-parietal reductions as a diagnostic marker, seven eligible studies with a total of 119 FTD subjects compared with 265 AD subjects were identified by Dougall et al. (Table 3) (73). The pooled weighted sensitivity was 71.5% against a specificity of 78.2% with a diagnostic odds ratio of 10.6 (95% CI 6.2 to 17.9). Using an additional marker such as fronto-temporal reductions may further improve diagnostic accuracy.

Summary

In the differential diagnosis of FTD from AD, the presence of frontal hypoperfusion is highly specific for FTD even when observed in combination with bilateral temporoparietal deficits. Anterior-posterior ratios appear more useful in younger age groups. Whereas posterior cingulate reductions have been reported as diagnostic for AD, conversely some evidence exists that anterior cingulate reductions are diagnostic of FTD.

Table 3 HMPAO-SPECT Studies Classifying Alzheimer's Disease from Frontotemporal Dementia (1985–2002 Inclusive)

First author	Year	Diagnosis confirmed by clinical follow-up	Number	Clinical definition of AD group	Age average (years)	MMSE mean score	Number	FTD group	Age average	MMSE mean score	Sensitivity (%)	Specificity (%)
Launes	1991	No	36	Assumed prob AD	64.9	NR	5	FTD	66	NR	63.9	80.0
Pasquier	1997	No	127	Probable AD	72.8	17.2	47	FTD	68	20.3	61.4	83.0
Pickut	1997	No	19	Probable AD	70	14.8	21	FTD	70	15.4	74.0	81.0
Sjogren	2000	No	52	Probable AD	67.4	NR	16	FTD	62	NR	88.5	87.5
Testa	1988	No	26	Probable AD	NR	NR	14	FTD	NR	NR	84.6	71.4
Varma	2002	Yes, 6 monthly for 1–3 years	22	Probable AD	62.8	18	21	FTD	63	21	77.3	66.6
Vela-koulis	1998	No	9	AD (clinical criteria NR)	63	NR	9	FTD	56	NR	88.9	67.0

Abbreviations: AD, alzheimer's disease; FTD, frontotemporal dementia; MMSE, mini mental state examination; NR, not reported; SPECT, single photon emission computed tomography.

DEMENTIA WITH LEWY BODIES

SPECT studies comparing dementia with Lewy bodies (DLB) with AD are rare. An early study by Varma et al. (84) reported posterior cortical reductions in both DLB and AD; both Pasquier et al. (85) and Talbot et al. (79) have concluded that classification is difficult. Ceravolo et al. (86) and Donnemiller et al. (87) found evidence exists for reductions in occipital lobe perfusion in DLB compared with AD and, conversely, reduced temporoparietal regions in AD relative to DLB. Ishii (88) found reduced perfusion in occipital areas, as well as relatively preserved medial temporal lobes in DLB compared with AD. These authors also reported that DLB and AD patients both had reduced parieto-temporal and posterior cingulate perfusion when compared with a group of normal controls.

Lobotesis et al. (89) used left occipital and right temporal reductions in perfusion to differentiate between DLB and AD and achieved a sensitivity of 64% against a specificity of 69.6% (Table 4). Colloby (90) re-analysed Lobotesis' data with SPM and found relative reductions in DLB relative to AD in right parietal, bilateral central parietal cortex, the precuneus, and the medial occipital gyri—and for DLB relative to normal controls, reductions in central and inferior parietal, left medial occipital, superior frontal regions, precuneus, and cingulate.

Summary

Occipital and posterior cingulate reductions and perhaps also the absence of medial temporal reductions are probable SPECT markers of DLB. Voxel-based techniques such as SPM may be more sensitive in earlier detection compared with ROI analysis.

MILD COGNITIVE IMPAIRMENT

Individuals presenting with cognitive impairment who do not meet clinical criteria for a dementing illness may qualify for a diagnosis of mild cognitive impairment (MCI). MCI is typically characterized by a decline from a previous level of memory functioning, which exceeds that expected by normal aging, with otherwise good functioning.

Predicting with SPECT whether individuals will make the transition from MCI to early AD or not may increase its value for planning appropriate early treatment interventions (91). Selected studies with accuracy measures investigating MCI, memory problems, as well as depression are summarized in Table 5.

One of the first published longitudinal studies by Celsis et al. (92) followed up subjects recruited from a memory clinic with a diagnosis of age related cognitive decline (ARCD) over a mean of two years. ^{133}Xe SPECT was used at baseline and during follow-up and compared with a normal comparison group

(Text continues on page 220.)

Table 4 HMPAO-SPECT Studies Classifying Alzheimer's Disease from Dementia with Lewy Bodies (1985–2002 Inclusive)

First author	Year	Diagnosis confirmed by clinical follow-up	Number	Clinical definition of AD patient group	Age average (years)	MMSE mean score	Number	Clinical definition of control group	Age average	MMSE mean score	Sensitivity (%)	Specificity (%)
Lee	2001	Yes, mean 11.1 months	58	Probable AD	NR	NR	12	Parkinsons disease with dementia	NR	NR	87.9	41.7
Pasquier[a]	1997	No	127	Probable AD	72.8	17.2	12	DLB	72.3	22.7	61.4	75
Pasquier[a]	1997	No	156	Mixed probable (n=127) and Possible AD (n=29)	70.6	20.8	12	DLB	72.3	22.7	57.1	75
Lobotesis	2001	NR	50	Definite (n=2) and prob (n=21) and poss (n=27) AD	81.6	17.3	23	DLB	79.4	16.0	64	69.6

[a] Same study.
Abbreviations: AD, Alzheimer's disease; DLB, dementia with Lewy bodies; MMSE, mini mental state examination; NR, not reported; SPECT, single photon emission computed tomography.

Table 5 Summary of Selected SPECT Studies Investigating Alzheimer's Disease, Mild Cognitive Impairment, and Memory Problems

First author (year)	Diagnosis confirmed by clinical follow-up	Number	Clinical definition of AD patient group	Age average (years)	MMSE mean score	Number	Definition of control group	Age average	MMSE mean score	Sensitivity (%)	Specificity (%)
Encinas (2003)	Every 6 months for 1–3 years	21	Progressed to probable AD from MCI	75.3	NR	21	Stable MCI	71.6	NR	79.0	76.0
Huang (2003)	Average of 26.4 months	82	Progressive MCI	63.4	25.7	20	Stable MCI	59.6	26.9	Area under ROC curve=0.75	
Okamura (2002)	Mean follow-up 3.1 years	22	Progression from MCI to AD on follow-up	71.9	25.6	8	Stable MCI	72.1	26.6	88.5	90.0
Knapp (1996)	NR	30	Probable AD	73.6	18.1	50	MCI	65.0	27.3	70.0	70.0
Johnson[a] (1998)	Yes, all subjects	56	Probable AD	77.4	18.0	27	Questionable AD (CDR=0.5)	72.4	NR	80.4	77.8
Johnson[a] (1998)	Yes, all subjects	56	Probable AD	77.4	18.0	18	Converters to AD on mean follow-up 16.7 m (n=18)	72.6	NR	80.4	94.4

(Continued)

Table 5 Summary of Selected SPECT Studies Investigating Alzheimer's Disease, Mild Cognitive Impairment, and Memory Problems (*Continued*)

First author (year)	Diagnosis confirmed by clinical follow-up	Number	Clinical definition of AD patient group	Age average (years)	MMSE mean score	Number	Definition of control group	Age average	MMSE mean score	Sensitivity (%)	Specificity (%)
Greene (1996)	Every 6 months for 2 years	31	Probable AD	69.9	23.5	24	Controls with memory problems	65.4	NR	80.6	66.7
Hashikawa (1995)	NR	12	Probable AD	57.7	NR	18	Controls with headaches or dizziness	58.7	NR	100.0	100.0
Mattman (1997)	NR	128	73 Probable and 55 possible AD	70.0	NR	48	Controls with memory problems	65.0	NR	78.9	64.6

Mielke (1994)	NR	20	Probable AD	68.8	20.9	13	Controls with memory problems	59.5	28.8	80.0	65.0
Muller (1999)	NR	116	AD (DSM-III-R)	66.0	19.9	20	Controls with memory problems	56.0	28.8	48.0	75.0
Launes (1991)	NR	36	Assumed probable AD	64.9	NR	62	Controls with memory problems including psychiatric disorder (depression or anxiety n=21)	NR	NR	63.9	83.8

[a] Johnson 1998 same study.

Abbreviations: AD, Alzheimer's disease; CDR, clinical dementia rating; MCI, mild cognitive impairment; MMSE, mini mental state examination; NR, not reported; ROC, receiver operating characteristic, SPECT, single photon emission computed tomography.

and a probable AD group with mild to moderate severity. ARCD subjects had pronounced asymmetrically decreased temporo-parietal perfusion at baseline compared with controls that declined further on follow up.

A large HMPAO-SPECT study by Johnson et al. (93) investigated differences between groups of normal cognition, questionable AD, converters to AD from questionable AD by two years follow-up, and probable AD (NINCDS-ADRDA) for preclinical predictors of developing AD. Singular value decomposition was used to reduce the SPECT data set to 20 vector scores, which were analyzed in turn by DFA. Probable AD could be differentiated from questionable AD with a sensitivity of 80% and specificity of 78%, and from converters to AD (mean 16.7 months) with a sensitivity of 80% against a specificity of 94%.

Using patients as their own controls, Kogure et al. (94) observed the changes of ECD-SPECT scans in 32 patients with MCI as they developed AD (mean follow-up 15 months). At baseline, MCI patients had bilateral reductions in posterior cingulate gyri and precunei compared with healthy volunteers— using SPM for analysis. Further decreases on follow-up and after conversion to AD were observed in left hippocampus and left parahippocampal gyrus. Selective perfusion decreases in posterior cingulate gyrus and precuneus in MCI as measured with sophisticated techniques of analysis may be a marker predicting future AD.

More recently, a follow-up study by Tanaka et al. (95) retrospectively examined non-demented subjects with memory loss of whom half converted to AD within two years. SPECT patterns at initial presentation suggested that both converters and non-converters had medial temporal and posterior cingulate reductions in perfusion (using SPM), with additional reductions in parietal and anterior cingulate in the individuals who later developed AD. SPECT could be useful in predicting conversion to AD, but typical AD perfusion deficits were also observed in subjects who did not convert to AD.

Posterior cingulate perfusion was again abnormal in an HMPAO study by Huang et al. (96) of 54 consecutively recruited MCI subjects, 17 of whom progressed to AD within two years (DSM-IV criteria). Activity in left posterior cingulate cortex was found to be decreased in those who progressed compared to those who retained a diagnosis of stable MCI. In a further SPM analysis of baseline HMPAO-SPECT images, Huang et al. (97) found bilateral prefrontal perfusion increases and parietal perfusion decreases (left more than the right) in the progressive group compared to the stable group and controls; the authors did not find any differences between groups in posterior cingulate—in contrast to their previous study.

An attempt to combine ^{123}I-IMP-SPECT and CSF tau protein levels to give higher predictive accuracy was reported by Okamura et al. (98). Perfusion in posterior cingulate was found to be lower in both progressive MCI and probable AD compared with cognitively normal subjects and the stable MCI group. In addition, CSF tau levels were higher in the progressive MCI and AD groups compared with normal subjects and stable MCI. Combining CSF and CBF data in a ratio [CSF (tau level)/CBF (posterior cingulate)], and using an optimum cut-off value, the authors achieved a sensitivity of 89% for progressive MCI and a specificity of 90% against stable MCI.

Encinas et al. (99) found that medial and anterior temporal perfusion deficits were of no value in predicting conversion to dementia since both stable and progressive MCI groups showed these deficits; this is in agreement with Tanaka et al. (95), who also found medial temporal deficits to be of no predictive value. In contrast, right and left pre-frontal deficits discriminated stable MCI from AD converters with accuracy measured by area under ROC curve of 75–78%.

El Fakhri et al. (100) extended the study of Johnson, this time comparing, both independently and in combination, MRI volume with HMPAO-SPECT perfusion estimates. Using DFA, both baseline SPECT and MRI were highly significant predictors of conversion to AD; they discriminated between questionable AD and converters to AD. Assessed by area under the ROC curve (AUC), MRI had relatively higher sensitivity and lower specificity than SPECT and vice versa. Taking MRI and SPECT in combination increased accuracy further—providing evidence that the two methods contribute independent information. For SPECT, Johnson reported that the best areas to discriminate between questionable AD and converters were: amygdala followed by superior temporal sulcus, basal forebrain, caudal anterior cingulate, hippocampus, and rostral anterior cingulate. In this study, the classification rules were derived from the study subjects themselves—testing these classification rules in a new group of patients would provide further insight as to the usefulness of the methodology.

Not all published SPECT studies have positive findings. A 3-year prospective study by McKelvey et al. (101) followed up MCI subjects at 9–12 monthly intervals and found that half progressed to probable AD. Of the MCI subjects, 36% were judged to have normal SPECT scans by visual assessment and 64% abnormal scans; 52% of those with abnormal scans progressed to dementia compared with 55% of those with normal scans. Since SPECT abnormalities did not predict cognitive decline (MMSE score) or conversion to dementia, McKelvey concluded that SPECT was not useful in predicting conversion—at least with visual inspection of images.

Summary

SPECT evidence demonstrates that the longitudinal spectrum of decline from normal cognitive function to MCI, and possible further decline to early AD is most likely associated with reductions in cingulate gyrus, in particular posterior cingulate, possible precuneus, hippocampal, and amygdala involvement as well as temporo-parietal cortex. It would appear that visual inspection of images does not discriminate between MCI and healthy volunteers. Regions of interest analysis is not as powerful or statistically robust as the technique of SPM for detecting subtle changes in small structures prone to partial volume effects.

CONCLUSION

Clinical criteria such as NINCDS-ADRDA for "probable AD" against the neuropathological gold standard have been estimated to have an average sensitivity of 81% and specificity of 70% (102). Comparing SPECT against clinical criteria in a meta-analysis finds it to be a test with relatively higher specificity than sensitivity. Therefore SPECT can be a useful adjunct to clinical criteria in the differential diagnosis of dementia. Diagnostic accuracy can be improved with SPECT for those demented patients not conforming with clinical criteria or who have possible co-morbid symptoms of vascular disease.

Recent research indicates that sophisticated multi-variate statistical processing of image data such as SPM enhances the diagnostic power of SPECT. Using such methods could help improve prognostic accuracy—for example, in patients presenting with memory problems or MCI. Visual inspection does not appear to be sufficient to discriminate between dementia sub-types in the early stages. While SPM is readily available and has been successfully implemented in clinical practice, subtle abnormalities associated with early disease are more likely to be identified with SPM or 3D-SSP (94,95).

To date most SPECT studies have been concerned with defining accurate markers for dementia sub-types that could be readily adopted in clinical use. Future research should investigate the value of SPECT in combination with other predictor variables, such as biological and cognitive markers, to optimize prediction and, by implication, therapeutic power.

REFERENCES

1. Patterson JC, Early TS, Martin A, Walker MZ, Russell JM, VillanuevaMeyer H. SPECT image analysis using statistical parametric mapping: Comparison of technetium-99m-HMPAO and technetium-99m-ECD. J Nucl Med 1997; 38:1721–1725.
2. Koyama M, Kawashima R, Ito H, et al. SPECT imaging of normal subjects with technetium-99m-HMPAO and technetium-99m-ECD. J Nucl Med 1997; 38:587–592.
3. Oku N, Matsumoto M, Hashikawa K, et al. Intra-individual differences between technetium-99m-HMPAO and technetium-99m-ECD in the normal medial temporal lobe. J Nucl Med 1997; 38:1109–1111.
4. Inoue K, Nakagawa M, Goto R, et al. Regional differences between Tc-99m-ECD and Tc-99m-HMPAO SPET in perfusion changes with age and gender in healthy adults. Eur J Nucl Med Mol Imaging 2003; 30:1489–1497.
5. Leveille J, Demonceau G, Walovitch RC. Intrasubject comparison between Technetium-99m-ECD and Technetium-99m-HMPAO in healthy human subjects. J Nucl Med 1992; 33:480–484.
6. Barthel H, Kampfer I, Seese A, et al. Improvement of brain SPECT by stabilization of Tc-99m-HMPAO with methylene blue or cobalt chloride—Comparison with Tc-99m-ECD. Nuklearmedizin 1999; 38:80–84.

7. Abdel-Dayem HM, Abu-Judeh H, Kumar M, et al. SPECT brain perfusion abnormalities in mild or moderate traumatic brain injury. Clin Nucl Med 1998; 23:309–317.

8. Makino K, Masuda Y, Gotoh S. Comparison of cerebral vasoreactivity to acetazolamide in normal volunteer among 123I-IMP, 99mTc-ECD and 99mTc-HMPAO. Kaku Igaku 1996; 33:551–555.

9. Dormehl IC, Oliver DW, Langen KJ, Hugo N, Croft SA. Technetium-99m-HMPAO, technetium-99m-ECD and iodine-123-IMP cerebral blood flow measurements with pharmacological interventions in primates. J Nucl Med 1997; 38:1897–1901.

10. JacquierSarlin MR, Polla BS, Slosman DO. Cellular basis of ECD brain retention. J Nucl Med 1996; 37:1694–1697.

11. Roth CA, Hoffman TJ, Corlija M, Volkert WA, Holmes RA. The effect of ligand structure on glutathione-mediated decomposition of propylene amine oxime derivatives. Nucl Med Biol 1992; 19:783–790.

12. Shishido F, Uemura K, Inugami A, Fujita H, Shimosegawa E, Nagata K. Discrepant 99mTc-ECD images of CBF in patients with subacute cerebral infarction: a comparison of CBF, CMRO2 and 99mTc-HMPAO imaging. Ann Nucl Med 1995; 9:161–166.

13. Miyazawa N, Koizumi K, Mitsuka S, Nukui H. Discrepancies in brain perfusion SPECT findings between Tc-99m HMPAO and Tc-99m ECD: Evaluation using dynamic SPECT in patients with hyperemia. Clin Nucl Med 1998; 23:686–690.

14. Moretti JL, Defer G, Tamgac F, Weinmann P, Belin C, Cesaro P. Comparison of brain SPECT using Tc-99m-Bicisate (l,l-ECD) and [I-123] IMP in cortical and subcortical strokes. J Cereb Blood Flow Metab 1994; 14:S84–S90.

15. Kashimada A, Machida K, Honda N, et al. A case of meningioma with non-accumulation of 99mTc-ECD and increased accumulation of 99mTc-HMPAO in the tumor. Kaku Igaku 1992; 29:1127–1131.

16. Fazekas F, Roob G, Payer F, Kapeller P, Strasser-Fuchs S, Aigner RM. Technetium-99m-ECD SPECT fails to show focal hyperemia of acute herpes encephalitis. J Nucl Med 1998; 39:790–792.

17. Lee DS, Lee SK, Kim YK, et al. Superiority of HMPAO ictal SPECT to ECD ictal SPECT in localizing the epileptogenic zone. Epilepsia 2002; 43:263–269.

18. Papazyan JP, Delavelle J, Burkhard P, et al. Discrepancies between HMPAO and ECD SPECT imaging in brain tumors. J Nuc Med 1997; 38:592–596.

19. Rieck H, Adelwohrer C, Lungenschmid K, Deisenhammer E. Discordance of technetium-99m-HMPAO and technetium-99m-ECD SPECT in herpes simplex encephalitis. J Nucl Med 1998; 39:1508–1510.

20. Tohyama Y, Sako K, Daita G, Yonemasu Y, Shuke N, Aburano T. Dissociation of Tc-99m-ECD and Tc-99m-HMPAO distributions in herpes simplex encephalitis. Childs Nerv Syst 1997; 13:352–355.

21. Lancman ME, Morris HH, Raja S, Sullivan MJ, Saha G, Go R. Usefulness of ictal and interictal Tc-99m ethyl cysteinate dimer single photon emission computed tomography in patients with refractory partial epilepsy. Epilepsia 1997; 38:466–471.

22. O'Brien TJ, Brinkmann BH, Mullan BP, et al. Comparative study of Tc-99m-ECD and Tc-99m-HMPAO for peri-ictal SPECT: qualitative and quantitative analysis. J Neurol Neurosurg Psychiatry 1999; 66:331–339.

23. Komatani A, Sugai Y, Watanabe N, Yamaguchi K, Kawakatsu S. Discrepancy between 99mTc-HMPAO and 99mTc-ECD in Alzheimer's disease: does the retention mechanism depend on the disease? Kaku Igaku 1998; 35:715–720.

24. Matsuda H, Li YM, Higashi S, et al. Comparative SPECT study of stroke using Tc-99m ECD, I-123 IMP, and TC-99m HMPAO. Clin Nucl Med 1993; 18:754–758.

25. vanDyck CH, Lin CH, Smith EO, et al. Comparison of technetium-99m-HMPAO and technetium-99m-ECD cerebral SPECT images in Alzheimer's disease. J Nucl Med 1996; 37:1749–1755.

26. Pohl P, Riccabona G, Hilty E, et al. Double-tracer SPECT in patients with AIDS encephalopathy - A comparison of I-123 IMP with TCm-99 HMPAO. Nucl Med Commun 1992; 13:586–592.

27. Small GW, Rabins PV, Barry PP, et al. Diagnosis and treatment of Alzheimer disease and related disorders. Consensus statement of the American Association for Geriatric Psychiatry, the Alzheimer's Association, and the American Geriatrics Society. JAMA 1997; 278:1363–1371.

28. Burns A, Philpot MP, Costa DC, Ell PJ, Levy R. The investigation of Alzheimers-disease with single photon-emission tomography. J Neurol Neurosurg Psychiatry 1989; 52:248–253.

29. Jagust WJ, Reed BR, Seab JP, Budinger TF. Alzheimer's disease. Age at onset and single-photon emission computed tomographic patterns of regional cerebral blood flow. Arch Neurol 1990; 47:628–633.

30. Caffarra P, Scaglioni A, Malvezzi L, Previdi P, Spreafico L, Salmaso D. Age at onset and SPECT imaging in Alzheimer's disease. Dementia 1993; 4:342–346.

31. OBrien JT, Eagger S, Syed GMS, Sahakian BJ, Levy R. A study of regional cerebral blood-flow and cognitive performance in Alzheimers-disease. J Neurol Neurosurg Psychiatry 1992; 55:1182–1187.

32. Habert MO, Spampinato U, Mas JL, et al. A comparative technetium 99m hexamethylpropylene amine oxime SPET study in different types of dementia. Eur J Nucl Med 1991; 18:3–11.

33. Hanyu H, Shimuzu T, Tanaka Y, Takasaki M, Koizumi K, Abe K. Effect of age on regional cerebral blood flow patterns in Alzheimer's disease patients. J Neurol Sci 2003; 209:25–30.

34. Kemp PM, Holmes C, Hoffmann SM, et al. Alzheimer's disease: differences in technetium-99m HMPAO SPECT scan findings between early onset and late onset dementia. J Neurol Neurosurg Psychiatry 2003; 74:715–719.

35. Nitrini R, Buchpiguel CA, Caramelli P, et al. SPECT in Alzheimer's disease: features associated with bilateral parietotemporal hypoperfusion. Acta Neurol Scand 2000; 101:172–176.

36. Dougall N, Nobili F, Ebmeier KP. Predicting the accuracy of a diagnosis of Alzheimer's disease with 99mTc HMPAO single photon emission computed tomography. Psychiatry Res Neuroimaging 2004; 131:157–168.

37. Kaneko K, Kuwabara Y, Sasaki M, et al. Posterior cingulate hypoperfusion in Alzheimer's disease, senile dementia of Alzheimer type, and other dementias evaluated by three-dimensional stereotactic surface projections using Tc-99m HMPAO SPECT. Clin Nucl Med 2004; 29:362–366.

38. Swartz RH, Black SE, Leibovitch FS, et al. Sex and mental status, but not apolipoprotein E, correlate with parietal and temporal hypoperfusion on SPECT in Alzheimer's disease. Neurology 1998; 50:03088.

39. Ott BR, Heindel WC, Tan Z, Noto RB. Lateralized cortical perfusion in women with Alzheimer's disease. J Gend Specif Med 2000; 3:29–35.

40. Lee YC, Liu RS, Liao YC, et al. Statistical parametric mapping of brain SPECT perfusion Abnormalities in patients with Alzheimer's disease. Eur Neurol 2003; 49:142–145.

41. Bonte FJ, Harris TS, Roney CA, Hynan LS. Differential diagnosis between Alzheimer's and frontotemporal disease by the posterior cingulate sign. J Nucl Med 2004; 45:771–774.

42. Ebmeier K, Darcourt J, Dougall N, et al. In: Ebmeier KP, ed. Voxel-Based Approaches in Clinical Imaging in Advances in Biological Psychiatry. Basel: Karger Verlag, 2003:72–85.

43. Soonawala D, Amin T, Ebmeier KP, et al. Statistical parametric mapping of 99mTc-HMPAO-SPECT images for the diagnosis of Alzheimer's disease: normalizing to cerebellar tracer uptake. Neuroimage 2002; 17:1193–1202.

44. Honda N, Machida K, Matsumoto T, et al. Three-dimensional stereotactic surface projection of brain perfusion SPECT improves diagnosis of Alzheimer's disease. Ann Nucl Med 2003; 17:641–648.

45. Yoshikawa T, Murase K, Oku N, et al. Statistical image analysis of cerebral blood flow in vascular dementia with small-vessel disease. J Nucl Med 2003; 44:505–511.

46. Yoshikawa T, Murase K, Oku N, et al. Quantification of the heterogeneity of cerebral blood flow in vascular dementia. J Neurol 2003; 250:194–200.

47. Nagao M, Murase K, Kikuchi T, et al. Fractal analysis of cerebral blood flow distribution in Alzheimer's disease. J Nucl Med 2001; 42:1446–1450.

48. Nagao M, Sugawara Y, Ikeda M, et al. Heterogeneity of cerebral blood flow in frontotemporal lobar degeneration and Alzheimer's disease. Eur J Nucl Med Mol Imaging 2004; 31:162–168.

49. Chan KH, Johnson KA, Becker JA, et al. A neural network classifier for cerebral perfusion imaging. J Nucl Med 1994; 35:771–774.

50. Dawson MR, Dobbs A, Hooper HR, McEwan AJ, Triscott J, Cooney J. Artificial neural networks that use single-photon emission tomography to identify patients with probable Alzheimer's disease. Eur J Nucl Med 1994; 21:1303–1311.

51. Page MP, Howard RJ, Brien JT, Buxton T, Pickering AD. Use of neural networks in brain SPECT to diagnose Alzheimer's disease. J Nucl Med 1996; 37:195–200.

52. Warkentin S, Ohlsson M, Wollmer P, Edenbrandt L, Minthon L. Regional cerebral blood flow in Alzheimer's disease: Classification and analysis of heterogeneity. Dement Geriatr Cogn Disord 2004; 17:207–214.

53. Mahony D, Coffey J, Murphy J, et al. The discriminant value of semiquantitative SPECT data in mild Alzheimer's disease. J Nucl Med 1994; 35:1450–1455.

54. O'Brien JT, Ames D, Desmond P, et al. Combined magnetic resonance imaging and single-photon emission tomography scanning in the discrimination of Alzheimer's disease from age-matched controls. Int Psychogeriatr 2001; 13:149–161.

55. Kanetaka H, Matsuda H, Ohnishi T, et al. Correction for partial volume effects elevates diagnostic performance of very early Alzheimer's disease in brain perfusion SPECT. J Nucl Med 2003; 44:830.

56. Masterman DL, Mendez MF, Fairbanks LA, Cummings JL. Sensitivity, specificity, and positive predictive value of technetium 99-HMPAO SPECT in discriminating Alzheimer's disease from other dementias. J Geriatr Psychiatry Neurol 1997; 10:15–21.

57. Launes J, Sulkava R, Erkinjuntti T, et al. 99 Tcm-HMPAO SPECT in suspected dementia. Nucl Med Commun 1991; 12:757–765.

58. Herminghaus S, Hertel A, Wittsack J, et al. Tc-99m-HMPAO-SPECT and proton MR spectroscopy in the diagnosis of Alzheimer's disease. Rivista di Neuroradiologia 1998; 11:27–30.

59. Pasquier F, Lavenu I, Lebert F, Jacob B, Steinling M, Petit H. The use of SPECT in a multidisciplinary memory clinic. Dement Geriatr Cogn Disord 1997; 8:85–91.

60. Lee BF, Liu CK, Tai CT, et al. Alzheimer's disease: scintigraphic appearance of Tc-99m HMPAO brain spect. Kaohsiung J Med Sci 2001; 17:394–400.

61. Velakoulis D, Lloyd JH. The role of SPECT scanning in a neuropsychiatry unit. Aust NZ J Psychiatry 1998; 32:511–522.

62. Villa G, Cappa A, Tavolozza M, et al. Neuropsychological tests and [99mTc]-HMPAO SPECT in the diagnosis of Alzheimer's dementia. J Neurol 1995; 242:359–366.

63. Smith FW, Gemmell HG, Sharp PF. The use of 99Tcm-HM-PAO for the diagnosis of dementia. Nucl Med Commun 1987; 8:525–533.

64. Battistin L, Pizzolato G, Dam M, et al. Regional cerebral blood flow study with 99mTc-hexamethyl-propyleneamine oxime single photon emission computed tomography in Alzheimer's and multi-infarct dementia. Eur Neurol 1990; 30:296–301.

65. Weinstein HC, Haan J, van R, et al. SPECT in the diagnosis of Alzheimer's disease and multi-infarct-dementia. Clin Neurol Neurosurg 1991; 93:39–43.

66. Butler RE, Costa DC, Greco A, Ell PJ, Katona CLE. Differentiation between Alzheimer's disease and multi-infarct dementia: SPECT vs MR imaging. Int J Geriatr Psychiatry 1995; 10:121–128.

67. McKeith IG, Bartholomew PH, Irvine EM, Cook J, Adams R, Simpson AE. Single photon emission computerised tomography in elderly patients with Alzheimer's disease and multi-infarct dementia. Regional uptake of technetium-labelled HMPAO related to clinical measurements. Br J Psychiatry 1993; 163:597–603.

68. deFigueiredo RJ, Shankle WR, Maccato A, et al. Neural-network-based classification of cognitively normal, demented, Alzheimer disease and vascular dementia from single photon emission with computed tomography image data from brain. Proc Natl Acad Sci USA 1995; 92:5530–5534.

69. Starkstein SE, Sabe L, Vazquez S, et al. Neuropsychological, psychiatric, and cerebral blood flow findings in vascular dementia and Alzheimer's disease. Stroke 1996; 27:408–414.

70. Bergman H, Chertkow H, Wolfson C, et al. HM-PAO (CERETEC) SPECT brain scanning in the diagnosis of Alzheimer's disease. J Am Geriatr Soc 1997; 45:15–20.

71. Varma AR, Adams W, Lloyd JJ, et al. Diagnostic patterns of regional atrophy on MRI and regional cerebral blood flow change on SPECT in young onset patients with Alzheimer's disease, frontotemporal dementia and vascular dementia. Acta Neurol Scand 2002; 105:261–269.

72. Yoshikawa T, Murase K, Oku N, Hatazawa J, et al. Heterogeneity of cerebral blood flow in Alzheimer disease and vascular dementia. Am J Neuroradiol 2003; 24:1341–1347.

73. Dougall NJ, Bruggink S, Ebmeier KP. Systematic review of the diagnostic accuracy of 99mTc-HMPAO-SPECT in dementia. Am J Geriatr Psychiatry 2004; 12:554–570.

74. Starkstein SE, Migliorelli R, Teson A, et al. Specificity of changes in cerebral blood flow in patients with frontal lobe dementia. J Neurol Neurosurg Psychiatry 1994; 57:790–796.

75. Read SL, Miller BL, Mena I, Kim R, Itabashi H, Darby A. SPECT in dementia: clinical and pathological correlation. J Am Geriatr Soc 1995; 43:1243–1247.

76. Frisoni GB, Pizzolato G, Geroldi C, Rossato A, Bianchetti A, Trabucchi M. Dementia of the frontal type: neuropsychological and [99Tc]-HM-PAO SPET features. J Geriatr Psychiatry Neurol 1995; 8:42–48.

77. Pickut BA, Saerens J, Marien P, et al. Discriminative use of SPECT in frontal lobe-type dementia versus (senile) dementia of the Alzheimer's type. J Nucl Med 1997; 38:929–934.

78. Charpentier P, Lavenu I, Defebvre L, et al. Alzheimer's disease and frontotemporal dementia are differentiated by discriminant analysis applied to 99(m)Tc HmPAO SPECT data. J Neurol Neurosurg Psychiatry 2000; 69:661–663.

79. Talbot PR, Lloyd JJ, Snowden JS, Neary D, Testa HJ. A clinical role for Tc-99m-HMPAO SPECT in the investigation of dementia? J Neurol Neurosurg Psychiatry 1998; 64:306–313.

80. Pagani M, Salmaso D, Ramstrom C, et al. Mapping pathological Tc-99m-d,I-hexamethylpropylene amine oxime uptake in Alzheimer's disease and frontal lobe dementia with SPECT. Dement Geriatr Cogn Disord 2001; 12:177–184.

81. Pagani M, Kovalev VA, Lundqvist R, Jacobsson H, Larsson SA, Thurfjell L. A new approach for improving diagnostic accuracy in Alzheimer's disease and frontal lobe dementia utilising the intrinsic properties of the SPET dataset. Eur J Nucl Med Mol Imaging 2003; 3:1481–1488.

82. Sjogren M, Gustafson L, Wikkelso C, Wallin A. Frontotemporal dementia can be distinguished from Alzheimer's disease and subcortical white matter dementia by an anterior-to-posterior rCBF-SPET ratio. Dement Geriatr Cogn Disord 2000; 11:275–285.

83. Varrone A, Pappata S, Caraco C, et al. Voxel-based comparison of rCBF SPET images in frontotemporal dementia and Alzheimer's disease highlights the involvement of different cortical networks. Eur J Nucl Med Mol Imaging 2002; 29:1447–1454.

84. Varma AR, Talbot PR, Snowden JS, Lloyd JJ, Testa HJ, Neary D. A 99mTc-HMPAO single-photon emission computed tomography study of Lewy body disease. J Neurol 1997; 244:349–359.

85. Pasquier J, Michel BF, Brenot-Rossi I, Hassan-Sebbag N, Sauvan R, Gastaut JL. Value of Tc-99m-ECD SPET for the diagnosis of dementia with Lewy bodies. Eur J Nucl Med Mol Imaging 2002; 29:1342–1348.

86. Ceravolo R, Volterrani D, Gambaccini G, et al. Dopaminergic degeneration and perfusional impairment in Lewy body dementia and Alzheimer's disease. Neurol Sci 2003; 24:162–163.

87. Donnemiller E, Heilmann J, Wenning GK, et al. Brain perfusion scintigraphy with Tc-99m-HMPAO or Tc-99m-ECD and I-123-beta-CIT single-photon emission tomography in dementia of the Alzheimer-type and diffuse Lewy body disease. Eur J Nucl Med 1997; 24:320–325.

88. Ishii K, Yamaji S, Kitagaki H, Imamura T, Hirono N, Mori E. Regional cerebral blood flow difference between dementia with Lewy bodies and AD. Neurology 1999; 53:413–416.
89. Lobotesis K, Fenwick JD, Phipps A, et al. Occipital hypoperfusion on SPECT in dementia with Lewy bodies but not AD. Neurology 2001; 56:643–649.
90. Colloby SJ, Fenwick JD, Williams ED, et al. A comparison of (99m)Tc-HMPAO SPET changes in dementia with Lewy bodies and Alzheimer's disease using statistical parametric mapping. Eur J Nucl Med 2002; 29:615–622.
91. Petersen RC, Stevens JC, Ganguli M, Tangalos EG, Cummings JL, DeKosky ST. Practice parameter: Early detection of dementia: Mild cognitive impairment (an evidence-based review): Report of the Quality Standards Subcommittee of the American Academy of Neurology. Neurology 2001; 56:1133–1142.
92. Celsis P, Agniel A, Cardebat D, Demonet JF, Ousset PJ, Puel M. Age related cognitive decline: a clinical entity? A longitudinal study of cerebral blood flow and memory performance J Neurol Neurosurg Psychiatry 1997; 62:601–608.
93. Johnson KA, Jones K, Holman BL, et al. Preclinical prediction of Alzheimer's disease using SPECT. Neurology 1998; 50:1563–1571.
94. Kogure D, Matsuda H, Ohnishi T, et al. Longitudinal evaluation of early Alzheimer's disease using brain perfusion SPECT. J Nucl Med 2000; 41:1155–1162.
95. Tanaka M, Fukuyama H, Yamauchi H, et al. Regional cerebral blood flow abnormalities in nondemented patients with memory impairment. J Neuroimaging 2002; 12:112–118.
96. Huang C, Wahlund LO, Svensson L, Winblad B, Julin P. Cingulate cortex hypoperfusion predicts Alzheimer's disease in mild cognitive impairment. BMC Neurology 2002; 2:9.
97. Huang CR, Wahlund LO, Almkvist O, et al. Voxel- and VOI-based analysis of SPECT CBF in relation to clinical and psychological heterogeneity of mild cognitive impairment. Neuroimage 2003; 19:1137–1144.
98. Okamura N, Arai H, Maruyama M, et al. Combined analysis of CSF Tau levels and [(123)]iodoamphetamine SPECT in mild cognitive impairment: Implications for a novel predictor of Alzheimer's disease. Am J Psychiatry 2002; 159:474–476.
99. Encinas M, de Juan R, Marcos A, et al. Regional cerebral blood flow assessed with Tc-99m-ECD SPET as a marker of progression of mild cognitive impairment to Alzheimer's disease. Eur J Nucl Med Mol Imaging 2003; 30:1473–1480.
100. El Fakhri G, Kijewski MF, Johnson KA, et al. MRI-guided SPECT perfusion measures and volumetric MRI in prodromal Alzheimer disease. Arch Neurol 2003; 60:1066–1072.
101. McKelvey R, Bergman H, Stern J, Rush C, Zahirney G, Chertkow H. Lack of prognostic significance of SPECT abnormalities in non- demented elderly subjects with memory loss. Can J Neurol Sci 1999; 26:23–28.
102. Knopman DS, DeKosky ST, Cummings JL, et al. Practice parameter: Diagnosis of dementia (an evidence-based review) - Report of the Quality Standards Subcommittee of the American Academy of Neurology. Neurology 2001; 56:1143–1153.

8

FDG PET: Imaging Cerebral Glucose Metabolism with Positron Emission Tomography

Karl Herholz

*Wolfson Molecular Imaging Centre, University of Manchester,
Manchester, U.K., and Department of Neurology,
University of Cologne, Cologne, Germany*

POSITRON EMISSION TOMOGRAPHY

Around 1975, positron emission tomography (PET) was used for the first time to image brain function (1). It remained primarily a research tool for the next 20 years, until its cost-effectiveness in oncology was proven and widely accepted (2). Since then, PET has become widely available in major hospitals, and therefore now also has the perspective for clinical use in neurology (3).

PET is based on the detection of coincident 511 keV gamma rays that originate from positron electron pair annihilation. At the core of PET scanners are scintillation detectors associated with coincidence electronics to detect the paired 511 keV gamma rays. Detectors made of scintillation crystals such as bismuth germanate (BGO), sodium iodide, cesium fluoride, barium fluoride, gadolinium, or lutetium oxyorthosilicate are typically arranged as hexagonal, octagonal, or circular rings. The width of the detector ring is larger in whole body scanners than in dedicated brain scanners, and both can be used for brain studies. Some older scanners had axial fields of view (FOV) of less than 12 cm, but modern scanners have an axial FOV of 12 to 15 cm at a nearly isotropic spatial resolution of 2.2 to 6 mm that allows scanning of the entire brain without repositioning. Image reconstruction from the recorded coincident events by filtered backprojection or iterative procedures needs to take into account corrections for gamma ray attenuation, scatter, and isotope decay.

Positron emitting isotopes typically have nuclear masses that are smaller than those of stable isotopes, and most of them are very short lived. Compared to other tracers that are commonly used in nuclear medicine, such as ^{99m}Tc (see Chapter 7), higher doses (typically 185 to 740 MBq) can be applied at rather low effective biological radiation doses (4). In addition, the efficiency of PET scanners is substantially higher than that of single-photon emission computed tomography (SPECT) scanners, resulting typically in high-count PET images with excellent signal-to-noise ratio.

The physical half-lives of oxygen-15 (^{15}O, 2 minutes) and carbon-11 (^{11}C, 20 minutes) require an on-site cyclotron for tracer preparation, and therefore the availability of these tracers usually is limited to highly specialized research laboratories. Tracers labeled by fluorine-18 (^{18}F, 109 minutes), however, can be reasonably well stored and transported over several hours and therefore increasingly become available by regional suppliers. The most widely used tracer, not only for brain studies but also for cancer studies, is ^{18}F-2-fluoro-2-deoxy-D-glucose (FDG) (5), which is usually synthesized in a radiochemistry laboratory by a stereospecific procedure based on nucleophilic substitution (6).

MEASUREMENT OF LOCAL CEREBRAL GLUCOSE METABOLISM

Glucose is the main substrate for energy supply of the brain. Measurement of local cerebral metabolic rates of glucose (lCMRglc) by PET are based on the fact that FDG is transported into tissue and phosphorylated to FDG phosphate, like glucose, but does not undergo significant further metabolism. It accumulates in the brain in proportion to lCMRglc, and after the first 10 to 20 minutes after i.v. bolus injection the distribution of FDG in brain approximates lCMRglc. Thus, images of FDG distribution recorded over 20 to 40 minutes within a time window of 20 to 90 minutes after tracer injection are suited to represent lCMRglc. Quantification of lCMRglc can be achieved by comparing measured cerebral activity with the plasma input function, obtained by multiple arterial or arterialized venous blood samples (7,8). FDG uptake of the brain is reduced in hyperglycemia, which leads to poor signal-to-noise and problems with measurement quantification. Thus, clinical FDG PET studies should be done under fasting conditions at normoglycemia (9).

In normal subjects, typical resting state gray matter CMRglc values are in the range of 40 to 60 µmol glucose/100 g/minute, and they are around 15 µmol glucose/100 g/minute in white matter. There are regional differences, with highest values in striatum and parietal cortex close to the parieto-occipital sulcus. Some phylogenetically old brain structures such as the mesial temporal cortex and cerebellum have metabolic rates below the gray matter average but are still higher than normal white matter. There is probably a slight decline of lCMRglc with age, most prominently seen in frontal cortex (10), but this has not been confirmed in all studies.

Local brain glucose metabolism depends on brain function. During functional activation lCMRglc increases, and it is decreased by sedation and during slow-wave sleep (11). Thus, a valid measurement of lCMRglc must include adherence to a defined functional state. Usually this is resting state characterized by lying comfortably in the scanner in supine position in a quiet examination room with dimmed lights. In many laboratories patients are asked to close their eyes before beginning the examination and to keep them closed. It is important to make subjects familiar with the surroundings prior to examination to avoid any unnecessary level of anxiety and restlessness.

MAIN FINDINGS IN ALZHEIMER'S DISEASE

A consistent finding that has been noted since the earliest PET studies in Alzheimer's disease (AD) is hypometabolism affecting the temporal and parietal association cortex (12–15), with the angular gyrus usually being the center of the metabolic impairment (Fig. 1). Frontolateral association cortex is also frequently involved to a variable degree (16–19). Primary motor, somatosensory, and visual cortical areas are relatively spared. This pattern corresponds in general to the clinical symptoms, with impairment of memory and associative thinking, including higher-order sensory processing and planning of action, but with relative preservation of primary motor and sensory function. These changes differ from those of normal aging, which leads to predominantly mesial frontal metabolic decline and may cause some apparent dorsal parietal and frontotemporal (perisylvian) metabolic reduction due to partial volume effects caused by atrophy (10,20–23).

More recent studies that used voxel-based comparisons to normal reference data clearly showed that the posterior cingulate cortex (PCC) and the precuneus are also impaired early in AD (24). The histochemical correlate of reduced FDG is a pronounced decline in cytochrome oxidase activity in AD relative to controls, whereas adjacent motor cortex does not show such differences (25). Metabolic impairment of the posterior cingulate gyrus is not directly obvious by inspection of FDG PET scans because metabolism in that area is typically above the normal cortical average level (26). When impairment develops, it decreases to the level of surrounding cortex but is not a visually apparent hypometabolic lesion. Thus, this potential diagnostic sign is easily missed by standard visual interpretation of FDG scans.

Automatic detection of abnormal metabolism on individual PET scans requires appropriate reference data sets, spatial normalization of scans, statistical algorithms to compare the voxels in scan data with normal reference data, and suitable display of the results (Fig. 2). Signorini et al. (27) demonstrated that this can be achieved by adapting the statistical parametric mapping software package that was developed at the Wellcome Institute, London, U.K., originally for

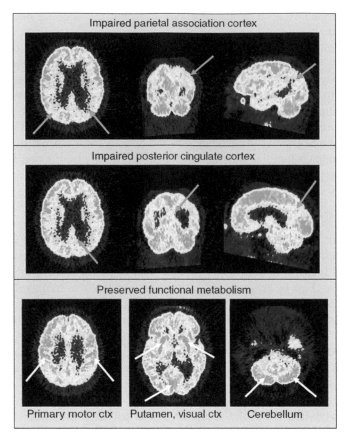

Figure 1   (*See color insert.*) Typical findings with FDG PET in Alzheimer's disease.

analysis of activation studies (28). Some commercial software packages provide similar approaches, but users should take care to check the validity of normal reference data, statistics, and normalization procedures. Special non-linear warping procedures for spatial normalization and surface renderings that provide a quick overview of abnormalities have been developed for diagnosis of AD by FDG PET scans by Minoshima et al. (29,30). This software package, 3D-SSP or NEUROSTAT, has since been used successfully to identify metabolic alterations in dementia and MCI by several groups (31–33).

Even more advanced approaches go beyond detection of abnormal voxels and aim at automatic recognition of the typical anatomical distribution of metabolic abnormalities in AD. Discriminant functions derived by multiple regression of regional data achieved 87% correct classification of AD patients versus controls (34), and a neural network classifier arrived at 90% accuracy (35). The sum of abnormal t-values in regions that are typically hypometabolic in AD

[t_map CLUSTER IMAGES (Up to 8)]

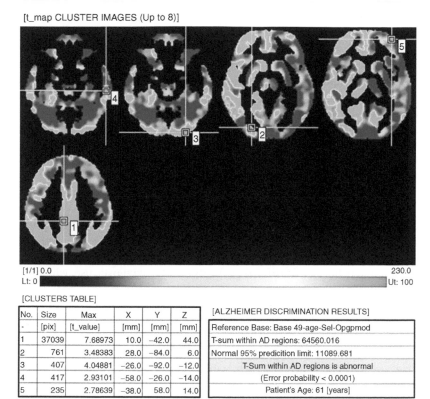

No.	Size	Max	X	Y	Z	[ALZHEIMER DISCRIMINATION RESULTS]
-	[pix]	[t_value]	[mm]	[mm]	[mm]	Reference Base: Base 49-age-Sel-Opgpmod
1	37039	7.68973	10.0	−42.0	44.0	T-sum within AD regions: 64560.016
2	761	3.48383	28.0	−84.0	6.0	Normal 95% predicition limit: 11089.681
3	407	4.04881	−26.0	−92.0	−12.0	T-Sum within AD regions is abnormal
4	417	2.93101	−58.0	−26.0	−14.0	(Error probability < 0.0001)
5	235	2.78639	−38.0	58.0	14.0	Patient's Age: 61 [years]

Figure 2 (*See color insert.*) Automatic detection of abnormal metabolism, including correction for age (PMOD Technologies Ltd., Adliswil, Switzerland).

has been used as an indicator with 93% accuracy (23). The same accuracy was achieved even without image reconstruction by a special pattern extraction technique from PET sinograms (36). Several discrimination functions combined with principal component analysis or partial least-squares have been tested for discrimination between AD and FTD in a sample of 48 patients with autopsy-confirmed diagnosis and achieved accuracies between 80% and 90% (37).

Use of FDG PET to diagnose AD rests on the typical distribution of these functional changes in brain. Impairment of local FDG uptake by itself, however, is not specific for AD pathology and could potentially be caused by many other disorders, e.g., ischemic lesions, when they just happen to affect those areas that are typically affected in AD. Correspondingly, a high sensitivity in the order of 90% to 95% for FDG PET to detect AD has been documented in several studies, but specificity for discrimination from other neurodegenerative disorders is lower and in the order of 65–75% (38). Patients with Parkinson's disease (PD) may show a very similar metabolic impairment (39,40), even in absence of major cognitive deficits (41). These changes may even be reversible with successful electrical stimulation of the subthalamic nucleus (42). With appropriate clinical information, the "pseudo-AD" metabolic pattern should not be a major problem because it is seen only in patients with long-standing PD who also have the clinical motor symptoms of PD. Thus FDG PET scans always need to be interpreted in the context of clinical history and symptoms. They also cannot replace structural imaging by computed tomography (CT) or magnetic resonance imaging (MRI), which are needed to recognize non-degenerative lesions such as infarcts, tumors, hematomas, or hydrocephalus that may also lead to focal or generalized cortical hypometabolism (43).

Patients with late-onset AD may show less difference between typically affected and non-affected brain regions than usually seen in early-onset AD, which could potentially lead to reduced diagnostic accuracy with FDG PET (44–46). This could reflect the fact that at older age multifactor damage to the brain is likely to accumulate, and, actually, also in neuropathological studies the proportion of unclassifiable dementia is highest in the oldest old (see Chapter 11). Thus, in very old multimorbid patients, FDG PET is probably of little diagnostic use, which is in accord with general clinical wisdom.

Atrophy of hippocampal and parahippocampal structures is a main finding of structural imaging in AD (see Chapter 6). Therefore one would expect also major functional changes of lCMRglc in this brain area, but this has not generally been the case (47). It is difficult to identify hippocampal metabolic impairment on FDG PET scans because it exhibits lower resting metabolism than neocortex and pathological changes are not obvious by visual image analysis. However, by coregistration of MRI and standardized placement regions of interest onto the hippocampus in FDG PET scans to increase spatial accuracy, a reduction, especially of entorhinal metabolism, has indeed been observed in mild cognitive impairment (MCI) and AD (48). In normal controls, lCMRglc in the neocortex is correlated with entorhinal cortex lCMRglc across both hemispheres, whereas in AD patients these functional metabolic correlations are largely lost (49). Metabolic impairment in the parahippocampal gyrus had also been noted in a previous study during activation using a simple memory task (50). As would be expected, hypometabolism in that region is associated with memory impairment (51).

Atrophy may cause an apparent reduction in local FDG uptake due to increased partial volume effects, even if local glucose metabolic rate in remaining cortex was constant. Algorithms to correct for that effect have been applied in AD (52,53) and concluded that partial volume effects contribute to apparent hypometabolism but also that in spite of that local glucose metabolism remains reduced in temporoparietal cortex even after correction. In contrast, the negative correlation between frontal and perisylvian apparent glucose metabolism and age seen in normal subjects could largely be resolved by partial volume correction (54). Partial volume correction is not usually applied to clinical data because it requires accurate coregistration with high-quality MRI, is very sensitive to slight mismatch potentially producing severe artifacts, increases image noise, and is not needed for diagnostic purposes because metabolic impairment and atrophy generally go in parallel in neurodegenerative diseases. Readers of clinical PET images, however, need to keep in mind that atrophy in otherwise healthy individuals, which most frequently is most pronounced in frontal and upper parietal cortex as well as adjacent to the major fissures (interhemispheric and Sylvian), may cause an apparent reduction of FDG uptake in those areas that should not be confused with AD.

Both local cerebral blood flow (CBF) and local cerebral glucose metabolism are coupled to neuronal function and are reduced in neuro-degenerative disease (55). Thus, regional reductions of CBF similar to the reductions of CMRglc can be observed with CBF imaging methods in AD and other dementias. In clinical practice, especially SPECT is widely used for that purpose (see Chapter 7) because it is less expensive and more widely available than PET. In direct comparisons of the two techniques (56,57), SPECT always showed inferior diagnostic discrimination which limits its power to detect early cases. O-15 water PET has also been used to measure CBF in AD, but in a clinical study its diagnostic power turned out to be much lower than in FDG studies (58). Several receptor ligands with high blood-brain transfer rates provide information about local CBF when early uptake is measured by appropriate kinetic modeling, in addition to measurements of receptor binding potential (see Chapter 9). This property of ^{11}C-dihydrotetrabenazine, a vesicular monoamine transporter ligand, has been used to demonstrate that it may also serve for detection of AD in addition to its ability to detect degeneration of aminergic pathways (59).

LONGITUDINAL STUDIES AND TRIALS

Longitudinal studies have shown that the severity and extent of metabolic impairment in temporal and parietal cortex increases as dementia progresses, and frontal involvement becomes more prominent (60,61). The decline of metabolism is in the order of 16% to 19% over three years in association cortices, which contrasts with an absence of significant decline in normal control subjects (62). Our own longitudinal data indicate that the total cortical metabolic impairment in AD increases at a constant rate to reach the maximum observed impairment after eight to nine years. Metabolic asymmetries and associated predominance of language or visuospatial impairment tends to persist during progression (63,64). Metabolic rates in basal ganglia and thalamus remain stable and are unrelated to progression (62). Thus in late dementia, there is typically a pattern of severe hypometabolism in temporoparietal and frontal association cortices, with a relative sparing of primary cortical areas.

In a few clinical trials, the effects of nootropic drugs on cerebral glucose metabolism in AD have been explored. An increase of CMRglc has been demonstrated with piracetam (a putative enhancer of cerebral metabolism) (65), propentofylline (an adenosine uptake blocker) (66), and metrifonate (a long-lasting cholinesterase inhibitor) (67); the latter two studies showed an associated improvement in certain cognitive measures. Reductions of CMRglc were found with physostigmine (68), however, in spite of improved attention. Studies with other centrally acting cholinergic drugs generally did not show a main treatment effect on cerebral glucose metabolism, but when subjects were divided into responders and non-responders the former showed a metabolic increase that was mostly located in frontal cortex and associated areas (69–71). These trials studied the effect of drugs on CMRglc but did not address whether drugs might slow disease progression. To perform such a trial, it has been estimated that 24 patients with Alzheimer's disease per active treatment and placebo group would be needed to detect a significant 33% treatment response with $p < 0.05$ and 80% power in a one-year, double-blind, placebo-controlled treatment study (72).

EARLY DIAGNOSIS OF ALZHEIMER'S DISEASE

The current main issue for diagnosis of AD with PET is early diagnosis when patients present with a mild cognitive deficit, but before clinical dementia arises. This may be of particular importance for subjects with a high premorbid cognitive level, who can experience a substantial decline of cognitive function before reaching the lower normal limit of standard neuropsychological tests. There are many indications that this will be possible with FDG PET. Even at an asymptomatic stage, impairment of cortical glucose metabolism has been observed in subjects at high risk for AD due to family history of AD and Apolipoprotein E (ApoE) ε4 homozygosity (73,74) and this abnormality is seen decades before the likely onset of dementia (75). In middle-aged and elderly asymptomatic ApoE ε4-positive subjects, temporoparietal and posterior cingulate lCMRglc declines by about 2% per year (76). The potential for primary intervention studies employing FDG PET as an outcome measure in samples of 50 and 115 cognitively normal ε4 heterozygotes has been documented (77). After onset of manifest dementia, ε4-positive patients still had more severe metabolic deficits in some studies (78,79). Mesial temporal hypometabolism is often seen in patients with severe memory impairment, including MCI and other amnesic disorders (48,80–82). Depending on subject selection, it may also have prognostic impact. A longitudinal study of cognitively normal subjects indicated that cognitive decline to MCI within three years, follow-up is related to metabolic reductions in entorhinal cortex at entry, independent of ε4 status (83). Progression to dementia usually is associated with additional metabolic impairment in temporoparietal and posterior cingulate cortex (82,84).

Nondemented patients with MCI may already show the metabolic impairment of association cortices that is characteristic of AD. MCI patient groups when compared to normal controls typically show significantly impaired metabolism (24,33). In our multicenter database (85), about one-third of patients clinically diagnosed as having MCI have significant metabolic impairment of association cortex. Severe impairment was observed in one subject with a presenilin-1 mutation (A431V) who clinically still was at the MCI stage of AD (86).

Data are accumulating that the presence of the AD metabolic pattern in MCI predicts conversion to clinical dementia of Alzheimer type, and therefore indicates "incipient AD." The predictive power of posterior cingulate metabolic impairment was documented by Minoshima and colleagues as early as 1997 (24). We studied 31 patients with cognitive deficits, mostly limited to the memory domain, with Mini-Mental State Examination (MMSE) scores of 24 or higher and not yet fulfilling the criteria of probable AD. They were therefore diagnosed as "possible AD," and most of these patients would have fulfilled the criteria of MCI (which were not yet used by us at that time). We found that 60–70% of those patients who already had moderate or severe metabolic impairment of association cortices in FDG PET declined on MMSE by three points or more within two years (mostly leading to clinical dementia), whereas only 10–20% of patients without such metabolic impairment had that decline (87). Similar conversion rates (seven of 10 within three years in subjects with abnormal metabolism, three of 10 with normal lCMRglc) were reported by Berent et al. (88). In a three-year follow-up study of 20 MCI patients, Arnaiz et al. (89) observed nine converters. The two variables that most effectively predicted future development of AD were lCMRglc from the left temporoparietal area and performance on the block design. These combined measures gave an optimal 90% correct classification rate, whereas only lCMRglc or neuropsychology alone gave 75% and 65% correct classification, respectively. In a one-year study of 22 patients, eight converters had reduced lCMRglc in PCC (compared to normal controls and non-converters) and temporoparietal cortex (32). After one year, additional bilateral reduction of lCMRglc in prefrontal areas along with a further progression of the abnormalities in the parietal and posterior cingulate cortex was observed in converters, whereas non-converters had unchanged metabolism. Among 17 patients followed for 18 months, seven converters had significantly lower lCMRglc in right temporoparietal cortex than non-converters (90). In a recent study, Anchisi et al. (91) have demonstrated that by neuropsychological testing alone one can identify subjects who are likely not to progress to dementia because their memory deficit is relatively mild, thus providing a high negative predictive value with regard to progression. However, prediction based on neuropsychological testing is less reliable for MCI patients with severe memory impairment. In these patients, FDG PET adds significant information by separating those who will progress within the next from those who will remain stable.

Few studies so far compared FDG PET with other biomarkers. The combination with ApoE ε4 has been addressed by Mosconi et al. (92) in 37 patients who were followed over one year. There were eight converters, and inferior parietal cortex lCMRglc predicted conversion with 84% accuracy, compared to 62% prediction accuracy of ε4 status. PET prediction accuracy was best (94%) within the ε4-positive group. In a series of 30 patients who were followed over 16 months, the positive and negative predictive values of FDG PET for progression to AD were 85% and 94%, respectively, whereas corresponding values for the ApoE4 genotype were 53% and 77% only (93). By combination of the two indicators, predictive values increased to 100% in subgroups of patients with concurrent genetic and metabolic findings. When comparing phosphorylated tau protein in CSF with FDG PET in MCI, Fellgiebl et al. found similar findings with both tests (94). Seven of 16 patients had increased phosphorylated tau levels, and six of them also had AD-typical FDG PET findings.

CLINICAL DIAGNOSTIC USE OF ^{18}F-2-FLUORO-2-DEOXY-D-GLUCOSE POSITRON EMISSION TOMOGRAPHY IN ALZHEIMER'S DISEASE

FDG PET is an expensive procedure, but with its broader use mainly in oncology, costs for the tracer and scanning have been declining from initial levels of several thousand dollars and are now in the order of US $1000 or even lower in some places. There have been model calculations indicating that it could be cost efficient under certain circumstances (95), but studies do not yet fulfill generally accepted standards. Although the promise of FDG PET in clinical diagnosis was recognized by the Quality Standards Subcommittee of the American Academy of Neurology (96) and other professional organizations (97,98), its routine use had not been recommended until 2004 in most countries. Meanwhile, the US Medicare and Medicaid services refund FDG PET studies in dementia if certain conditions are met, including difficulty of clinical diagnosis because of atypical cause or presentation and FDG PET (99). Similar regulations are active in Switzerland, whereas many other countries do not yet have obligatory refunding regulations.

DEMENTIA WITH LEWY BODIES

Patients with dementia with Lewy bodies (DLB) often clinically have fluctuating levels of attention and consciousness, visual hallucinations, and may develop the motor features of Parkinson's disease (100,101). Reduced FDG uptake is found to be very similar to AD, but also in primary visual cortex which is usually spared in AD (Fig. 3) (102–105). The impairment of glucose metabolism in visual cortex may well be the correlate of the impairment of visual processing and visual hallucinations. The diagnostic reliability of the finding is not yet clear and could potentially be confounded by reduced occipital FDG uptake secondary to vision impairment. Another characteristic finding in DLB is the reduction of F-18-DOPA uptake in the putamen that has been described in DLB (106,107) but is absent in AD (108).

FRONTOTEMPORAL DEMENTIA

Frontotemporal dementia (FTD) is characterized clinically by leading changes in personality and behavior, such as apathy or disinhibition, whereas memory impairment may be absent or less prominent (109). In practice, FTD is readily identified on FDG PET scans by a distinct frontal or frontotemporal metabolic

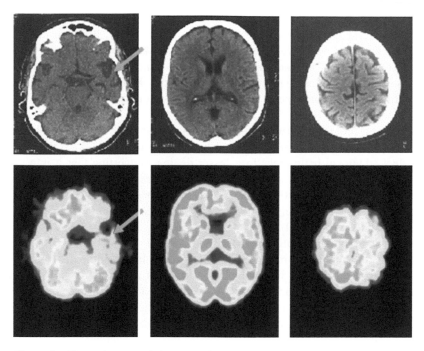

Figure 3 (*See color insert.*) Asymmetric frontotemporal atrophy and metabolic impairment in frontotemporal dementia.

impairment that typically is quite asymmetrically centered in frontolateral cortex and the anterior pole of the temporal lobe from where it may extend to other association areas (110–113). Mesial frontal metabolic impairment can be found in nearly every case of FTD (114). Apathy was found to be associated with a prevalent dorsolateral and frontal medial hypometabolism, whereas disinhibition demonstrated a more severe hypometabolism in limbic structures (115). Frequently there is also unilateral focal atrophy of the frontal and temporal lobe corresponding to the metabolic deficit.

Automatic methods have been explored in order to distinguish between FTD and AD. An analysis using multivariate methods such as principal components analysis and partial least squares regression achieved over 90% accuracy in a sample of 48 patients (116). Preliminary results of a prospective study indicated that FDG PET may be more accurate than clinical judgment in predicting histopathological diagnosis (117). This discrimination is of primary interest in dementia patients with presenile onset, whereas there may be substantial overlap of the FTD pattern with frontotemporal impairment and the AD pattern with predominant temporoparietal impairment, especially in senile dementia patients (118).

Semantic dementia is usually regarded as a variant of FTD with similar histopathological features and tau protein deposition (119). Its main clinical symptoms are the progressive inability to comprehend common concepts, often associated with fluent aphasia, but there are less emotional disturbances and repetitive, compulsive behaviors than in FTD (120). Metabolic impairment is similar to FTD (121) but appears to be more focused on the left temporal rather than the frontal lobes (122).

Primary progressive (non-fluent) aphasia is another related syndrome associated with left frontal and temporal hypometabolism (123–127) that may also affect additional brain areas to a lesser degree, suggesting that it is not a strictly focal impairment. A similar condition also seems to exist for the right hemisphere, clinically consisting of progressive prosopagnosia (128). Some cases seem to be histopathologically related to FTD, whereas others may represent a posterior variant of AD (129).

FTD can be differentiated from corticobasal degeneration with predominant parietal metabolic reduction (130), although histopathological features may overlap (131). Frontal metabolic impairment is also part of many other diseases and conditions, including progressive supranuclear palsy (in combination with midbrain impairment) (132), spinocerebellar atrophy (133), and cocaine abuse (134). Moderate frontal dysfunction and hypometabolism is also observed in many psychiatric disorders, and therefore cannot be regarded as a specific diagnostic feature.

VASCULAR DEMENTIA

Diagnosis of vascular dementia (VaD) is easily made in the case of multiple cortical infarcts multi-infarct dementia, but may be a difficult issue in cases with severe microvascular changes but without major cortical infarcts. There is currently no consensus about clinical criteria, and correspondence between existing criteria (e.g., ICD-10, DSM-IV, NINDS-AIREN, CAMDEX) is poor (135,136). Several studies have suggested that a diffuse global reduction of cerebral glucose metabolism is a typical finding in VaD (Fig. 4), and that the degree of that reduction in association cortex is similar to that seen in AD (137,138). In cases without gross cortical infarcts, the effects of WML are generalized and frontal hypometabolism correlates with memory and global impairment, cognitive as well as executive function. The effects of subcortical cerebrovascular disease appear to converge on the frontal lobes but are diffuse, complex, and of modest magnitude (139). Thus, the contrast between metabolic impairment in association areas and preserved metabolism in primary areas, basal ganglia, and cerebellum, which is typical for AD but not for VaD, seems to provide some distinction with FDG PET between these two types of dementia (137). Only large white matter lesions may cause moderate focal reductions of overlying cortical blood flow and metabolism (140), and it therefore is likely that presence of the typical metabolic AD pattern in demented patients with multiple deep white matter lesions does

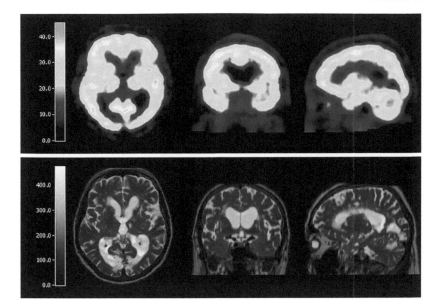

Figure 4 *(See color insert.)* Global reduction of cerebral glucose metabolism in vascular dementia.

indicate that this is predominant AD rather than VaD (141). However, a definitive distinction between VaD and AD or the relative importance of vascular and Alzheimer-type lesions in patients who have signs of both often remains uncertain, even after autopsy and histopathological examination (see Chapter 11).

VaD may also be caused by strategic infarcts in structures that are essential for integrating higher cognitive functions, especially the thalamus. Even small thalamic lesions may lead to considerable deactivation of cortex, as demonstrated by FDG PET (142–144).

CREUTZFELDT–JAKOB DISEASE

Clinically, this disease is characterized by rapidly progressive dementia, often accompanied by insomnia, myoclonus, and other extrapyramidal disorders. In all cases reported so far, cerebral glucose metabolism was severely reduced in a multifocal fashion (145–149).

SUMMARY

Imaging cerebral glucose metabolism with PET has a proven potential for early diagnosis of AD at the clinical stage of MCI. The typical regional pattern of metabolic impairment differs between major neurodegenerative diseases that may cause dementia. Thus, FDG PET also has the potential to improve early and differential diagnosis, and it may be used to monitor disease progression and treatment effects. Because of its widespread use in oncology it is now available in most major hospitals. Due to its high cost it can currently not be recommended as a routine diagnostic tool, but PET continues playing a major role in clinical and scientific studies and as a supplementary diagnostic test in selected cases.

REFERENCES

1. Phelps ME, Hoffman EJ, Coleman RE, et al. Tomographic images of blood pool and perfusion in brain and heart. J Nucl Med 1976; 17:603–612.
2. Valk PE, Pounds TR, Tesar RD, Hopkins DM, Haseman MK. Cost-effectiveness of PET imaging in clinical oncology. Nucl Med Biol 1996; 23:737–743.
3. Herholz K, Herscovitch P, Heiss WD. NeuroPET. Berlin/Heidelberg/New York: Springer, 2004.
4. Gatley SJ. Estimation of upper limits on human radiation absorbed doses from carbon-11-labeled compounds. J Nucl Med 1993; 34:2208–2215.
5. Reivich M, Kuhl D, Wolf A, et al. The [18F]fluorodeoxyglucose method for the measurement of local cerebral glucose utilization in man. Circ Res 1979; 44:127–137.
6. Hamacher K, Coenen HH, Stocklin G. Efficient stereospecific synthesis of no-carrier-added 2-[18F]-fluoro-2-deoxy-D-glucose using aminopolyether supported nucleophilic substitution. J Nucl Med 1986; 27:235–238.
7. Sokoloff L, Reivich M, Kennedy C, et al. The [14C]deoxyglucose method for the measurement of local cerebral glucose utilization: theory, procedure, and normal values in the conscious and anesthetized albino rat. J Neurochem 1977; 28:897–916.
8. Wienhard K, Pawlik G, Herholz K, Wagner R, Heiss WD. Estimation of local cerebral glucose utilization by positron emission tomography of [18F]2-fluoro-2-deoxy-D-glucose: a critical appraisal of optimization procedures. J Cereb Blood Flow Metab 1985; 5:115–125.
9. Bartenstein P, Asenbaum S, Catafau A, et al. European association of nuclear medicine procedure guidelines for brain imaging using [18F]FDG. Eur J Nucl Med Mol Imaging 2002; 29:BP43–BP48.
10. Zundorf G, Kerrouche N, Herholz K, Baron JC. An efficient principal component analysis for multivariate 3D voxel-based mapping of brain functional imaging data sets as applied to FDG-PET and normal aging. Hum Brain Mapp 2003; 18:13–21.
11. Phelps ME, Kuhl DE, Mazziotta JC. Metabolic mapping of the brain's response to visual stimulation: studies in humans. Science 1981; 211:1445–1448.
12. Benson DF, Kuhl DE, Hawkins RA, Phelps ME, Cummings JL, Tsai SY. The fluorodeoxyglucose 18F scan in Alzheimer's disease and multi- infarct dementia. Arch Neurol 1983; 40:711–714.
13. DeLeon MJ, Ferris SH, George AE, et al. Computed tomography and positron emission transaxial tomography evaluations of normal aging and Alzheimer's disease. J Cereb Blood Flow Metab 1983; 3:391–394.

14. Foster NL, Chase TN, Fedio P, Patronas NJ, Brooks RA, Di Chiro G. Alzheimer's disease: focal cortical changes shown by positron emission tomography. Neurology 1983; 33:961–965.

15. Friedland RP, Budinger TF, Ganz E, et al. Regional cerebral metabolic alterations in dementia of the Alzheimer type: positron emission tomography with [18F]fluorodeoxyglucose. J Comput Assist Tomogr 1983; 7:590–598.

16. Chase TN, Foster NL, Fedio P, Brooks R, Mansi L, Di Chiro G. Regional cortical dysfunction in Alzheimer's disease as determined by positron emission tomography. Ann Neurol 1984; 15:S170–S174.

17. Haxby JV, Grady CL, Koss E, et al. Heterogeneous anterior-posterior metabolic patterns in dementia of the Alzheimer type. Neurology 1988; 38:1853–1863.

18. Grady CL, Haxby JV, Schapiro MB, et al. Subgroups in dementia of the Alzheimer type identified using positron emission tomography. J Neuropsychiatry Clin Neurosci 1990; 2:373–384.

19. Salmon E, Sadzot B, Maquet P, et al. Differential diagnosis of Alzheimer's disease with PET. J Nucl Med 1994; 35:391–398.

20. Kuhl DE, Metter EJ, Riege WH, Phelps ME. Effects of human aging on patterns of local cerebral glucose utilization determined by the [18F]fluorodeoxyglucose method. J Cerebral Blood Flow Metab 1982; 2:163–171.

21. Moeller JR, Ishikawa T, Dhawan V, et al. The metabolic topography of normal aging. J Cereb Blood Flow Metab 1996; 16:385–398.

22. Petit-Taboue MC, Landeau B, Desson JF, Desgranges B, Baron JC. Effects of healthy aging on the regional cerebral metabolic rate of glucose assessed with statistical parametric mapping. Neuroimage 1998; 7:176–184.

23. Herholz K, Salmon E, Perani D, et al. Discrimination between Alzheimer dementia and controls by automated analysis of multicenter FDG PET. Neuroimage 2002; 17:302–316.

24. Minoshima S, Giordani B, Berent S, Frey KA, Foster NL, Kuhl DE. Metabolic reduction in the posterior cingulate cortex in very early Alzheimer's disease. Ann Neurol 1997; 42:85–94.

25. Valla J, Berndt JD, Gonzalez-Lima F. Energy hypometabolism in posterior cingulate cortex of Alzheimer's patients: superficial laminar cytochrome oxidase associated with disease duration. J Neurosci 2001; 21:4923–4930.

26. Gusnard DA, Raichle ME, Raichle ME. Searching for a baseline: functional imaging and the resting human brain. Nat Rev Neurosci 2001; 2:685–694.

27. Signorini M, Paulesu E, Friston K, et al. Rapid assessment of regional cerebral metabolic abnormalities in single subjects with quantitative and nonquantitative [18F]FDG PET: a clinical validation of statistical parametric mapping. Neuroimage 1999; 9:63–80.

28. Friston KJ. Imaging cognitive anatomy. Trends Cogn Sci 1997; 1:21–27.

29. Minoshima S, Koeppe RA, Frey KA, Kuhl DE. Anatomic standardization: linear scaling and nonlinear warping of functional brain images. J Nucl Med 1994; 35:1528–1537.

30. Minoshima S, Frey KA, Koeppe RA, Foster NL, Kuhl DE. A diagnostic approach in Alzheimer's disease using three- dimensional stereotactic surface projections of fluorine-18-FDG PET. J Nucl Med 1995; 36:1238–1248.

31. Ishii K, Willoch F, Minoshima S, et al. Statistical brain mapping of 18F-FDG PET in Alzheimer's disease: validation of anatomic standardization for atrophied brains. J Nucl Med 2001; 42:548–557.

32. Drzezga A, Lautenschlager N, Siebner H, et al. Cerebral metabolic changes accompanying conversion of mild cognitive impairment into Alzheimer's disease: a PET follow-up study. Eur J Nucl Med Mol Imaging 2003; 30:1104–1113.

33. Ishii K, Mori T, Hirono N, Mori E. Glucose metabolic dysfunction in subjects with a clinical dementia rating of 0.5. J Neurol Sci 2003; 215:71–74.

34. Azari NP, Pettigrew KD, Schapiro MB, et al. Early detection of Alzheimer's disease: a statistical approach using positron emission tomographic data. J Cereb Blood Flow Metab 1993; 13:438–447.

35. Kippenhan JS, Barker WW, Nagel J, Grady C, Duara R. Neural-network classification of normal and Alzheimer's disease subjects using high-resolution and low-resolution PET cameras. J Nucl Med 1994; 35:7–15.

36. Sayeed A, Petrou M, Spyrou N, Kadyrov A, Spinks T. Diagnostic features of Alzheimer's disease extracted from PET sinograms. Phys Med Biol 2002; 47:137–148.

37. Higdon R, Foster NL, Koeppe RA, et al. A comparison of classification methods for differentiating fronto-temporal dementia from Alzheimer's disease using FDG-PET imaging. Stat Med 2004; 23:315–326.

38. Silverman DH, Small GW, Chang CY, et al. Positron emission tomography in evaluation of dementia: regional brain metabolism and long-term outcome. JAMA 2001; 286:2120–2127.

39. Kuhl DE, Metter EJ, Riege WH, Markham CH. Patterns of cerebral glucose utilization in Parkinson's disease and Huntington's disease. Ann Neurol 1984; 15:S119–S125.

40. Schapiro MB, Pietrini P, Grady CL, et al. Reductions in parietal and temporal cerebral metabolic rates for glucose are not specific for Alzheimer's disease. J Neurol Neurosurg Psychiatry 1993; 56:859–864.

41. Eidelberg D, Moeller JR, Ishikawa T, et al. Early differential diagnosis of Parkinson's disease with 18F-fluorodeoxyglucose and positron emission tomography. Neurology 1995; 45:1995–2004.

42. Hilker R, Voges J, Thiel A, et al. Deep brain stimulation of the subthalamic nucleus versus levodopa challenge in Parkinson's disease: measuring the on- and off-conditions with FDG-PET. J Neural Transm 2002; 10:1257–1264.

43. Hejl A, Hogh P, Waldemar G. Potentially reversible conditions in 1000 consecutive memory clinic patients. J Neurol Neurosurg Psychiatry 2002; 73:390–394.

44. Grady CL, Haxby JV, Horwitz B, Berg G, Rapoport SI. Neuropsychological and cerebral metabolic function in early vs late onset dementia of the Alzheimer type. Neuropsychologia 1987; 25:807–816.

45. Mielke R, Herholz K, Grond M, Kessler J, Heiss WD. Differences of regional cerebral glucose metabolism between presenile and senile dementia of Alzheimer type. Neurobiol Aging 1992; 13:93–98.

46. Mosconi L, Herholz K, Prohovnik I, et al. Metabolic interaction between ApoE genotype and onset age in Alzheimer's disease: implications for brain reserve. J Neurol Neurosurg Psychiatry 2005; 76:15–23.

47. Ishii K, Sasaki M, Yamaji S, Sakamoto S, Kitagaki H, Mori E. Relatively preserved hippocampal glucose metabolism in mild Alzheimer's disease. Dement Geriatr Cogn Disord 1998; 9:317–322.
48. Mosconi L, Tsui WH, DeSanti S, et al. Reduced hippocampal metabolism in MCI and AD: automated FDG-PET image analysis. Neurology, 2005; In press.
49. Mosconi L, Pupi A, De Cristofaro MT, Fayyaz M, Sorbi S, Herholz K. Functional interactions of the entorhinal cortex: an 18F-FDG PET study on normal aging and Alzheimer's disease. J Nucl Med 2004; 45:382–392.
50. Stein DJ, Buchsbaum MS, Hof PR, Siegel BV, Jr., Shihabuddin L. Greater metabolic rate decreases in hippocampal formation and proisocortex than in neocortex in Alzheimer's disease. Neuropsychobiology 1998; 37:10–19.
51. Desgranges B, Baron JC, Giffard B, et al. The neural basis of intrusions in free recall and cued recall: a PET study in Alzheimer's disease. Neuroimage 2002; 17:1658–1664.
52. Meltzer CC, Zubieta JK, Brandt J, Tune LE, Mayberg HS, Frost JJ. Regional hypometabolism in Alzheimer's disease as measured by positron emission tomography after correction for effects of partial volume averaging. Neurology 1996; 47:454–461.
53. Ibanez V, Pietrini P, Alexander GE, et al. Regional glucose metabolic abnormalities are not the result of atrophy in Alzheimer's disease. Neurology 1998; 50:1585–1593.
54. Yanase D, Matsunari I, Yajima K, et al. Brain FDG PET study of normal aging in Japanese: effect of atrophy correction. Eur J Nucl Med Mol Imaging 2005; epub.
55. Toga AW, Mazziotta JC, Frackowiak RSJ. Brain Mapping: The Disorders. San Diego: Academic Press, 2000.
56. Herholz K, Schopphoff H, Schmidt M, et al. Direct comparison of spatially normalized PET and SPECT scans in Alzheimer disease. J Nucl Med 2002; 43:21–26.
57. Messa C, Perani D, Lucignani G, et al. High-resolution technetium-99m-HMPAO SPECT in patients with probable Alzheimer's disease: comparison with fluorine-18-FDG PET. J Nucl Med 1994; 35:210–216.
58. Powers WJ, Perlmutter JS, Videen TO, et al. Blinded clinical evaluation of positron emission tomography for diagnosis of probable Alzheimer's disease. Neurology 1992; 42:765–770.
59. Koeppe RA, Gilman S, Joshi A, et al. 11C-DTBZ and 18F-FDG PET measures in differentiating dementias. J Nucl Med 2005; 46:936–944.
60. Jagust WJ, Friedland RP, Budinger TF, Koss E, Ober B. Longitudinal studies of regional cerebral metabolism in Alzheimer's disease. Neurology 1988; 38:909–912.
61. Mielke R, Herholz K, Grond M, Kessler J, Heiss WD. Clinical deterioration in probable Alzheimer's disease correlates with progressive metabolic impairment of association areas. Dementia 1994; 5:36–41.
62. Smith GS, de Leon MJ, George AE, et al. Topography of cross-sectional and longitudinal glucose metabolic deficits in Alzheimer's disease. Pathophysiologic implications. Arch Neurol 1992; 49:1142–1150.
63. Grady CL, Haxby JV, Schlageter NL, Berg G, Rapoport SI. Stability of metabolic and neuropsychological asymmetries in dementia of the Alzheimer type. Neurology 1986; 36:1390–1392.

64. Haxby JV, Grady CL, Koss E, et al. Longitudinal study of cerebral metabolic asymmetries and associated neuropsychological patterns in early dementia of the Alzheimer type. Arch Neurol 1990; 47:753–760.
65. Heiss WD, Hebold I, Klinkhammer P, et al. Effect of piracetam on cerebral glucose metabolism in Alzheimer's disease as measured by positron emission tomography. J Cerebral Blood Flow Metab 1988; 8:613–617.
66. Mielke R, Kittner B, Ghaemi M, et al. Propentofylline improves regional cerebral glucose metabolism and neuropsychologic performance in vascular dementia. J Neurol Sci 1996; 141:59–64.
67. Mega MS, Cummings JL, O'Connor SM, et al. Cognitive and metabolic responses to metrifonate therapy in Alzheimer disease. Neuropsychiatry Neuropsychol Behav Neurol 2001; 14:63–68.
68. Blin J, Ivanoiu A, De Volder A, et al. Physostigmine results in an increased decrement in brain glucose consumption in Alzheimer's disease. Psychopharmacology (Berl) 1998; 136:256–263.
69. Szelies B, Herholz K, Pawlik G, Beil C, Wienhard K, Heiss WD. [Cerebral glucose metabolism in presenile dementia of the Alzheimer type—follow-up of therapy with muscarinergic choline agonists] [German]. Fortschritte der Neurologie-Psychiatrie 1986; 54:364–373.
70. Potkin SG, Anand R, Fleming K, et al. Brain metabolic and clinical effects of rivastigmine in Alzheimer's disease. Int J Neuropsychopharmacol 2001; 4:223–230.
71. Mega MS, Dinov ID, Porter V, et al. Metabolic patterns associated with the clinical response to galantamine therapy: a fludeoxyglucose F 18 positron emission tomographic study. Arch Neurol 2005; 62:721–728.
72. Alexander GE, Chen K, Pietrini P, Rapoport SI, Reiman EM, Longitudinal PET. Evaluation of cerebral metabolic decline in dementia: a potential outcome measure in Alzheimer's disease treatment studies. Am J Psychiatry 2002; 159:738–745.
73. Small GW, Mazziotta JC, Collins MT, et al. Apolipoprotein E type 4 allele and cerebral glucose metabolism in relatives at risk for familial Alzheimer disease. JAMA 1995; 273:942–947.
74. Reiman EM, Caselli RJ, Yun LS, et al. Preclinical evidence of Alzheimer's disease in persons homozygous for the epsilon 4 allele for apolipoprotein E. N Engl J Med 1996; 334:752–758.
75. Reiman EM, Chen K, Alexander GE, et al. Functional brain abnormalities in young adults at genetic risk for late-onset Alzheimer's dementia. Proc Natl Acad Sci USA 2004; 101:284–289.
76. Small GW, Ercoli LM, Silverman DH, et al. Cerebral metabolic and cognitive decline in persons at genetic risk for Alzheimer's disease. Proc Natl Acad Sci USA 2000; 97:6037–6042.
77. Reiman EM, Caselli RJ, Chen K, Alexander GE, Bandy D, Frost J. Declining brain activity in cognitively normal apolipoprotein E epsilon 4 heterozygotes: a foundation for using positron emission tomography to efficiently test treatments to prevent Alzheimer's disease. Proc Natl Acad Sci USA 2001; 98:3334–3339.
78. Mielke R, Zerres K, Uhlhaas S, Kessler J, Heiss WD. Apolipoprotein E polymorphism influences the cerebral metabolic pattern in Alzheimer's disease. Neurosci Lett 1998; 254:49–52.

79. Mosconi L, Nacmias B, Sorbi S, et al. Brain metabolic decreases related to the dose of the ApoE e4 allele in Alzheimer's disease. J Neurol Neurosurg Psychiatry 2004; 75:370–376.

80. Perani D, Bressi S, Cappa SF, et al. Evidence of multiple memory systems in the human brain. A [18F]FDG PET metabolic study. Brain 1993; 116:903–919.

81. Heiss WD, Pawlik G, Holthoff V, Kessler J, Szelies B. PET correlates of normal and impaired memory functions. Cerebrovasc Brain Metab Rev 1992; 4:1–27.

82. Nestor PJ, Fryer TD, Smielewski P, Hodges JR. Limbic hypometabolism in Alzheimer's disease and mild cognitive impairment. Ann Neurol 2003; 54:343–351.

83. de Leon MJ, Convit A, Wolf OT, et al. Prediction of cognitive decline in normal elderly subjects with 2-F-18-fluoro-2-deoxy-D-glucose positron-emission tomography (FDG PET). Proc Natl Acad Sci USA 2001; 98:10966–10971.

84. De Santi S, de Leon MJ, Rusinek H, et al. Hippocampal formation glucose metabolism and volume losses in MCI and AD. Neurobiol Aging 2001; 22:529–539.

85. Herholz K. PET studies in dementia. Ann Nucl Med 2003; 17:79–89.

86. Matsushita S, Arai H, Okamura N, et al. Clinical and biomarker investigation of a patient with a novel presenilin-1 mutation (A431V) in the mild cognitive impairment stage of Alzheimer's Disease. Biol Psychiatry 2002; 52:907–910.

87. Herholz K, Nordberg A, Salmon E, et al. Metabolic impairment of association cortex predicts progression in Alzheimer's disease: a prospective multicenter positron emission tomography (PET) study. Eur J Neurol 1998; 5:S24.

88. Berent S, Giordani B, Foster N, et al. Neuropsychological function and cerebral glucose utilization in isolated memory impairment and Alzheimer's disease. J Psychiatr Res 1999; 33:7–16.

89. Arnaiz E, Jelic V, Almkvist O, et al. Impaired cerebral glucose metabolism and cognitive functioning predict deterioration in mild cognitive impairment. Neuroreport 2001; 12:851–855.

90. Chetelat G, Desgranges B, de la Sayette V, Viader F, Eustache F, Baron JC. Mild cognitive impairment: Can FDG-PET predict who is to rapidly convert to Alzheimer's disease? Neurology 2003; 60:1374–1377.

91. Anchisi D, Borroni B, Francheschi M, et al. Heterogeneity of glucose brain metabolism in mild cognitive impairment predicts clinical progression to Alzheimer's disease. Arch Neurol, 2005; 62:1728–1733.

92. Mosconi L, Perani D, Sorbi S, et al. MCI conversion to dementia and the APOE genotype: A prediction study with FDG-PET. Neurology 2004; 63:2332–2340.

93. Drzezga A, Grimmer T, Riemenschneider M, et al. Prediction of individual clinical outcome in MCI by means of genetic assessment and FDG-PET imaging. J Nucl Med 2005; 46:1625–1632.

94. Fellgiebel A, Siessmeier T, Scheurich A, et al. Association of elevated phospho-tau levels with Alzheimer-typical 18F-Fluoro-2-Deoxy-D-Glucose positron emission tomography findings in patients with mild cognitive impairment. Biol Psychiatry 2004; 56:279–283.

95. Silverman DH, Gambhir SS, Huang HW, et al. Evaluating early dementia with and without assessment of regional cerebral metabolism by PET: a comparison of predicted costs and benefits. J Nucl Med 2002; 43:253–266.

96. Knopman DS, DeKosky ST, Cummings JL, et al. Practice parameter: diagnosis of dementia (an evidence-based review). Report of the quality standards sub-committee of the American academy of neurology. Neurology 2001; 56:1143–1153.
97. Deutsche Gesellschaft fur Psychiatrie, Psychotherapie and Nervenheilkunde. Behandlungsleitlinie Demenz. Steinkopff: Darmstadt, 2000.
98. Forstl H, Herholz K, Lang C, et al. Diagnostik degenerativer Demenzen (Morbus Alzheimer-Demenz, Frontotemporale Demenz, Lewy-Koerperchen-Demenz). In: Diener HC, ed. Leitlinien fuer Diagnostik und Therapie in der Neurologie. 3rd ed. Stuttgart: Thieme, 2005.
99. Society of Nuclear Medicine Summary of Coverage Criteria/Guidelines for AD and FTD PET Studies Effective September 15, 2004. Soc Nucl Med 2004.
100. Perry RH, Irving D, Blessed G, Fairbairn A, Perry EK. Senile dementia of Lewy body type. A clinically and neuropathologically distinct form of Lewy body dementia in the elderly. J Neurol Sci 1990; 95:119–139.
101. Verghese J, Crystal HA, Dickson DW, Lipton RB. Validity of clinical criteria for the diagnosis of dementia with Lewy bodies. Neurology 1999; 53:1974–1982.
102. Ishii K, Imamura T, Sasaki M, et al. Regional cerebral glucose metabolism in dementia with Lewy bodies and Alzheimer's disease. Neurology 1998; 51:125–130.
103. Higuchi M, Tashiro M, Arai H, et al. Glucose hypometabolism and neuropathological correlates in brains of dementia with Lewy bodies. Exp Neurol 2000; 162:247–256.
104. Minoshima S, Foster NL, Sima AA, Frey KA, Albin RL, Kuhl DE. Alzheimer's disease versus dementia with Lewy bodies: cerebral metabolic distinction with autopsy confirmation. Ann Neurol 2001; 50:358–365.
105. Mirzaei S, Knoll P, Koehn H, Bruecke T. Assessment of diffuse Lewy body disease by 2-[18F]fluoro-2-deoxy-D-glucose positron emission tomography (FDG PET). BMC Nucl Med 2003; 3:1.
106. Hu XS, Okamura N, Arai H, et al. 18F-fluorodopa PET study of striatal dopamine uptake in the diagnosis of dementia with lewy bodies. Neurology 2000; 55:1575–1577.
107. Hisanaga K, Suzuki H, Tanji H, et al. Fluoro-DOPA and FDG positron emission tomography in a case of pathologically verified pure diffuse lewy body disease. J Neurol 2001; 248:905–906.
108. Tyrrell PJ, Sawle GV, Ibanez V, et al. Clinical and positron emission tomographic studies in the 'extrapyramidal syndrome' of dementia of the Alzheimer type. Arch Neurol 1990; 47:1318–1323.
109. Neary D, Snowden JS, Gustafson L, et al. Frontotemporal lobar degeneration: a consensus on clinical diagnostic criteria. Neurology 1998; 51:1546–1554.
110. Kamo H, McGeer PL, Harrop R, et al. Positron emission tomography and histopathology in Pick's disease. Neurology 1987; 37:439–445.
111. Friedland RP, Koss E, Lerner A, et al. Functional imaging, the frontal lobes, and dementia. Dementia 1993; 4:192–203.
112. Jauss M, Herholz K, Kracht L, et al. Frontotemporal dementia: clinical, neuroimaging, and molecular biological findings in 6 patients. Eur Arch Psychiatry Clin Neurosci 2001; 251:225–231.

113. Grimmer T, Diehl J, Drzezga A, Forstl H, Kurz A. Region-specific decline of cerebral glucose metabolism in patients with frontotemporal dementia: a prospective 18F-FDG-PET study. Dement Geriatr Cogn Disord 2004; 18:32–36.

114. Salmon E, Garraux G, Delbeuck X, et al. Predominant ventromedial frontopolar metabolic impairment in frontotemporal dementia. Neuroimage 2003; 20:435–440.

115. Franceschi M, Anchisi D, Pelati O, et al. Glucose metabolism and serotonin receptors in the frontotemporal lobe degeneration. Ann Neurol 2005; 57:216–225.

116. Higdon R, Foster NL, Koeppe RA, et al. A comparison of classification methods for differentiating fronto-temporal dementia from Alzheimer's disease using FDG-PET imaging. Stat Med 2004; 23:315–326.

117. Foster NL, Barbas NR, Heidebrink JL, et al. Adding FDG-PET to clinical history and examination improves the accuracy of dementia diagnosis. Neurobiol Aging 2004; 25:372.

118. Herholz K, Salmon E, Perani D, Holthoff VA, Pupi A, Heiss WD. Prospective multicenter study of the discrimination between dementia of Alzheimer and frontotemporal type by automatic pattern detection on FDG PET scans. J Nucl Med 2004; 45:66.

119. Kertesz A, Munoz D. Pick's disease, frontotemporal dementia, and pick complex: emerging concepts. Arch Neurol 1998; 55:302–304.

120. Hodges JR, Patterson K, Oxbury S, Funnell E. Semantic dementia. Progressive fluent aphasia with temporal lobe atrophy. Brain 1992; 115:1783–1806.

121. Ibach B, Poljansky S, Marienhagen J, Sommer M, Manner P, Hajak G. Contrasting metabolic impairment in frontotemporal degeneration and early onset Alzheimer's disease. Neuroimage 2004; 23:739–743.

122. Diehl J, Grimmer T, Drzezga A, Riemenschneider M, Forstl H, Kurz A. Cerebral metabolic patterns at early stages of frontotemporal dementia and semantic dementia. A PET study. Neurobiol Aging 2004; 25:1051–1056.

123. Chawluk JB, Mesulam MM, Hurtig H, et al. Slowly progressive aphasia without generalized dementia: studies with positron emission tomography. Ann Neurol 1986; 19:68–74.

124. De Oliveira SA, Castro MJ, Bittencourt PR. Slowly progressive aphasia followed by Alzheimer's dementia: a case report. Arq Neuropsiquiatr 1989; 47:72–75.

125. Kempler D, Metter EJ, Riege WH, Jackson CA, Benson DF, Hanson WR. Slowly progressive aphasia: three cases with language, memory, CT and PET data. J Neurol Neurosurg Psychiatry 1990; 53:987–993.

126. Cappa SF, Perani D, Messa C, Miozzo A, Fazio F. Varieties of progressive non-fluent aphasia. Ann N Y Acad Sci 1996; 777:243–248.

127. Nagy TG, Jelencsik I, Szirmai I. Primary progressive aphasia: a case report. Eur J Neurol 1999; 6:515–519.

128. Tyrrell PJ, Warrington EK, Frackowiak RS, Rossor MN. Progressive degeneration of the right temporal lobe studied with positron emission tomography. J Neurol Neurosurg Psychiatry 1990; 53:1046–1050.

129. Nestor PJ, Caine D, Fryer TD, Clarke J, Hodges JR. The topography of metabolic deficits in posterior cortical atrophy (the visual variant of Alzheimer's disease) with FDG-PET. J Neurol Neurosurg Psychiatry 2003; 74:1521–1529.

130. Hosaka K, Ishii K, Sakamoto S, et al. Voxel-based comparison of regional cerebral glucose metabolism between PSP and corticobasal degeneration. J Neurol Sci 2002; 199:67–71.

131. Feany MB, Mattiace LA, Dickson DW. Neuropathologic overlap of progressive supranuclear palsy, Pick's disease and corticobasal degeneration. J Neuropathol Exp Neurol 1996; 55:53–67.

132. Karbe H, Grond M, Huber M, Herholz K, Kessler J, Heiss WD. Subcortical damage and cortical dysfunction in progressive supranuclear palsy demonstrated by positron emission tomography. J Neurol 1992; 239:98–102.

133. Soong B, Liu R, Wu L, Lu Y, Lee H. Metabolic characterization of spinocerebellar ataxia type 6. Arch Neurol 2001; 58:300–304.

134. Volkow ND, Hitzemann R, Wang GJ, et al. Long-term frontal brain metabolic changes in cocaine abusers. Synapse 1992; 11:184–190.

135. Erkinjuntti T, Ostbye T, Steenhuis R, Hachinski V. The effect of different diagnostic criteria on the prevalence of dementia. N Engl J Med 1997; 337:1667–1674.

136. Chui HC, Mack W, Jackson JE, et al. Clinical criteria for the diagnosis of vascular dementia: a multicenter study of comparability and interrater reliability. Arch Neurol 2000; 57:191–196.

137. Mielke R, Herholz K, Grond M, Kessler J, Heiss WD. Severity of vascular dementia is related to volume of metabolically impaired tissue. Arch Neurol 1992; 49:909–913.

138. Sultzer DL, Mahler ME, Cummings JL, Van Gorp WG, Hinkin CH, Brown C. Cortical abnormalities associated with subcortical lesions in vascular dementia. Clinical and position emission tomographic findings. Arch Neurol 1995; 52:773–780.

139. Reed BR, Eberling JL, Mungas D, Weiner M, Kramer JH, Jagust WJ. Effects of white matter lesions and lacunes on cortical function. Arch Neurol 2004; 61:1545–1550.

140. Herholz K, Heindel W, Rackl A, et al. Regional cerebral blood flow in patients with leuko-araiosis and atherosclerotic carotid artery disease. Arch Neurol 1990; 47:392–396.

141. Mendez MF, Ottowitz W, Brown CV, Cummings JL, Perryman KM, Mandelkern MA. Dementia with leukoaraiosis: clinical differentiation by temporoparietal hypometabolism on (18)FDG-PET imaging. Dement Geriatr Cogn Disord 1999; 10:518–525.

142. Szelies B, Herholz K, Pawlik G, Karbe H, Hebold I, Heiss WD. Widespread functional effects of discrete thalamic infarction. Arch Neurol 1991; 48:178–182.

143. Baron JC, Levasseur M, Mazoyer B, et al. Thalamocortical diaschisis: positron emission tomography in humans. J Neurol Neurosurg Psychiatry 1992; 55:935–942.

144. Pappata S, Mazoyer B, Tran Dinh S, Cambon H, Levasseur M, Baron JC. Effects of capsular or thalamic stroke on metabolism in the cortex and cerebellum: a positron tomography study. Stroke 1990; 21:519–524.

145. Holthoff VA, Sandmann J, Pawlik G, Schroder R, Heiss WD. Positron emission tomography in Creutzfeldt-Jakob disease. Arch Neurol 1990; 47:1035–1038.

146. Goldman S, Laird A, Flament-Durand J, et al. Positron emission tomography and histopathology in Creutzfeldt- Jakob disease. Neurology 1993; 43:1828–1830.

147. Ogawa T, Inugami A, Fujita H, et al. Serial positron emission tomography with fludeoxyglucose F 18 in Creutzfeldt-Jakob disease. AJNR Am J Neuroradiol 1995; 16:978–981.
148. Matochik JA, Molchan SE, Zametkin AJ, Warden DL, Sunderland T, Cohen RM. Regional cerebral glucose metabolism in autopsy-confirmed Creutzfeldt-Jakob disease. Acta Neurologica Scandinavica 1995; 91:153–157.
149. Engler H, Lundberg PO, Ekbom K, et al. Multitracer study with positron emission tomography in Creutzfeldt-Jakob disease. Eur J Nucl Med Mol Imaging 2003; 30:85–95.

9

Imaging of Neurotransmitter Systems in Dementia

Steen G. Hasselbalch

*Neurobiology Research Unit and Memory Disorders Research Group,
Copenhagen University Hospital, Rigshospitalet, Copenhagen, Denmark*

Gitte M. Knudsen

*Neurobiology Research Unit, Copenhagen University Hospital,
Rigshospitalet, Copenhagen, Denmark*

INTRODUCTION

Chemical neurotransmission as a tool for cell communication in the human brain relies on the interaction of neurotransmitters acting on their target receptors. At the moment, over 100 neurotransmitters with 300 corresponding receptors have been identified. Malfunction of some of these neurotransmitter systems in degenerative disorders may provide part of the pathophysiological basis for the varying symptomatology found in these disorders.

Animal models, peripheral measures of receptors, neurotransmitters and their metabolites, and clinical effects of neuropharmacological treatment are crucial to improving our understanding of the underlying pharmacology involved in aging and cognitive dysfunction. As opposed to these indirect approaches, molecular imaging of the neurotransmitter systems with positron emission tomography (PET) or single photon emission computed tomography (SPECT) is able to characterize the functional state of human central receptor systems in vivo. PET is a powerful technique for investigating human brain physiology and pathophysiology. When used with appropriate radioligands, PET can reveal the distribution of neuroreceptors in the living human brain, and their interactions with neurotransmitters or administered drugs. PET radioligands suitable for these purposes give large signals that are quantifiable in terms of robust measures of regional receptor concentration. They should also be selective and sensitive to occupancy of receptors by administered psychoactive drugs, and some of them are even sensitive to competition with an endogenously released neurotransmitter. Though some receptors have been imaged successfully with PET, many others lack effective radioligands. An overview of published data on some radiopharmaceuticals that with reasonable success have been applied in humans is given in Table 1.

Table 1 Examples of Ligands Used for Neuroreceptor Imaging in Humans

Transmitter involved	Target	Examples of ligands
Monoamines	Vesicular monoamine transporter 2	$(+)^{11}$C-DTBZ
	Monoamine oxidase A	^{11}C-clorgyline
	Monoamine oxidase B	^{11}C-L-deprenyl
Dopamine	Dopa synthesis	^{18}F-dopa
	Dopamine reuptake site	^{11}C-CFT
		^{123}I-PE2I/^{11}C-PE2I
	D1	^{11}C-NNC112
		^{11}C-SCH23390
		$[^{11}$C]-NNC 756
	D2-like	^{11}C-raclopride
		^{123}I-IBZM
Serotonin	Serotonin synthesis	^{11}C-5-hydroxytryptophan
	Serotonin reuptake site	^{11}C-DASB
	5HT$_{1A}$	^{11}C-WAY-100635
	5HT$_{2A}$	^{11}C-MDL100907
		^{18}F-altanserin
		^{123}I-R91150
Acetylcholine	Vesicular acetylcholine transporter	^{123}I-IBVM
	Cholinesterase activity	^{11}C-MP4A
		^{11}C-PMP
	Muscarinic	^{11}C-NMPB
		^{11}C-TRB
	M2 selective	^{18}F-FP-TZTP
	Nicotinic	^{11}C-nicotine
	α4β2	6-^{18}Fluoro-A-85380
Opioid	Mu	^{11}C-carfentanyl
	Mu/delta/kappa	^{11}C-diprenorphine
Histamine	H1	^{11}C-pyrilanine
		^{11}C-doxepine
GABA	α1	^{11}C-flumazenil
		^{123}I-iomazenil
	α5	^{11}C-Ro154513
Glutamate	NMDA	^{11}C-MK801
Microglia activation	τ_3-benzodiazepine	^{11}C-PK 11195

Molecular imaging is likely to provide a better insight into the malfunction of the different transmitter systems, and at some point it may also lend itself to detection of gene expression and monitoring of gene therapy, thereby holding a promising potential for future research areas with the ultimate goal to better understand and treat the underlying pathophysiology in different neuro-degenerative disorders.

The interaction between the functioning receptor systems render it likely that the affection of one transmitter system is associated with malfunction of other receptor systems. Very little is, however, known about such interactions and their impact for the clinical picture of different neurodegenerative disorders.

In the following, a review of neurotransmitter dysfunction in the most prevalent dementia disorders will be given. We focus on Alzheimer's disease (AD), but will briefly touch upon dementia with Lewy bodies (DLB) and frontotemporal dementia (FTD). Neurotransmitter imaging shows great potential in diagnosing Parkinson's disease (PD) and related disorders. Although several of these movement disorders are associated with cognitive dysfunction, they fall outside the scope of this chapter. In the daily clinical practice, differential diagnosis between primary neurodegenerative diseases and cognitive dysfunction due to cerebrovascular disease is often difficult, and clinical application of neurotransmitter imaging will also briefly be touched upon.

NORMAL AGING

Although the amount of receptors varies considerably between individuals (1) it is well established that a number of different receptor systems decline with age—frequently at a rate that varies between the different brain areas. This has been demonstrated both in postmortem human and in brain imaging studies.

Postmortem studies have shown a loss of dopamine transporters amounting to 5–7% per decade in striatum (2) and that dopaminergic D_1 and D_2 receptors in striatum also decline with age (3). These findings have been corroborated in imaging studies where van Dyck et al. found a 6.6% decrease per decade in striatal dopamine transporters (Fig. 1) (4), and postsynaptically, dopamine D_1 and D_2 receptors in the same areas seem to decrease at the same rate (5,6).

For the serotonergic system, postmortem studies showed evidence for a decrease in $5\text{-}HT_{2A}$ receptor binding with age (7). A gender-specific effect of age on $5\text{-}HT_{1A}$ receptor density was initially reported with an inverse relationship between $5\text{-}HT_{1A}$ receptor density and age in men, but not in women (8). PET data from a large sample of healthy control subjects have, however, not been able to confirm this finding, and the density of $5\text{-}HT_{1A}$ receptors seemed to be remarkably constant within the age span from 23 to 54 years (9). Neocortical $5\text{-}HT_{2A}$ receptor binding, by contrast, was found to decline by 6% per decade in a large group of healthy controls aged between 21 and 79 years (Fig. 2) (10), corroborating previous findings in a smaller sample (11).

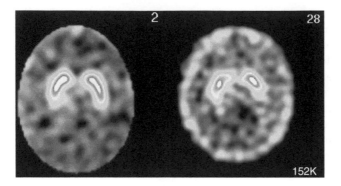

Figure 1 (*See color insert.*) Loss of dopamine transporters with age. Dopamine transporters measured using SPECT and [^{123}I]-PE2I in a 21-year-old healthy male (*left*) and in a 70-year-old healthy male (*right*). *Source*: Courtesy of the Neurobiology Research Unit, Copenhagen, Denmark.

For the glutamatergic NMDA receptor complex a similar decrease has been reported in postmortem frontal cortex (12,13). Since no appropriate glutamatergic PET tracers are available yet, imaging data cannot add any further information.

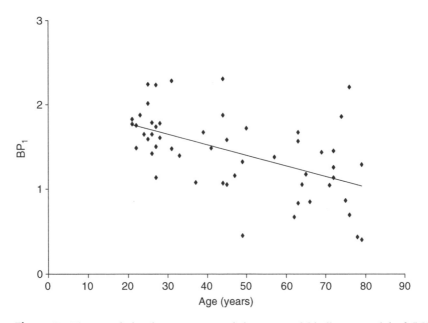

Figure 2 The correlation between age and the averaged binding potential of 5-HT$_{2A}$ receptors for all cortical brain regions (measured with PET and [^{18}F]-altanserin in healthy controls). The regression coefficient corresponds to an average decrease of 5-HT$_{2A}$ receptors of about 6% per decade. *Source*: From Ref. 10.

Postmortem data have shown a significant decrease in M1 and M2 receptors as well as in nicotinic receptors in the cerebral cortex (14,15), whereas one PET study using [18]FP-TZTP as a selective ligand for the M2 receptor found a higher binding throughout the brain in older controls as compared to younger controls (16). One possible explanation for this could be a lower concentration of acetylcholine in the synapse in older controls. Data have been less consistent for the presynaptic marker choline acetyltransferase (ChAT) that catalyzes the biogenesis of acetylcholine (17,18). Thus in general, it seems that several—but not all—receptor systems decline with age, but the rate of decline varies between systems. Further, within one system it may also differ between different brain regions, which necessitates a close matching between control and patient groups. Event though most imaging studies so far have not taken into account that brain atrophy associated with age invariably will be associated with the so-called partial volume effect and thereby a tendency for underestimation of the receptor binding in a given brain region, the decrease in receptor binding with age is not explained fully by these effects.

ALZHEIMER'S DISEASE

The earliest and most prominent symptom of AD is problems with episodic memory due to failure of learning and retention of new material. Therefore neurotransmitter systems involved in memory processes, such as the cholinergic system, have generally been studied in more detail than other systems, although lack of specific ligands for this system have hampered in vivo imaging data. However, behavioural and neuropsychiatric symptoms are frequently occurring in the course of AD, and even extrapyramidal symptoms are encountered in the disease, sometimes rendering a firm diagnosis difficult. One of the purposes of past and recent neurotransmitter imaging studies has been to aid clinicians in improving diagnostic accuracy by revealing disease-specific neurotransmitter changes in the most prevalent neurodegenerative disorders, including AD. Another purpose has been to better understand the pathophysiology behind certain symptoms with the ultimate goal of improving treatment. In the following, only receptor systems considered of importance for AD are included. A summary of these main findings is given in Table 2. Data based both on postmortem studies and in vivo emission tomography studies will be reviewed and the potential impact of disturbances within the receptor systems discussed.

Cholinergic Transmitter System

The most prominent and specific neurotransmitter deficit in AD is found in the cholinergic system. According to current concepts, cholinergic neurons are involved in specific forms of attention, thereby serving a modulatory function in cognition by optimizing cortical information processing (47). Cholinergic receptors comprise transmitter-gated ion channels [nicotinic acetylcholine

Table 2 Single Photon Emission Computed Tomography and Positron Emission Tomography Neuroreceptor Studies in Alzheimer's Disease

Receptor system	Number of controls	Number of patients	Ligand	Results	Author
Cholinergic					
Muscarinic receptors	11	14	[^{123}I]-QNB	↓	Weinberger 1991 (19)
	4	8	[^{123}I]-QNB	↔ (↓)	Wyper 1993 (20)
	5	5	[^{123}I]-IDEX	↓	Claus 1997 (21)
	18	18	[^{11}C]-NMPB	↓	Yoshida 1998 (22)
	18	6	[^{11}C]-NMPB	↔	Zubieta 2001 (23)
Cholinergic					
Nicotinic receptors	3	8	[^{11}C]-nicotine	↓ (high affinity)	Nordberg 1995 (24)
Cholinergic					
Acetylcholin-esterase	8	5	[^{11}C]-MP4A	↓	Iyo 1997 (25)
	4	4	[^{11}C]-MP4A	↓	Herholz 2000 (26)
	14	28	[^{11}C]-MP4A	↓	Shinotoh 2000 (27)
	26	14	[^{11}C]-PMP	↓	Kuhl DE 1999 (28)
GABAergic					
GABA$_A$ receptors (central benzodiazepine receptors)	5	6	[^{123}I]-iomazenil	↓	Soricelli 1996 (29)
	4	8	[^{123}I]-iomazenil	↓	Fukuchi 1997 (30)
	6	13	[^{11}C]-flumazenil	↔	Meyer 1995 (31)
	5	5	[^{11}C]-flumazenil	↔	Ohyama 1999 (32)

Serotonergic					
5-HT$_{2A}$ receptors	37	9	[^{11}C]-setoperone	→	Blin 1993 (33)
	10	9	[^{18}F]-altanserin	→	Meltzer 1999 (34)
	26	9	[^{123}I]-R91150	→	Versijpt 2003 (35)
Glutamatergic					
NMDA receptors	5	5	[^{11}C]-MK 801	(↑)	Brown 1997 (36)
Microglia marker (peripheral benzodiazepine receptors)	8	8	[^{11}C]-PK11195	↔	Groom 1995 (37)
	15	8	[^{11}C]-PK11195	←	Cagnin 2001 (38)
	9	10	[^{123}I]-PK11195	←	Versijpt 2003 (39)
Dopaminergic					
D2 (striatum)	9	15	[^{123}I]-IBZM	→	Pizzolato 1996 (40)
	10	10	[^{11}C]-raclopride	↔	Kemppainen 2000 (41)
	5	10	[^{11}C]-raclopride	→	Tanaka 2003 (42)
D2(D3) (hippocampus)	11	14	[^{11}C]-FLB 457	→	Kemppainen 2003 (43)
Dopaminergic					
D1 (striatum)	8	10	[^{11}C]-NNC 756	→	Kemppainen 2000 (41)
Dopaminergic					
DAT	12	15	[^{18}F]-dopa	↔	Tyrrell 1990 (44)
	15	12	[^{11}C]-betaCFT	→	Rinne 1998 (45)
	33	34	[^{123}I]-FP-CIT	↔	O'Brien 2004 (46)

receptors (nAChR)] and G protein-coupled muscarinic acetylcholine receptors (mAChR), which are located both presynaptically and postsynaptically. nAChRs belong to a superfamily of homologous receptors including GABA, glycine, and 5-HT$_3$ receptors. Each nAChR consists of five membrane spanning subunits arranged around an aqueous channel in the center. So far, nine different types have been identified and cloned (48). In vitro studies of human autopsy brain tissue suggest heterogeneity regarding nAChRs which can be rationalized into three different types of binding sites: super-high, high, and low affinity sites corresponding to the $\alpha 3$, $\alpha 4$, and $\alpha 7$ subunits (15,49,50). The nAChRs are expressed in low density in the human brain, as compared to the muscarinic receptors. The distribution of nAChRs is relatively homogenous and not restricted to defined cholinergic pathways, although it is more dense in some brain regions including thalamus, cortex, and basal ganglia. Nicotinic receptors are distributed to influence many neurotransmitter systems at more than one location, and the broad, but sparse, cholinergic innervation throughout the brain enables nAChRs to become important modulators of neuronal excitability (51). An abundant amount of research has provided evidence that the nAChRs are involved in several important functional processes including cognition, learning, memory, and arousal (52). Substantial evidence also indicates the involvement of the nicotinic cholinergic system in the pathology of AD (53). Drugs targeting these sites may not only have a positive effect on cognitive function, but also have additional therapeutic benefits in terms of restoring the hypoactivity in the excitatory amino acid pyramidal system and even slowing the emergence of AD pathology.

Nicotinic Receptors

A consistent and severe loss of nicotinic receptors in AD was reported in early postmortem studies (54,55). The major loss in cortical nAChRs in AD appears to occur in the $\alpha 4$-$\beta 2$ nAChR subtype (56), and a study on nAChR expression in the frontal and temporal cortex of AD patients has demonstrated that both the numbers of $\alpha 4$- and $\alpha 7$-immunoreactive neurons and the quantitative amount, in particular of the $\alpha 4$ protein, are markedly decreased in AD (57).

Until recently only one tracer ligand was available for PET studies, namely ^{11}C-nicotine (58). ^{11}C-nicotine imaging suffers from high nonspecific binding and rapid metabolism; but even so, ^{11}C-nicotine binding seems to agree well with the distribution of nAChR observed in vitro in human postmortem brain tissue (24,59,60). Significant reductions in ^{11}C-nicotine binding were found in AD patients in frontal and temporal cortices and in hippocampus when compared to age-matched controls, and the changes were associated with cognitive function (24,61). ^{11}C-nicotine-PET has also been used to evaluate the effect of cholinergic drug treatment: after three months of treatment with the AChE inhibitor tacrine, the binding of ^{11}C-nicotine was increased in temporal cortex in AD patients (61) suggesting a restoration of nAChR with treatment, which may explain part of the therapeutic benefit of AChE inhibitors (62). Recent reports point towards the $\alpha 7$

subtype as a target for specific amyloid binding (63), but at present there are no suitable tracers available for in vivo imaging of this subtype. Recently, radiohalogenated analogs of 3-(2(S)-azetidinylmethoxy)pyridine (A-85380) were used successfully for the in vivo visualization of alpha4beta2 nicotinic receptors in the human brain with PET/SPECT (64), but so far, data for 6-^{18}F-fluoro-A-85380 PET imaging in AD are still missing.

Muscarinic Receptors

Although some biopsy and autopsy studies point to nAChR as the receptor subtype most affected in AD with relative sparing of the mAChR subtype (55,65), a selective loss of the subtype M2 compared to M1 has been shown (66,67). Recent studies suggesting a role for muscarinic agonists in regulating the production of Aβ-amyloid raise the possibility that selective M1 agonists could be useful in treating not only the symptoms, but also the underlying cause(s) of AD. Unfortunately, due to several methodological problems, imaging of mAChR has so far revealed contradictory results, and has not been able to demonstrate the selective loss of M2 as compared to M1 receptors obtained from postmortem studies. Using non-selective M1/M2 mACh receptor tracers, PET and SPECT studies have rather consistently shown a reduction in mAChR in AD (19–22). Thus, using ^{11}C-NMPB and PET, Yoshida et al. found significant reductions in mAChR binding in the parietal cortex of AD patients as compared to controls. However, taking some of several methodological problems into account, Zubieta et al. could not demonstrate a reduction in mAChR in six mild to moderate AD patients (23). In healthy *APOE* ε4-positive subjects, a higher M2 receptor binding as assessed with ^{18}F-TZTP PET has been demonstrated as compared to *APOE* ε4-negative subjects, presumably because of a lower synaptic concentration of acetylcholine in these individuals (16). So far, no studies have been conducted with selective muscarinic tracers in AD, but future studies should reveal mAChR subtypes are differentially affected in vivo in AD.

Choline Acetyltransferase and Acetylcholinesterase

Marked reductions in the enzymes ChAT and acetylcholinesterase (AChE) and cholinergic neuronal loss have been reported in postmortem studies as well as in biopsies from AD brains, and this cholinergic dysfunction correlates with the cognitive function (65,68,69). Currently, there are no tracers to map the key cholinergic enzyme ChAT, but AChE tracers are in use. Pappata et al. used a labeled inhibitor of AChE (^{11}C-physostigmine) in normal subjects to demonstrate tracer distribution corresponding to that found in postmortem studies (70). The PET tracer ^{11}C-MP4A serves as an in vivo AChE substrate so that the local rate of radiotracer hydrolysis can be followed by PET. Based on this methodology, AChE levels were reported to be decreased by 30–40%, especially in temporoparietal regions in 1997 by Iyo et al. (25), and this finding was later confirmed by Kuhl and coworkers using ^{11}C-PMP in patients with mild to moderate AD (28). These data agreed with earlier postmortem data with regard to normal relative cerebral distributions, absence of large age-effect in normal aging, and deficits in AD (see above). AChE activity has, however, been found to be more globally reduced in the brain in contrast to the more selective reductions in CMRGlc and CBF in the temporoparietal association areas (Fig. 3) (26). Further, Kuhl et al. demonstrated a 50% displacement of the radiolabeled ligand following acute treatment with physostigmine, suggesting that this tracer can be used to assess the efficacy of AChE inhibitors which currently are the most widely used drugs in AD (28). Using the same method as Iyo et al. Shinotoh et al. found significantly reduced AChE activity in neocortex, hippocampus, and amygdala in 28 AD patients (71). In seven of these patients where PET scans were repeated after two years, a progressive loss of AChE activity was found (27). Thus, PET studies using AChE tracers might be used to evaluate and monitor the concentration of AChE in AD patients, thereby assessing drug efficacy objectively. In particular, the objective demonstration of a lack of efficacy of AChE inhibitors in some patients and in different disease severity states could be useful knowledge to guide the clinician.

Elucidation of whether AChE acting drugs applied in AD exert their effect by an inhibitory activity on AChE or by other complex actions may be investigated by following the pharmacokinetics of the drug in the target organ by PET. [11C]N-methyl-labeled tacrine (MTHA) has for example been shown to cross the blood-brain barrier easily in healthy human volunteers and to be highly concentrated in the brain, though the regional brain distribution of [11C]MTHA does not correspond to that of in vivo AChE concentrations (72).

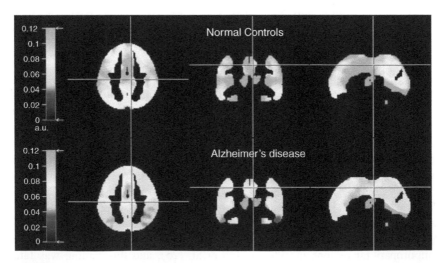

Figure 3 (*See color insert.*) Acetylcholinesterase activity in the central nervous system evaluated with C11-MP4A. *Source*: From Ref. 26.

Central Benzodiazepine Receptor Imaging

The central benzodiazepine receptor (BZR) is part of the major inhibitory neurotransmitter system γ-aminobutyric acid (GABA$_A$) receptor complex. GABA$_A$ is widely expressed in cortical neurons, and is considered a marker for neuronal integrity and viability.

Although one study found a modest 22% reduction in frontal cortex (73), most postmortem studies have found GABA$_A$ receptor subtypes relatively preserved in the hippocampus in AD patients in different disease stages, despite marked loss of neurons in this area (74,75). On the other hand, SPECT studies using [I-123]labeled iomazenil have shown reduced cortical BZR in temporo-parietal areas (76,77), and iomazenil may even be a more sensitive marker for cortical dysfunction than the cerebral blood flow tracer [Tc-99m]HMPAO (30,78). In contrast, a PET and [C-11]-flumazenil study by Meyer et al. showed relatively preserved benzodiazepine binding sites in AD (31). In a later PET-flumazenil study it was also found that the BZR reduction was less prominent than the CBF suppression as measured by [15-O]H$_2$O (32). The apparent discrepancy between the PET and SPECT results of BZRs may be caused by differences in the two tracers, and at this time it is not clear whether the moderate reductions in BZR density is more sensitive or specific than conventional cerebral blood flow imaging in the differential diagnosis between different degenerative disorders.

Serotonergic Transmitter System

Animal and human studies suggest that serotonin (5-HT) is linked to many functions, such as cognition, body temperature, hormonal release, mood, aggression, feeding, and sleep. Modulation for cholinergic neuronal activity by 5-HT may play a role in higher cognitive processes such as memory and learning. 5-HT$_{1A}$ receptor antagonism appears to enhance activation and signaling through neuronal circuits known to be involved in cognitive processes (79). There is also substantial evidence from postmortem studies on human brain, clinical pharmacology, animals studies, and recently PET studies in humans to implicate this transmitter in several major neuropsychiatric disorders, including depression (80). This observation is of contextual interest because depression is commonly seen in AD patients and may further interfere with cognitive function. The relationship between dementia and depression in elderly people is incompletely understood and probably complex. A large fraction of elderly depressives have evidence of significant cognitive dysfunction, which may be reversible ("pseudodementia"). On the other hand, depression may be the initial sign of a neurodegenerative disease and is known to constitute a nearly five-fold increased risk for later development of dementia (81), and depression complicates AD in about one-fifth of patients (82).

In postmortem frontal cortical brain samples it has been found that serotonin levels correlate negatively and 5-HT$_{1A}$ receptor density correlates positively with the rate of cognitive decline in patients with AD (83). By contrast, in younger individuals with major depressive disorder, a PET study has revealed a more widespread reduction in 5-HT_{1A} receptor binding (80).

The 5-HT_{2A} receptors are highly expressed in neocortex but less so in limbic cortex and basal ganglia (84). 5-HT_{2A} receptors are also associated with cholinergic nerve terminals in the cerebral cortex and hippocampus. In a postmortem study of hippocampus receptor binding, the largest decrease was found for 5-HT_2 binding, with N-methyl-D-aspartate (including glutamate, phencyclidine, and glycine binding sites), quisqualate, kainic acid, adenosine A1, benzodiazepine, 5-HT_1, muscarinic cholinergic, beta-adrenergic, neurotensin, and opioid receptors showing parallel but less pronounced reductions in binding (85). Bowen et al. also showed that 5-HT_1 and 5-HT_2 receptors (7,86) and serotonin reuptake sites (87) were decreased in postmortem AD studies with 5-HT_{2A} receptors preferentially affected over 5-HT_{1A} receptors (86,88). Using ^{18}F-setoperone and PET in moderately to severely demented AD patients, Blin et al. demonstrated large reductions in 5-HT_{2A} receptor binding in frontal, temporal, parietal, and occipital cortices (33). This finding was corroborated in a more recent study by Meltzer et al. (34). They studied 5-HT_{2A} receptor binding using ^{18}F-altanserin in patients with depression and in patients with mild to moderate AD, including three with concurrent depression, and compared these results to age-matched controls after controlling for partial volume effects. No differences were, however, found between AD patients with and without depression, but the limited sample size prevented any examination of relations between neuropsychiatric symptoms and 5-HT_{2A} receptor binding. Likewise, using SPECT in nine AD patients, Versijpt et al. found a generally decreased 5-HT_{2A} receptor density in the orbitofrontal, prefrontal, lateral frontal, cingulate, sensorimotor, parietal inferior, and occipital regions (35). In very early AD (mild cognitive impairment of the amnestic type), reduction in 5-HT_{2A} density has been demonstrated, suggesting that the 5-HT_{2A} receptors are affected early in the course of the disease (Hasselbalch et al., unpublished data).

The 5-HT_4 receptor is highly expressed in cortex and hippocampus and seems to enhance memory formation through its action on cholinergic neurons (89). One postmortem study found significant reductions of 5-HT_4 receptors in hippocampus (67%), and smaller reductions in the neocortex in postmortem AD brains (90), whereas another study did not find 5-HT_4 receptor density affected in the frontal and temporal cortex in AD (91).

A more widespread decrease in 5-HT transporter sites was also found in brain tissue from AD patients with depressive symptoms as compared to AD patients without depressive symptoms (92).

In conclusion, both postmortem and imaging studies have consistently found evidence for serotonergic dysfunction in AD with 5-HT_{2A} receptors most prominently affected. Although there is substantial evidence for a serotonergic dysfunction in AD, no PET studies have so far addressed the relationship between on one hand the serotonergic system, and on the other hand neuropsychiatric and behavioral symptoms in AD. In particular, the question of to what extent deficits in serotonergic function are linked to coexisting depression in AD needs to be clarified in larger human studies.

Peripheral Benzodiazepine Receptor Imaging

It is well established that glial cells play an important role during injury and neurodegenerative processes in the central nervous system. There is no global glial proliferation in normal aging, but reactive gliosis has been described in specific areas of the limbic system and neocortex in non-demented elderly persons. In contrast to the relatively moderate overall glial changes in normal aging, the close association of activated astrocytes and microglial cells with neuritic plaques and cells undergoing neurofibrillary degeneration in AD, the expression of receptors for complement by glial cells, and the release of soluble cytokines strongly suggest that inflammatory processes may play an important part in the complex pathophysiological interactions that occur in AD (93). Visualization of the extent of microgliosis in age-associated neurodegenerative disorders may provide new tools to detect and monitor the disease process. In an early report on the peripheral BZR ligand PK11195, it was concluded that the peripheral BZR binding sites associated with microgliosis and cellular inflammation in AD at postmortem are undetectable by PET using ^{11}C-PK-11195 in patients with mild to moderate dementia (37). A more recent paper did, however, possibly due to improvements in quantification methods and in scanner sensitivity, show an increased binding in the entorhinal cortex, temporoparietal, and cingulate (94). Further evidence for increased microgliosis in AD was obtained recently by a SPECT study using ^{123}I-iodo-PK11195, where significant increases were found in frontal and mesotemporal cortex in AD (39). Whether ^{11}C-PK11195 turns out to be specific enough for the diagnosis of early AD and whether it holds potential as a prognostic tool still needs to be clarified.

Dopaminergic Transmitter System

Dopamine is well known as a neurotransmitter with an important regulatory role for motor and limbic functions. It may, however, also be involved in cognition and attentional processes, and since it is considered a key neuroregulator in behavioral adaptation (95), alterations in the dopaminergic transmission could, therefore, be associated with cognitive disturbances.

Postmortem receptor studies have generally failed to show any changes in D1, D2, or D3 receptors in AD (96–98). In patients with combined AD and Lewy body pathology or with significant extrapyramidal symptoms, however, D1 receptors are upregulated, whereas D2 receptors are downregulated (96,98). In a PET study of mild to moderate AD patients with only mild extrapyramidal symptoms, Kemppainen et al. found a selective loss of D1 receptors in striatum, whereas D2 receptor density was unchanged (41). Also, in AD patients without overt extrapyramidal symptoms, SPECT scanning showed a significant reduction in striatal D2-like receptors as compared to healthy controls (40), suggesting that the dopamine system may be affected in AD patients without clinical signs of motor abnormalities. The role of dopamine in neuropsychiatric symptoms in AD has also been explored. Using ^{11}C-raclopride and PET, Tanaka et al. found that striatal D_2 receptor density correlated inversely with behavioral symptoms in severely affected AD patients (42). Further, in AD patients with psychotic symptoms, D3 receptors have, in postmortem tissue, been found to be upregulated as compared to AD patients without psychosis (98). Finally, an implication of the dopamine system in cognitive function was suggested by Kemppainen et al., who found a bilateral reduction in hippocampal D_2/D_3 receptor density in AD patients which correlated positively with memory performance (43).

In a postmortem study by the same group, Kemppainen and co-workers found a 30–50% reduction in the number of dopamine transporters in the striatum of patients dying of, or with, AD (2), with the putamen being more severely affected as compared to normal aging, where dopamine transporter density in the caudate nucleus seemed to decline more rapidly with age. By contrast, in a PET study, Rinne et al. found a less pronounced decline (20%) in putamen and caudate dopamine transporter density in AD patients (45), even though the same tracer was used. Interestingly, the reduction in [11C]beta-CFT uptake correlated with the severity of the extrapyramidal symptoms of the patients. In another PET study of presynaptic dopaminergic function (striatal dopa synthesis measured by ^{18}F-dopa), no significant differences were found in AD patients with rigidity as compared to healthy controls (44).

Thus, part of the apparently contradicting data obtained from postmortem studies and the few PET studies may be explained by the clinical classification of patients and differences in the severity of extrapyramidal and behavioral symptoms in the AD groups. Further, at the moment it is not clear whether significant dopaminergic dysfunction exists in early "pure AD," and if so, whether the profile of this dysfunction differs from that of DLB.

LEWY BODY DEMENTIA

Core symptoms of DLB consist of a mixed cortical/subcortical dementia, extrapyramidal symptoms, a fluctuating course with episodes of disturbed consciousness, and recurrent detailed visual hallucinations (99). Because differential diagnosis between DLB and AD can be difficult, neuroimaging may be of importance by increasing the diagnostic accuracy of these disorders. Due to the nature of the symptoms in DLB, several studies have looked for dysfunction in the dopaminergic system, but also profound changes in the cholinergic system have been demonstrated.

Neurochemically, the decline of cholinergic (ChAT) activity has been shown to be greater than that of AD (100) and to occur early in the course of the disease (101). As in AD, loss of nAChR occurs in parietal cortex, but in contrast to AD, loss of nAChR is also evident in putamen, probably reflecting loss of nicotinic receptors from dopaminergic neuronal projections to striatum as found in PD (102).

In a postmortem study comparing AD, DLB, and PD, Piggott et al. found dopamine transporter activity reduced by 57% in DLB, by 75% in PD, and normal in AD when compared to controls (97). Further, D_2 receptor density was more reduced in striatum in DLB than in PD, whereas D_1 and D_3 receptor density was unchanged. Similarly, in AD patients additional Lewy body pathology has been associated with decreases in D_2 and D_3 receptor density (97). Some of these findings have been corroborated in SPECT and PET studies. Using the dopamine transporter ligand ^{123}I-FP-CIT and SPECT, significantly lower uptake in striatum has been found in DLB and PD when compared to AD and to controls (103,104). Using the same tracer, similar findings were obtained by O'Brien et al. (46), but they also demonstrated a more uniform tracer distribution in striatum in DLB as compared to PD (Fig. 4). Likewise, in a PET study Hu et al. found pronounced

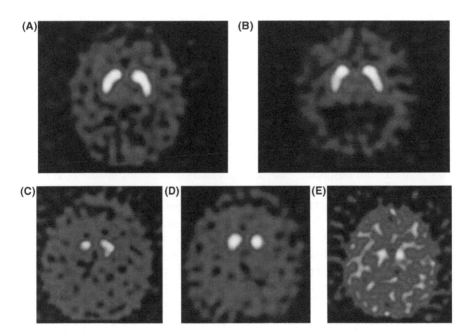

Figure 4 (*See color insert.*) Dopamine transporter loss visualized with FP-CIT SPECT in the differential diagnosis of dementia with Lewy bodies (DLB). Reductions in FP-CIT binding occurred in the caudate and anterior and posterior putamens in subjects with DLB compared with subjects with Alzheimer's disease and controls. Transporter loss in DLBs was of similar magnitude to that seen in Parkinson's disease (PD), while the greatest loss in all three areas was seen in those who had PD and dementia. In Parkinson's disease, there was a greater selective reduction in putamen uptake compared with DLB and PD and dementia. *Source*: From Ref. 46.

reductions in striatal ^{18}F-dopa uptake in moderately demented DLB patients when compared to moderate AD (105). Using a tracer that binds to the presynaptic monoamine vesicular transporter, Gilman et al. found striatal mean binding potential decreased by 45% to 67% in a group of DLB patients, as compared to both controls and AD patients (106). Interestingly, in a few AD patients binding values were below the range of the controls, and in one of these patients autopsy showed neuropathological features of both DLB and AD, although the patient had no extrapyramidal symptoms (Fig. 4). In line with this, the PET study by Rinne et al. suggests that decreases in striatal dopamine transporter density correlate with the severity of extrapyramidal symptoms (45), perhaps due to concomitant Lewy body pathology in AD patients. Studying postsynaptic D2 receptor density in striatum with IBZM-SPECT, similar reductions were found in DLB and AD when compared to controls; although the reduction was somewhat more pronounced in DLB, a considerable overlap between AD and DLB was found (107). These few neuroimaging studies suggest that presynaptic dopamine imaging might prove useful in the differential diagnosis between AD and DLB, and that imaging may be sensitive to Lewy body pathology already in the very early stages of the disease.

FRONTOTEMPORAL DEMENTIA

With regard to neuroreceptor imaging, FTD is the least studied progressive neurodegenerative disorder. Furthermore, FTD comprise a group of disorders with different neuropathological findings, and therefore neurochemical post-mortem studies might reflect this heterogeneity.

In a postmortem study of 16 FTD patients (10 Pick pathology patients, and six patients with unspecific changes), cholinergic activity (measured as ChAT activity and M1 receptors) was not significantly reduced in cortical areas in FTD as compared to controls (108). This data supports the empirical clinical finding of no effect of cholinergic drugs in FTD. By contrast, in the same study both 5-HT$_{1A}$ and 5-HT$_{2A}$ receptors were reduced in temporal and frontal cortices in FTD as compared to controls. Interestingly, serotonergic receptors were also lost in AD, but only in temporal and parietal areas. Thus, there might be regional differences in the serotonergic dysfunction in FTD and AD, but whether imaging of serotonergic receptors might be helpful in the differential diagnosis remains to be settled, since no imaging studies have explored this possibility.

Since extrapyramidal symptoms are relatively common in FTD, the expected dopaminergic dysfunction has indeed been supported by one post-mortem study in which neuronal loss in the substantia nigra was found (109). In familial FTD with parkinsonism due to a mutation in chromosome 17, one SPECT study (110) and one PET study (111) have found evidence for a reduced dopamine transporter binding. In the latter study, striatal D2 receptors were preserved much in line with what is found in PD. In a ^{11}C-CFT PET study, dopamine transporter binding was reduced by 18% and 14% in putamen and in

(A) **(B)**

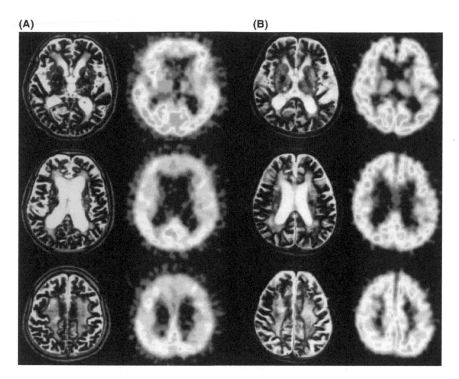

Figure 5 (*See color insert.*) Differences in cortical GABA$_A$ receptor density between patients with leukoaraiosis and dementia (**A**) and patients with leukoaraiosis without dementia (**B**), indicating that severe white matter ischemic lesions may cause cortico-subcortical disruption, which may augment cognitive dysfunction. *Source*: From Ref. 116.

caudate, and the reductions correlated with extrapyramidal symptoms (112). In the differential diagnosis between AD, DLB, and FTD, these findings suggest that dopamine transporter imaging might not be very helpful, since reductions have been found in all three disorders, and seem to be related to extrapyramidal symptoms, rather than to a specific neurodegenerative disorder.

COGNITIVE DYSFUNCTION DUE TO CEREBROVASCULAR DISEASE

The concept of vascular dementia is currently changing since it is increasingly understood that cerebrovascular disease leading to cognitive dysfunction cannot be categorized under one disease, but results from different pathophysiological processes. Structural imaging, especially magnetic resonance imaging (MRI), has increased our understanding of cerebrovascular disease and cognitive dysfunction considerably over the last decades. With regard to neurotransmitter imaging, research has focused on neuronal dysfunction due to ischemic stroke (113), where markers of neuronal integrity, such as $GABA_A$ ligands, combined with measurements of cerebral blood flow, oxygen metabolism, and oxygen extraction may determine the extent of tissue damage (114). Few studies have investigated more global cortical or subcortical neurotransmitter changes (outside ischemia injured tissue) in cerebrovascular disease. One study found that cortical $5-HT_2$ receptor binding positively correlated with cognitive performance in post-stroke patients, suggesting that alterations in the serotonergic system following stroke may affect cognition (115). Ihara et al. demonstrated significant differences in cortical $GABA_A$ receptor between patients with leukoaraiosis and dementia and patients with leukoaraiosis without dementia, indicating that severe white matter ischemic lesions may cause cortico-subcortical disruption, which may augment cognitive dysfunction (Fig. 5) (116).

In conclusion, few studies have addressed the relationship between cognitive dysfunction and neurotransmitter changes in cerebrovascular disease in vivo. In particular, it would be interesting to look further into the pathophysiological background for the specific symptomatology found in subcortical vascular dementia.

CONCLUSIONS

Among the primary degenerative disorders, AD is the most extensively investigated when it comes to neuroreceptor studies. In postmortem studies, marked reductions in some of the receptor systems, in particular $5-HT_2$ receptors, nicotinic $\alpha4-\beta2$, and a preferential loss of M2 as compared to M1 muscarinic receptors have been found. Studies of muscarinic and dopaminergic receptors have shown conflicting results. Some of these findings have been partially replicated in in vivo imaging studies: a decrease in $5-HT_2$, nicotinic, and possibly muscarinic receptors.

In DLB cholinergic and dopaminergic dysfunctions have been established, and in FTD reductions in serotonergic receptors and dopamine reuptake are among the neurochemical changes. Some of these results have been replicated in vivo in neuroimaging studies, and imaging of neurotransmitters may prove useful in the differential diagnosis between the primary neurodegenerative disorders.

Generally, the development of more selective radiotracers that are accurately quantifying receptor binding would greatly enhance our knowledge on in vivo changes in the transmitter systems in dementia disorders. Neurotransmission imaging has an enormous potential for increasing our understanding of the complex relationship between neurochemical processes and cognitive and neuropsychiatric symptoms in dementia.

REFERENCES

1. Farde L, Hall H, Pauli S, Halldin C. Variability in D2-dopamine receptor density and affinity: a PET study with [11C]-raclopride in man. Synapse 1995; 20:200–208.

2. Kemppainen N, Marjamaki P, Roytta M, Rinne JO. Different pattern of reduction of striatal dopamine reuptake sites in Alzheimer's disease and ageing. J Neural Transm 2001; 108:827–836.

3. Rinne JO, Lonnberg P, Marjamaki P. Age-dependent decline in human brain dopamine D1 and D2 receptors. Brain Res 1990; 508:349–352.

4. van Dyck CH, Seibyl JP, Malison RT, et al. Age-related decline in dopamine transporters: analysis of striatal subregions, nonlinear effects, and hemispheric asymmetries. Am J Geriatr Psychiatry 2002; 10:36–43.

5. Wang Y, Chan GL, Holden JE, et al. Age-dependent decline of dopamine D1 receptors in human brain: a PET study. Synapse 1998; 30:56–61.

6. Antonini A, Leenders KL, Reist H, Thomann R, Beer HF, Locher J. Effect of age on D2 dopamine receptors in normal human brain measured by positron emission tomography and 11C-raclopride. Arch Neurol 1993; 50:474–480.

7. Bowen DM, Najlerahim A, Procter AW, Francis PT, Murphy E. Circumscribed changes of the cerebral cortex in neuropsychiatric disorders of later life. Proc Natl Acad Sci USA 1989; 86:9504–9508.

8. Cidis Meltzer C, Drevets WC, Price JC, et al. Gender-specific aging effects on the serotonin 1A receptor. Brain Res 2001; 895:9–17.

9. Rabiner EA, Messa C, Sargent PA, et al. A database of [(11)C]WAY-100635 binding to 5-HT(1A) receptors in normal male volunteers: normative data and relationship to methodological, demographic, physiological, and behavioral variables. Neuroimage 2002; 15:620–632.

10. Adams KH, Pinborg LH, Svarer C, et al. A database of (18)F-altanserin binding to 5-HT(2A) receptors in normal volunteers: normative data and relationship to physiological and demographic variables. Neuroimage 2004; 21:1105–1113.

11. Meltzer CC, Smith G, Price JC, et al. Reduced binding of [18F]altanserin to serotonin type 2A receptors in aging: persistence of effect after partial volume correction. Brain Res 1998; 813:167–171.

12. Piggott MA, Perry EK, Perry RH, Court JA. [3H]MK-801 binding to the NMDA receptor complex, and its modulation in human frontal cortex during development and aging. Brain Res 1992; 588:277–286.

13. Magnusson KR. The aging of the NMDA receptor complex. Front Biosci 1998; 3:e70–e80.

14. Nordberg A, Alafuzoff I, Winblad B. Nicotinic and muscarinic subtypes in the human brain: changes with aging and dementia. J Neurosci Res 1992; 31:103–111.

15. Marutle A, Warpman U, Bogdanovic N, Nordberg A. Regional distribution of subtypes of nicotinic receptors in human brain and effect of aging studied by (+/−)-[3H]epibatidine. Brain Res 1998; 801:143–149.

16. Cohen RM, Podruchny TA, Bokde AL, et al. Higher in vivo muscarinic-2 receptor distribution volumes in aging subjects with an apolipoprotein E-epsilon4 allele. Synapse 2003; 49:150–156.

17. Perry EK, Piggott MA, Court JA, Johnson M, Perry RH. Transmitters in the developing and senescent human brain. Ann NY Acad Sci 1993; 695:69–72.

18. Wu CK, Mesulam MM, Geula C. Age-related loss of calbindin from human basal forebrain cholinergic neurons. Neuroreport 1997; 8:2209–2213.

19. Weinberger DR, Gibson R, Coppola R, et al. The distribution of cerebral muscarinic acetylcholine receptors in vivo in patients with dementia. A controlled study with

123IQNB and single photon emission computed tomography. Arch Neurol 1991; 48:169–176.

20. Wyper DJ, Brown D, Patterson J, et al. Deficits in iodine-labelled 3-quinuclidinyl benzilate binding in relation to cerebral blood flow in patients with Alzheimer's disease. Eur J Nucl Med 1993; 20:379–386.

21. Claus JJ, Dubois EA, Booij J, et al. Demonstration of a reduction in muscarinic receptor binding in early Alzheimer's disease using iodine-123 dexetimide single-photon emission tomography. Eur J Nucl Med 1997; 24:602–608.

22. Yoshida T, Kuwabara Y, Ichiya Y, et al. Cerebral muscarinic acetylcholinergic receptor measurement in Alzheimer's disease patients on 11C-N-methyl-4-piperidyl benzilate—comparison with cerebral blood flow and cerebral glucose metabolism. Ann Nucl Med 1998; 12:35–42.

23. Zubieta JK, Koeppe RA, Frey KA, et al. Assessment of muscarinic receptor concentrations in aging and Alzheimer disease with [11C]NMPB and PET. Synapse 2001; 39:275–287.

24. Nordberg A, Lundqvist H, Hartvig P, Lilja A, Langstrom B. Kinetic analysis of regional (S)(-)11C-nicotine binding in normal and Alzheimer brains—in vivo assessment using positron emission tomography. Alzheimer Dis Assoc Disord 1995; 9:21–27.

25. Iyo M, Namba H, Fukushi K, et al. Measurement of acetylcholinesterase by positron emission tomography in the brains of healthy controls and patients with Alzheimer's disease. Lancet 1997; 349:1805–1809.

26. Herholz K, Bauer B, Wienhard K, et al. In-vivo measurements of regional acetylcholine esterase activity in degenerative dementia: comparison with blood flow and glucose metabolism. J Neural Transm 2000; 107:1457–1468.

27. Shinotoh H, Namba H, Fukushi K, et al. Progressive loss of cortical acetylcholinesterase activity in association with cognitive decline in Alzheimer's disease: a positron emission tomography study. Ann Neurol 2000; 48:194–200.

28. Kuhl DE, Koeppe RA, Minoshima S, et al. In vivo mapping of cerebral acetylcholinesterase activity in aging and Alzheimer's disease. Neurology 1999; 52:691–699.

29. Soricelli A, Postiglione A, Grivet-Fojaja MR, et al. Reduced cortical distribution volume of iodine-123 iomazenil in Alzheimer's disease as a measure of loss of synapses. Eur J Nucl Med 1996; 23:1323–1328.

30. Fukuchi K, Hashikawa K, Seike Y, et al. Comparison of iodine-123-iomazenil SPECT and technetium-99m-HMPAO-SPECT in Alzheimer's disease. J Nucl Med 1997; 38:467–470.

31. Meyer M, Koeppe RA, Frey KA, Foster NL, Kuhl DE. Positron emission tomography measures of benzodiazepine binding in Alzheimer's disease. Arch Neurol 1995; 52:314–317.

32. Ohyama M, Senda M, Ishiwata K, et al. Preserved benzodiazepine receptors in Alzheimer's disease measured with C-11 flumazenil PET and I-123 iomazenil SPECT in comparison with CBF. Ann Nucl Med 1999; 13:309–315.

33. Blin J, Baron JC, Dubois B, et al. Loss of brain 5-HT2 receptors in Alzheimer's disease. In vivo assessment with positron emission tomography and [18F]setoperone. Brain 1993; 116:497–510.

34. Meltzer CC, Price JC, Mathis CA, et al. PET imaging of serotonin type 2A receptors in late-life neuropsychiatric disorders. Am J Psychiatry 1999; 156:1871–1878.
35. Versijpt J, Van Laere KJ, Dumont F, et al. Imaging of the 5-HT2A system: age-, gender-, and Alzheimer's disease-related findings. Neurobiol Aging 2003; 24:553–561.
36. Brown DR, Wyper DJ, Owens J, et al. 123Iodo-MK-801: a spect agent for imaging the pattern and extent of glutamate (NMDA) receptor activation in Alzheimer's disease. J Psychiatr Res 1997; 31:605–619.
37. Groom GN, Junck L, Foster NL, Frey KA, Kuhl DE. PET of peripheral benzodiazepine binding sites in the microgliosis of Alzheimer's disease. J Nucl Med 1995; 36:2207–2210.
38. Cagnin A, Brooks DJ, Kennedy AM, et al. In-vivo measurement of activated microglia in dementia. Lancet 2001; 358:461–467.
39. Versijpt JJ, Dumont F, Van Laere KJ, et al. Assessment of neuroinflammation and microglial activation in Alzheimer's disease with radiolabelled PK11195 and single photon emission computed tomography. A pilot study. Eur Neurol 2003; 50:39–47.
40. Pizzolato G, Chierichetti F, Fabbri M, et al. Reduced striatal dopamine receptors in Alzheimer's disease: single photon emission tomography study with the D2 tracer. Neurology 1996; 47:1065–1068.
41. Kemppainen N, Ruottinen H, Nagren K, Rinne JO. PET shows that striatal dopamine D1 and D2 receptors are differentially affected in AD. Neurology 2000; 55:205–209.
42. Tanaka Y, Meguro K, Yamaguchi S, et al. Decreased striatal D2 receptor density associated with severe behavioral abnormality in Alzheimer's disease. Ann Nucl Med 2003; 17:567–573.
43. Kemppainen N, Laine M, Laakso MP, et al. Hippocampal dopamine D2 receptors correlate with memory functions in Alzheimer's disease. Eur J Neurosci 2003; 18:149–154.
44. Tyrrell PJ, Sawle GV, Ibanez V, et al. Clinical and positron emission tomographic studies in the 'extrapyramidal syndrome' of dementia of the Alzheimer type. Arch Neurol 1990; 47:1318–1323.
45. Rinne JO, Sahlberg N, Ruottinen H, Nagren K, Lehikoinen P. Striatal uptake of the dopamine reuptake ligand [11C]beta-CFT is reduced in Alzheimer's disease assessed by positron emission tomography. Neurology 1998; 50:152–156.
46. O'Brien JT, Colloby S, Fenwick J, et al. Dopamine transporter loss visualized with FP-CIT SPECT in the differential diagnosis of dementia with Lewy bodies. Arch Neurol 2004; 61:919–925.
47. Baxter MG, Chiba AA. Cognitive functions of the basal forebrain. Curr Opin Neurobiol 1999; 9:178–183.
48. Paterson D, Nordberg A. Neuronal nicotinic receptors in the human brain. Prog Neurobiol 2000; 61:75–111.
49. Nordberg A, Adem A, Hardy J, Winblad B. Change in nicotinic receptor subtypes in temporal cortex of Alzheimer brains. Neurosci Lett 1988; 86:317–321.
50. Sihver W, Gillberg PG, Nordberg A. Laminar distribution of nicotinic receptor subtypes in human cerebral cortex as determined by. Neuroscience 1998; 85:1121–1133.

51. Bednar I, Zhang X, Dastranj-Sedghi R, Nordberg A. Differential changes of nicotinic receptors in the rat brain following ibotenic acid and 192-IgG saporin lesions of the nucleus basalis magnocellularis. Int J Dev Neurosci 1998; 16:661–668.

52. Mesulam M. The cholinergic lesion of Alzheimer's disease: pivotal factor or side show? Learn Mem 2004; 11:43–49.

53. Auld DS, Kornecook TJ, Bastianetto S, Quirion R. Alzheimer's disease and the basal forebrain cholinergic system: relations to beta-amyloid peptides, cognition, and treatment strategies. Prog Neurobiol 2002; 68:209–245.

54. Whitehouse PJ, Martino AM, Antuono PG, et al. Nicotinic acetylcholine binding sites in Alzheimer's disease. Brain Res 1986; 371:146–151.

55. Nordberg A, Winblad B. Reduced number of [3H]nicotine and [3H]acetylcholine binding sites in the frontal cortex of Alzheimer brains. Neurosci Lett 1986; 72:115–119.

56. Warpman U, Nordberg A. Epibaaatidine and ABT 418 reveal selective losses of alpha 4 beta 2 nicotinic receptors in Alzheimer brains. Neuroreport 1995; 6:2419–2423.

57. Wevers A, Burghaus L, Moser N, et al. Expression of nicotinic acetylcholine receptors in Alzheimer's disease: postmortem investigations and experimental approaches. Behav Brain Res 2000; 13:207–215.

58. Sihver W, Langstrom B, Nordberg A. Ligands for in vivo imaging of nicotinic receptor subtypes in Alzheimer brain. Acta Neurol Scand Suppl 2000; 176:27–33.

59. Nordberg A. PET studies and cholinergic therapy in Alzheimer's disease. Rev Neurol (Paris) 1999; 155:S53–S63.

60. Nordberg A, Hartvig P, Lilja A, et al. Decreased uptake and binding of 11C-nicotine in brain of Alzheimer patients as visualized by positron emission tomography. J Neural Transm Park Dis Dement Sect 1990; 2:215–224.

61. Nordberg A, Lundqvist H, Hartvig P, et al. Imaging of nicotinic and muscarinic receptors in Alzheimer's disease: effect of tacrine treatment. Dement Geriatr Cogn Disord 1997; 8:78–84.

62. Maelicke A, Albuquerque EX. Allosteric modulation of nicotinic acetylcholine receptors as a treatment strategy for Alzheimer's disease. Eur J Pharmacol 2000; 393:165–170.

63. Liu Q, Kawai H, Berg DK. beta -Amyloid peptide blocks the response of alpha 7-containing nicotinic receptors on hippocampal neurons. Proc Natl Acad Sci USA 2001; 98:4734–4739.

64. Ding YS, Fowler JS, Logan J, et al. 6-[18F]Fluoro-A-85380, a new PET tracer for the nicotinic acetylcholine receptor: studies in the human brain and in vivo demonstration of specific binding in white matter. Synapse 2004; 53:184–189.

65. DeKosky ST, Harbaugh RE, Schmitt FA, et al. Cortical biopsy in Alzheimer's disease: diagnostic accuracy and neurochemical, neuropathological, and cognitive correlations. Intraventricular Bethanecol Study Group. Ann Neurol 1992; 32:625–632.

66. Mash DC, Flynn DD, Potter LT. Loss of M2 muscarine receptors in the cerebral cortex in Alzheimer's disease and experimental cholinergic denervation. Science 1985; 228:1115–1117.

67. Vanderheyden P, Ebinger G, Dierckx R, Vauquelin G. Muscarinic cholinergic receptor subtypes in normal human brain and Alzheimer's presenile dementia. J Neurol Sci 1987; 82:257–269.

68. Perry EK, Perry RH, Blessed G, Tomlinson BE. Changes in brain cholinesterases in senile dementia of Alzheimer type. Neuropathol Appl Neurobiol 1978; 4:273–277.

69. DeKosky ST, Scheff SW. Synapse loss in frontal cortex biopsies in Alzheimer's disease: correlation with cognitive severity. Ann Neurol 1990; 27:457–464.

70. Pappata S, Tavitian B, Traykov L, et al. In vivo imaging of human cerebral acetylcholinesterase. J Neurochem 1996; 67:876–879.

71. Shinotoh H, Namba H, Fukushi K, et al. Brain acetylcholinesterase activity in Alzheimer disease measured by positron emission tomography. Alzheimer Dis Assoc Disord 2000; 14:S114–S118.

72. Traykov L, Tavitian B, Jobert A, et al. In vivo PET study of cerebral [11C] methyl-tetrahydroaminoacridine distribution and kinetics in healthy human subjects. Eur J Neurol 1999; 6:273–278.

73. Lloyd GK, Lowenthal A, Javoy-Agid F, Constantidinis J. GABAA receptor complex function in frontal cortex membranes from control and neurological patients. Eur J Pharmacol 1991; 197:33–39.

74. Howell O, Atack JR, Dewar D, McKernan RM, Sur C. Density and pharmacology of alpha5 subunit-containing GABA(A) receptors are preserved in hippocampus of Alzheimer's disease patients. Neuroscience 2000; 98:669–675.

75. Armstrong DM, Sheffield R, Mishizen-Eberz AJ, et al. Plasticity of glutamate and GABAA receptors in the hippocampus of patients with Alzheimer's disease. Cell Mol Neurobiol 2003; 23:491–505.

76. Schubiger PA, Hasler PH, Beer-Wohlfahrt H, et al. Evaluation of a multicenter study with Iomazenil—a benzodiazepine receptor ligand. Nucl Med Commun 1991; 12:569–582.

77. Soricelli A, Postiglione A, Grivet-Fojaja MR, et al. Reduced cortical distribution volume of iodine-123 iomazenil in Alzheimer's disease as a measure of loss of synapses. Eur J Nucl Med 1996; 23:1323–1328.

78. Varrone A, Soricelli A, Postiglione A, Salvatore M. Comparison between cortical distribution of I-123 iomazenil and Tc-99m HMPAO in patients with Alzheimer's disease using SPECT. Clin Nucl Med 1999; 24:660–665.

79. Schechter LE, Dawson LA, Harder JA. The potential utility of 5-HT1A receptor antagonists in the treatment of cognitive dysfunction associated with Alzheimer s disease. Curr Pharm Des 2002; 8:139–145.

80. Sargent PA, Kjaer KH, Bench CJ, et al. Brain serotonin1A receptor binding measured by positron emission tomography with. Arch Gen Psychiatry 2000; 57:174–180.

81. Alexopoulos GS, Meyers BS, Young RC, Mattis S, Kakuma T. The course of geriatric depression with "reversible dementia": a controlled study. Am J Psychiatry 1993; 150:1693–1699.

82. Komahashi T, Ohmori K, Nakano T, et al. Epidemiological survey of dementia and depression among the aged living in the community in Japan. Jpn J Psychiatry Neurol 1994; 48:517–526.

83. Lai MK, Tsang SW, Francis PT, et al. Postmortem serotoninergic correlates of cognitive decline in Alzheimer's disease. Neuroreport 2002; 13:1175–1178.

84. Dwivedi Y, Pandey GN. Quantitation of 5HT2A receptor mRNA in human postmortem brain using competitive RT-PCR. Neuroreport 1998; 9:3761–3765.

85. Jansen KL, Faull RL, Dragunow M, Synek BL. Alzheimer's disease: changes in hippocampal N-methyl-D-aspartate, quisqualate, neurotensin, adenosine, benzodiazepine, serotonin and opioid receptors—an autoradiographic study. Neuroscience 1990; 39:613–627.

86. Reynolds GP, Arnold L, Rossor MN, Iversen LL, Mountjoy CQ, Roth M. Reduced binding of ketanserin to cortical 5-ht2 receptors in senile dementia of the Alzheimer type. Neurosci Lett 1984; 44:47–51.

87. Palmer AM, Francis PT, Benton JS, et al. Presynaptic serotonergic dysfunction in patients with Alzheimer's disease. J Neurochem 1987; 48:8–15.

88. Cheng AV, Ferrier IN, Morris CM, et al. Cortical serotonin-S2 receptor binding in Lewy body dementia, Alzheimer's and Parkinson's diseases. J Neurol Sci 1991; 106:50–55.

89. Bockaert J, Claeysen S, Compan V, Dumuis A. 5-HT4 receptors. Curr Drug Targets CNS Neurol Disord 2004; 3:39–51.

90. Wong EH, Reynolds GP, Bonhaus DW, Hsu S, Eglen RM. Characterization of GR 113808 binding to 5-HT4 receptors in brain tissues from patients with neurodegenerative disorders. Behav Brain Res 1996; 73:249–252.

91. Lai MK, Tsang SW, Francis PT, et al. [3H]GR113808 binding to serotonin 5-HT(4) receptors in the postmortem neocortex of Alzheimer disease: a clinicopathological study. J Neural Transm 2003; 110:779–788.

92. Chen CP, Alder JT, Bowen DM, et al. Presynaptic serotonergic markers in community-acquired cases of Alzheimer's disease: correlations with depression and neuroleptic medication. J Neurochem 1996; 66:1592–1598.

93. McGeer PL, McGeer EG. The possible role of complement activation in Alzheimer disease. Trends Mol Med 2002; 8:519–523.

94. Cagnin A, Brooks DJ, Kennedy AM, et al. In-vivo measurement of activated microglia in dementia. Lancet 2001; 358:461–467.

95. Nieoullon A. Dopamine and the regulation of cognition and attention. Prog Neurobiol 2002; 67:53–83.

96. Joyce JN, Murray AM, Hurtig HI, Gottlieb GL, Trojanowski JQ. Loss of dopamine D2 receptors in Alzheimer's disease with parkinsonism but not Parkinson's or Alzheimer's disease. Neuropsychopharmacology 1998; 19:472–480.

97. Piggott MA, Marshall EF, Thomas N, et al. Striatal dopaminergic markers in dementia with Lewy bodies, Alzheimer's and Parkinson's diseases: rostrocaudal distribution. Brain 1999; 122:1449–1468.

98. Sweet RA, Hamilton RL, Healy MT, et al. Alterations of striatal dopamine receptor binding in Alzheimer disease are associated with Lewy body pathology and antemortem psychosis. Arch Neurol 2001; 58:466–472.

99. McKeith IG, Burn DJ, Ballard CG, et al. Dementia with lewy bodies. Semin Clin Neuropsychiatry 2003; 8:46–57.

100. Tiraboschi P, Hansen LA, Alford M, et al. Cholinergic dysfunction in diseases with lewy bodies. Neurology 2000; 54:407–411.

101. Tiraboschi P, Hansen LA, Alford M, et al. Early and widespread cholinergic losses differentiate dementia with lewy bodies from Alzheimer disease. Arch Gen Psychiatry 2002; 59:946–951.

102. Perry E, Martin-Ruiz C, Lee M, et al. Nicotinic receptor subtypes in human brain ageing, Alzheimer and Lewy body diseases. Eur J Pharmacol 2000; 393:215–222.

103. Walker Z, Costa DC, Walker RW, et al. Differentiation of dementia with lewy bodies from Alzheimer's disease using a dopaminergic presynaptic ligand. J Neurol Neurosurg Psychiatry 2002; 73:134–140.

104. Ransmayrl G, Seppi K, Donnemiller E, et al. Striatal dopamine transporter function in dementia with lewy bodies and Parkinson's disease. Eur J Nucl Med 2001; 28:1523–1528.

105. Hu XS, Okamura N, Arai H, et al. 18F-fluorodopa PET study of striatal dopamine uptake in the diagnosis of dementia with lewy bodies. Neurology 2000; 55:1575–1577.

106. Gilman S, Koeppe RA, Little R, et al. Striatal monoamine terminals in Lewy body dementia and Alzheimer's disease. Ann Neurol 2004; 55:774–780.

107. Walker Z, Costa DC, Janssen AG, Walker RW, Livingstone G, Katona CL. Dementia with lewy bodies: a study of post-synaptic dopaminergic receptors with iodine-123 iodobenzamide single-photon emission tomography. Eur J Nucl Med 1997; 24:609–614.

108. Procter AW, Qurne M, Francis PT. Neurochemical features of frontotemporal dementia. Dement Geriatr Cogn Disord 1999; 10:80–84.

109. Mann DM, South PW, Snowden JS, Neary D. Dementia of frontal lobe type: neuropathology and immunohistochemistry. J Neurol Neurosurg Psychiatry 1993; 56:605–614.

110. Sperfeld AD, Collatz MB, Baier H, et al. FTDP-17: an early-onset phenotype with parkinsonism and epileptic seizures caused by a novel mutation. Ann Neurol 1999; 46:708–715.

111. Pal PK, Wszolek ZK, Kishore A, et al. Positron emission tomography in pallido-ponto-nigral degeneration (PPND) family (frontotemporal dementia with parkinsonism linked to chromosome 17 and point mutation in tau gene. Parkinsonism Relat Disord 2001; 7:81–88.

112. Rinne JO, Laine M, Kaasinen V, Norvasuo-Heila MK, Nagren K, Helenius H. Striatal dopamine transporter and extrapyramidal symptoms in frontotemporal dementia. Neurology 2002; 58:1489–1493.

113. Powers WJ, Zazulia AR. The use of positron emission tomography in cerebrovascular disease. Neuroimaging Clin N Am 2003; 13:741–758.

114. Heiss WD, Kracht L, Grond M, et al. Early [11-C]-Flumazenil/H(2)O positron emission tomography predicts irreversible ischemic cortical damage in stroke patients receiving acute thrombolytic therapy. Stroke 2000; 31:366–369.

115. Morris PL, Mayberg HS, Bolla K, et al. A preliminary study of cortical S2 serotonin receptors and cognitive performance following stroke. J Neuropsychiatry Clin Neurosci 1993; 5:395–400.

116. Ihara M, Tomimoto H, Ishizu K, et al. Decrease in cortical benzodiazepine receptors in symptomatic patients with leukoaraiosis: a positron emission tomography study. Stroke 2004; 35:942–947.

10

Development and Application of β-Amyloid Imaging Agents in Alzheimer's Disease

William E. Klunk, Robert D. Nebes, and Nicholas Tsopelas
Department of Psychiatry, University of Pittsburgh, Pittsburgh, Pennsylvania, U.S.A.

Brian J. Lopresti and Julie C. Price
Department of Radiology, University of Pittsburgh, Pittsburgh, Pennsylvania, U.S.A.

Steven T. DeKosky
Departments of Psychiatry and Neurology, University of Pittsburgh, Pittsburgh, Pennsylvania, U.S.A.

Chester A. Mathis
Departments of Radiology, Pharmacology, and Pharmaceutical Sciences, University of Pittsburgh, Pittsburgh, Pennsylvania, U.S.A.

INTRODUCTION

The ability to localize and quantify amyloid deposition in the living brain can advance the study and management of Alzheimer's disease (AD) in several important ways. This chapter describes some recent progress in the development and application of amyloid imaging agents. Sensitive in vivo detection of amyloid deposition could aid in early, perhaps even pre-clinical, diagnosis. Longitudinal studies of amyloid deposition could shed new light onto the controversial "amyloid cascade hypothesis." The ability to assess amyloid deposition pre- and post-treatment with anti-amyloid therapies could significantly facilitate the development of these promising experimental treatments. Surrogate marker questions must await clinical trials in which amyloid imaging is performed before and after treatment with anti-amyloid therapies. While the results of initial studies are promising, they must be followed by larger studies, employing a wider range of disease severity, incorporating longitudinal studies, and examining amyloid imaging agent retention in dementias other than AD.

Neuropathology of Alzheimer's Disease

The definitive diagnosis of AD relies on the demonstration of amyloid plaques and neurofibrillary tangles (NFT) at autopsy (1) (see Chapter 11). Amyloid plaques are composed of 40–42 amino acid amyloid-beta (Aβ) peptides (2), while NFT are composed mainly of a hyperphosphorylated form of the microtubule-associated protein, tau (3). Frequently, α-synuclein deposits in the form of Lewy bodies or threads also are present making the Lewy body variant of AD a "triple amyloidosis." Plaques occur earliest in neocortex, where they are relatively evenly distributed (2), and tangles appear first in limbic areas, such as the transentorhinal cortex, and progress in a predictable pattern of regional distribution to the neocortex (3). Arnold et al. (4) mapped the distribution of NFT and neuritic plaques (amyloid plaques surrounded by dystrophic neurites) in the brains of patients with AD. Compared to NFT, neuritic plaques were generally more evenly distributed throughout the cortex, with the exceptions of notably fewer neuritic plaques in limbic periallocortex and allocortex (the areas with greatest NFT density such as the hippocampus). This is supported by the findings of Price and Morris (5), who found little amyloid pathology in the hippocampus of amyloid-positive controls or very mild AD patients. Thus, while limbic areas have early and severe tangle pathology, the medial temporal lobe has relatively little neuritic plaque pathology early in the disease. The cerebellum is notably free of neuritic plaques in AD, although diffuse amyloid deposits that do not label with fibrillar dyes, such as Congo red, are commonly observed (6,7).

The following facts support the use of amyloid plaque imaging for the study of AD. First, while small degrees of AD-like pathology can be found in cognitively normal individuals over the age of 75, large deposits of these pathological entities or deposits prior to that age appear specific to AD (5). Second, although the time course of amyloid deposition in AD has not been elucidated, evidence gained through postmortem study of Down syndrome (DS) (a condition in which Aβ amyloid deposition is always present by age 40 and dementia is very common) suggests that amyloid deposition begins over a decade prior to the clinical symptoms of dementia (8).

The Central Role of Aβ in the Pathophysiology of Alzheimer's Disease

A growing consensus points to Aβ deposition as a central event in the pathogenesis of AD. The single, most important piece of evidence for this "amyloid cascade hypothesis" of AD is the demonstration that mutations in the Aβ precursor protein (APP) gene on chromosome 21 cause early onset AD (9). While there are a very small number of families affected with this form of AD, the disease is phenotypically indistinguishable from the more common sporadic form of AD, save only for its early age of onset. Further genetic support for the amyloid cascade hypothesis comes from the finding that the most common form of autosomal dominant AD is caused by mutations in the presenilin-1 gene on chromosome 14, which codes for a protein that is strongly suggested to be an essential component of the "gamma-secretase" enzyme complex (10).

Aβ Deposition as a Therapeutic Target in Alzheimer's Disease

It is not surprising that the metabolism of Aβ has become an important therapeutic target in AD research. A corollary of the amyloid cascade hypothesis is that prevention of Aβ accumulation in oligomers or plaques should prevent AD. Approaches to "anti-amyloid" therapy have focused both on decreasing production and increasing clearance of Aβ. Attempts to decrease Aβ production involve inhibition of two distinct "secretase" enzymes responsible for cleavage of Aβ from its much larger precursor protein (11). The β-secretase or β-amyloid cleaving enzyme cleaves the N-terminus of Aβ, and the γ-secretase enzyme complex cleaves the C-terminus (12). Studies with transgenic mice that deposit Aβ plaques in their brains have shown that γ-secretase inhibitors can prevent amyloid deposition (13). Human studies have begun with γ-secretase inhibitors, although few details have yet been released.

A second "anti-amyloid" approach makes use of immunotherapy against Aβ. It is generally regarded that this approach lowers Aβ levels by augmenting clearance of Aβ. The first iteration of the immunotherapeutic approach involved active immunization with fibrillar Aβ itself. This approach had marked anti-amyloid effects in amyloid-depositing transgenic mice (14). Much interest was given to the first human trials of this approach, sometimes referred to as the "Alzheimer's vaccine." Unfortunately, this trial was suspended due to a 6% incidence of a serious adverse event of meningoencephalitis (15). Follow-up of the initially treated cases continues, and a preliminary report on a subset of patients suggests that successful immunization against Aβ slows cognitive decline (16). Analysis of the full cohort showed a modest effect on slowing cognitive decline that appeared to be related to the level of antibody response to the immunizations (17). Proof-of-concept evidence supporting the removal of amyloid deposits from the human brain emerged from three autopsy studies from the Aβ-immunization trials (18–20). While all of these cases showed evidence of significant amyloid clearance, it is interesting that this was typically a very focal finding. This focality underscores the need to have an in vivo method capable of measuring amyloid burden in the entire brain when assessing the effects of immunotherapy. The promising findings from the Aβ-immunization trial have prompted more intense interest in further refinements of the immunotherapeutic anti-amyloid approach such as passive immunization with anti-Aβ antibodies (21,22) that should avoid many untoward effects of active immunization including meningoencephalitis. These passive immunization trials have now entered early-phase human studies.

Need for In Vivo Quantitation of Aβ

The advent of anti-amyloid therapies clearly demonstrates one of the most pressing needs for a technology that would allow non-invasive, in vivo quantitation of amyloid deposition in human brain. For example, even though the autopsy cases reported from the vaccine study appeared to show decreased amyloid load, some have pointed out that we can not be sure that these were not just anomalous cases since no measures of pre-treatment amyloid load were available. In addition, the authors of the preliminary study that suggested cognitive slowing due to Aβ immunization stated, "We do not know whether brain Aβ-amyloid load was reduced in our study patients; in vivo imaging techniques will be required to answer this question" (16). These anti-amyloid therapies are among the most promising in the current pharmaceutical industry pipeline, and the ability to quantify amyloid load before treatment and then follow the effects of treatment is critical to the efficient development of this class of drugs. The success of these or any preventive therapy for AD will require an accurate means of early, and ideally pre-symptomatic, detection of those with the disease or at high risk for the disease. The significant overlap of symptoms among various forms of dementia can make diagnosis challenging, and clinicians would benefit from a method to detect the neuropathology of AD in vivo. Amyloid imaging could thus become an important diagnostic tool to clinicians. Finally, the ability to follow the natural history of amyloid deposition beginning in pre-symptomatic stages in subjects at very high risk for AD (e.g., carriers of mutations causing early onset familial AD) should yield important pathophysio-logical insights regarding the accuracy of the amyloid cascade hypothesis of AD.

DEVELOPMENT OF AMYLOID IMAGING TECHNOLOGIES

Preclinical Development

A number of groups have worked to develop radiolabeled amyloid-specific imaging agents, but early efforts were limited by poor brain entry, high levels of non-specific binding, or low levels of specific binding in brain regions known to contain high concentrations of Aβ (23). Most groups used postmortem tissue dyes known to bind amyloid as the starting point. We reported that Chrysamine G (CG), a lipophilic analog of the amyloid dye Congo red, possessed high affinity for Aβ fibrils and plaques (24), but the penetration of an I-125-labeled CG derivative into normal rat brain was low (25). Similar results were reported using a Tc-99 m-labeled CG derivative (26). Other more chemically distant analogs of CG comprised of styrylbenzene salicylic acids, such as X-34, provided similar results of high in vitro binding affinity to aggregated Aβ but low brain penetration in normal rodent brain (23,27–29). Further modification of the structure by removing the carboxylic acid groups to provide Methoxy-X04 resulted in improved brain entry, but not to the degree typically necessary to provide a good non-invasive positron emission tomography (PET) imaging agent (27). To overcome the low brain penetration of the styrylbenzenes, we developed neutral carbon-11-labeled derivatives of another amyloid dye, thioflavin-T. Modification of the amyloid-binding histologic dye, thioflavin-T, led to the finding that neutral benzothiazole-anilines (or BTAs) bound to amyloid with high affinity and crossed the blood-brain barrier (BBB) very well (30). The basic properties of the prototypical benzothiazole amyloid binding agent, termed BTA-1, and related derivatives have been described in detail (23,31–33). These studies showed that these compounds could bind to amyloid with low nanomolar affinity, enter brain in amounts sufficient for imaging with PET, and clear rapidly from normal brain tissue. At the low nanomolar concentrations typically used in PET studies, the binding of BTA-1 to postmortem human brain was shown to be a good indication of Aβ amyloid deposition, but did not appear to detect the presence of NFT (34). These postmortem data suggested benzothiazole derivatives could be good in vivo PET amyloid imaging agents. A structure-activity study of a series of benzothiazoles suggested that a hydroxylated BTA-1 derivative had brain clearance properties typical of many useful PET radiotracers (32). Therefore, this hydroxybenzothiazole was chosen as the lead compound for the first human trial of benzothiazole amyloid imaging agents performed in Uppsala, Sweden (35). The compound, {N-methyl-[^{11}C]}2-(4'-methylaminophenyl)-6-hydroxyben-zothiazole, was given the Uppsala University PET Center code of "Pittsburgh compound-B" or PIB. Pre-clinical studies showed that PIB bound to AD brain with a Kd of 1–2 nM entered the brain rapidly ($\sim$7%ID/g two minutes post IV injection in mice), and cleared rapidly from normal mouse brain and baboon brain (32). Using real-time in vivo multiphoton microscopy, BTA amyloid-imaging agents have been shown to label individual amyloid plaques in transgenic mouse models of AD within three minutes following IV injection and clear rapidly from normal brain parenchyma (36).

Kung and co-workers developed similar radioiodinated thioflavin-T derivatives as potential Aβ imaging agents for single photon emission computed tomography (SPECT), and several of these compounds (e.g., IMPY) show promise for this purpose with high binding affinities for aggregated Aβ and good penetration in mouse brain (37–39). This same group, working in collaboration with researchers from the University of Toronto, has reported C-11-labeled stilbene derivatives for amyloid imaging in human studies (see below) (40).

Barrio and co-workers reported the synthesis of a lipophilic F-18-radiolabeled tracer for PET imaging of plaques and NFTs in the brains of AD patients (41,42). This tracer is a fluorinated derivative of a non-specific cellular membrane dye, 1,1-dicyano-2-[6-(dimethylamino)naphthalen-2-yl]propene (DDNP). This agent is capable of crossing the BBB and entering brain tissue, and the nature and degree of its specific binding to β-amyloid and NFTs has been partially characterized (43). [F-18]FDDNP was used in one of the early human amyloid imaging studies (see below).

Several groups have taken a large biomolecule approach to amyloid imaging using either antibodies to Aβ (44–47) or labeled Aβ itself (48–51). All of these approaches have met with the problem of achieving substantial penetration of the BBB (23).

In addition to these PET and SPECT radiotracer approaches, several groups have sought to image amyloid using magnetic resonance imaging (MRI) or spectroscopy (MRS). These earliest of these approaches utilized gadolinium-labeled putrescine modified Aβ (52) or monocrystalline iron oxide nanoparticle (MION)-labeled Aβ (53). The MION approach required mannitol infusion to temporarily open the BBB to allow passage of the large modified Aβ probe. The gadolinium-labeled Aβ approach suffered from similar brain uptake difficulties. More recently, another group has reported using a fluorine-labeled derivative of X-34 with fluorine-MRS (54). Interestingly, Jack et al. (55) have shown that it is possible to use MRI to resolve individual plaques in living transgenic mice without MRI contrast agents. Unfortunately, current MRI technical limitations do not allow either the fluorine-MRS or the no-contrast approach to be applied to human studies. It is possible that refinements of MRI technology will allow human MRI amyloid imaging studies in the future, and this would be advantageous given the widespread availability of MRI.

Human Amyloid Imaging Studies

Radiolabeled Monoclonal Antibody Fragments

The first attempt to non-invasively image brain amyloid deposits in probable AD patients was made using 10H3, a monoclonal antibody fragment targeting the Aβ$_{1-28}$ residues, which was labeled with technetium-99 m for SPECT imaging (45). While this agent showed specific binding to senile plaques and cerebrovascular amyloid in postmortem tissue sections (46), only non-specific retention in scalp was observed in human subjects in a manner that did not distinguish AD and control subjects. A major limitation of this approach is the inability of such large molecules to readily enter brain and achieve concentrations sufficient for detection by standard molecular imaging techniques. It may be possible to achieve detectable brain concentrations of this and other antibody fragments over a protracted period of observation of days or weeks, although the relatively short biologic half-life of this injected antibody fragment (two to three hours) and the half-life of the radionuclide would render such an approach impractical for in vivo investigations in human subjects.

[^{18}F]FDDNP

The second agent for the in vivo visualization of amyloid deposits was a radiofluorinated derivative of the solvent and viscosity sensitive fluorophore 2-{1-[6-(dimethylamino)-2-naphthyl]ethylidene}malononitrile (DDNP), termed [^{18}F]FDDNP. In vitro characterization of FDDNP demonstrated that it bound to amyloid-beta fibrils with high affinity and fluorescently stained both plaques and NFTs at high concentrations (43,56). Human studies in AD patients ($n = 9$) and controls ($n = 7$) showed slightly greater retention of [^{18}F]FDDNP in frontal, parietal, temporal, and occipital cortices at steady-state (60–120 minutes post injection), though this increased cortical retention was shown to exceed the reference region (pons) by only a margin of 10–15%. The area of highest retention at equilibrium was a region encompassing hippocampus/amygdala/entorhinal (h-a-e) cortex region, which was shown to exceed retention in the pons by ~30% (57). Interestingly, autopsy studies (4) showed that neuritic plaques are more densely concentrated in neocortex, while the mesial temporal lobe structures, including the h-a-e cortex region, contain the fewest neuritic plaques. NFTs, in contrast, are densely concentrated in the mesial temporal lobe where [^{18}F]FDDNP retention is greatest (3).

Initial analyses of [^{18}F]FDDNP PET data were performed using a novel kinetic analysis method, termed the relative residence time (RRT), which relates specific radiotracer binding to the negative net difference between the reciprocal of the tissue clearance constants (k_2) for the reference and target tissues. The authors demonstrated significantly longer h-a-e RRT values for AD patients as compared to controls, and that the value of the RRT parameter was significantly correlated with Mini-Mental State Examination (MMSE) (58). A concern with this method of analysis is that it is sensitive to both peak and steady-state levels of [^{18}F]FDDNP in tissue, which could potentially result in aberrations of the outcome measure by blood flow and transport phenomenon. For instance, brain areas with nearly identical equilibrium levels of tracer, such as temporal cortex and occipital cortex, produced RRT estimates that differed by more than a factor of 15. Additional analyses of [^{18}F]FDDNP have been reported in a preliminary form comparing 13 AD subjects (age: 76 ± 8 years; MMSE: 18 ± 6) and 10 controls (age: 63 ± 10 years; MMSE: all scored 30). The method used a standard uptake value (SUV) computed from 60–120 minutes tissue radioactivity concentrations that were normalized to a reference region devoid of specific binding (SUVR), such as cerebellum. These analyses have shown significant differences ($p < 0.001$) in the retention of [^{18}F]FDDNP between control and AD subjects in regions such as the medial temporal, parietal, and prefrontal cortices, although the magnitude of the signal in the AD subjects did not exceed the control value by more than 15% in any region (59). The applicability of conventional quantitative analysis methodologies, such as compartmental modeling and graphical analyses, to dynamic [^{18}F]FDDNP PET data remains to be demonstrated. These studies are necessary to fully understand the nature of [^{18}F]FDDNP retention and to assess the overall sensitivity and specificity of the compound for the detection of AD pathology in vivo.

[^{11}C]SB-13

The properties of a stilbene derivative, 4-N-methylamino-4'-hydroxystilbene or SB-13, were recently reported (60). In vitro, [^{3}H]SB-13 was shown to bind specifically and with high affinity (Kd = 2.4 ± 0.2 nM) to cortical homogenates prepared from postmortem brain tissue samples of four patients with a pathological confirmation of AD. In contrast, homogenates of cerebellar and white matter tissues prepared from both AD or control elderly brain tissue did not represent significant sources of [^{3}H]SB-13 specific binding. In vitro competition binding studies demonstrated comparable potencies in the low nanomolar range (Ki = 6.9 nM) for BTA-1 displacement of [^{3}H]SB-13. FDDNP exhibited less competition with [^{3}H]SB-13 (Ki = 294 nM) as compared to BTA-1. This suggested that benzothiazoles, such as BTA-1 and PIB, share a binding site on the Aβ peptide with SB-13, while FDDNP does not (61). [^{3}H]SB-13 was shown to label Aβ plaques in sections of human AD cortex, but not in control brain. These favorable in vitro properties supported the continued investigation of SB-13 as a potential molecular imaging probe for the non-invasive assessment of brain amyloid deposition in human subjects.

SB-13 was labeled with carbon-11 for in vivo investigations in five female AD subjects and six healthy controls (HCs) using PET (60). These same subjects were imaged with PIB, in order to provide a basis of comparison for [^{11}C]SB-13. Venous blood samples were drawn throughout the first 70 minutes of PET data acquisition to characterize the metabolism of [^{11}C]SB-13 and to provide an approximation of the arterial input function for quantitative data analysis. To estimate non-specific binding of [^{11}C]SB-13, the cerebellum was selected as a reference region as it has been shown to contain a relative paucity of fibrillar amyloid deposits in AD and can be assumed to be nearly devoid of [^{11}C]SB-13 specific binding. Following the injection of [^{11}C]SB-13, cerebellar time-activity data showed similar retention characteristics between AD patients and controls. Clearance of cerebellar radioactivity after injection of [^{11}C]SB-13 was somewhat slower than that observed for PIB in the same subjects, with [^{11}C]SB-13 exhibiting a ~3:1 ratio in the peak to 90 minutes radioactivity concentrations as compared to ~8:1 for PIB. Increased retention of [^{11}C]SB-13 was observed in AD subjects compared to controls in cortical areas known to contain significant amyloid deposits in AD, such as the frontal cortex (FRC). Across the four cortical areas included in this investigation (frontal, temporal, parietal, occipital), SUVs were determined from 40–120 minutes post-injection emission data and AD cortical averages were shown to exceed control averages by a ratio of 1.44–1.75, with the greatest distinction observed in left FRC. In the same subjects, the ratio of AD to control SUV values for PIB ranged from 1.96 to 2.52, which was also maximal in the left FRC. It is likely that the improved distinction between AD and control subjects using PIB is a result of more rapid clearance of non-specific binding. While the pattern of retention of [^{11}C]SB-13 appears to mirror that of PIB, the latter provides a greater dynamic range and improved distinction of AD subjects from controls.

Pittsburgh Compound-B

The first human studies with PIB were presented in preliminary form in 2002 (35) and were followed by a full report in 2004 (62). The initial study included 16 probable AD patients (65.9 $\pm$ 11 years; 12.3 $\pm$ 4 years education), six elderly age-matched controls (69.0 $\pm$ 7 years; 12.7 $\pm$ 4 years education), and three 21-year-old controls (young controls). The young controls were included in the study because of the near certainty that these young subjects would represent true plaque-negative controls. Dementia severity in the probable AD subject group, as evaluated by the MMSE, varied from mild (MMSE = 18) to very mild/questionable (MMSE = 29) with a mean MMSE of 24.9 $\pm$ 3.4. Subjects were administered ∼ 300 MBq (8 mCi) of PIB, and dynamic PET data were acquired for 60 minutes. In this study, neither MRI images nor arterial blood samples were obtained for anatomical co-registration and input function determination, and analyses of these studies were limited to semi-quantitative SUV measures of PIB uptake. Nevertheless, striking differences in PIB retention were observed between control and AD subjects in brain areas known to contain significant amyloid deposits in AD [e.g., FRC, and parietal cortex (PAR)]. The six elderly control subjects showed a brain entry and clearance pattern that was indistinguishable from that of the three young control subjects. This permitted young and elderly control groups to be combined to form a unified (HC) group for comparison to the AD patients. As a group, the control subjects showed rapid entry and clearance of PIB from all cortical and subcortical gray matter areas, including the cerebellar cortex (Fig. 1). Cerebellum, an area generally lacking fibrillar amyloid plaques in AD, showed nearly identical uptake and clearance of PIB in the cerebellum of HC and AD groups (Fig. 1A). Subcortical white matter showed relatively lower entry and slower clearance in both HC subjects and AD patients compared to cortical and subcortical gray matter areas (Fig. 1B). In contrast, the AD patients showed a markedly enhanced retention of PIB compared to HC subjects in areas of the brain known to contain high levels of amyloid deposits in AD (Figs. 1C, D, and E), such as parietal and frontal cortices (2,4).

The regional distribution of PIB retention was clearly different in AD patients compared to the HC subjects (Fig. 2). PIB accumulation in AD patients as a group was most prominent in cortical association areas and lower in white matter areas, a pattern consistent with that described in postmortem studies of amyloid deposition in AD brain (2). PIB images from HC subjects showed little or no PIB retention in cortical areas, leaving the subcortical white matter regions highest in relative terms. In absolute terms, the accumulation of PIB in white matter was essentially the same in AD patients and HC subjects (Fig. 1B). A series of axial and sagittal SUV images provides a three-dimensional sense of

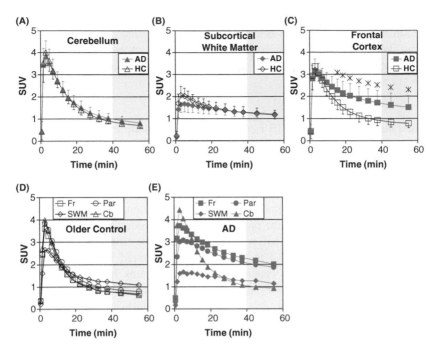

Figure 1 Pittsburgh compound-B (PIB) is differentially retained only in amyloid-laden cortical areas of the Alzheimer's disease (AD) brain. Standardized uptake values (SUV) demonstrating brain entry and clearance of PIB. (**A–C**) represent averaged SUV values for all HC subjects (*open symbols*; $n = 9$) and all AD patients (*filled symbols*; $n = 15$) in cerebellum, subcortical white matter, and frontal cortex. (**D**) and (**E**) show brain entry and clearance in cerebellum (*triangles*), subcortical white matter (*diamonds*), frontal cortex (*squares*), and parietal cortex (*circles*) for an older control subject (**D**) and an AD patient (**E**). Error bars represent one standard deviation (SD) and are too small to be seen in some of the HC subject data in (**A–C**). Asterisks indicate a significant difference between AD and HC values ($p < 0.006$). Shaded areas highlight the 40–60 minute time period used for the summed SUV data displayed in Figures 2–4. *Source*: From Ref. 62.

the regional distribution of PIB retention (Fig. 3). The marked difference between PIB retention in the AD patient and the HC subject is apparent throughout most of the forebrain. FRC was widely affected in the AD patient, but intense PIB retention also was observed in temporal and parietal cortices, part of the occipital cortex, and in the striatum. Lateral temporal cortex (LTC) appeared to have greater PIB accumulation than mesial temporal areas. Consistent with previous reports of extensive amyloid deposition in the striatum of virtually all AD patients (63–66), the striatum was found to have significantly higher PIB retention in AD patients than in HC subjects. Cerebellar cortex (Fig. 3) showed little PIB retention and was similar in AD patients and HC subjects. In general, the observed pattern of PIB retention in AD subjects was found to be consistent

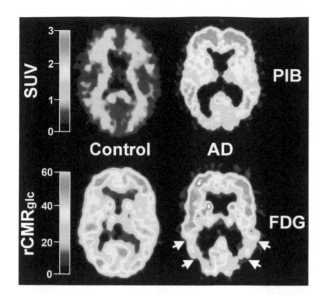

Figure 2 (*See color insert.*) Pittsburgh compound-B (PIB) standard uptake value (SUV) images demonstrate a marked difference between PIB retention in Alzheimer's disease (AD) patients and HC subjects. PET images of a 67-year-old HC subject (*left*) and a 79-year-old AD patient [AD6; Mini-Mental State Examination = 21; (*right*)]. (*Top*) PIB SUV images summed over 40–60 minutes; (*bottom*): fluorodeoxyglucose (FDG) $rCMR_{glc}$ images (μmol/min/100 ml). The left column shows lack of PIB retention in the entire gray matter of the HC subject (*top left*) and normal FDG uptake (*bottom left*). Nonspecific PIB retention is seen in the white matter (*top left*). The right column shows high PIB retention in the frontal and temporoparietal cortices of the AD patient (*top right*) and a typical pattern of FDG hypometabolism present in the temporoparietal cortex [*arrows*; (*bottom right*)] along with preserved metabolic rate in the frontal cortex. PIB and FDG scans were obtained within three days of each other. *Source*: From Ref. 62.

with the pattern of amyloid plaque deposition described in postmortem studies of AD brain (2,4). PIB retention typically predominated in FRC, but it should be noted that FRC did not always show the highest PIB retention in a given subject and mean levels of frontal PIB retention exceed parietal levels by less than 10%.

Three patients diagnosed as probable AD had high MMSE scores (28–29) and showed no significant deterioration over the two-to-four year follow-up period (i.e., MMSE remained 28–29). These atypical subjects had levels of PIB retention in cortical regions typical of controls (open triangles in Fig. 4), though they were retained in the AD group for all analyses. Other mild AD patients with similar clinical profiles showed typical AD-like changes in PIB retention and rCMRglc. It was unclear whether PIB was simply insensitive to the amount of amyloid deposits in the brains of these three atypical AD patients with MMSE scores of 28–29 or whether PIB imaging had correctly identified subjects without

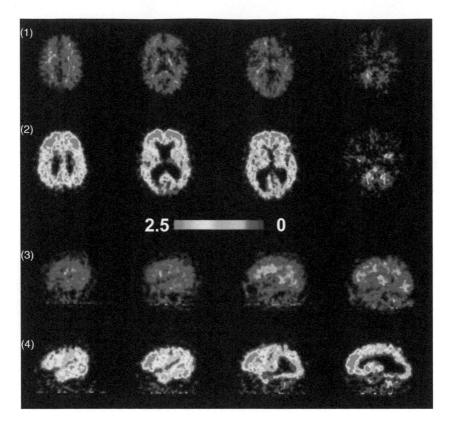

Figure 3 (*See color insert.*) Serial planes demonstrate the topography of Pittsburgh compound-B (PIB) retention. Axial (*top two rows*) and sagittal (*bottom two rows*) PIB standard uptake value (SUV) images of the subjects shown in Figure 2. The HC subject data is shown in rows (**1**) and (**3**). The AD patient data is shown in rows (**2**) and (**4**). The reference region, the cerebellum, can best be appreciated in the images at the far right. The cerebellar peduncles (white matter) show some nonspecific retention, but the cerebellar cortex shows negligible retention. Scale bar indicates relative levels of PIB SUV values. *Source*: From Ref. 62.

amyloid deposits in whom the clinical diagnosis of AD was incorrect and would not be confirmed by postmortem evaluation. In the elderly control group, the oldest subject (76 years old) consistently showed the highest cortical PIB retention and the lowest cortical rCMRglc (boxed circles in Fig. 4). This subject had not expressed any subjective memory complaints and performed within the normal range on the neuropsychological test battery except for difficulty copying a complex cube. This type of case, which could be described as an asymptomatic amyloid-positive case, highlights the issue of specificity versus early detection. One possibility could be that a high PIB signal was obtained in the absence of amyloid deposits (i.e., a false-positive). If this finding does represent the true

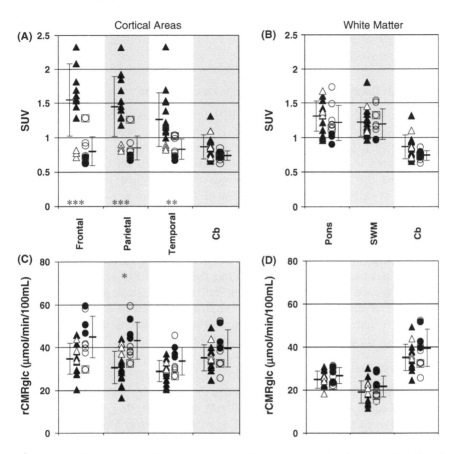

Figure 4 Differences in Pittsburgh compound-B (PIB) retention between Alzheimer's disease (AD) patients and HC subjects can be quantified and are statistically significant. Accumulation of PIB and rCMRglc in selected regions. Average PIB standard uptake values (SUV) were summed over 40–60 minutes in cortical areas (**A**) or white matter areas (**B**) and compared to cerebellum. Values for fluorodeoxyglucose (FDG) uptake were calculated with the Gjedde-Patlak method in cortical areas (**C**) or white matter areas (**D**) and compared to cerebellum. The mean and one SD are indicated with the error bars beside the individual points. HC subjects (*circles*, $n=9$): filled circles represent the three young HC subjects; boxed circle represents the outlier in the HC group (oldest subject). AD patients [*triangles*, $n=15$ (SUV) or $n=16$ (FDG)]: open triangles represent the three outliers in the AD group. AD mean and SD values include all 15 (SUV) or 16 (FDG) AD subjects; $p < 0.01$ (*); $p < 0.002$ (**); $p < 0.0002$ (***). *Source*: From Ref. 62.

presence of amyloid in an asymptomatic individual, the question becomes whether substantial amyloid deposition can be found as part of the normal aging process in subjects who will never develop AD (67) or is increased amyloid deposition always a sign of pre-clinical AD (68–70). The ability to longitudinally follow PIB retention as an in vivo measure of amyloid deposition provides a new tool through which we may be able to answer this question in a manner that postmortem studies can not.

Pittsburgh Compound-B Methodology Development

Since the initial report detailing the PIB proof-of-concept studies, additional studies conducted at the University of Pittsburgh have sought to extend these studies to include in vitro analyses of PIB binding kinetics, fully quantitative imaging, and a third group of subjects with a diagnosis of mild cognitive impairment (MCI). Significant extensions of the original imaging paradigm included: (1) MRI image acquisition (for PET image co-registration, region-of-interest definition, and partial volume correction), (2) the determination of the arterial input function, and (3) the collection of 90 minutes of PET emission data. The ultimate goal of these studies was to apply quantitative imaging techniques, such as compartmental modeling, to identify a suitable method for the analysis of PIB PET data that could be used to validate the utility of PIB across the spectrum of AD. A second goal of these fully quantitative studies was to provide a basis for which to evaluate the performance of simplified methods of analysis applied to human PIB studies in AD, MCI, and control subjects, such as the substitution of reference tissue data in place of an arterial input function.

Fully Quantitative Analyses

The initial quantitative studies conducted at the University of Pittsburgh included five subjects with mild to moderate AD (5M; age: 68 ± 10 years; MMSE 18–26), five control subjects (3F, 2M; age: 59 ± 16 years; MMSE 28–30), and five subjects characterized as MCI (5M; age 71 ± 10 years; MMSE 23–29). All AD subjects met NINDS-ADRDA criteria for Probable AD and DSM-IV criteria for Dementia of the Alzheimer's type (71,72). MRI was performed on all subjects, and a volumetric spoiled gradient recalled sequence optimized for contrast between gray matter, white matter, and cerebrospinal fluid was obtained. Ninety minutes of PET data were acquired following the injection of 370–555 MBq (10–15 mCi) of PIB. Arterial blood samples were withdrawn from a catheter placed in the radial artery for the purposes of input function determination. Radiolabeled metabolites in plasma were determined using a combination of high-performance liquid chromatography and a liquid-liquid extraction technique. Details of the methods used in these studies are described elsewhere (73).

PET emission data were analysed using a variety of techniques routinely employed for the analysis of PET receptor studies using reversibly binding radioligands. These techniques included spectral analysis, a data driven method that does not assume an underlying model configuration (74,75), conventional 2- and 3- compartment pharmacokinetic models (76), and regression methods such as the Logan graphical analysis (77). These models of radioligand binding assume reversible in vivo kinetics and provide outcome measures, such as the binding potential (BP, unitless), distribution volume, and the distribution volume ratio (DVR), which are related to Bmax, the concentration of free receptors, and the ligand dissociation constant Kd.

Determination of the PIB tissue-to-plasma ratios for a variety of cortical and subcortical regions showed that a constant ratio (plateau) was achieved after approximately 20 minutes in the cerebellar regions of both AD and control subjects. Tissue-to-plasma ratios in regions known to contain significant amyloid deposits in AD, such as the posterior cingulate gyrus (PCG), also achieved a constant ratio that was greater than threefold higher than that observed for controls, though the time to plateau was considerably delayed (45–50 minutes). Furthermore, the specific binding of [^{3}H]PIB to human AD brain tissue homogenates was shown to be clearly reversible with an off-rate (k_{off}) of 0.0027/min, or a clearance half-life of 252 minutes (73). These observations were consistent with reversible radioligand binding and supported the use of models of reversible radioligand binding.

Compartmental modeling of PIB data showed that PIB kinetics were best described by a model that allowed for influx and efflux from two tissue compartments (2T-4k) for all subject groups and regions, including cerebellum. Nonspecific PIB retention was found to be similar across subjects, as no significant group differences in the cerebellar 2T-4k DV were observed. In cortical regions, the 2T-4k DVR value showed greater PIB retention in PCG, PAR, LTC, and FRC relative to control subjects.

The Logan graphical analysis, a regression method for describing reversible radioligand binding, was applied to regional and cerebellar PIB data over the 35–90 minutes post-injection interval. Linear regression of the graphical variables yields slope values that are equivalent to the 2T-4k radiotracer DV (77). Good agreement between compartmental and Logan DVR values (e.g., PCG: $r = 0.89$, slope $= 0.91$) was observed, although the Logan results were considerably less variable. Statistically significant differences ($p < 0.05$) in Logan DVR values were observed for AD subject relative to controls in cortical areas after correction for multiple comparisons. The Logan DVR measure also demonstrated favorable intrasubject variability, as assessed in five subjects (2AD, 1 MCI, 2C) who returned for a repeat PIB PET scan 8–20 days later. Test-retest variability averaged $8.4 \pm 5.4\%$ across 11 cortical and subcortical regions-of-interest, and $6.1 \pm 1.5\%$ across the five areas with the highest PIB retention in AD: PCG, PAR, FRC, LTC, and caudate. The intersubject variability was greatest in regions dominated by non-specific PIB retention, such as the subcortical white matter and pons.

In general, mean MCI Logan DVR values fell between control and AD means in brain areas that showed high PIB retention in AD. Figure 5 shows that individual MCI subjects do not fall as a group into an area that is intermediate between the control and AD ranges, but, instead, MCI subjects are either indistinguishable from controls, or indistinguishable from AD subjects. This was equally true for SUV and compartmental analyses (data not shown).

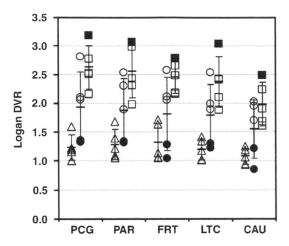

Figure 5   Scatter-plot showing the distribution of individual subject Logan distribution volume ratio values. Control (*triangles*, $n = 5$), mild cognitive impairment (MCI) (*circles*, $n = 5$) and Alzheimer's disease (AD) subject (*squares*, $n = 5$) data in the five brain regions showing the highest Pittsburgh compound-B (PIB) retention in AD subjects are shown. The two MCI subjects that had relatively stable clinical courses (MCI-2 and MCI-5) are shown with filled circles. Note that MCI-2 and MCI-5 are indistinguishable from controls in all five brain areas while the other MCI subjects are essentially indistinguishable from the AD subjects. The AD subject with the highest PIB retention in the posterior cingulate gyrus (*filled squares*) also had the highest retention in the other brain areas. *Source*: From Ref. 62.

Figure 6 shows examples of parametric Logan DVR images that were generated for a control (C-5), a "control-like" MCI subject (MCI-2), an "AD-like" MCI subject (MCI-4), and the AD subject with the highest PIB retention (AD-1). The parametric images show greatest PIB retention in cortical areas of the AD brain and the "AD-like" MCI brain consistent with known patterns of amyloid deposition (2,4,78), with comparatively minimal retention in the control and MCI-2 subjects.

Overall, this initial quantitative assessment of PIB binding yielded differences between AD subjects and controls that were consistent with the distribution of amyloid deposition over the AD disease spectrum. The quantitative results were found to be entirely consistent with the data obtained in the proof-of-concept study (see above), and supported the use of arterial blood sampling and 90 minutes of data acquisition. Most importantly, the study demonstrated that conventional modeling approaches that assume reversible binding kinetics (i.e., the Logan graphical method) can be employed in the analysis of PIB data and produce results that agree with SUV-based analyses. The Logan graphical analysis and the DVR were identified as the preferred method and outcome measure, due to its favorable level of inter- and intra-subject variability across regions, high correlation with compartmental 2T-4k outcome measures, and ease of implementation. The data support the

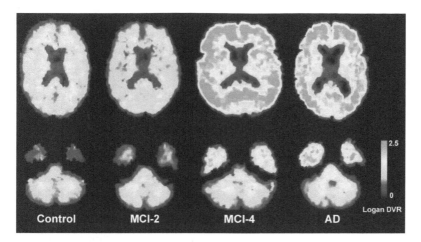

Figure 6 (*See color insert.*) Examples of Pittsburgh compound-B (PIB) Logan distribution volume ratio (DVR) images. Shown are a control (C-5), a "control-like" mild cognitive impairment (MCI) (MCI-2), an "Alzheimer's disease (AD)-like" MCI (MCI-4), and the AD subject with highest PIB retention. Images were generated using arterial plasma data and a 90-minute analysis. The DVR images reflect greater PIB binding in many cortical areas of the AD subject and MCI-4, with background levels in the control and MCI-2 subjects. Similar DVR values were measured in the cerebellum across all subject groups.

feasibility of performing multiple fully-quantitative PET studies in AD subjects, and provide a basis to validate simplified methods of analysis for routine use across the AD disease spectrum.

Simplified Analysis Methods

Ongoing studies at the University of Pittsburgh seek to extend the quantitative PIB studies of Price et al. (73) to include an evaluation of simplified methods for PIB PET imaging, with the ultimate goal of identifying a methodology that can be simply and reliably applied across the AD disease spectrum. PIB PET scans were conducted in 24 subjects (6 AD, 10 MCI, 8 controls) with arterial blood sampling. Repeat scans were performed in eight subjects (3 AD, 1 MCI, 4 controls) within 28 days. Data were analyzed over 60 and 90 minutes using the Logan analysis and (1) metabolite-corrected input functions based on arterial plasma, (2) input functions based on carotid artery time-activity data with a population average metabolite correction applied, and (3) cerebellar reference tissue. Data also were analyzed using the simplified reference tissue method and a single-scan method based on late-scan ratios of SUV.

All simplified methods of analysis effectively discerned regional differences between AD and control subjects in amyloid-laden cortical regions ($p < 0.001$), although the performance of the simplified methods varied in terms of bias, test-retest variability, and Cohen's effect size (AD vs. control) (79). Carotid volume-of-interest-based methods showed the lowest bias of any method relative to the metabolite-corrected arterial methods. Although the test-retest variability was the poorest of all the simplified methods examined, the carotid-based methods demonstrated acceptable test-retest variability ($\pm 7.1\%$ across 11 regions). Cerebellar input methods showed negative biases relative to the metabolite-corrected arterial methods that were greater in subjects with higher levels of PIB retention, although these cerebellar reference-based methods showed the lowest test-retest variability of any method ($\pm 4.5\%$ across 11 regions) and a large effect size [~ 6.5 for PCG]. The single-scan SUV-based methods showed the largest effect sizes for AD and control group differences (6.9 for PCG) and performed very well in terms of inter-subject and test-retest variability ($\pm 5.0\%$), although the SUV measures were positively biased relative to the arterial methods. While the results of the comparison of simplified methods of PIB analysis are preliminary, they suggest that several simplified methods of analysis may be applicable to human PIB PET data, some requiring only a 20 minutes PET scanning session.

Pattern of PIB Retention in Alzheimer's Disease, Mild Cognitive Impairment, and Controls

The finding of Price et al. (73) that MCI subjects may have as much amyloid as AD patients must be interpreted with caution due to the small number of subjects ($n = 5$), but this is a finding with potentially important implications. At some point in the development of AD pathology, there must be a stage at which amyloid levels are midway between typical controls and typical AD patients. It would be expected that anti-amyloid therapeutic approaches (e.g., passive immunization, secretase inhibitors, etc.) would be optimally effective at these earliest stages of amyloid buildup. These findings suggest that, at the very least, MCI patients do not uniformly represent a homogeneous group that is at the very beginning or middle stages of amyloid deposition. Although the numbers are small, these findings hint that a significant percentage of MCI subjects will have amyloid pathology nearly as well established as mild-moderate AD subjects. This finding of AD-like levels of PIB retention in MCI is not particularly surprising in light of the previous postmortem reports of AD-like levels of amyloid deposition in some MCI subjects and in some elderly subjects with normal cognition (67–69,80). It should be noted that the findings of Price et al. (73) in MCI patients do not appear to be due to an unusually severe cohort of subjects since the least impaired MCI subject (MCI-4; MMSE $= 27$) actually showed the greatest PIB retention. In addition, the fact that 40% of the MCI subjects in the Price et al. study had no evidence of amyloid deposition compared to controls (73) is entirely consistent with the fact that 40–50% of clinically diagnosed MCI subjects do not develop AD over a 10-year period of follow-up and may revert to a diagnosis of "normal" (81,82).

FUTURE APPLICATIONS OF AMYLOID IMAGING

The studies described above suggest that amyloid load can be accurately and reproducibly measured in living human brain. As with all new imaging technologies, the challenge that lies ahead will be to discover the unique advantages of this technology as well as its limitations. Amyloid imaging will not serve all purposes in neuroimaging studies of AD, but will likely find a niche alongside the current standards, FDG PET, and structural MRI.

Improved and Earlier Diagnosis

Most imaging techniques have been used with the intent of identifying preclinical pathology and developing a predictive diagnostic method (i.e., an antecedent biomarker). Amyloid imaging holds potential as an antecedent biomarker if detectable amyloid deposition occurs before the onset of clinical symptoms. Evidence for pre-clinical amyloid deposition comes from postmortem histological studies in AD and cognitively normal controls (69) and from the "Nun Study" (66), in which preliminary data suggests that the prevalence of amyloid in clinically unimpaired elderly may be on the order of 25–40%. Perhaps the strongest indication of the time course of preclinical amyloid deposition comes from postmortem studies of DS patients. Having three copies of the APP gene on chromosome 21, nearly all DS patients develop amyloid pathology by their 30s or 40s and a large percentage later show clinical dementia in their 40s and 50s. Although the time course of amyloid deposition in AD is not known, evidence gained through postmortem study of DS suggests that amyloid deposition begins over a decade prior to the clinical symptoms of dementia (8,83).

The question for amyloid imaging is when in this possible 10-year prodromal phase can preclinical amyloid deposition be detected? It is possible that detectable fibrillar amyloid deposits would occur only late in the preclinical phase or even only after the onset of clinical symptoms. Existing data from the application of PIB imaging to MCI subjects certainly shows that amyloid deposition is easily detectable at this very early clinical stage and is already well-established (73). Early PIB studies (62,73) also suggest that increased PIB retention can be detected in cognitively normal control subjects. Natural history studies are underway in subjects who carry early-onset, autosomal dominant familial AD gene mutations in efforts to define when in the course of the illness amyloid deposition can be detected. Similar PIB PET studies in other populations with predictable amyloid deposition, such as DS, could be similarly useful.

In addition to improved early diagnosis, amyloid imaging could play a role in the differential diagnosis of dementias other than AD or when an AD component is suspected. In this context, we might think of defining dementia syndromes as "dementia with β-amyloidosis" and "dementia without β-amyloidosis." Dementia with β-amyloidosis would presumably be equivalent to the presence of AD (alone or in combination with another dementing disorder). A large variety of dementias could make up the group of dementias without β-amyloidosis. In particular, the finding of a negative PIB PET study could be very useful in defining pure frontotemporal dementia. One might be able to identify cases of "pure" dementia with Lewy bodies (DLB) and "pure" vascular dementia (VaD), although they may be relatively rare as neuropathological studies indicate that many patients with DLB and VaD also have amyloid deposits.

Prediction of Mild Cognitive Impairment Conversion to Alzheimer's Disease

A closely related application of imaging technology in AD research is the prediction of which MCI patients will progress to a diagnosis of AD. On average, patients diagnosed with MCI progress to AD at a rate of about 10–15% per year, but nearly half do not develop AD even after follow-up periods as long as five years (81,84). It would be very useful to accurately distinguish these two types of MCI patients, particularly for inclusion in clinical trials of anti-amyloid drugs. In the only group of MCI subjects thus far reported ($n = 5$), PIB imaging has been able to distinguish MCI patients with AD-like retention patterns from patients diagnosed with MCI but who have control-like PIB retention. While this is promising, it is too early to tell if this distinction will accurately predict conversion to AD, and if so, how many years before the clinical diagnosis of AD can an AD-like pattern of PIB retention be detected.

Natural History of Amyloid Deposition

The use of amyloid imaging as an antecedent biomarker and for prediction of conversion from MCI to AD can be thought of in the wider context of the natural history of amyloid deposition. To optimally achieve preclinical diagnosis or prediction of MCI progression to clinical AD, we should ideally understand the entire process of amyloid deposition. This understanding will require a coupling of detailed cognitive assessment with the amyloid imaging studies. Correlations between mild though specific cognitive deficits and early focal amyloid deposition can then be made. These natural history studies are critical to fully understand the still controversial role of amyloid deposition in the pathogenesis of AD. For example, deposition of Aβ protein in the brain has been postulated to be the cause of AD (9). However, the finding of postmortem amyloid plaque deposition in the brains of individuals in whom the *absence* of clinical AD was well documented prior to their death (85) has been interpreted to both support (68) and refute (86) the amyloid cascade hypothesis. This wide range of interpretations exists partly because of the lack of in vivo longitudinal data on the natural history of amyloid deposition. Such data could clarify whether cognitively normal individuals with brain amyloid deposition are destined to develop clinical dementia.

In ongoing amyloid imaging studies, we are assessing the in vivo prevalence of brain amyloid deposition in cognitively "normal" elderly subjects who do not meet clinical criteria for MCI or AD. With increasing age, the cognitive performance of many individuals will decline while still not meeting criteria for MCI or AD (i.e., cognitive decline below the threshold of clinical impairment). We prefer to refer to these subjects as "clinically unimpaired." Although these elderly subjects do not meet clinical diagnostic criteria for cognitive impairment, previous studies have shown that a high percentage of these clinically unimpaired elderly will have cognitive performance below that of young subjects with equal education (Fig. 7A) (87). We refer to these subjects as "low-normal performers" (Fig. 7A). We have recently initiated studies aimed to assess whether in vivo evidence of amyloid deposition is associated with cognitive performance in the lower end of this "normal" range (i.e., being a "low-normal performer" Fig. 7A). In these studies, we will assess whether evidence of amyloid deposition is associated with greater decrements in cognitive performance which could ultimately lead to conversion to MCI or AD over time (Fig. 7B).

There are at least three reasons to relate cognition and amyloid deposition in clinically unimpaired elderly: (1) definition of the prevalence of amyloid deposition in clinically unimpaired elderly, (2) determination of whether the greater variability of cognitive performance in the clinically unimpaired elderly (compared to the young) is explained by the presence or absence of amyloid deposition, and (3) assessment of whether clinically unimpaired individuals with substantial amyloid deposition will invariably progress to clinical dementia.

Studies have attempted to address the first two questions with postmortem assessment of amyloid deposition, but there are obvious weaknesses to this approach. First, it is difficult to acquire cognitive testing close to the time of death—when the amyloid assessment is made. The time period between cognitive testing and death can vary by over a year in some studies. Even cognitive testing occurring very close to the time of death is problematic since any cognitive impairment present could be due to effects of the disease that led to the individual's death. Second, there is an additional selection bias added by the decision to agree to autopsy. This means that not all of the cognitively assessed group will be represented in the amyloid assessment. Finally, many of these studies involve cognitive testing that was not performed for the specific purposes of the study, but was retrospectively gathered to the best degree possible. Much of the cognitive data available comes from cognitive screening tests such as the MMSE (58) and not measures that examine the specific components of cognition thought to be particularly affected by aging (e.g., information processing speed, working memory, inhibitory efficiency). Even when longitudinal data on cognitive performance are available [e.g., (88,89)], it is not possible to link an age-related decrease in cognitive performance to an increase in amyloid load (i.e., to establish causality) because amyloid load could only be determined at one time point—after death. All of these factors have hindered attempts to determine the role that

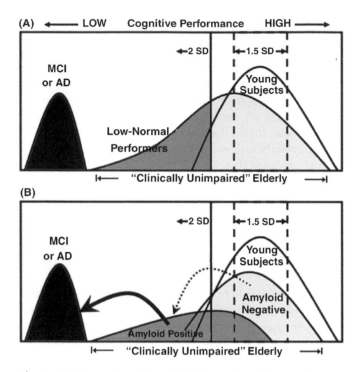

Figure 7 Schematic of the distribution of cognitive performance measures in young subjects, "clinically unimpaired" elderly, and clinically affected individuals who meet criteria for mild cognitive impairment (MCI) or Alzheimer's disease (AD). (**A**) Clinically unimpaired elderly show increased variability compared to young subjects, skewed towards poorer performance, but not reaching clinical criteria for MCI or AD. (**B**) We hypothesize that much of the poorer performance of the elderly is explained by a subset who have amyloid deposition and that this "amyloid-positive" subset contains those individuals who may convert to MCI or AD over time (i.e., amyloid-negative subjects will become amyloid-positive before converting to MCI or AD).

amyloid deposition may play in the various cognitive decrements found in the "normal" old. The availability of amyloid imaging techniques that can measure the amyloid load at multiple time points in living individuals who are not close to death is thus a major advantage.

Natural History in Early-Onset, Autosomal Dominant Familial Alzheimer's Disease

Discussion of the three issues described above regarding the natural history of amyloid deposition presumes that, in a person destined to demonstrate clinical symptoms of AD, amyloid deposition precedes these clinical symptoms and can be detected by in vivo amyloid imaging. This can be a difficult assumption to demonstrate in normal aging studies due to the difficulty in identifying with certainty people who will develop clinical AD. Although tragic, the predictable clinical outcome of individuals who carry an early-onset autosomal dominant familial AD mutation offers an opportunity to efficiently gain insights into the natural history of amyloid deposition in general. In addition, the clinical time course can also be reasonably predicted by the family history. Therefore, studies can be designed with relatively few subjects that can be known with certainty to be on a predictable course toward the development of clinical AD. The imaging studies can be timed to occur at points before pathological changes are expected and be continued through the onset of clinical symptoms. Studies such as these have previously been performed using volumetric MRI (90).

Knowledge of this natural history has implications not only for early onset familial AD, but for typical late-onset sporadic AD as well. Information from early-onset familial AD studies could help address the natural history issue regarding the validity of the amyloid cascade hypothesis. If possible, definition of a particular distribution or amount of amyloid deposition which heralds clinical decline in early-onset familial AD could add important information to the design of studies aimed to determine whether non-demented individuals with substantial amyloid deposition (with or without an early-onset familial AD mutation) invariably progress to clinical dementia. This issue is key to the amyloid cascade hypothesis and to health care policy decisions regarding the need to treat asymptomatic individuals with evidence of amyloid deposition when and if effective anti-amyloid therapies are successfully developed. This in turn could lead to more effective treatments, not only for those with early onset familial AD, but also for those destined to develop sporadic AD.

Amyloid Imaging in Clinical Trials of Anti-amyloid Drugs

One of the most important uses of amyloid imaging technology may be in the facilitation of new drug development. While amyloid imaging may or may not have a general role to play in the development of the so-called "disease modifying" therapies, it is relatively easy to envision its role in the evaluation of drugs aimed specifically at amyloid production (e.g., secretase inhibitors) or amyloid clearance (e.g., plaque breakers and immunotherapies). For the optimal evaluation of these anti-amyloid therapies, it will first be essential to define homogeneous trial populations that have some identifiable baseline level of amyloid deposition. In other words, it would make little sense to use anti-amyloid drugs in subjects who have no brain amyloid deposits to begin with. Furthermore, since effects on amyloid deposition are not likely to be an all-or-none phenomenon, it will be essential to quantitatively and precisely define the baseline status of amyloid deposition for the purposes of comparison to post-treatment outcomes. Early studies suggest that amyloid imaging with PIB is a very stable and reproducible measure over short time periods with test-retest variability of only 5–10% (73). Therefore, reductions in amyloid load of 20% or more should be easily measurable, once corrected for the increase in amyloid load over the time period of the study determined from natural history studies.

One must consider whether imaging large fibrillar Aβ deposits is the appropriate method for assessing the efficacy of anti-amyloid therapies. Evidence is accumulating to suggest that small, soluble oligomers may be the toxic species of Aβ in the human brain (91,92). Some would even suggest that large insoluble aggregates of Aβ are beneficial in that they serve to "detoxify" these soluble oligomers. This concept appears to have some support from in vitro studies of other amyloid-related pathologies (e.g., prion protein accumulator in yeast) in which large intracellular aggregates of the protein in discrete cellular organelles appear to be related to cell survival (93). However, plaques are *extracellular* aggregates and are very different from the carefully managed *intracellular* "detoxification" programs seen in cellular models of prion disease that use both the cell membrane and organelle membrane to control the toxic waste. Plaques are more akin to an unmanaged dumping of barrels of toxic waste into a land fill. Even when the soluble/free toxin is removed, the plaque serves as a source from which more toxin can leach into the surrounding extracellular environment. To keep the potential danger of the insoluble Aβ deposits in perspective, we must remember that in AD brain, soluble forms of Aβ make up less than 1% of total brain Aβ (94). In addition, it is almost certain that soluble and insoluble Aβ pools are in equilibrium. This is supported by the fact that it is extremely difficult to separate soluble and insoluble Aβ in the laboratory, because even after ultracentrifugation and removal of soluble Aβ, resuspension of the "insoluble" Aβ results in the appearance of more soluble Aβ (unpublished observation). Other support for this equilibrium comes from the observation that immunization of amyloid-depositing transgenic mice in a manner that produces antibodies specific for oligomeric Aβ leads to marked reduction of not only oligomeric forms of Aβ, but also results in clearance of thioflavin-S positive plaque forms of Aβ as well (95,96). This suggests that any meaningful anti-amyloid therapy will need to have a significant impact on insoluble brain Aβ deposits for there to be a long-lasting lowering of soluble Aβ. Such an effect should be detectable with agents that bind to fibrillar amyloid.

SUMMARY

In vivo amyloid imaging technology has largely overcome the hurdle of achieving sufficient brain entry while retaining adequate affinity for the Aβ target. Brain clearance and the resulting specific labeling of Aβ deposits also appears sufficient in some of the existing tracers, but future radiopharmaceutical development may result in tracers with even better signal-to-noise ratio and sensitivity. Existing tracers all appear to target aggregated β-sheet forms of Aβ, but further work is necessary to precisely define the subtypes of Aβ deposits that are labeled by each tracer. The early proof-of-concept phase has produced convincing evidence that amyloid load can be quantitatively assessed in living humans. Future challenges lie in the application of amyloid imaging to increase the understanding of the natural history of amyloid deposition and its relationship to cognitive change. Perhaps the most important impact of amyloid imaging technology will be in the facilitation of the development of anti-amyloid therapies, early (even preclinical) identification of cognitively normal individuals with amyloid deposition who would be good candidates for anti-amyloid therapy, and individual patient follow-up to monitor the success of anti-amyloid treatment regimens.

ACKNOWLEDGMENTS

This work was supported by grants from The National Institutes of Health (R01 AG018402, P50 AG005133, K02 AG001039, R01 AG020226, R01 MH070729, K01 MH001976), The Alzheimer's Association (TLL-01-3381), The U.S. Department of Energy (DE-FD02-03 ER63590), and GE Healthcare, Inc. GE Healthcare entered into a license agreement with the University of Pittsburgh based on some of the technology described in this manuscript. Drs. Klunk and Mathis arc co-inventors of PIB and, as such, have a financial interest in this license agreement.

REFERENCES

1. Mirra SS, Heyman A, McKeel D, et al. The Consortium to Establish a Registry for Alzheimer's Disease (CERAD). Part II. Standardization of the neuropathologic assessment of Alzheimer's disease. Neurology 1991; 41:479–486.
2. Thal DR, Rub U, Orantes M, Braak H. Phases of Aβ-deposition in the human brain and its relevance for the development of AD. Neurology 2002; 58:1791–1800.
3. Braak H, Braak E. Neuropathological staging of Alzheimer-related changes. Acta Neuropathol 1991; 82:239–259.
4. Arnold SE, Hyman BT, Flory J, Damasio AR, Van Hoesen GW. The topographical and neuroanatomical distribution of neurofibrillary tangles and neuritic plaques in the cerebral cortex of patients with Alzheimer's disease. Cereb Cortex 1991; 1:103–116.
5. Price JL, Davis PB, Morris JC, White DL. The distribution of tangles, plaques and related immunohistochemical markers in healthy aging and Alzheimer's disease. Neurobiol Aging 1991; 12:295–312.
6. Joachim CL, Morris JH, Selkoe DJ. Diffuse senile plaques occur commonly in the cerebellum in Alzheimer's disease. Am J Pathol 1989; 135:309–319.
7. Yamaguchi H, Hirai S, Morimatsu M, Shoji M, Nakazato Y. Diffuse type of senile plaques in the cerebellum of Alzheimer- type dementia demonstrated by beta protein immunostain. Acta Neuropathol 1989; 77:314–319.

8. Hyman BT, West HL, Rebeck GW, Lai F, Mann DM. Neuropathological changes in Down's syndrome hippocampal formation. Effect of age and apolipoprotein E genotype. Arch Neurol 1995; 52:373–378.

9. Hardy JA, Higgins GA. Alzheimer's disease: the amyloid cascade hypothesis. Science 1992; 256:184–185.

10. Xia W, Ostaszewski BL, Kimberly WT, et al. FAD mutations in presenilin-1 or amyloid precursor protein decrease the efficacy of a gamma-secretase inhibitor: evidence for direct involvement of PS1 in the gamma-secretase cleavage complex. Neurobiol Dis 2000; 7:673–681.

11. Olson RE, Copeland RA, Seiffert D. Progress towards testing the amyloid hypothesis: inhibitors of APP processing. Curr Opin Drug Discov Devel 2001; 4:390–401.

12. Nunan J, Small DH. Regulation of APP cleavage by alpha-, beta- and gamma-secretases. FEBS Lett 2000; 483:6–10.

13. Dovey HF, John V, Anderson JP, et al. Functional gamma-secretase inhibitors reduce beta-amyloid peptide levels in brain. J Neurochem 2001; 76:173–181.

14. Schenk D, Barbour R, Dunn W, et al. Immunization with amyloid-beta attenuates Alzheimer-disease-like pathology in the PDAPP mouse. Nature 1999; 400:173–177.

15. Birmingham KF. Set back to Alzheimer vaccine studies. Nature Med 2002; 8:199–200.

16. Hock C, Konietzko U, Streffer JR, et al. Antibodies against β-amyloid slow cognitive decline in Alzheimer's disease. Neuron 2003; 38:547–554.

17. Gilman S, Koller M, Black RS, et al. Clinical effects of Aβ immunization (AN1792) in patients with AD in an interrupted trial. Neurology 2005; 64:1553–1562.

18. Nicoll JA, Wilkinson D, Holmes C, Steart P, Markham H, Weller RO. Neuropathology of human Alzheimer disease after immunization with amyloid-β peptide: a case report. Nature Med 2003; 9:448–452.

19. Ferrer I, Boada R, Sanchez G, Rey MJ, Costa-Jussa F. Neuropathology and pathogenesis of encephalitis following amyloid-beta immunization in Alzheimer's disease. Brain Pathol 2004; 14:11–20.

20. Masliah E, Hansen L, Adame A, et al. Aβ vaccination effects on plaque pathology in the absence of encephalitis in Alzheimer disease. Neurology 2005; 64:129–131.

21. Bard F, Cannon C, Barbour R, et al. Peripherally administered antibodies against amyloid β-peptide enter the central nervous system and reduce pathology in a mouse model of Alzheimer disease. Nat Med 2000; 6:916–919.

22. DeMattos RB, Bales KR, Cummins DJ, Dodart JC, Paul SM, Holtzman DM. Peripheral anti-Aβ antibody alters CNS and plasma Aβ clearance and decreases brain Aβ burden in a mouse model of Alzheimer's disease. Proc Natl Acad Sci USA 2001; 98:8850–8855.

23. Mathis CA, Wang Y, Klunk WE. Imaging beta-amyloid plaques and neurofibrillary tangles in the aging human brain. Curr Pharm Des 2004; 10:1469–1492.

24. Klunk WE, Debnath ML, Pettegrew JW. Chrysamine-G binding to Alzheimer and control brain: autopsy study of a new amyloid probe. Neurobiol Aging 1995; 16:541–548.

25. Mathis CA, Mahmood K, Debnath ML, Klunk WE. Synthesis of a lipophilic radioiodinated ligand with high affinity to amyloid protein in Alzheimer's disease brain tissue. J Label Compd Radiopharm 1997; 40:94–95.

26. Dezutter NA, Dom RJ, de Groot TJ, Bormans GM, Verbruggen AM 99mTc-MAMA-chrysamine G. A probe for beta-amyloid protein of Alzheimer's disease. Eur J Nucl Med 1999; 26:1392–1399.

27. Klunk WE, Bacskai BJ, Mathis CA, et al. Imaging Abeta plaques in living transgenic mice with multiphoton microscopy and methoxy-X04, a systemically administered Congo red derivative. J Neuropathol Exp Neurol 2002; 61:797–805.

28. Wang Y, Mathis CA, Huang G-F, Holt DP, Debnath ML, Klunk WE. Synthesis and ^{11}C-labelling of (E,E)-1-(3′,4′-dihydroxystyryl)-4-(3′-methoxy-4′-hydroxystyryl) benzene for PET imaging of amyloid deposits. J Label Comp Radiopharm 2002; 45:647–664.

29. Styren SD, Hamilton RL, Styren GC, Klunk WE. X-34, a fluorescent derivative of Congo red: a novel histochemical stain for Alzheimer's disease pathology. J Histochem Cytochem 2000; 48:1223–1232.

30. Klunk WE, Wang Y, Huang GF, Debnath ML, Holt DP, Mathis CA. Uncharged thioflavin-T derivatives bind to amyloid-beta protein with high affinity and readily enter the brain. Life Sci 2001; 69:1471–1484.

31. Mathis CA, Bacskai BJ, Kajdasz ST, et al. A lipophilic thioflavin-T derivative for positron emission tomography (PET) imaging of amyloid in brain. Bioorg Med Chem Lett 2002; 12:295–298.

32. Mathis CA, Wang Y, Holt DP, Huang GF, Debnath ML, Klunk WE. Synthesis and evaluation of 11C-labeled 6-substituted 2-arylbenzothiazoles as amyloid imaging agents. J Med Chem 2003; 46:2740–2754.

33. Wang Y, Klunk WE, Huang GF, Debnath ML, Holt DP, Mathis CA. Synthesis and evaluation of 2-(3′-iodo-4′-aminophenyl)-6-hydroxybenzothiazole for in vivo quantitation of amyloid deposits in Alzheimer's disease. J Mol Neurosci 2002; 19:11–16.

34. Klunk WE, Wang Y, Huang GF, et al. The binding of 2-(4′-methylaminophenyl)-benzothiazole to postmortem brain homogenates is dominated by the amyloid component. J Neurosci 2003; 23:2086–2092.

35. Engler H, Nordberg A, Blomqvist G, et al. First human study with a benzothiazole amyloid-imaging agent in Alzheimer's disease and control subjects. Neurobiol Aging 2002; 23:S429.

36. Bacskai BJ, Hickey GA, Skoch J, et al. Four-dimensional multiphoton imaging of brain entry, amyloid binding, and clearance of an amyloid-beta ligand in transgenic mice. Proc Natl Acad Sci USA 2003; 100:12462–12467.

37. Zhuang ZP, Kung MP, Hou C, et al. IBOX[2-(4′-dimethylaminophenyl)-6-iodobenzoxazole]: a ligand for imaging amyloid plaques in the brain. Nucl Med Biol 2001; 28:887–894.

38. Zhuang ZP, Kung MP, Hou C, et al. Radioiodinated styrylbenzenes and thioflavins as probes for amyloid aggregates. J Med Chem 2001; 44:1905–1914.

39. Zhuang ZP, Kung MP, Wilson A, et al. Structure-activity relationship of imidazo[1,2-a]pyridines as ligands for detecting beta-amyloid plaques in the brain. J Med Chem 2003; 46:237–243.

40. Ono M, Wilson A, Nobrega J, et al. 11C-labeled stilbene derivatives as Abeta-aggregate-specific PET imaging agents for Alzheimer's disease. Nucl Med Biol 2003; 30:565–571.

41. Barrio JR, Huang SC, Cole GM, et al. PET imaging of tangles and plaques in Alzheimer's disease. J Nucl Med 1999; 40:70.
42. Barrio JR, Huang SC, Cole GM, et al. PET imaging of tangles and plaques in Alzheimer's disease with a highly hydrophilic probe. J Label Comp Radiopharm 1999; 42:S194–S195.
43. Agdeppa ED, Kepe V, Liu J, et al. Binding characteristics of radiofluorinated 6-dialkylamino-2- naphthylethylidene derivatives as positron emission tomography imaging probes for beta-amyloid plaques in Alzheimer's disease. J Neurosci 2001; 21:RC189.
44. Bickel U, Lee VM, Trojanowski JQ, Pardridge WM. Development and in vitro characterization of a cationized monoclonal antibody against beta A4 protein: a potential probe for Alzheimer's disease. Bioconjug Chem 1994; 5:119–125.
45. Friedland RP, Kalaria R, Berridge M, et al. Neuroimaging of vessel amyloid in Alzheimer's disease. Ann NY Acad Sci 1997; 826:242–247.
46. Friedland RP, Majocha RE, Reno JM, Lyle LR, Marotta CA. Development of an anti-A beta monoclonal antibody for in vivo imaging of amyloid angiopathy in Alzheimer's disease. Mol Neurobiol 1994; 9:107–113.
47. Majocha RE, Reno JM, Friedland RP, VanHaight C, Lyle LR, Marotta CA. Development of a monoclonal antibody specific for beta/A4 amyloid in Alzheimer's disease brain for application to in vivo imaging of amyloid angiopathy. J Nucl Med 1992; 33:2184–2189.
48. Ghilardi JR, Catton M, Stimson ER, et al. Intra-arterial infusion of [125I]A beta 1–40 labels amyloid deposits in the aged primate brain in vivo. Neuroreport 1996; 7:2607–2611.
49. Maggio JE, Stimson ER, Ghilardi JR, et al. Reversible in vitro growth of Alzheimer disease beta-amyloid plaques by deposition of labeled amyloid peptide. Proc Natl Acad Sci USA 1992; 89:5462–5466.
50. Saito Y, Buciak J, Yang J, Pardridge WM. Vector-mediated delivery of 125I-labeled beta-amyloid peptide A beta 1–40 through the blood-brain barrier and binding to Alzheimer disease amyloid of the A beta 1-40/vector complex. Proc Natl Acad Sci USA 1995; 95:10227–10231.
51. Wengenack TM, Curran GL, Poduslo JF. Targeting Alzheimer amyloid plaques in vivo. Nat Biotechnol 2000; 18:868–872.
52. Poduslo JF, Wengenack TM, Curran GL, et al. Molecular targeting of Alzheimer's amyloid plaques for contrast-enhanced magnetic resonance imaging. Neurobiol Dis 2002; 11:315–329.
53. Wadghiri YZ, Sigurdsson EM, Sadowski M, et al. Detection of Alzheimer's amyloid in transgenic mice using magnetic resonance microimaging. Magn Reson Med 2003; 50:293–302.
54. Higuchi M, Iwata N, Matsuba Y, Sato K, Sasamoto K, Saido TC. ^{19}F and ^{1}H MRI detection of amyloid beta plaques in vivo. Nat Neurosci 2005; 8:527–533.
55. Jack CR, Jr., Garwood M, Wengenack TM, et al. In vivo visualization of Alzheimer's amyloid plaques by magnetic resonance imaging in transgenic mice without a contrast agent. Magn Reson Med 2004; 52:1263–1271.
56. Agdeppa ED, Kepe V, Liu J, et al. 2-Dialkylamino-6-acylmalononitrile substituted naphthalenes (DDNP analogs): novel diagnostic and therapeutic tools in Alzheimer's disease. Mol Imaging Biol 2003; 5:404–417.

57. Shoghi-Jadid K, Small GW, Agdeppa ED, et al. Localization of neurofibrillary tangles and beta-amyloid plaques in the brains of living patients with Alzheimer disease. Am J Geriatr Psychiatry 2002; 10:24–35.
58. Folstein M, Folstein S, McHugh PR. Mini-mental state: a practical method for grading the cognitive state of patients for the clinician. J Psychiatr Res 1975; 12:189–198.
59. Small G, Kepe V, Huang SC, et al. Plaque and tangle brain imaging using [F-18]FDDNP PET differentiates Alzheimer's disease, mild cognitive impairment and older controls. Neuropsychopharmacology 2004; 29:S8.
60. Verhoeff NP, Wilson AA, Takeshita S, et al. In-vivo imaging of Alzheimer disease beta-amyloid with [11C]SB-13 PET. Am J Geriatr Psychiatry 2004; 12:584–595.
61. Kung MP, Hou C, Zhuang ZP, Skovronsky D, Kung HF. Binding of two potential imaging agents targeting amyloid plaques in postmortem brain tissues of patients with Alzheimer's disease. Brain Res 2004; 1025:98–105.
62. Klunk WE, Engler H, Nordberg A, et al. Imaging brain amyloid in Alzheimer's disease with Pittsburgh compound-B. Ann Neurol 2004; 55:306–319.
63. Braak H, Braak E. Alzheimer's disease: striatal amyloid deposits and neurofibrillary changes. J Neuropathol Exp Neurol 1990; 49:215–224.
64. Brilliant MJ, Elble RJ, Ghobrial M, Struble RG. The distribution of amyloid beta protein deposition in the corpus striatum of patients with Alzheimer's disease. Neuropathol Appl Neurobiol 1997; 23:322–325.
65. Suenaga T, Hirano A, Llena JF, Yen SH, Dickson DW. Modified Bielschowsky stain and immunohistochemical studies on striatal plaques in Alzheimer's disease. Acta Neuropathol 1990; 80:280–286.
66. Wolf DS, Gearing M, Snowdon DA, Mori H, Markesbery WR, Mirra SS. Progression of regional neuropathology in Alzheimer disease and normal elderly: findings from the nun study. Alzheimer Dis Assoc Disord 1999; 13:226–231.
67. Morris JC, Storandt M, McKeel DW, Jr., et al. Cerebral amyloid deposition and diffuse plaques in "normal" aging: Evidence for presymptomatic and very mild Alzheimer's disease. Neurology 1996; 46:707–719.
68. Goldman WP, Price JL, Storandt M, et al. Absence of cognitive impairment or decline in preclinical Alzheimer's disease. Neurology 2001; 56:361–367.
69. Morris JC, Price AL. Pathologic correlates of nondemented aging, mild cognitive impairment, and early-stage Alzheimer's disease. J Mol Neurosci 2001; 17:101–118.
70. Schmitt FA, Davis DG, Wekstein DR, Smith CD, Ashford JW, Markesbery WR. "Preclinical" AD revisited: neuropathology of cognitively normal older adults. Neurology 2000; 55:370–376.
71. DSM-IV: DSM-IV Diagnostic and Statistical Manual of Mental Disorders. Washington D.C., American Psychiatric Association, 1995.
72. McKhann G, Drachman D, Folstein M, Katzman R, Price D, Stadlan EM. Clinical diagnosis of Alzheimer's disease: report of the NINCDS-ADRDA work group under the auspices of the department of health and human services task force on Alzheimer's disease. Neurology 1984; 34:939–944.
73. Price JC, Klunk WE, Lopresti BJ, et al. Kinetic modeling of amyloid binding in humans using PET imaging and Pittsburgh Compound-B. J Cereb Blood Flow Metab (advance online publication) ; doi. 2005 10.1038/sj.jcbfm.9600146

74. Cunningham V, Jones T. Spectral analysis of dynamic PET studies. J Cereb Blood Flow Metab 1993; 13:15–23.
75. Meikle SR, Matthews JC, Brock CS, et al. Pharmacokinetic assessment of novel anti-cancer drugs using spectral analysis and positron emission tomography: a feasibility study. Cancer Chemother Pharmacol 1998; 42:183–193.
76. Koeppe RA, Frey KA, Mulholland GK, et al. [11C]tropanyl benzilate-binding to muscarinic cholinergic receptors: methodology and kinetic modeling alternatives. J Cereb Blood Flow Metab 1994; 14:85–99.
77. Logan J, Fowler JS, Volkow ND, et al. Graphical analysis of reversible radioligand binding from time-activity measurements applied to [N-^{11}C-methyl]-(-)-cocaine PET studies in human subjects. J Cereb Blood Flow Metab 1990; 10:740–747.
78. Braak H, Braak E. Frequency of stages of Alzheimer-related lesions in different age categories. Neurobiol Aging 1997; 18:351–357.
79. Cohen J. Statistical Power Analyses for the Behavioral Sciences. Hillsdale, NJ: Lawrence Erlbaum Associates, 1988.
80. Crystal H, Dickson D, Fuld P, et al. Clinico-pathologic studies in dementia: nondemented subjects with pathologically confirmed Alzheimer's disease. Neurology 1988; 38:1682–1687.
81. Larrieu S, Letenneur L, Orgogozo JM, et al. Incidence and outcome of mild cognitive impairment in a population-based prospective cohort. Neurology 2002; 59:1594–1599.
82. Ganguli M, Dodge HH, Shen C, DeKosky ST. Mild cognitive impairment, amnestic type: an epidemiologic study. Neurology 2004; 63:115–121.
83. Hyman BT. Down syndrome and Alzheimer disease. Prog Clin Biol Res 1992; 379:123–142.
84. Yesavage JA, O'Hara R, Kraemer H, et al. Modeling the prevalence and incidence of Alzheimer's disease and mild cognitive impairment. J Psychiatr Res 2002; 36:281–286.
85. Dickson DW, Crystal HA, Mattiace LA, et al. Identification of normal and pathological aging in prospectively studied nondemented elderly humans. Neurobiol Aging 1992; 13:179–189.
86. Terry RD, Masliah E, Salmon DP, et al. Physical basis of cognitive alterations in Alzheimer's disease: synapse loss is the major correlate of cognitive impairment. Ann Neurol 1991; 30:572–580.
87. Rabbitt P. Does it all go together when it goes? The nineteenth bartlett memorial lecture Q J Exp Psychol A. 1993; 46:385–434.
88. Green MS, Kaye JA, Ball MJ. The Oregon brain aging study: neuropathology accompanying healthy aging in the oldest old. Neurology 2000; 54:105–113.
89. Davis DG, Schmitt FA, Wekstein DR, Markesbery WR. Alzheimer neuropathologic alterations in aged cognitively normal subjects. J Neuropathol Exp Neurol 1999; 58:376–388.
90. Fox NC, Black RS, Gilman S, et al. Effects of Aβ immunization (AN1792) on MRI measures of cerebral volume in Alzheimer disease. Neurology 2005; 64:1563–1572.
91. Caughey B, Lansbury PT. Protofibrils, pores, fibrils, and neurodegeneration: separating the responsible protein aggregates from the innocent bystanders. Annu Rev Neurosci 2003; 26:267–298.

92. Walsh DM, Klyubin I, Fadeeva JV, Rowan MJ, Selkoe DJ. Amyloid-beta oligomers: their production, toxicity and therapeutic inhibition. Biochem Soc Trans 2002; 30:552–573.

93. Serio TR, Lindquist SL. The yeast prion [PSI+]: molecular insights and functional consequences. Adv Protein Chem 2001; 59:391–412.

94. Lue LF, Kuo YM, Roher AE, et al. Soluble amyloid beta peptide concentration as a predictor of synaptic change in Alzheimer's disease. Am J Pathol 1999; 155:853–862.

95. Glabe CG. Conformation-dependent antibodies target diseases of protein misfolding. Trends Biochem Sci 2004; 29:542–547.

96. Zhou J, Fonseca MI, Glabe CG, Cribbs DH, Tenner AJ. Age-related decline in the clearance of plaques by Aβ-immunotherapy in murine model of Alzheimer's disease using either fibrillar or a novel oligomeric Aβ as an immunogen. Soc Neurosci Abstr 2004; 716:9.

11

A View on Early Diagnosis of Dementias from Neuropathology

Kurt A. Jellinger

Institute of Clinical Neurobiology, Vienna, Austria

INTRODUCTION

With an increasingly elderly population the incidence of dementing disorders is rapidly increasing in frequency and represents a major scientific, humanitarian, and socioeconomic problem. Due to recent progress in genetic, molecular biological, imaging, and neuropsychological techniques, and detection of disease specific biological markers, the diagnosis and classification of these processes have increased in accuracy. However, despite the establishment of diagnostic guidelines and consensus criteria, a definite diagnosis still depends on neuropathological examination of the brain at autopsy and, rarely, by biopsy. This is particularly true for early stages of such processes, in which the validity of clinical and neuroimaging criteria is limited. Studies of the brains of elderly individuals without cognitive changes and in those with Alzheimer's disease (AD) and other dementias have provided a major input for progress in our understanding of brain aging and the lesion thresholds for mild cognitive impairment (MCI) and initial stages of dementia (1–16).

The quality and pattern of brain lesions in aging and AD, their spreading along well-defined anatomical pathways, and the consecutive biochemical changes have been described and correlations with cognitive function and clinical course have been performed. Recent insights into the cell biology of protein misfolding and its consequences for neuronal (dys)function offer hope for a better understanding of the underlying molecular processes (17–21). However, many questions concerning the pathology of dementia, its relations to clinical phenotypes, and the lesion threshold for cognitive impairment remain unanswered. Additional difficulties arise from the multimorbidity of aged individuals and frequent concurrence of age-related brain lesions with other pathologies that may interact in "unmasking" or promoting mental impairment.

The majority of demented patients die in advanced stages of the disorder, and only in a few instances is postmortem examination possible in early stages when death occurs under acute and unforeseen circumstances, e.g., due to fatal trauma, suicide, or intercurrent diseases.

The present chapter aims to give a brief update of the neuropathology of major dementia disorders and an outline of the current pathological guidelines for their diagnosis. Regarding the possibilities of early diagnosis, the available morphological data in cognitively normal aged subjects and the lesion threshold between physiological aging and MCI as a pre- or subclinical stage of AD and other dementias (22–28) are reviewed. The few available and partly contradicting results of comparative biopsy and autopsy studies in the same patients have provided some opportunities to follow the progression of AD. Early morphological changes in other diseases have hardly been described and only can be suggested from their full-blown pathology. The relations between disease morphology and various biomarkers will be discussed, and a conclusion will critically summarize the current possibilities for early diagnosis of dementing disorders from the view of neuropathology.

CLASSIFICATION OF DEMENTIA DISORDERS

Dementia has recently been redefined as the differential manifestation of deteriorating brain functions over time as a part of aging due to cell deaths in the brain caused by neurodegeneration or any other disease (29). Currently, dementing disorders are classified according to their principal underlying molecular biological and genetic changes (Table 1). Here only the morphology of the major types of dementia will be reviewed.

BASIC PATHOLOGY OF MAJOR DEMENTING DISORDERS

Alzheimer's Disease

The morphological features of AD include extracellular deposition of amyloid β peptide (Aβ) in plaques and cerebral vasculature [cerebral amyloid angiopathy (CAA)] and accumulation of microtubule-associated hyperphosphorylated tau-protein forming paired helical filaments (PHF) in neurons [neurofibrillary tangles (NFT)], dendrites [neuropil threads (NT)] , and around plaques [neuritic plaques (NP)]. Although most of these changes are nonspecific, the diagnosis of AD depends on their semiquantitative assessment. Other lesions are loss of synapses, synaptic proteins, and neurons causing cerebral volume loss (atrophy)

Table 1 Classification of Dementing Disorders According to Hitherto Known Cause

Degenerative dementias (biomolecular types)
  Proteinopathies
    Tauopathies (secondary)
      Alzheimer's disease (AD) $(3+4$-R tau-triplet$+\beta$-amyloid deposition)
    Tauopathies (primary)
      Progressive supranuclear palsy (PSP) (4-R tau doublet$+$Exon 10)
      Corticobasal degeneration (similar to PSP)
      Tangle-predominant dementia (NFTs, no/little amyloid)
      Argyrophilic grain disease (4-R tau with/without AD lesions)
      Frontotemporal dementia and Parkinsonism linked to chromosome 17 (FTDP-17T)
        (mutations Exon 9, 10, 12, 13 of tau gene)
      Pick disease (3-R tau without exon 10)
      Familial progressive subcortical gliosis (tau mutation on chromosome 17q)
      Multisystem tauopathy with presenile dementia (4-R tau)
    α-Synucleinopathies
      Dementia with lewy bodies (DLB)
      Parkinson disease with dementia (PDD)
      LB-variant of AD (LBV/AD) (DLB$+$AD)
    Ubiquitinopathies
      Familial frontotemporal dementia (FTD) with Ub-positive cell inclusions (FTD-U)
      FTD with motoneuron disease (FTD-MND)
    Lobar atrophies
      Frontotemporal lobar degeneration (FTLD) without tau pathology
    Polyglutamic disorders
      Huntington disease (CA6-trinucleotid repeat disorder)
    Prion disease (transmissible spongiform encephalopathies)
      Creutzfeldt–Jakob disease (sporadic)
      Creutzfeldt–Jakob disease (familial)
      Creutzfeldt–Jakob disease (iatrogenic)
      Creutzfeldt–Jakob disease (new variant)
      Gerstmann-Sträussler-Scheinker disease
      Fetal insomnia
Vascular-ischemic dementias (VID)
      Vascular cognitive impairment (VCI)
      Multiinfarct encephalopathy (MIE)
      Subcortical atherosclerotic encephalopathy (SAE)
      Strategic infarct dementia (SID)
      Postanoxic-hypoxic encephalopathy
"Mixed dementias"
      Combination AD$+$VID
      Combination AD$+$other pathologies
Infectious-inflammatory disorders
  Viral
      HIV dementia
      Herpes encephalitis (residual)

(Continued)

Table 1 Classification of Dementing Disorders According to Hitherto Known Cause (*Continued*)

Progressive multifocal leukoencephalopathy (PML)
Neurosyphilis (paretic dementia)
Demyelinating disorders
    Multiple sclerosis
    Subacute sclerosing panencephalopathy (SSPE)
    Leukodystrophies
Neoplasia
    Primary and secondary brain tumors
    (Para-) neoplastic processes
Internal hydrocephalus
    Obstructive vs. non-obstructive
    Normal-pressure hydrocephalus
Head injuries
    Sequelae of brain trauma
    Subdural hematoma
    Boxer's encephalopathy (dementia pugilistica)
Toxic injuries
    Alcohol
    Drugs
    Metals, other chemicals
Nutritional and metabolic disorders
    Vitamine deficiencies
    Systemic metabolic disease (endocrine, kidney, liver, etc.)
    Lysosomal/peroxisomal disorders (gangliosidoses, leukodystrophies)
    Mitochondrial encephalopathies (MELAS, etc.)

and progressive disruption/disconnection of neuronal circuits as major substrates of dementia (30–33), microglial activation (inflammatory cascades) (34,35), astroglial proliferation, granulovacuolar degeneration, and Lewy bodies (LBs) (Table 2). Neuron loss, particularly affecting glutamatergic neurons, is prominent in the neocortex and hippocampus, areas of importance in memory and cognition, as well as in some subcortical regions, e.g., in the cholinergic and GABAergic systems (36).

Amyloid or Tau Pathology—Chicken or Egg?

It is generally accepted that β-amyloid precursor protein (APP) functioning, metabolism, and intraneuronal transport are key factors in the pathogenesis of AD (37). Aβ is considered central to the pathogenesis of AD (38–42). Aβ derived from the proteolysis of a large transmembrane glycoprotein precursor, the APP, is released as soluble peptides of 39 to 46 residues, with Aβ 40 as the most abundantly produced isoform. The balance between biogenesis versus catabolism of Aβ may be an important factor in the pathogenesis of AD. The balance is disturbed between overproduction of Aβ through enhancement of β- and γ-secretase activity, which

Table 2 Histopathology of Alzheimer's Disease—Diagnostic Markers

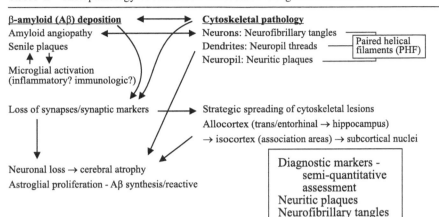

appears to be constantly expressed in normal tissues, or an altered conformation of substrate found in some inherited mutations of APP, and failure to adequately degrade or clear Aβ from its intracellular and extracellular compartment in the brain (43). It has been proposed that the Aβ pathology seen in AD is a continuous process from an initial abnormal Aβ intracellular accumulation to the well-established extracellular Aβ aggregation, culminating in the formation of amyloid plaques and dystrophic neurites (44). Water-soluble Aβ (wsAβ) is present in cerebral cortex of subjects at risk of AD as well as in normal elderly subjects as a mixture of three major species: 1-42, py3-42, and py11-42. The three wsAβ species are not detectable in the brains of young people, free of immunohistochemically detectable APs. In the brains of Down syndrome (DS) and APP-mutant tg mice, wsAβ appears a long time before amyloid deposition, indicating that it represents the first form of Aβ aggregation and accumulation. In the normal brain, wsAβ is bound to apolipoprotein E (ApoE) which favours its degradation by proteases. The composition of wsAβ, in terms of the ratio between the full-length 1-42 and the py3-42 peptides, correlates with the severity of clinical and pathological phenotype in familial early onset AD. Water-soluble Aβ is the native counterpart of the Aβ small aggregates (soluble oligomers) that show, in vitro, an early and high neuronal toxicity (45). They localize to axons and axon terminals with a higher density in AD than in non-demented brains and might be related to synaptic dysfunction in AD (46). The central questions in AD focus on whether cerebral and cerebrovascular Aβ accumulation is (1) a final neurotoxic pathway, common to all forms of AD; (2) a toxic by-product of an independent primary metabolic lesion that, by itself, is also neurotoxic; or (3) an inert by-product of an independent primary neurotoxic reaction (47). In late onset AD, there are compelling reasons that a failure of degradation or clearance of Aβ from the brain underlies its accumulation. Clearance of aggregated Aβ is a complex process, for which microglia, macrophages, and bulk flow across the blood-brain barrier (BBB) are important. Aβ42 can form fibrils more rapidly and at lower concentrations than Aβ40 (48). The most abundant form of Aβ42 fibril exhibits a nodular structure with a 100-nm periodicity. This length is very similar (1) to the length of protofibril bundles that are the dominant feature at earlier stages in the aggregation process, (2) to the period of helical structures that have been observed in the core of fibrils, and (3) to the distance between regularly spaced, structurally weak fibril points. Taken together, these data are consistent with the existence of an approximately similar to 100-nm long basic protofibril unit that is a key fibril building block (49). Cleavage of APP by α- and β-secretase is determined by dynamic interactions with lipid rafts (50), that are also associated with the active γ-secretase complex (51). Hence, lipid rafts play an important role in APP processing, in the generation, aggregation, and degradation of Aβ (52), and are a common component of human extracellular amyloid fibrils (53). A fraction of these Aβ molecules never leave the membrane lipid bilayer after they are generated, but instead exert their toxic effects by competing with and compromising the functions of intramembranous segments of membrane-bound proteins that serve many critical functions. Based on the presence of shared amino acid sequences it was speculated that accumulations of intramembranous Aβ might affect the functions of APP itself and the assembly of the PSEN1, Aph1, Pen 2, Nicastrin complex (54).

Clouds and fine diffuse plaques (DP), initial stages of Aβ deposition with accumulation of nonfibrillary Aβ42, are followed by deposition of Aβ40 (55) that is inserted into lipid layers (56), and oligomerization of both (57), later evolving into primitive plaques containing fibrillary Aβ, tau-positive dystrophic neurites, activated glia, and subsequent development of NFTs (58). Aβ42 plays a more important role in the pathogenesis of AD since its aggregative ability and neurotoxicity are considerably greater than those of Aβ40 (59). Increased concentrations of Aβ lead to the formation of insoluble Aβ plaques (60). Evidence that synaptically released Aβ accumulates as extracellular deposits in the hippocampus of transgenic (tg) mice suggests that these are dynamic structures and a perforant path lesion alters the equilibrium between Aβ production/deposition towards clearance as a consequence of blocked APP transport from the entorhinal cortex to terminal fields in the hippocampus (61,62). Intracellular Aβ42 increases with aging and accumulates in multi-vesicular bodies within presynaptic and postsynaptic compartments (63,64) in the endoplasmic reticulum (ER), mitochondria, and Nissl bodies (65), and a positive feedback mechanism between Aβ production and intracellular APP levels has been described (66); deposition of Aβ fibrils promotes cell-surface accumulation of APP (67).

Brain-derived neurotrophic factor (BDNF) induces APP expression in vivo, but a significant reduction of BDNF in AD brain suggests that cellular APP expression is mainly modulated by other factors (68). There is growing evidence that reduced neurotrophic support is a significant factor in the pathogenesis of AD and other neurodegenerative diseases (69). ER-localized Aβ is degraded in the cytosol (70). Intracellular accumulation of Aβ42, detected in human brain (71–73) and in APP and presenilin-1 (PSEN1) double-tg mice (74–76) and rats (77), is associated with abnormal synaptic morphology before Aβ pathology, and synaptic alterations predominate in tg mice where amyloid is primarily targeted (78–80). Recently, Aβ peptides, whether added to cultures or produced by neurons, have been shown to decrease the number and activity of synaptic glutamate receptors (81,82). This confirms the critical role of intraneuronal A42 for synaptic plasticity and neuronal loss and may provide alternative explications for the early pathogenesis of AD, other than the conventional extracellular Aβ deposition hypothesis (83–85). Co-localization of intraneuronal phosphorylated APP and tau has been observed in very early AD (86). Important synaptic loss may take place even in the absence of amyloid plaques (87,88), implying that the major causative synaptotoxic insult in AD occurs during the early steps of amyloid processing and fibrillar aggregation. Another possible way of plaque-independent neurotoxicity might be membrane permeabilization or disruption (89,90). In AD, endosome abnormalities are among the earliest neuropathologic features to develop and have now been closely linked to genetic risk factors for AD, including APP triplication in Trisomy 21 (DS) and *APOE* ε4 and ε2 genotype in sporadic AD. Recent findings on endosome regulation and developmental and late-onset neurodegenerative disease disorders are beginning to reveal how endocytic pathway impairment may lead to neuronal dysfunction and cell death in these disorders and may also promote amyloidogenesis in AD (91).

Animal Models

The identification of genes and pathways implicated in the pathogenesis of AD led to the production of tg models of Aβ amyloidosis, which recapitulate many of the neuropathological features of AD, including progressive accumulation of SPs, synaptic loss, and gliosis, associated with learning and memory deficits (92,93). The molecular basis of the disease phenotype in the majority of these tg animals is probably enhanced production of Aβ species. Furthermore, the mechanisms by which additional factors implicated in Aβ metabolism and AD, such as ApoE, cholesterol, and inflammatory mediators, have been explored (92). In some triple-tg models, ultrastructural changes, such as dystrophic neurites and behavioural changes, precede Aβ deposition, which in turn precedes tangle formation (94–96), while tg mice expressing the β-cleaved C-terminal APP show no alterations of hippocampal neuronal and synaptic bouton numbers (97), but dynamin-1 depletion in hippocampal neurons, a potential mechanism for early cognitive loss without a major decline in synapse number (98). However, tg animals overexpressing Aβ lacking tau pathology and showing little or no neuronal damage (99) are an incomplete model of AD (100). In APP/PSEN1 double-tg mice, Aβ pathology does not correlate with synaptic and cognitive deficits, hippocampal cell loss, or central cholinergic function, which occur only at a later age as amyloid burden increases, suggesting that Aβ levels are not a marker of memory decline that is related to disease progression (101–103), whereas in the APP^{SL}PS1KI mice massive CA1/2 neuronal loss correlates with strong accumulation of intraneuronal Aβ42 (104), and APP/tau double-tg mice show accelerated Aβ deposition, neurofibrillary degeneration, and neuronal loss suggesting a reciprocal interaction between Aβ and tau (105). In triple-tg (3xTgAD) mice harboring PSEN1, APP, and tau (P301L) antigens and progressively developing SPs and NFTs, synaptic dysfunction manifests in an age-related manner before plaque and tangle pathology (96), suggesting that plaque or tangle pathology contribute to cognitive dysfunction at later time points. APP(SL) PSEN1 tg mice develop age-related synaptophysin-IR presynaptic boutons within the hippocampus, which supports their role in neurodegeneration (106). Clearance of the intraneuronal AD pathology by immunotherapy rescues the early cognitive deficits on a hippocampal-dependent task, strongly implicating intraneuronal Aβ in the onset of cognitive dysfunction (107). This AD model and APP(SL) PS1 K1 mice show massive CA1/2 neuronal loss with intraneuronal and N-terminal truncated Aβ42 accumulation (104). The introduction of Aβ into tau-tg mice has led to enhanced tau pathology with no change in Aβ deposition, further supporting the amyloid cascade hypothesis (92,95,108). Tangle formation in tg mice expressing mutant human tau is accompanied by extensive axonal and neuronal damage (109).

Aβ Neurotoxicity

Amyloid proteins appear as a subgroup of misfolded proteins, where misfolding leads to subsequent aggregation. This aggregation may be a generic property of polypeptide chains possibly linked to their common peptide backbone that does not depend on specific amino acid sequences. And, in fact, many proteins can, in vitro, form amyloid-like aggregates, while in vivo, only 20 amyloid proteins have been so far identified. Although misfolding and aggregation are quite well studied in vitro, the last step of amyloid deposition, i.e., anchorage to the extracellular matrix, cannot be so easily approached. Proteoglycans and serum amyloid P component have nevertheless been identified as key elements involved in extracellular deposition of amyloid (110).

Mounting data suggest that soluble Aβ oligomers (protofibrils), intraneuronal and spherical aggregates of Aβ42 (amylospheroids), rather than Aβ fibrils, may be the primary toxic species and the principal cause of synaptotoxicity (111–118). Aβ cytotoxicity is mediated by p38 inducing oxidative stress (119). Soluble Aβ oligomers ultrastructurally localize to cell processes and might be related to synaptic dysfunction in AD brain (46). These soluble neurotoxins [known as "amyloid β-derived diffusible ligands" (ADDLs) (120,121) and protofibrils] seem likely to account for the imperfect correlation between insoluble fibrillar amyloid deposits and AD progression. ADDLs are known to be potent inhibitors of hippocampal long-term potentiation in vivo, which is a paradigm for synaptic plasticity, and have been linked to synapse loss and reversible memory failure in tg mouse AD models (111), and binding occurs predominantly at synapses (117). If such oligomers were to build up in human brain, their neurological impact could provide the missing link that accounts for the poor correlation between AD dementia and amyloid plaques. Oligomers in AD reach levels up to 70-fold over control brains. Brain-derived and synthetic oligomers exhibit the same striking patterns of attachment to cultured hippocampal neurons, binding on dendrite surfaces in small clusters with ligand-like specificity. Binding assays using solubilized membranes show oligomers to be high-affinity ligands for a small number of low abundance proteins. Current results confirm the prediction that soluble oligomeric Aβ ligands are intrinsic to AD pathology (121). Recent experiments have detected the presence of ADDLs in AD-afflicted brain tissue and in tg models of AD. The presence of high affinity ADDL binding proteins in hippocampus and frontal cortex parallels the regional specificity of AD pathology and suggests involvement of a toxin receptor-mediated mechanism. The properties of ADDLs and their presence in AD-afflicted brain are consistent with their putative role even in the earliest stages of AD (116). The strong correlation between soluble Aβ brain concentrations and severity of neural circuitry dysfunction (122) and early aggregates of nondisease-associated proteins are potent cytotoxics, whereas their final fibrillar aggregates (indistinguishable from AD fibrils) are not (123). The presence of misfolded proteins in the ER triggers a cellular stress response called the unfolded protein response (UPR) that may protect the cell against the toxic buildup of misfolded proteins. Phosphorylated (activated) pancreatic ER kinase (p-PERK), which is activated during the UPR, was observed in neurons in AD patients, but not in nondemented controls and did not co-localize with AT8-positive tangles. These data show that the UPR is activated in AD, and the increased occurrence of p-PERK in cytologically normal-appearing neurons suggests a role for the UPR early in AD neuro-degeneration. Although the initial participation of the UPR in AD pathogenesis might be neuroprotective, sustained activation of the UPR in AD might initiate or mediate neurodegeneration (124).

On the other hand, recent data suggest that synapse-associated Aβ is prominent in regions relatively unaffected by AD lesions, and that amyloid accumulation in surviving terminals is accompanied by gliosis and alteration in the postsynaptic structure (125). In accordance, single systemic administration of an antibody against Aβ produces rapid improvement in behavioural performance of APP-tg mice without affecting total amyloid levels, obviously because of blockage of a diffusible Aβ species (126). The binding of Aβ to membrane lipids facilitates Aβ fibrillation which in turn disturbs the structure and function of neuronal membranes (127). Fibrillary Aβ deposition has been shown to be more detrimental to neuronal circuitry than previously thought (128). Aβ toxicity mediated by the formation of APP complexes (129) but not by secreted Aβ (130) and mitochondrial dysfunction (131,132) induce oxidative stress-mediated

(133–136), apoptotic neuronal death in vitro and in vivo (137). Aβ further induces impairment of endothelial function causing vascular disorders and disorders of the BBB (138). An increased influx of circulatory Aβ into the CNS across the BBB may result in accumulation of soluble neurotoxic Aβ in brain interstitial fluid and/or its subsequent aggregation and deposition in the CNS (139). All these changes were previously suggested to be caspase-independent (140), but recent studies indicate that Aβ could function as a key suicide molecule through caspase-3 in AD (141). Aβ further induces activation of the p38, JNK pathways, and NF-κB in control cybrids and offers protection against the neurotoxic effects of Aβ. Expression of AD mitochondrial genes in cybrids activates stress-related signaling pathways and reduces viability. This AD phenotype is produced by endogenously generated Aβ and can be replicated by exogenous Aβ acting through AGEs (142). Proteins are modified by oxidation, glycoxidation, and lipoxidation, an early event in MCI (143), supporting an important role for lipid-peroxidation-derived protein modifications in AD pathogenesis (144,145). On the other hand, in tg animal models of AD, brain oxidative damage precedes Aβ formation (146). Both extracellular Aβ deposits and intraneuronal Aβ42 production triggered by sustained increase of cytosolic calcium concentration resulting from Aβ ion channel-like structures in the cellular lipid-bilayer, allowing calcium uptake (147,148), may activate caspases leading to cleavage of nuclear and cytoskeletal proteins, induce neuronal death, and underlie disruptions of neuronal signaling in the early stages of AD. Thus, Aβ channels may provide a direct pathway for calcium-dependent Aβ toxicity in AD, which can be prevented by zinc, an Aβ-channel blocker and by the removal of extracellular calcium (147) or a γ-secretase inhibitor (148–150).

Mechanisms of Cell Death in AD

Aging renders the brain vulnerable to Aβ neurotoxicity (151), and DNA replication precedes neuronal death in AD (152). Recent evidence suggests that two intrinsic pathways, mitochondrial dysfunction and ER stress, are central in the execution of apoptosis in AD, mediated by organelle dysfunction (153). In particular, the cleavage of cytoskeletal components, which clearly alters cell morphology, may either activate death signals or disrupt survival signals necessary to suppress cell death (154). Accumulation of both Aβ42 and p53 was found in some neurons with degenerative morphology in both tg mice and human AD cases. Thus, the intracellular Aβ42/p53 pathway may be directly relevant to neuronal loss in AD. Although neurotoxicity of extracellular Aβ is well known and both synaptic and mitochondrial dysfunction by intracellular Aβ42 has been suggested, intracellular Aβ42 may cause p53-dependent neuronal apoptosis through activation of the p53 promoter, thus demonstrating an alternative pathogenesis in AD (155). Furthermore, Aβ induces cell death by an apoptotic process due to activation of the caspase-3 apoptotic cascade regulated by calcineurin dephosphorylation. Calcineurin inhibitors were also effective by preventing loss of mitochondrial membrane potential induced by Aβ, not allowing cytochrome c release from mitochondria and subsequently caspase-3 activation. Thus calcineurin activation and BAD dephosphorylation are are upstream in premitochondrial signaling events leading to caspase-3 activation in Aβ-treated cells (156). The detection of active caspases and the accumulation of cleaved substrates, such as fodrin, actin, and APP, in postmortem AD brain tissue support the hypothesis that apoptosis-like mechanisms may contribute to neuronal loss in AD (157–159), and studies indicate that caspase-mediated cleavage of critical proteins contributes to neuronal degeneration in AD (160,161). Although an in vivo model suggests that a relation between apoptosis and AD may exist, apoptosis, at least in human postmortem AD brains, is rare (162–164). A complex cascade involving immune reactive cells, cytokines, chemokines, and neurotransmitters may contribute to Aβ-induced toxicity and may be related to the delay of Aβ-induced neuronal cell death in vivo (85,142,165). It has been suggested that the presence of a disordered BBB and the presence of immunoglobuline in neurons (166) is associated with microglial activation and neuroinflammation, this being subsequent to AP formation (35,167). Misfolded Aβ, via a disturbance of signaling pathways, may lead to cycles of synapse loss and aberrant sprouting (168). However, the mechanisms by which the toxic form of Aβ acts remain to be elucidated. Aβ leads to internalization of NMDA receptors, reducing their availability at synapses (169). Paradoxical effects occur when Aβ forms complexes with metal ions (iron, zinc, or copper), where Aβ-metal complexes are capable of being neurotoxic or neuroprotective (170,171). Amorphous plaques in the cerebral cortex of AD patients and nondemented subjects are associated with glial Aβ (111,172–175), which may be related to glial clearance of non-fibrillary Aβ, whereas expression of the β-site APP-cleaving enzyme (BACE1) by reactive astrocytes may contribute to developing AD (176). ApoE promotes Aβ aggregation as well as senile plaque (SP) and astrocyte colocalization and degradation of deposited Aβ (177). Aβ42 accumulation and the selective lysis of Aβ-burdened neurons and astrocytes make a major contribution to the formation of SPs (178,179). Astrocytes can protect neurons from Aβ toxicity, but when they interact with Aβ, neuronal damage is enhanced and the expression of synaptic vesicle proteins is decreased (180). Cortical synaptic integration in vivo is disrupted by amyloid plaques (APs) (181). The levels of both Aβ40 and Aβ42 are elevated early in dementia and are correlated with the severity of cortical AD changes and with cognitive decline (182–186), this being confirmed in a *Drosophila* model (187). Elevation of Aβ in the frontal cortex demonstrated in vivo supports the importance of Aβ in early AD (188,189).

However, in support of a physiological role for Aβ was the demonstration that its production is important for neuronal viability and modulation of synaptic functions, protection against oxidative stress, and surveillance against toxins and pathogens (190,191), and blockade of endogenous rodent Aβ production enhances spontaneous neuronal activity and synaptic plasticity. For this regulatory feedback loop that is broken in AD, resulting in unchecked accumulation of Aβ and neurotoxicity, two possible scenarios were proposed: either neurons might fail to be depressed by Aβ, leading to a gradual build-up of neuronal activity and further Aβ secretion, or the machinery for Aβ production becomes independent from neuronal activity (41). Different causes may underlie the familial and sporadic forms of AD. These studies have challenged our traditional perception of Aβ in the pathological processes. Originally thought of as a toxic waste product, it has now been revealed as an endogenous regulator of synaptic structure/plasticity, and neuronal activity (192). Amyloid may also be beneficial, in this case, following neuronal stress or disease. Although controversial, a protective function for Aβ is supported by the available literature (66) and also explains why many aged individuals, despite the presence of high numbers of SPs, show little or no cognitive decline (193).

Tau Pathology and AD

Cytoskeletal lesions, resulting from accumulation of phosphorylated (p)-tau protein (194), include NFTs in the neuronal cell soma, pretangles, defined as non-fibrillar accumulations of tau and considered to be premature NFTs (195,196), and NTs, which account for 85–90% of cortical tau pathology in aging and early AD (197). The vast majority of NTs occurs in dendrites, while a small proportion is present in axons (198). In early stages, NTs occur occasionally in the cerebral cortex, corresponding to a dendritic tree that is arborized from a tau-positive neuron (199). There is an argument that NFTs in the cell soma and NTs in the cell processes are formed simultaneously (196); however, it has been argued that more than half of the NTs arise from neurons without NFTs (200). P-tau accumulates simultaneously in the cell soma and processes in early stages of AD and in nondemented aged subjects. NFTs and NTs contain either 3-repeat tau, 4-repeat tau, or both (201,202). Sections CA 2–4 of the Amon's horn show predominantly 4-R NFTs containing the pSer422 epitope, while pSer262 may detect the process of transformation from p-NFT to intracellular NFT and extracellular NFT consisting predominantly of 3-R tau (202a). This shift in 3-R to 4-R tau may lead to NFT formation. Such isoform differences may depend on the nature of individual neurons bearing NFTs and NTs, though the process of aging and AD is not likely to be tau isoform-specific (199). The most established and the most compelling cause of dysfunctional tau in AD is its abnormal hyperphosphorylation. It not only results in the loss of tau function in promoting assembly and stabilizing microtubules but also in a gain of a toxic function whereby the pathological tau sequesters normal tau and mitogen-activated proteins (MAP1A or MAP1B) and causes inhibition and disruption of microtubules (203). In addition changes in phosphorylation state, tau undergoes multiple truncations and shifts in conformation as it transforms from an unfolded monomer to the structured polymer characteristic of NFT (204). Truncations at both the amino- and carboxy-termini directly influence the conformation into which the molecule folds, and hence the ability of tau to polymerize into fibrils.

Certain of these truncations may be due to cleavage by caspases as part of the apoptotic cascade (205). Although to date no mutations or changes of the splicing regulation of the tau gene and the relative expression of tau isoforms have been found in sporadic cases of the disease, differential expression of tau isoforms in temporal cortex might underlie the susceptibility of certain brain areas to NFT formation (206,207).

Alzheimer-specific epitopes of tau representing lipid peroxidation-induced conformations support the idea that oxidative stress is involved in NFT formation in AD brain (208). Creation of the Tau-C3 epitope specific for tau cleavage of aspartic acid 421 appears to occur relatively early in the disease state, at the same time as the initial Alz50 folding event that heralds the appearance of filamentous tau in NFTs, NTs, and the dystrophic neurites surrounding APs (209). Quantification of tau-positive regional NFT density showed that the AD-associated phosphorylation process progresses from the C-terminus to the N-terminus of the amino acid sequence, and correlation of the Gallyas (silver) stained NFT density was more significant in the limbic cortices than in neocortices with a heterogenous pattern, suggesting that stereotypical phosphorylation occurs in the limbic structures (210).

Recent biochemical studies on brains from elderly people at Braak stages I to III showed a steep rise in the levels of tau and possibly Aβ42 in the enterlinal cortex (EC) at approximately 75 years of age. The levels of insoluble tau increased as the Braak stage increased from I to II, but had a tendency to remain stable between stages II and III. Aβ42 showed a small increase with increasing SPs, while Aβ40 increased continuously with advancing Braak stage. There was no significant correlation between the levels of insoluble tau and Aβ in the EC. Even if Aβ did not accumulate to a significant extent, substantial accumulation of insoluble tau occurred. These data clearly indicate that accumulation of tau and Aβ occur independently in the EC (211).

In AD, phosphorylated tau proteins are considered a control mediator of disease pathogenesis. On the other hand, it has been proposed that tau phophorylation represents a compensatory response mounted by neurons against oxidative stress and serves a protective function. In a new tau-tg mouse in which the overexpression of mutant human tau can be regulated by doxycycline, turning off tau expression after deposits have formed halts neuronal loss and reverses memory deficits. But surprisingly, NFTs continue to accumulate, suggesting that they are not responsible for neurodegeneration (212). These findings provide compelling evidence that perikaryal tau inclusions alone may not cause disease and do not directly serve a role in neuronal loss or cognitive impairment (213). This is consistent with a recent report that neurofibrillary pathology was not correlated with neuronal death in a human tau-tg model displaying neurodegeneration (214). The study by SantaCruz et al. (212) also provides the exciting prospective that recovery of cognitive function is possible even after significant progression of neurodegeneration. These findings have implications in the understanding of AD and other tauopathies. This novel concept, which can also be applied to protein aggregates in other neurodegenerative diseases, opens a new window of knowledge with broad implications for the understanding of mechanisms underlying disease pathophysiology (215).

Spreading Patterns of AD Pathologies

The cytoskeletal lesions that are associated with conformational changes of tau-protein (216,217) show a distinct and predictable spreading pattern from the (trans)entorhinal cortex in the mediobasal temporal lobe via the hippocampus to neocortical association areas and, later, to subcortical nuclei (218,219). This pattern correlates with early memory disorders due to synaptic dysfunction and deafferentiation of the hippocampus by dissection of the GABAergic "perforant pathway" (220,221), followed by disturbances of higher cortical functions due to disorganization of cortico-cortical circuitry (222). However, due to considerable overlap particulary in intermediate (limbic) stages and deviations from the stereotypic expansion pattern, this model is of limited value (223–226). Different populations of neurons prone to NFT formation are lost at different rates. In the prefrontal cortex non-phosphorylated NF protein-enriched neurons represent a vulnerable subpopulation. Their preferential involvement suggests that neurons providing specific cortico-cortical connections between association areas predict cognitive impairment in AD (227). Involvement of the primary motor and association cortices, affected only in late stages of AD, provide significant morphologic markers for dementia (219,228).

The extension of tau pathology is different from the phases of Aβ deposition (Fig. 1A and B). Diffusion of soluble Aβ in the extracellular space is involved in the spread of Aβ pathology and can lead to neurodegeneration (230). Amyloidosis usually begins in the neocortex and later progresses to allocortical regions expanding anterogradely into regions that receive neuronal projections from already affected brain areas (229,231). In contrast to the usually precise pathway of tau pathology, Aβ pathology is more diffusely and less predictably distributed. Both lesions start before symptoms become apparent (10,229), and clinically manifest AD is considered to be a late stage of these processes. While AP variants are present in both early and late AD, disease progression is associated with both a shift to a higher proportion of fibrillar plaques that induce local neuritic alterations, and transformation of cytoskeletal proteins within associated neuronal processes (232). Increased Aβ correlates with cognitive decline in early AD, and demented individuals usually show higher Aβ loads than nondemented ones (185,233), but the individual variability and independence of equilibrium distribution of Aβ40 and Aβ42 may explain the inconsistent and weak correlations between disease progression, neuronal loss, and Aβ phases (229,234–236), while tau pathology is strongly correlated with disease progression and the degree of dementia (6,22,237–239). However, while large numbers of NFTs exist in neocortical projection neurons late into the course of AD, it is not possible to assess whether these neurons are dead or functional and may respond to therapeutic strategies (240).

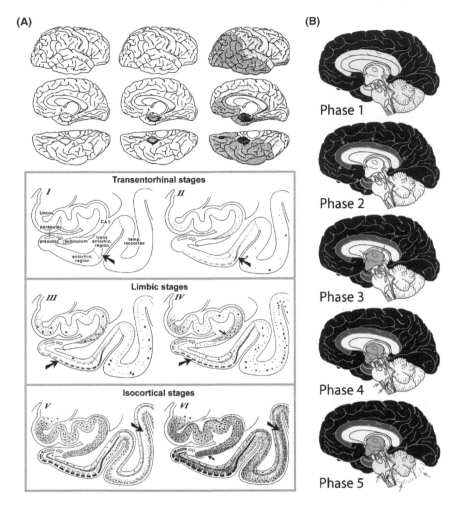

Figure 1 (*See color insert.*) Spreading pattern of (**A**) cytoskeletal/tau pathology and (**B**) of Aβ deposition. *Source*: From Refs. 218, 229.

Interaction Between Aβ and Tau

Although it is now widely believed that an increase in the production of Aβ is central to the pathogenesis of AD, little is known about the relationship between APP/Aβ and tau changes (150,241,242). In the rare familial forms of AD, pathogenic mutations have been identified in both the gene encoding the precursor of the Aβ peptide, *APP* gene itself, and in the presenilin genes which encode part of the APP-protease complex, supporting the "amyloid cascase hypothesis" (48,243) which claims that Aβ causes the imbalance between Aβ generation and clearance as the basis of AD or enhances the tau pathology. For the more frequent sporadic form of AD, the pathogenic trigger has not been unambiguously identified. Whether Aβ is again the main cause remains to be determined, although tau-tg mice and tissue-culture models provide insight into the biochemical mechanisms of tau aggregation and nerve cell degeneration (244,245). Chronic activation of microglia, via the secretion of cytokines and reactive molecules, may exacerbate plaque pathology and enhance the hyperphosphorylation of tau and the subsequent development of NFTs. Suppression of microglial activity in AD brain has been considered as a potential treatment of AD and may slow disease progression (246). Recent results clearly indicate that $A\beta_{25-35}$, the peptide region to which the cytotoxic properties of Aβ can be assigned, interacts with the peptide region of tau protein involved in microtubule binding; intracellular binding of Aβ oligomeres to soluble tau may promote tau phosphorylation. This interaction produces the aggregation of tau peptide and the concomitant disassembly of $A\beta_{25-35}$, offering an explanation for the lack of co-localization of NFTs and SPs in AD, and suggesting the possibility that tau protein may have a protective action by preventing Aβ from adopting the cytotoxic, aggregated form (247).

Recent data indicate nonoverlapping but synergistic actions of both pathologies in sporadic AD (248,249). APP dysfunction/mismetabolism inducing Aβ accumulation in the brain is believed to be the primary influence driving AD pathology due to a failure of an autoregulation feedback reducing neuronal activity and could contribute to cognitive decline in early AD and to disease progression (41,250). Tau colocalizes with Aβ42 and is induced by Aβ42 in vitro. Recent evidence suggests that plaques, NFTs, and caspases share a common pathway (251). Caspases cleavage of APP and tau has been demonstrated in AD (158,252,253). Aβ accumulation triggers caspase activation which, in turn, leads to caspase-cleavage of tau which is an early event that precedes hyperphosphorylation in the evolution of AD tangle pathology (252,254,255). Caspase-cleaved tau (Δtau) may initiate or accelerate the development of tangle pathology (164,253). Its accumulation may represent a common pathway associated with abnormal intracellular accumulation of tau or α-synuclein (AS) and may be less dependent on the extracellular accumulation of Aβ in non-AD dementias (256). Δtau occurs early in the development of tangle pathology within AD brains and in a tg mouse AD model, suggesting that caspase cleavage of tau plays an important role in the development of NFT pathology. Alterations in tau phosphorylation and cleavage by caspases have been reported in neuronal apoptosis. The presence of activated caspase-6 in pre-tangles suggests that it occurs early and supports previous studies demonstrating caspase activation in MCI but not in AD subjects. While caspase-6-cleaved tau was found in NPs, NTs, and NFTs, active caspase-6 localized primarily to neurites (161). This is consistent with the hypothesis that apoptosic-like mechanisms can damage synapses, axons, and dendrites, without causing overt neuronal death. These results also lend support to the hypothesis that the activation of apoptosis-like mechanisms may be involved in AD pathogenesis (160,251). Caspase inhibition prevents tau cleavage without reversing changes in tau phosphorylation linked to apoptosis. The microtubule depolymerizing agent, colchicine, induces tau dephosphorylation and caspase-independent tau cleavage and degradation. Both phenomena are blocked by inhibiting protein phosphatase 2A (PP2A) by okadaic acid (257). Thus, caspase cleavage of tau provides a mechanistic link between the development of amyloid and tangle pathologies in AD (251). However, others suggest that tau is essential for Aβ-induced neurotoxicity (258), and precedes the occurrence of Aβ deposits (259,260). Elevated tau inhibits the axonal transport of APP, suggesting a possible link between the two key proteins in AD (261,262), and is likely to be independent of amyloidosis or APP dysfunction. Both APP and tau are implicated in axonal transport. Dysregulation of APP and tau metabolism by abnormalities in APP, PSEN, ApoE, and tau can cause impairment of fast axonal transport, leading to axonal depletion of critical components and neurodegeneration (263,264). The suggestion that both processes evolve systematically in parallel and that APP amplifies tau pathology (248) is supported by findings that Aβ induces PHF-like tau filaments in tissue culture (265), and a reciprocal interaction between Aβ and tau in vivo is supported by tg mouse findings (265a).

AD lesions in the primary visual cortex (Brodmann area 17), which is affected only late in AD, were scored into 4 grades. At grade 1 only deposits of Aβ were noticed. Grade 2 showed congo red positive deposits and processes containing Ub and cathepsin D immunoreactivity around plaque cores. At grade 3, NPs and NTs were present, and NFTs at grade 4. The density of all lesions drastically increased at grade 4 (266). This sequence is believed to be compatible with a cascade of events beginning with deposition of Aβ and ending with NFT pathology (267) but awaits further confirmation. The spatial relationship in early AD stages indicating that SPs lie in the terminal fields of NFT-bearing neurons suggests that NFTs either antecede plaques or, less likely, are independently formed (268). An explanation for the current results of independent accumulation of tau and Aβ in the human EC (211) is that the amyloid cascade hypothesis is valid in the neocortex but not in the hippocampus or the EC. This cannot explain accelerated alterations in both regions of the brain affected by familial AD (FAD). Another possibility would be an additional effect(s) of mutant *APP* and *PSEN* 1/2. In addition to increased production of Aβ42, this may lead to premature NFT formation and degeneration in the hippocampus and entorhinal cortex and could have a significant role for enhanced neuronal degeneration in the hippocampus and EC in FAD. There is evidence that the massive neurodegeneration at an early age in FAD patients could be a consequence of an increased vulnerability of neurons by mitochondrial abnormalities resulting in activation of different apoptotic pathways as a consequence of elevated oxidative stress. A hypothetical sequence of the pathogenic steps linking sporadic AD, FAD, Aβ production, mitochondrial dysfunction with caspase pathway activation, and neuronal loss has been proposed (269). There is a correlation of the duration of dementia with the degree of NFT formation and synapse loss (31), but not with any Aβ measures. The accumulation of Aβ is markedly increased in AD brain independent of disease duration, even in cases of short duration (270). Others suggest a sequence of events whereby the effect of Aβ deposition on cognitive impairment is mediated by NFTs (271). NF triplet and α-internexin immunoreactive neurites were localized to plaques densely packed with Aβ fibrils in preclinical AD cases, indicating that certain plaques may cause structural injury or impediment of local axonal transport. However, α-internexin, and not NF triplet, ring-like reactive neurites were present in end-stage AD cases, indicating the relatively late involvement of neurons that selectively contain α-internexin. These results implicate the expression of specific intermediate filament proteins in a distinct hierarchy of differential neuronal vulnerability to AD (272).

Although the relationship between SP, NFTs, and neuronal/synapse loss remains to be elucidated, there is a cascade of reactions (273), and most clinico-pathological studies have shown that both lesions, if present in sufficient amounts, particularly in the neocortex, are considered the best markers for dementia, and that all clinically defined AD cases have huge amounts of amyloid deposits and widespread tau pathology (7,228,274). On the other hand, widely distributed diffuse and neuritic plaques in allocortex are frequently present in both nondemented old subjects and those with MCI. Thus, they often do not permit a distinction between questionable and definite dementia, although preclinical (CERAD) "possible" AD or "pathological aging" often has more neuritic pathology mainly in hippocampus than "normal" aging with no or single Aβ deposits and no to moderate NFTs in hippocampus and frontal cortex (7,238). They also differ in both PHF-tau and Aβ biochemistry (219,248). However, some highly functioning seniors may show severe Aβ deposition (275–277). Breakdown of white matter is seen in normal aging but is exagerated in AD due to Aβ deposition and toxicity resulting in "disconnection" of widely distributed neuronal networks (278).

Guidelines for the Neuropathological Diagnosis of AD

Current criteria for the neuropathological diagnosis of AD are based on (semi)quantitative assessment of plaques and tangles, considered to be histological hallmarks of the disease (Table 3). Several guidelines have been suggested:

1. National Institute of Aging (NIA) criteria emphasizing neocortical SPs per unit corrected for age which could include diffuse as well as neuritic types (279).
2. Criteria based on the semiquantitative assessment of plaques and NFTs in neocortex and hippocampus (280).
3. The Consortium to Establish a Registry for Alzheimer's Disease (CERAD) criteria, using semiquantitative NP counts with adjustment for age together with clinical history (dementia) to give the level of likelihood of AD (281).

Table 3 Currently Used Consensus Criteria for the Pathological Diagnosis of AD

Criteria according to Khachaturian (1985) (279)

    Senile (SP) or neuritic plaques (NP) in the presence of neurofibrillary degeneration (NFT) in neocortex (any region)

        Age < 50 a: $2\text{--}5/\text{mm}^2$

        Age 50–60 a: $\geq 8/\text{mm}^2$

        Age 66–75 a: $> 10/\text{mm}^2$

        Age > 75 a: $> 15/\text{mm}^2$

Criteria according to Tierney et al. (1988) (280) Lesion/x25 field

    A1: one/several SP+NFT in hippocampus (without neocortex)

    A2: one/several SP+NFT in neocortex + hippocampus

    A3: one/several SP+NFT in neocortex (without hippocampus)

CERAD criteria (Mirra et al., 1993) (281)

    Method

        Semiquantitative assessment of neuritic plaque density, graded by "cartoon" comparison as sparse, moderate, and frequent. Sampling of multiple cortical areas and midbrain

        Generation of "age-related plaque score"

            Definite AD: "C" age-adapted plaque score[a], clinical dementia

            Probable AD: "B" age-adapted plaque score, clinical dementia presence/absence of other lesions causing or related to dementia

    Potential disadvantages: Neurites in plaques do not have to display tail immunoreactivity

Braak & Braak scheme (1991) (218)

    Topographic pattern of neurofibrillary tangle spreading (stage I—VI)

NIA-Reagan Institute Criteria (1997) (282)

    Probability statements based upon topographic "staging" of NFT and SP

    All lesions considered (amyloid deposits, neuritic plaques, neuropil threads, and NFT)

    "Age-related plaque score" and topographic staging of NFT combined with clinical information

    Probabilistic approach for diagnosis of dementia

        Low probability: CERAD "sparse" and Braak stage I/II

        Intermediate probability: CERAD "moderate" and Braak stage III/IV

        High probability: CERAD "frequent" and Braak stage V/VI

        Disadvantage: Other possible combinations of CERAD and Braak scores not considered.

    Uncertainty over application when no clinical details

Specific recommendations—routine diagnosis

    Semi-quantitative methodologies (i.e., the CERAD approach) should be used to assess neuritic plaques and neurofibrillary tangles

    Examination of the hippocampus and the neocortex for the presence of neurofibrillary tangles is essential

[a]Age-adapted plaque score:

Age at death	Frequency of plaques			
	None	Few	Moderate	Numerous
<50 a	0	C	C	C
50–75 a	0	B	C	C
>75 a	0	A	B	C

Abbreviations: 0, no evidence; A, uncertain evidence of AD; B, suggestive of AD; C, indicative of AD.
Source: From Refs. 218, 279–282.

4. Topographic staging of neuritic (neurofibrillary) changes, distinguishing six different stages—entorhinal (1 & 2), hippocampal (3 & 4), and neocortical (5 & 6) (218);

5. The Washington University quantitative criteria for diagnosis of AD (5,6,283). These criteria are a modification of the 1985 NIA consensus criteria (279). The main modifications are: 1) a modified Bielschowsky silver stain that better visualizes the whole range of SPs, including the diffuse variety (284); and 2) a counting protocol that evaluates the total number of SPs in 10 contiguous 1 mm^2 microscopic fields in each brain region. This strategy was designed to assess total average plaque distribution across a 10 mm^2 expanse of cortex, thus precluding a diagnosis of AD based on only one to three selected fields. The counting protocol differs from the 1985 NIA consensus quantitative method where SP density in only one single microscopic field has to meet or exceed criteria, and from the CERAD semiquantitative counting strategy in which only NPs are evaluated and maximal plaque counts in any three microscopic fields are averaged and compared to cartoons that depict mild, moderate, and severe plaque numbers in one field.

6. The guidelines of the NIA and the Ronald and Nancy Reagan Institute of the Alzheimer's Association (RI) for making the postmortem diagnosis of AD, combining the CERAD and the Braak scores (285,282). Assessment by NIA-RI guidelines leads to a probability statement for a *low* (CERAD 0-A, Braak stages 1–2), *intermediate* (CERAD B, Braak 3–4), or *high likelihood* (CERAD C, Braak 5–6) that dementia is due to AD. These categories apply only to individuals with dementia, but the underlying guiding principle was that any degree of Alzheimer changes is abnormal.

These algorithms that only consider the classical "plaque and tangle" phenotype of AD have some weaknesses and do not recognize other dementias and AD subtypes, e.g., the "plaque predominant" type with abundant APs, no or very little neuritic AD pathology restricted to the hippocampus (Braak stages 4 or less), and abnormal p-tau in neocortical pyramidal neurons but lacking overt tangle formation, accounting for 3.5–8% of demented subjects over age 85 years (286–288), the "tangle-predominant type" with NFT pathology in the limbic areas, absence of NPs and no or very little amyloidosis, accounting for 5–7% of oldest-olds with female predominance (288,289), and the Lewy body variant of AD (LBV/AD), displaying cortical and subcortical LBs with severe AD pathology (290). Although the interlaboratory comparison of neuropathological assessment of AD when using standardized criteria showed reasonable interrater agreement (291–294), it is important to recognize that pathological diagnosis merely represents the association of a pattern of pathological changes with a clinical phenotype. Therefore, it should be acknowledged that, although Aβ detection and semiquantification have some diagnostic utility, the simple presence of APs, as with proteinaceous accumulations in essentially all neurodegenerative diseases, does not presume aetiology. The major morphological lesions differentiating AD from other neurodegenerative dementing disorders are given in Table 4.

The evaluation of the NIA-RI criteria demonstrated fairly good correlations with clinical dementia and good agreement with pathological methods, and their easy and rapid use in AD and nondemented subjects, but much less reliability for other dementing disorders. Comparison of these criteria with clinical scores identified almost all cases with severe dementia, but often failed in mild to moderate dementias. However, use of these criteria would result in many of CDR 0.5 and some CDR 1 cases being classified as "low probability" AD despite convincing clinical and psychometric data that indicate that they have recognizable progressive dementia, distinct from cognitive changes associated with nondemented aging (25). This suggests that NFT-based neuropathologic criteria will be weighted toward diagnosing AD in its moderate and severe stages, because neocortical neurofibrillary pathology—although present—is relatively modest in early-stage AD (i.e., very mild and mild DAT). Most nondemented cases were assigned to the low or intermediate categories, but several studies in those with no or only MCI showed a wide range of AD-related pathology, and even the combined use of all current criteria often cannot distinguish between questionable and definite dementia (Table 5). Although the sensitivity and specificity of the above algorithm is suggested to be 90%, 40–50% of the brains of patients with the clinical diagnosis of AD show "pure" AD pathology (Table 6). Thus, their predictive value may be reduced to 38–44% (299). It should be borne in mind that all additional pathologies may interact in inducing cognitive impairment. Therefore, the reliability and clinical relevance of the current diagnostic criteria need better qualification and validation.

Dementia with Lewy Bodies vs. Parkinson's Disease with Dementia

Dementia with Lewy bodies (DLB), a relatively new term for a progressive dementia syndrome, is associated clinically with the core neuropsychiatric features of fluctuating cognition and visual hallucinations with parkinsonian features. It represents the second most frequent cause of dementia in the elderly after AD, accounting for 7–30% with means of 15–25% in several autopsy series (300–302). An early-onset case of an atypical form of DLB developing neurological signs at 13 years of age was reported recently (303). DLB is characterized by a variable burden of α-synucleinopathy and AD pathology (300,304). Morphological hallmarks are LB and Lewy neurites (LN) in the brainstem, basal ganglia, limbic cortex, and neocortex, which are scored semiquantitatively according to the severity and anatomical distribution, separating brainstem predominant (i.e., PD), limbic (or transitional), and neocortical types (Table 7a). Case validation is compromised by the lack of

Table 4 Morphological Differential Diagnosis of Alzheimer's Disease

Major morphological lesions	AD disease	Plaque only AD	Tangle dementia	Vascular dementia	MIX type dementia	LBV/AD	Diffuse LBD	FTD	Pick's disease	PSP	CBD	MSA	Prion disease
Brain atrophy, diffuse	+++/++	++	+	±	++	++	±	+	+	+	±	+	++
Brain atrophy, focal	++	−	−	+	+	−	−	+++	+++	+/+++	++	±	±
Amyloid plaques	+++	+++	−/±	±/+	+++	+++	+/++	±/+	±/+	±	+	±/+	+
Neuritic plaques + tangles limbic/temporal	+++	±	±	−	+++	+++	−	−	±	++	+/++	−	−
Neocortex	+++	−	−/+	−	+++	+++	−	−	±	+	±/+	−	−
Tangles subcortical	+/+++	−	+++	−	±/+	+/++	−	−	−	+++	+++	−	−
Lewy bodies cortical	±	+	−	−	−	+++	+++	−	−	−	−	−	−
Lewy bodies subcortical	±	±	−	−	−	+++	+++	−	−	±/+	−	−	−

Pick bodies	−	−	−	−	−	−	−	−	−	−
Spongy changes	±	−	−	+	+	+	+++	+	−	++/+++
Ballooned neurons	−	−	−	−	−/+	+	+	+/++	+++	−
GCIs	−	−	−	−	−	−	−	−	+++	−
Glial tau + inclusions	±	+	+	+	±/+	++	++	+/++	+	−
Glial plaques	−	−	−	−	−	−	−	+++	−	−
Vascular lesions subcortical	±	−	+++	−	−	−	−	−	−	−
Vascular lesions large/cortical	±	−	±/+	+++	−	−	−	−	−	−
Prion (anti-PrP) immuno-histochemistry	−	−	−	−	−	−	−	−	−	+++

Key: −, lacking; ±, rare; +, occasional; ++, moderate; +++, severe.

Abbreviations: AD, Alzheimer's disease; CBD, corticobasal degeneration; DLB, dementia with Lewy bodies; FTD, frontotemporal dementia; GCIs, glial cytoplasmic inclusions; LBV/AD, Lewy body variant of Alzheimer's disease; MSA, multiple system atrophy; PSP, progressive supranuclear palsy.

Table 5 Likelihood of Dementia (in Percent) Due to Alzheimer's Disease According to NIA-R-Institute Criteria in Various Autopsy Series

Disorder CERAD/Braak	Low A/0-II	Interm. B/III-IV	High C/V/VI	Mean age (years)
Cochran et al. (1998) (295)				
Demented (n = 17)	47	41	12	?
Nondemented (n = 40)	72.5	22.5	5	?
Newell et al. (1999) (23)				
AD (n = 33)	0	3	97	83
DLB (n = 15)	48	26	26	81
PSP (n = 12)	75	17	8	68
Controls (n = 17)	76	24	0	77
Harding et al. (1999) (296)				
AD (n = 31/22-no LB) (CDR 1–3)	26/13	20/27	54/60	77
DLB, neocort. (n = 11)	73	18	9	76
PD (n = 7) (CDR 0–0.5)	83	17	0	79
Controls (n = 18) (CDR 0–0.5)	83	17	0	79
Davis et al. (1999) (297)				
Controls (n = 57, MMSE 27–29)	88	–	12	84
McKee et al. (2002) (298)				
AD (n = 12) (CDR 1–3)	0	17	83	81
Cogn. normal (n = 23) (CDR 0)	62	38	0	83
Jellinger (2003 f) (277)				
AD (n = 100) (MMSE 0–17)	0	24	76	85
DLB (n = 36) (MMSE 0–20)	25	33	42	77
PSP (n = 10)	70	20	10	72
PD dem. (n = 20, MMSE 0–20)	25	50	25	83
PD nondem. (n = 17, MMSE > 20)	70	30	0	72
Controls (n = 20, MMSE 28–30)	100	0	0	81

Abbreviations: AD, Alzheimer's disease; DLB, dementia with Lewy bodies; MMSE, Mini-Mental State Examination; PSP, progressive supra nuclear palsy; PD, Pick's disease.
Source: From Refs. 23, 277, 295–298.

defined neuropathological criteria for DLB and the presence of LBs in many cases at autopsy with non-DLB clinical presentations. The distribution of cortical LBs in DLB does not follow the spread of NFTs (196), while the spreading pattern of AS pathology with onset in the lower brainstem and progression to the midbrain, dorsal forebrain, amygdala, limbic cortex, and final extension to the neocortex is similar to that in sporadic PD (306). The late stages 5 and 6 of LB pathology (involvement of sensory association and prefrontal, primary sensory, and motor areas) suggest transition between PD and DLB (275,307,308). DLB was classified into the limbic type and neocortical type according to the degree of Lewy pathology, including LBs and LNs, and, on the other hand, into the pure form, common form, and AD form according to the degree of Alzheimer

Table 6 Morphological Diagnosis in Consecutive Vienna Autopsy Series (1985–2004) **(A)** of Demented Individuals, 541 Males, 899 Females, Age 50–103 (Mean 83.3 ± 6.0) Years; and **(B)** of Patients with Clinical Diagnosis of Probable or Possible Alzheimer's Disease (Mean Age 81.3 ± 6.0 Years)

Morphological diagnosis	(A)		(B)	
	n	%	n	%
"Pure" AD (CERAD pos., Braak V-VI)	623	41.5	432	52.0
Alzheimer type path, (plaque, limbic, NFT/SD) (26/53/28, 12/22/24)	107	7.1	58	7.0
AD + CVD (lacunar state, old/acute infarcts old, AH-sclerosis (129/66/37/4, 97/18/41/11)	236	15.7	167	20.1
AD + cerebral hemorrhage (CAA)	44	2.9	17	2.0
Lewy body variant AD/Diff, LB disease (33/33, 22/7)	66	4.4	29	3.5
AD + Parkinson pathol., PD, Incid, LBD, SN lesions (51/14/8, 21/14/8)	73	4.8	43	5.2
MIX type dem, (AD + MIE, + SAE, + SID) (39/22/7, 12/7/1)	68	4.6	20	2.4
AD + other pathol. (tumors, MS, MSA, etc.)	39	2.6	13	1.6
Alzheimer pathology total	1256	83.7	779	93.9
Vascular dementia (MIE, SAE, SID) (61/79/22, 5/6/6)	162	10.8	17	2.0
Other disorders (Huntington disease, FTD, CJD, others)	67	4.5	28	3.4
Nothing abnormal beyond age	15	1.0	6	0.7
Non-Alzheimer pathologies	244	16.3	51	6.1
Total	1500	100.0	830	100.0

Abbreviations: AD, Alzheimer's disease; AH, Amon's horn; CVD, cerebrovascular disease; CAA, cerebral amyloid angiopathy; CJD, Creutzfeldt–Jakob disease; FTD, frontotemporal dementia; LBD, Lewy body disease; MIE, multi-infarct encephalopathy; NFT, neurofibrillary tangles; SAE, subcortical atherosclerotic encephalopathy; SID, strategic infarct dementia; SD, senile dementia; SN, substantia nigra.

pathology including NFT and amyloid deposits by Braak staging (218). These combined subtypes were lined up on a spectrum not only with Lewy pathology but also with other DLB-related lesions including Alzheimer pathology, neuronal loss in the SN, spongiform changes in the transentorhinal cortex, and LNs in the CA2-3 region. There were some similarities in the extent of Lewy pathology between PD and DLB, although Lewy pathology of PD was below the lowest stage of Lewy pathology. In contrast, AD did not meet the stages of DLB Lewy pathology, and there were also no similarities in other DLB-related pathologies between AD and DLB. In addition, LBs of AD showed characteristics different from those of DLB in the coexistence of LBs with NFTs. These findings suggest that DLB has pathological continuity with PD, but can be pathologically differentiated from AD. While this would suggest that DLB exists as a discrete pathological entity, as with AD and PD (309), others showed no (310) or only

Table 7a Consensus Pathological Guidelines for Scoring Cortical Lewy
Body Deposition

Cortical region	Brodmann area	Anatomy	Score		
Entorhinal cortex	29	Medial flank of collateral sulcus	0	1	2
Cingulate gyrus	24	Whole gyral cortex	0	1	2
Mid-frontal cortex	8/9	Lateral flank of superior frontal sulcus	0	1	2
Mid-temporal cortex	21	Inferior surface of superior temporal sulcus	0	1	2
Inferior parietal lobule	40	Lateral flank of parietal sulcus	0	1	2

For each region Lewy bodies are counted from the depth of the sulcus to the lip. Counts are not made over the crest of the gyri except for the cingulate gyrus. Lewy bodies are predominantly located in deeper cortical layers (layers 5 and 6). In each region a count of up to five Lewy bodies in the cortical ribbon gives a score of 1 in the table. Counts greater than five score as 2. The sum of the five areas is used to derive the category of cortical spread (maximum score 10). Cortical Lewy body score: 0–2, brainstem-predominant; 3–6, limbic or "transitional"; 7–10, neocortical.
Source: From Ref. 305.

little difference between Parkinson's disease with dementia (PDD) and DLB (310a), in particular, more frequent involvement of the amygdala-limbic system, and neocortex in DLB (308).

LB pathology may progress in a systematic fashion through the brain regardless of the clinical phenotype. Except for some deviations in the severity and distribution of lesions in substantia nigra pars compacta (SNc) and a more frequent involvement of the CA2-3 region of hippocampus in DLB, these similarities suggest morphological and pathogenetic relations between both disorders. DLB is frequently associated with AD pathology of variable intensity and extent. A subgroup with diffuse Aβ deposition and neuritic AD lesions absent or restricted to the hippocampus is referred to as "pure" DLB, while those showing significant neuritic pathology that fits with the diagnosis of definite AD (281) have been classified as LBV/AD (290,311). They occupy higher Braak stages of AD pathology than age-matched controls, but lower stages than pure AD (290,312). Among 96 autopsy cases, 62% were classified as "pure" DLB and 37% had severe additional AD pathology (Braak stages 5 and 6). LBV/AD was present in 33% each of the limbic and neocortical subtypes (276,313). "Pure" DLB shows no significant differences in neocortical synapse density and synaptophysin immunoreactivity compared to controls, while severe synapse loss comparable to AD is seen in LBV/AD (314). Although neuronal loss in the cholinergic basal forebrain is consistently found in DLB, PDD, and AD (1), early and more widespread cholinergic decline differentiates DLB from AD (300), while LBV/AD shows an increase of cortical M1 muscarinic cholinergic receptors compared to both AD and controls (315).

Selective neuronal loss in the presubiculum in DLB (296), decreased expression of BDNF in hippocampal neurons and increased activated microglia producing neurotrophic cytokines, eg. interleukin-6 (IL-6), in PD and DLB brain may be related to functional changes affecting cognitive function (316,317). The clinical diagnostic accuracy was higher in DLB cases with low (75%) compared to high (39%) Braak stages (318). Unlike AD, neurochemical markers [synaptophysin and choline acetyl transferase (ChAT)] often do not correlate with cognitive decline in DLB (319) that showed a significant inverse association between NFT burden and psychosis (320). Microvascular disease due to hypotension related to carotid sinus syndrome may be a (reversible) substrate of cognitive impairment in DLB (321). Patients with AD alone or with LB pathology usually have more severe memory impairment than those with DLB alone that is associated with more severe executive dysfunctions. AD with LB pathology has the most rapid rate of cognitive decline (322). However, there is neither correlation between LB density in any brain area among DLB patients with cognitive changes or parkinsonism, nor between LB density and neuritic Braak stages or frequency of NPs, nor between LBs in cortex and SN (323), and no correlation betweeen the distribution pattern of NFTs, AP, and AS-positive structures, and ChAT activity (324).

Whereas cortical LB densities, in general, cannot separate DLB from PDD, the severity and duration of dementia appears to be related to both increasing parahippocampal LB densities and NP grade. Both LB and AD pathology contribute to dementia severity, but there may be considerable overlap between demented and nondemented patients. LBs appear to be a major determinant of dementia severity in DLB cases with milder AD pathology (Braak 3–4), but not in those with severe AD pathology (Braak 5–6). Advanced AD pathology may facilitate LB formation and, reciprocally, neocortical LBs may promote secondary AD pathology. It was concluded that the same neuronal circuits within the hippocampal formation are involved by both pathologies in AD and DLB and may contribute to cognitive impairment in both diseases (325). The relatively more severe executive impairment in DLB than in PDD may relate to the loss of frontohippocampal projections in DLB (326). Despite the morphological similarity of α-synucleinopathy in different types of LBD, indicating its coexistence with both PD and AD, their pathogenic relationship remains to be clarified (300,301,327). DLB and PDD could be so similar at a biological level that a categorical distinction is difficult or inappropriate (328–330).

Recent biochemical studies of tau, Aβ, and AS deposition showed an overlap of all three pathologies in sporadic AD with similar progression from the limbic system to the neocortex. Tau pathology and Aβ deposits were biochemically identical in both AD and DLB, but, corroborating neuropathological findings, tau pathology was usually less severe in sporadic DLB than in AD, the mean Braak scores being 4.1 versus 5.1 in AD, and the tau stages according to Delacourte et al. (248) were 7.3 versus 9.3 in DLB, respectively. These studies suggest that Aβ may stimulate progression of cortical synucleinopathy in sporadic DLB, while "pure" DLB without essential AD lesions was found only in a single familial PD case (331). The presence of AS-positive lesions in 7–71% of sporadic and familial AD in the amygdala, even in the absence of subcortical LBs (332–336), associated with the *APOE* ε4 and ε2 allele (337), and involvement of other brain areas (275,308,338,339), the co-localization of tau and AS epitopes in LBs (340) as well as clinical, biochemical and morphological overlaps between PD, DLB, and AD suggest that the process of LB formation is triggered, at least in part, by AD pathology (307,341). This collision of two processes may occur within the same region or within a single cell in the human brain (336,341) and in tg mice (342), though in an early-onset case of DLB no co-localization of tau and AS was found (303). The upregulation of the PD-associated protein DJ-1 in tau neuronal inclusions in Pick's disease (PiD), progressive supranuclear palsy (PSP), corticobasal degeneration (CBD), and AD and in glial inclusions in PSP, CBD, and multiple system atrophy (MSA) also suggests a common reaction, but human LBs and LB-like inclusions in AS-tg mice were negative (343). In vitro, AS promotes tau aggregation (fibrillation) and vice versa (344), suggesting a synergy between tau and AS (345). Furthermore, the presence of Aβ deposits in the cerebral cortex was often associated with extensive AS lesions and higher levels of insoluble AS. This suggests that Aβ enhances the development of cortical AS lesions in LB disorders (346). This evidence challenges the view of DLB as a distinct entity and suggests that in neurodegeneration certain neurons display fibrillary aggregates that are typical of two or more different disease processes (double or triple amyloidosis). It is unclear whether there is a common underlying pathological mechanism or if these lesions represent a common final pathology leading to neuronal degeneration.

Guidelines for the Diagnosis of DLB

The pathological guidelines, intended to provide a method of scoring the severity and distribution of LBs in the cerebral cortex (300,305), do not provide diagnostic criteria. Since they were formulated prior to the introduction of specific AS immunohistochemistry for the detection of LBs (347), the scores for LBs per region are based on ubiquitin (Ub) or conventional H & E staining. Inclusion of this method into the CERAD protocol (281) has not been achieved. The LB scoring system is based on five cortical areas, chosen on the basis of their frequent involvement. A simplified protocol by excluding the frontal region has been proposed because of the common finding of occasional LBs in this region in PD (312) (Table 7b). Another screening algorithm suggested that semiquantitative LB density thresholds in the parahippocampus may distinguish PDD and demented from nondemented DLB cases independent from other pathologies (348). Within pathological studies of patients with clinically diagnosed DLB and PDD, there is heterogeneity in terms of Alzheimer's and LB pathology. There do not seem to be obvious neuropathological differences between DLB and PDD, so a descriptive clinicopathological approach to their classification will probably be most productive, with specificity both about clinical terms (DLB or

Table 7b Modified Criteria of Dementia with Lewy Bodies, Cases Without Brainstem Lewy Bodies Excluded

Maximum number of Lewy bodies per field	Rating score for each region
0	0
1–5	1
6+	2

	Region sampled			
Category	Temporal cortex	Cingulate cortex	Transentorhinal cortex + hippocampus	Total
Brainstem predominant	0	0–1	0–1	0–2
Limbic (transitional)	1	1–2	1	3–4
Neocortical	1–2	2	2	5–6

Source: From Ref. 312.

PDD, largely determined by the temporal order of symptoms) and also about pathological findings (LBD, AD). The latter "categories" will need to be further illustrated by details of lesion density and distribution (330). Thus, a practical consensus for the diagnosis of DLB at present is not available.

Frontotemporal Dementias and Related Tauopathies

The heterogeneous group of frontotemporal dementias (FTD) or—neuropathologically more correct—frontotemporal lobar degeneration (FTLD), previously subsumed as PiD or Pick complex (349), represents the third most frequent cause of dementia (10–20%) (350,351). Clinico-pathological correlates in FTD have recently been summarized (352,353), and with awareness of the unique clinical manifestation of FTD, accurate antemortem diagnosis appears feasible (354). The temporal variant of FTD follows a characteristic cognitive and behavioral progression that suggests early spread from one anterior temporal lobe to the other. Later symptoms implicate ventromedial frontal, insular, and inferoposterior temporal regions, but their precise anatomic correlates await confirmation (355). Morphologically it is featured by focal atrophy of the frontal and temporal lobes with neuronal loss, microvacuolar (spongiform) changes, and gliosis, with or without tau or Ub pathology (356). Neurodegenerative mechanisms in FTD may be assisted or precipitated by the loss of astrocytic support (357). Constantinidis (358) distinguished type A, classic PiD with Pick bodies (Pib) and cells, and type B, with frontal and parietal atrophy, ballooned neurons, but no Pibs (359). Most cases of type B are now considered as CBD or FTD and parkinsonism related to chromosome 17 (FTDP-17) (353). Phenotype C without Pib or tau pathology is now classified as dementia lacking distinctive histopathology (DLDH) (360). Updated classifications of FTD suggest the following diagnoses (361,362):

1. Tau-positive lesions with predominantly insoluble 3-repeat tau:
   (*i*) PiD
   (*ii*) FTDP-17
2. Tau-positive lesions with predominantly insoluble 4-repeat tau:
   (*i*) CBD
   (*ii*) PSP
   (*iii*) FTDP-17
3. Tau-positive inclusions and insoluble 3- and 4-repeat tau:
   (*i*) NFT dementia
   (*ii*) FTDP-17
4. Frontotemporal neuronal loss and gliosis without tau/ubiquitin-positive inclusions, no insoluble and reduced soluble tau:
   (*i*) DLDH
5. Ub-positive, tau-negative inclusions without detectable tau, with or without motoneuron disease (MND), but MND-type inclusions:
   (*i*) FTD with MND that may be closely linked to ALS with dementia (363)
   (*ii*) FTD with MND-type inclusions without clinical MND presenting as semantic dementia (364)
   (*iii*) Motoneuron disease inclusion dementia (MNDID) related to chromosome areas 9 and 11

Ub intraneuronal inclusions and dendrites have also been reported in familial FTD (365,366), in FTD-17 (367), in familial and non-familial cases of FTD-MND (368), and a few sporadic FTD cases in the absence of MND (369–371), while neuronal intranuclear inclusions distinguish familial FTD-MND type from sporadic cases (372). There is a close relationship between CBD, PSP, and FTD (373,374), but, despite the identical composition of tau isoforms, different proteolytic processing of abnormal tau distinguishes PSP from CBD (375). Tau mutations have not been identified in sporadic FTD cases (376) and in some FTD families showing genetic linkage to the tau locus (377).

Specific subtypes of FTD that deserve description in detail are:

Pick's Disease

PiD is a rare variant FTD that accounts for 1–2% of all elderly dementia cases; its classical type shows frontotemporal lobe and limbic atrophy with neuronal loss, spongiosis, and gliosis including microglial activation, achromatic (Pick) cells, and intraneuronal globose inclusions (Pib) in hippocampus, in particular in dentate granule neurons, in cerebral cortex, and in selected brainstem nuclei. Ultrastructurally, they are composed of straight and long-period twisted filaments, made up of 3-repeat tau doublets (60 and 64 kDa) and a minor

68 kDa band (332,378). Tau-positive glial inclusions, mainly in the white matter, NFTs, and a network of dystrophic neurites differentiate PiD from FTD with tau-negative astrocytes (379). In sporadic PiD cases, in addition to 3- repeat tau deposits, isolated filaments formed from 3- and 4-repeat tau isoforms, and tau phosphorylation-dependent and exon 10-specific epitopes are found. Thus, accumulation of Pibs with 3- and 4-repeat tau pathology distinguish PiD from other tauopathies (380) along with a lack of any association with the tau H2 haplotype (381). A novel presenilin 1 mutation with familial Pick-type tauopathy without tau gene mutation and without Aβ plaques (382), a familial FTD with Pick-like pathology associated with Q336R mutation of the tau gene (383), another phenotype with a missense mutation of S305N (384), and a family with the R406W mutation and pathology consistent with NFTD (362) have been reported recently.

Frontotemporal Dementia Without Specific Lesions

FTD, without disease-specific lesions or DLDH, is a sporadic or familial "tau-less" tauopathy with no insoluble or fibrillary tau inclusions, and reduction of soluble tau but normal tau mRNA levels (385). Similar brain pathology was seen in a US family without known genetic background (386) and in a pedigree known as hereditary dysphasia disinhibition dementia (HDDD2) with linkage to chromosome 17q21–22, but no tau mutation. Reduction of soluble tau in most brains with DLDH and in some HDDD2 brains differs from previous FTD cases containing substantial mounts of insoluble tau (376,385). The phenotypic heterogenity of HDDD2 parallels that of other hereditary FTDs caused by tau gene mutation (387,388). No tau mutations have been identified in sporadic FTD cases (376) and in FTD families showing genetic linkage to the tau locus (377).

Familial Tauopathies

Several genetically distinct groups of inherited FTD have been identified: (1) FTDP-17; (2) FTD-MND linked to chromosome 3; and (3) FTD linked to chromosome 3 (FTD-3). Tau mutations have been found in 25% of familial cases of dominantly inherited FTD, but only in 4% of sporadic cases (389). Tau on chromosome 17 is the only gene where mutations have been identified, while Ub and tau inclusions have been found in the frontal cortex of patients from a Danish family with FTD-MND that shows more diffuse cortical involvement than other forms of FTD (390,391). Autosomal-dominantly inherited disorders linked to chromosome 17q21–22 show diverse but overlapping phenotypes (392), with tau pathology in neurons and glia, but no Aβ deposits or other disease-specific brain lesions (393). Two classes of tau mutations have been found in 10–40% of familial FTD cases—those directly affecting the microtubule-binding sites of tau and those that alter tau splicing (378,387). The majority of the currently known tau mutations are located in exons 9 to 13. P301L mutation was detected in 11% of familial FTD cases. The H1 haplotype was not overrepresented, but the P301L mutation appeared in the background of the H2 tau haplotype. Single nuclear polymorphisms in intron 9 and deletion in other introns upstream from exon 10 were increased in FTD cases with an increase in exon 10-containing tau transcripts (388). Thus, sequence variations in regulatory regions may lead to tau dysfunction and neurodegeneration (394). The aggregation of tau protein produces a significant accumulation of intracellular $A\beta42$ in cortical neurons, which, however, does not reach the critical concentrations needed for AP formation (395). A San Francisco family of 17q-linked FTD-amyotrophic lateral sclerosis (ALS) with AS and tau inclusions (4-R/ON isoform) but without tau mutations is different from other familial forms of FTD and ALS (396).

A study of 55 autopsy cases of FTD revealed tau pathology in 14, and tau-positive PiD inclusions in four, while 60% showed no tau pathology in the brain, except for rare NFTs. The 33 non-tau cases showed variable loss of soluble tau protein, broadly comparable with the extent of neuronal loss (397). In other series there was a predominance of FTLD-MND (398) and non-tauopathies with FTLD with Ub-only neuronal changes (FTLD-U) (370,399).

Neurochemical changes in FTD contrast with those of AD: a much lower cholinergic deficit and more serotonergic disturbance is linked with impulsivity, irritability, and affective change which are common features of FTD (400,401).

Consensus criteria for the postmortem diagnosis of FTDs: A recent pathological classification of FTDs suggests (402):

1. 3-repeat tauopathies—PiD.
2. 4-repeat tauopathies—CBD.
    PSP.
    Argyrophilic grain disease (AGD).
3. 3- and 4-repeat tauopathies; tangle-predominant dementia.
4. DLDH.
5. Diseases with motor neuron disease-type inclusions (DMNDI).

Another classification distinguishes pathological subtypes of FTD (352):

- with tau-immunopositive inclusions (with and without Pib)—CBD and AGD
- with Ub-immunopositive inclusions—FTD-MND/FTLD-U
- lacking distinctive histology (DLDH).

FTLD-U or FTLD-MND should be considered in the differential diagnosis of progressive FTD with an akinetic-rigid syndrome and PSP (399). An additional, recently described form is neuronal intermediate filament inclusion disease (NIFID) (372,403), representing a neuropathologically distinct, clinically heterogenous variant of FTD that may include parkinsonism or MND and is distinct from other FTDs (405). Genetic alterations can give rise to phentoypes more or less similar to any of the above. Tau mice recapitulate the key phenotypic hallmarks of human tauopathies (404).

Other Tauopathies

Hippocampal Sclerosis Dementia (with Tauopathy)

In a subset of elderly individuals, hippocampal sclerosis (HS) is the only remarkable morphological finding (406–412). Its frequency in autopsy series of elderly demented ranged from 0.4 to 26% (413), while it is almost never seen in nondemented oldest-olds (414,415). HS shows a wide range of severity and distribution, with damage of the hippocampus and subiculum ranging from neuronal loss and gliosis to frank infarction. It is occasionally accompanied by multiple small infarcts in other brain regions or leukoencephalopathy or both, while only rarely such brains show additional AD lesions (410,413). The cause of HS has been suggested to be due to occult hypoxic-ischemic episodes (408,409) or as a sequela of limbic encephalitis (416). Classical HS dementia (HSD), clinically being more similar to FTD than to AD (417), is morphologically characterized by severe loss of neurons and gliosis in the hippocampal CA1 region and subiculum. The EC, temporal pole, inferior frontal neocortex, and frontal pole may also be affected. Frequent tau-positive neurons and/or glial cells in neocortex, basal ganglia, thalamus and/or limbic regions, resembling to FDTP-17 and a mixture of 3- and 4-repeat tau isoforms, suggested the term "HSD with taupathy" (HSDT) (413). "Pure" HSD (406), where no other cause of dementia could be identified, shows morphological similarities to DLDH or ubiquitinated neuronal inclusions, similar to those of MNDID (363,418), but with brain levels of soluble and insoluble tau being normal, suggesting that "pure HSD" may represent FTD and, in particular, its MNDID variant (419). In addition, several cases had argyrophilic grains (413) that are also seen in argyrophilic grain disease (AGD). Selective degeneration of the CA2 sector of the hippocampus is rare, but when detected, it is associated with 4-repeat tauopathies, particularly AGD (420).

Argyrophilic Grain Disease

This neurodegenerative disorder of the elderly is seen in about 5% of demented patients and in subjects progressing from MCI to dementia (421–423). It may or may not be associated with a cognitive decline in the presence of only moderate amounts of AD-related pathology (424) and may be associated with anxiety, restlessness or depression (422) or may present with FTD (425). Morphologically AGD displays abnormal argyrophilic grains (AG), coiled bodies, and "pre-tangles" mainly in the limbic system (medial temporal lobe, amygdala) and insular cortex containing 4-repeat tau deposits with isoforms of 64 and 69 kDa (380,426–428). It shows genetic differences to other tauopathies (422,429). AGD is frequently associated with AD-related changes, low Aβ-load, and mild to moderate NFT pathology. A recent comparative morphological study showed that demented AGD cases showed lower stages of AD-related pathology, but higher ones than non-demented AGD patients. AGD associated dementia was associated with Braak stages 2–4 and Aβ phases 2–3, while those stages were not associated with dementia in the absence of AGD (424). Another recent study showed that the distribution of AGs follows a stereotypic regional pattern: in stage I, they are restricted to the ambient gyrus; in stage II they appear in the anterior and medial temporal lobe, subiculum, and entorhinal cortex; in stage III abundant AGs involve the septum, insular cortex, and anterior cingulate cortex, accompanying spongy degeneration of the ambient gyrus. 97% of AGD stage III cases without other pathology showed CDR> =0.5 (430). These data suggest that AGD is a clinically relevant neurodegenerative age-related tauopathy that independently contributes to the development of dementia by lowering the threshold for cognitive deficits in the presence of moderate degrees of AD-pathology (424,430). Since patients with AGD-associated dementia exhibit significant morphological and genetic differences from patients with "pure" AD, (431) they should be excluded from the AD group in future studies, although their clinical and morphological distinction may be very difficult, and recent studies using 4-repeat tau-specific immunohistochemistry detected AGD in 26% of neuropathologically confirmed AD cases (427).

Vascular-Ischemic Dementia—Vascular Cognitive Impairment

Vascular dementia (VaD) is a heterogeneous group due to lesions caused by different pathophysiological mechanisms and with different combinations of brain pathologies. It is therefore necessary to identify the various types of vascular brain lesions in order to correlate correlation with clinical symptoms and for diagnostic purposes to search for risk factors and therapeutic strategies. Dementias related to cerebrovascular disease (CVD) and ischemic brain damage were previously considered to be the second most common type of dementia (432–436) in the Western world after AD and DLB, with a possible incidence of 8–15% (415). Clinical diagnostic criteria for VaD–ICD-10 [WHO 93 (437)] exists: DSM-IV (438), the SCADDTC (439), and NINDS-AIREN criteria (440), supported by the Hachinski Ischemic score (HIS) (441,442), show variable sensitivity (average 50%) and specificity (range 64–98%) (443–446) and may exclude a number of subjects with VaD (447). NINDS-AIREN neuroimaging criteria have been found not to distinguish stroke patients with and without dementia (448). In an interobserver study, use of the operational definitions for the NINDS-AIREN criteria improved agreement but only for already experienced observers (449), whereas in another study none of the currently used clinical criteria identified the same group of incidentally demented subjects (450). On the other hand, integration of neuropsychological and neuroimaging data was suggested to be sufficient for the diagnosis of subcortical VaD (451). The classification may be based on: 1) primary vascular etiology, 2) primary type of ischemic brain lesions, 3) primary location of the brain lesions, and 4) primary clinical syndrome. Subcortical ischemic VaD is an example of such a subgroup. Vascular cognitive disorder (VCD) has been recently limited to cases without dementia, i.e., vascular cognitive impairment–no dementia (VCI-ND), but there are no universally accepted criteria for VCI (452–454). Other subgroups include post-stroke dementia (PSD) and mixed AD plus CVD (455). The Mayo Clinic criteria (temporal relationship between stroke and dementia or worsening of cognition, or bilateral infarction in specific regions) had 75% sensitivity and 81% specificity for autopsy-proven VaD (444). While the validity and liability of clinical diagnostic criteria is a matter of discussion (452), generally accepted and validated neuropathological criteria for VaD have not been established so far.

Morphological lesions associated with vascular cognitive disorder include focal and multifocal CVD (415,433,456–463):

1. Multifocal lesions with large territorial or borderline infarcts, microinfarcts and lacunar lesions in subcortical regions, cortical and cortico-subcortical infarcts, cortical pseudolaminar necrosis, granular cortical atrophy, and white matter lesions (WMLs) (Binswanger type of subcortical arteriosclerotic leukoencephalopathy), resulting from chronic ischemia, hypoperfusion, and other mechanisms (464–467), and multiple postischemic lesions.
2. Focal disease with strategically placed infarcts, i.e., in functionally important brain areas and neuronal circuits (see below).

Another classification distinguishes large and small vessel disease:

1. Large vessel dementia (LVD): classical multi-infarct encephalopathy/ large vessel disease—rather rare.
2. Small vessel dementia (SVD): microangiopathic (small vessel infarct) dementia with lacunes, strategic infarcts mainly in subcortical areas, WMLs (468–473).
3. Other types of VaD. Although cause-relationships between CVD and dementia evade strict classification, brain lesions associated with cognitive impairment are summarized in Tables 8 and 9.

Silent and symptomatic infarcts are related to an increased rate of dementia (474), and the presence of an *APOE E*4 and *E*2 allele is associated with greater progression of cognitive decline (475). Impairment of cognitive function is less related to the volume of brain destruction (476) than to the location of cerebrovascular lesions (CVLs), in particular to involvement of the hippocampus, entorhinal area, thalamus, basal forebrain, and interruption of corticothalamic and other important neuronal circuits (409,460,461,477–480). Cognitive impairment has been found in 20–41% of patients with ischemic stroke (473,481–483) and 40% with recurrent transient ischemic attacks (484). It is also associated with asymptomatic high-grade stenosis of the left internal carotid artery (485), and common carotid artery media thickness (486), although many patients with dementia identified after stroke already had dementia before (487). Older age, prestroke cognitive decline, stroke recurrence, hypoxic-ischaemic disorders,

Table 8   Major Morphological Types of Vascular Dementia

Classical multi-infarct encephalopathy (MIE)
   Multiple large (sub/territorial) infarcts in cortex and white matter/basal ganglia in
      territories of large cerebral arteries, MCA, MCA + PCA; involving the left or both
      hemispheres
Strategic infarct dementia (SID)
   Small or medium-sized infarcts/ischemic scars in functionally important brain regions:
      thalamus, hippocampus (PCA), basal forebrain angular gyrus (ACA), bilaterally or
      dominant hemispheres
Microangiopathic (small vessel infarct) dementia (SMVA)
   Subcortical arteriosclerotic leukoencephalopathy Binswanger (SAE)
      Multiple small infarcts in basal ganglia + white matter with preservation of cortex
   Multilacunar state
      Multiple microinfarcts (scars up to 1.5 cm Ø); basal ganglia, hemisphereal white
      matter, pontine basis
      Multiple cortico-subcortical microinfarctions (mixed encephalopathies)
   Granular cortical atrophy
      Multiple small scars within border zones ACA/MCA in one/both hemispheres
Subcortical microvascular leukoencephalopathy
      (acquired/genetically determined)
Gliosis or hippocampal sclerosis
Inflammatory angiopathy and other mechanisms

Abbreviations: ACA, anterior cerebral artery; MCA, middle cerebral artery; PCA, posterior cerebral
artery.
Source: From Refs. 440, 456, 463.

left-side infarcts, strategic infarcts, and white matter lesions appear to be the main
predictive factors of PSD (488). During a four-year follow-up the incidence of
PSD increased gradually, shifting from an initial AD-type picture to a VaD-type
later (489). Many patients with lacunar infarcts have a good functional outcome
at five years. For older patients, for patients with an initial severe stroke, and with
additional vascular risk factors, however, the prognosis is more severe, with an
increased risk for mortality, stroke recurrence, and physical and cognitive decline
(490). Dementia showed a correlation with widespread small ischemic lesions
throughout the CNS, mainly lacunes, microinfarcts, and hippocampal injury, and
much less with larger infarcts, many brains showing more than one type of CVLs,
although in cognitively normal aged controls similar lesions were present
(297,415,460,461,491). The size of WMLs in the elderly may progress with time
and may relate to clinical symptoms (492–494) and thus can be regarded as a risk
factor for cognitive impairment (495), whereas others may show territorial
infarcts and older age as predictors of cognitive impairment in the first year after
stroke (496). They impair frontal functions regardless of their location (497),
are associated with cortical more than entorhinal and hippocampal atrophy (498),
and increase the risk of dementia (499), particularly in patients with lacunar

Table 9 Pathophysiological Classification of Vascular Dementia

---

Multifocal/diffuse disease
Large vessel dementia (LVD)
  Multiple infarct dementia (MID)
    Multiple large artery/borderline infarcts, cortical and subcortical, with perifocal
      incomplete infarcts, especially in white matter
Small vessel dementia (SVD)
  Subcortical infarct dementia
    Multiple small lacunar infarcts with perifocal lesions in white matter
      "Granular atrophy" of cortex (multifocal cortical microinfarcts)
      Lacunar state
      Binswanger subcortical leukoencephalopathy (BSLE)
      Hereditary angiopathies — CADASIL (cerebral autosomal dominant arteriopathy
        with subcortical infarcts and leukoencephalopathy)
  Cortical plus subcortical infarct dementia
    Multiple, restricted small infarcts due to:
      Hypertensive and arteriolosclerotic angiopathy
      Amyloid angiopathy, with/without hemorrhages
      Collagen or inflammatory vascular disease (angiitis, PCNSA, FMD)
      Hereditary forms
 Hypoperfusive, hypoxic-ischemic dementia (HHD)
      Incomplete white matter infarcts
      Anti-PL related ischemia
      Diffuse hypoxic-ischemic encephalopathy (cortical lacunar necrosis, post cardiac
        arrest, hypotension)
Venous infarct dementia
  Large hemorrhagic, congestive symmetric infarcts due to thrombosis of the sagittal
    sinus or the great vein of Galen
Hemorrhagic dementia
  Subdural hemorrhage
  Subarachnoid hemorrhage
  Intracerebral hemorrhage
Focal disease/strategic infarct dementia (SID)
Few infarcts restricted to functional important regions
  Mesial temporal (including hippocampal) infarcts/ischemia/sclerosis
  Caudate and thalamic infarcts (especially DM nucleus, bilateral damage)
  Fronto-cingulate infarcts (basal forebrain, ACA territory)
  Angular gyrus infarct (dominant cerebral hemisphere—ACA and MCA territories)
  White matter key areas

Abbreviations: Anti-PL, anti-phospholipid; PCNSA, primary angiitis/arteritis of the central nervous system; FMD, fibromuscular dysplasia; ACA, anterior cerebral artery; DM, dorsomedial; MCA, middle cerebral artery.
Source: From Ref. 470.

infarcts (500,501), but WMLs and lacunes may be independently associated with cognitive dysfunction (502). Other studies showed that subcortical vascular disease on computed tomography (CT) is frequent in older patients with MCI, but does not appear to be associated with the severity of cognitive deficits (503). Postmortem detection of WMLs by MRI was less sensitive than pathology (504). These and recent neuroimaging data indicate that subcortical lacunes, WMLs, and multiple disseminated microinfarcts resulting from small vessel disease that damage structures of the prefrontal-subcortical circuits (505) are the most common pathological features of VCI/VaD, whereas large infarcts are less frequent (506).

Guidelines for the Morphological Diagnosis of Vascuar-Ischemic Dementia

While most of the currently used clinical guidelines for diagnosis of vascular-ischemic dementia (VID)/VCI show variable sensitivity and specificity, and the recent Mayo Clinic criteria (444) await validation by further clinicopathological studies, at present, no generally accepted and validated neuropathological criteria are available. Cognitive impairment appears to correlate with widespread ischemic and/or vascular lesions throughout the brain with particular involvement of functionally important areas and neuronal loops. "Pure" VaD/VCI should only be diagnosed in the absence of AD lesions beyond age-related levels or other concomitant pathologies (462). However, the postmortem diagnosis of VaD/VCI currently is a subjective one and a matter of discussion.

Mixed Dementias

Mixed type dementia (MD) is characterized by combined pathologies of both AD and VaD or other dementing disorders, but the distinction between these two pathological diseases is controversial (356,434,460,507–509). Recent emphasis on co-morbidity of AD and CVD (510–512), the link between AD and atherosclerosis (513), cognitive impairment associated with amyloid angiopathy (514,515), significant cerebral microvascular pathology (516,517), and deficient clearance of Aβ across the BBB in AD (518,519) all indicate that vascular disorder is an important feature of the chronic neurodegeneration in AD. Therefore, neurovascular dysfunction could have a major role in the pathogenesis of AD (140,520). ApoE E4 and E2 with its potential amyloidogenic role may be responsible for some of the microvascular changes found in AD (521). Many patients with dementia have radiological and neuropathological features of AD and VaD, with the classical NFTs and Aβ plaques of AD together with the cerebral infarcts of VaD. A close relationship between AD and VaD has been suggested since the age-related changes in cerebral blood vessels that are the basis of CVD and VaD may also be responsible for the failure of elimination of Aβ from the brain in AD (522). Neuronal overexpression of human APP renders the brain more vulnerable to ischemic injury and describes the factors that are involved in increased neuronal susceptibility to ischemic stroke (523). Criteria for the clinical diagnosis of mixed dementia are variable (439,440,524–528), and it has been questioned whether mixed dementia really exists as a separate entity (529,530). Generally accepted and validated histopathological criteria for the diagnosis of MD are currently not available, and its true frequency is unknown. Its prevalence rate in autopsy series showed a wide range from 2 to 56% in retrospective studies and 2.9 to 54.2% in prospective studies with means around 15% (13,460,461,477,531). Complicating the studies, many persons exhibit neuropathologic changes similar to AD, VaD, or mixed dementia, but do not meet clinical criteria for dementia (2,532).

Patients with AD frequently have other concomitant pathological lesions (533) and strokes are common and increase with age (534). Elderly people with silent brain infarcts have an increased risk of dementia and a steeper decline in cognitive function than those without such lesions (535). The severity of cognitive impairment was correlated to the total volume of infarcts with impact on lesions in limbic and medial association areas, frontal cortex, and white matter (536). In the Nun study, patients with autopsy-confirmed AD and CVLs had a higher prevalence of dementia than those without infarcts (24). The risk of being demented was 20-fold higher in subjects with AD and lacunar infarcts, but much lower and non-significant when a large territorial infarct was present (525,527,537). Other studies, however, showed lower Mini-Mental State Examination (MMSE) scores in AD patients without than in those with concomitant CVLs, the latter having a significantly more frequent history of strokes (Table 10). The presence of cerebral infarcts in AD increases significantly with age, but has little influence on the clinical features, and cannot be predicted from common vascular risk factors. In spite of a trend, there are no major differences in neurodegenerative lesion load (Aβ and NFT) between AD and AD with cerebral infarcts groups, except when cerebral infarcts are located in the temporal lobe (including hippocampus) where AD pathology was frequently lower, suggesting that this location may be important in the pathophysiology of mixed vascular and AD dementia (538). In a population-based study in the UK among 209 autopsies of elderly subjects, 48% being demented, 78% with CVD, and 70% AD pathology, the proportion of multiple vascular pathology was higher in the demented group (539), in which only 21% showed "pure" AD (471). In a health maintenance organization dementia registry, only 36% of patients had AD and no other findings, while 45% had pathologically definite AD plus coexistent CVLs, and 22% had AD plus DLB features (540). Comparison of 186 AD cases and 13 individuals with no cognitive impairment (NCI) suggested that neocortical core plaques were more related to dementia severity than the density of total SPs and NPs, while diffuse SPs were not. In those patients with infarcts, hemorrhages, or PD, NFT and SP densities were lower despite the presence of dementia (6). Among 333 autopsied men in the Honolulu-Asian Aging Study (120 demented, 115 marginal, 96 normal cognition), 24% of all dementias were linked with CVLs, and dementia frequency more than doubled with coexistent CVLs (45% vs. 20%). Findings suggest CVLs are associated with a marked excess of dementia in cases with low neuritic plaque

Table 10 Relation Between Cognitive State and Vascular Lesions in
Alzheimer's Disease

Disorder	n (M/F)	Age at death	Braak stage (mean)	Final MMSE (n)	History of stroke (%)
"Pure" AD	400 (159/241)	80.3 ± 8.9	5.2	1.1 (77)[a]	10.0
AD with lacunar state	133 (37/96)	83.2 ± 6.2	5.0	4.9 (19)	21.0[b]
AD with old infarcts (<10 mL)	37 (12/25)	84.6 ± 6.7	4.8	7.0 (5)	33.0[b]
AD with hippocampal sclerosis	16 (9/7)	86.1 ± 6.7[c]	4.7	5.0 (5)	NG
MIX (AD + CVD) infarcts >10 mL	33 (7/26)	82.7 ± 5.9	4.8	7.3 (4)	95.0[b]

[a]$p < 0.01$ vs. other groups.
[b]$p < 0.01$ vs. other groups.
[c]$p < 0.05$ vs. "pure" AD.
Abbreviations: AD, Alzheimer's disease; CVD, cerebrovascular disease; MMSE, Mini-Mental State Examination; M/F, male/female; NG, not given.

frequency. Prevention of CVLs may be critically important in preserving late-life cognitive function (541). A consecutive autopsy series of 1500 demented aged subjects showed AD-type pathology in 83.7%, but "pure" or atypical AD only in 48.6%, while 23% had additional CVLs, 9.2% α-synucleinopathy, and 2.6% other pathologies. Other disorders were seen in 16%, almost two thirds of them classified as "pure" VaD. Similar results were seen in 830 cases of the same autopsy cohort with the clinical diagnosis of probable or possible AD (Table 6). These and other studies indicate that most elderly patients with or without cognitive impairment have *mixed* disease.

There appears to be a close relationship between AD, atherosclerosis (542), and vascular pathology (460,510,512,543). Amyloid deposits in the vessel walls in aging and AD may be linked to consecutive CVLs and development of dementia (507,544–546). Soluble Aβ has a toxic effect on vascular endothelium via NOS phosphorylation, Ca^{2+} leakage, and other mechanisms causing vascular dysfunction (139), and CAA may be an independent risk factor for vascular cognitive impairment (471,514). CAA and hypertension are considered important contributors to mixed dementia (547), while severe CAA, more extensive than in AD and causing cortical infarctions, was seen in VaD (548).

Persons with hypertension have increased NFTs and brain atrophy at autopsy (549,550), and large vessel CVD, or atherosclerosis, is strongly associated with the presence of plaques (542). In autopsy series of demented patients, 18–80% had AD with CVLs (460,551–553). In a recent study the prevalence of vascular pathology in AD was significantly higher than in age-matched controls (48.0% vs. 32.8%, $p < 0.01$), in particular the presence of severe CVLs (old and recent infarcts and hemorrhages). The brain weight and severity of dementia did not correspond to the degree of vascular pathology, but higher Braak scores contributed to cognitive impairment (554). Another study of a consecutive series of autopsy-proven AD cases and age-matched controls revealed a higher frequency of CVLs and CAA in AD [57.4% vs. 33.2% and 94.5% vs. 33.3%, respectively (552)]. Concomitant cerebral infarction and, in particular, strategic lesions may have synergistic effects, lowering the threshold of AD pathology required for the development of dementia, and thus may aggravate cognitive impairment (525,527,533,555–558). In patients with CVD, the densities of plaques and neuritic AD lesions were significantly lower than in "pure" AD for every given level of cognitive deficit (6,546).

The contribution of small concomitant infarcts to cognitive decline in AD is unclear. In a cohort of longitudinally followed autopsy cases, significantly higher age and lower Braak stages were seen in patients with small infarcts of < 10 mL volume compared to those with "pure" AD, but small infarcts had no impact on cognitive decline (559). These data were at variance with others, suggesting a contribution of CVLs to cognitive decline in AD even with volumes of < 1 mL (508,536) but were confirmed by another autopsy study (526). This study indicated that coexistent small CVLs do not significantly influence the rate of progression of dementia in AD, although a concomitant vascular pathology may modulate both cognitive and non-cognitive features (560). In AD with minor CVLs, the majority of lesions were lacunes in basal ganglia and/or white matter and multiple microinfarcts, while in MD large lobar infarcts or multiple infarcts in the left or both hemispheres were more frequent, suggesting different pathogenic mechanisms between VaD, AD with small CVLs, and MD (460,461). The relevance of WMLs is a matter of discussion. WMLs in AD are significantly correlated with cortical atrophy and cognitive impairment (561), and together with cortical microinfarcts may contribute to the progression of cognitive deficits, but they do not contribute to the progression of AD (562). No interactions between WMLs and AD were found (563), and the neuropathological evaluation of focal cortical and white matter gliosis had no clinical validity (564). On the other hand, regional WML volumetry may be helpful in correlating subcortical pathology and cognitive impairment (565). In patients with subclinical AD and little functional brain reserve, additional cerebral infarcts independently contribute to cognitive decline, but do not interact with AD pathology to increase the likelihood of dementia beyond their additive effect (557). On the other hand, CVD has been suggested to be the most important cause in the elderly for the conversion of low-grade AD to dementia either by itself or acting as a catalyst (433). In full-blown AD with small CVLs, frequently observed by modern neuroimaging methods, cognitive decline is mainly related to the severity and extent of AD pathology (Table 10). Hence, the combination of two or more pathologic processes may influence the severity of cognitive deficits and represents a major diagnostic challenge.

Guidelines for the Diagnosis of Mixed Dementia

At present, there are no generally accepted and validated clinical or neuro-pathological guidelines for the diagnosis of MD. Criteria for AD and VaD are of limited value for the diagnosis of MD, and more distinct criteria for this diagnostic category are necessary.

Other Dementias

The pathological findings and diagnostic criteria for other types of dementia will not be discussed here (292,566).

EARLY PATHOLOGY OF AD AND CLINICAL CORRELATES

Longitudinal clinico-pathological studies have enhanced our understanding of early AD changes and their relationship to cognitive function (566a). Here we review (1) the most important studies comparing neuropathology of normal brain aging to AD, (2) morphological differences between MCI/early AD and AD dementia, (3) the role of hippocampus and the cholinergic system in early AD, (4) early involvement of the olfactory system, (5) comparison between biopsy and later autopsy findings, and (6) the value of biopsy demonstration of CAA.

Neuropathology in Cognitively Normal Aged Subjects (and AD)

Universally accepted neuropathologic criteria for differentiating AD from healthy brain aging do not exist. Older studies in small autopsy samples reported numerous SPs in 9–100% of nondemented elderly, but none of them met pathological criteria of AD (567). These and other data suggest that (1) $A\beta$ and diffuse SPs in the absence of neuritic pathology either appear to be part of normal aging with no clinical significance or may represent an early stage of AD, and (2) $A\beta$ deposits appear to be necessary but not a sufficient condition for inducing neuritic components and thus may not be, per se, markers of incipient AD (7,568,569). AD and controls could be distinguished from each other by mean NP and NFT counts, but sufficient overlap caused difficulty in diagnosing any individual case. Abundant diffuse SPs and NPs in the neocortex were seen only in AD cases (570), while in the neocortex of cognitively normal subjects, plaques are either absent or present as diffuse plaques only in scattered patches (571). Thus, both plaque burden and plaque morphology appear to be useful in distinguishing the earliest detectable form of AD from nondementing aging. In contrast, the slow accumulation of NFTs restricted to entorhinal cortex and related medial temporal lobe structures occurs as a function of age and appears not to reliably distinguish AD from aging (14,238).

Other studies of nondemented elderly individuals reveal at least a few NFT and SPs in ento- and perirhinal cortex, and the CA1 of hippocampus but with less involvement of the neocortex. The distribution of NFTs follows a similar pattern to that of AD, while the number of SPs was not related to the severity of NFTs (15). Only 17% of cognitively normal individuals (mean age 83.9 years) had no or few SPs and few hippocampal and entorhinal NFTs. Sixty-nine percent showed variable numbers of NPs in neocortex, amygdala, and EC. Forty-eight percent met Khachaturian criteria for AD, 25.4–27% CERAD, 11% intermediate NIA-RI criteria, and almost 9% Braak stages 5 or 6. Only NFTs in hippocampal CA1 region correlated with higher Braak stages and autopsy age, suggesting that they are associated with normal brain aging. Although many subjects had AD-like changes, they showed no differences in mental performance, suggesting compensatory mechanisms (298,572,573).

Among 39 nondemented elderly (mean age 85 years) only one brain was without NFTs, 56% had Braak stages 1 or 2, 28% stage 3, and 13% stage 4 or higher. Eighty-two percent and 95% had less than moderate numbers of cored SPs or NPs, 49% had moderate to frequent DPs, with 23% having a typical Braak staging in one region discordant from the scheme. 18% were CERAD positive for AD, 49% Khachaturian positive, and 13% had LBs, but only one with numerous neocortical LBs. Small, old infarcts were seen in 46%, with 23% having more than one, most of those being subcortical, rarely cortical, and none had a large infarct. Thus, the majority of cognitively normal individuals had minimal neuritic tau pathology (Braak stage <4 and NPs <6/100 field) in most affected neocortical regions (574). These and other studies, e.g., the Nun study, demonstrate a broad spectrum of neuropathology in the elderly cognitively normal. Several studies have indicated that the densities of total neocortical SPs (neuritic and diffuse), although correlating moderately and not as robustly as neocortical NFTs with dementia severity, constitute the best marker to differentiate AD, even in the earliest symptomatic stage (CDR 0.5), from nondemented controls (5,6,238). Neither neocortical nor hippocampal NFTs discriminated nearly as well between the nondemented and demented AD groups (282).

Brain Morphology in MCI Compared to Cognitively Normal Controls and AD

MCI is the term commonly used for a prominent memory impairment and relative sparing of other cognitive domains that is intermediate between CNS aging and very early dementia, particularly AD, and is a high-risk predementia state (26,503,574–582). Its clinical representation and morphological basis are heterogenous and include patients with both early AD and significant CVD, in whom memory and executive performance impairment predict likelihood of developing dementia (583–588).

Few NFTs in anterior olfactory nucleus and parahippocampal gyrus were seen in young nondemented individuals, with more NFTs in these areas and in the hippocampal area CA1 in older ones (73–89 years), while MCI cases had more NFTs in the same areas. Severely demented patients had large numbers of NFTs in neocortex, while only part of the nondemented group showed a few primitive plaques, and all the MCI to mildly demented groups had large numbers of primitive or mature SPs. Unlike NFTs they were not considered a feature of aging up to 80 years (14).

In another cohort, all nondemented individuals had NFTs in (para)-hippocampal areas, their mean density showing an exponential increase with age, even in the absence of SPs. A group of nondemented elderly showed widely distributed DPs and NPs in the neocortex and limbic areas; those with NPs were suggested to represent preclinical AD, CDR 0.5 in this particular study being the threshold of very mild dementia. NFTs in EC, suggested to be the earliest stages of AD, closely paralled cell loss in very mild demented subjects, but NFT formation was not associated with age-related cell loss, which was not found in nondemented subjects (237,238,589).

In another study, no clear differences in the frequence of NFTs between cognitively normal persons and CERAD "possible" AD cases were seen. Cognitively normal individuals had Braak stages 1 or 2 while "possible" AD cases had Braak stages 1–3 (590).

In a further study, diffuse SPs were seen in all cases with moderate dementia (mean age 60 years), in 65% with mild dementia, and in 58% with questionable or no dementia. SP density increased as a function of dementia severity and was correlated with NP and NFT formation (4). Diffuse SPs may not be part of normal aging but instead represent presymptomatic AD. The high density of DPs in controls just at the threshold of detectable dementia is consistent with the hypothesis that Aβ deposition is an initial event in development of AD (237).

This was confirmed in a 74-year-old female with advanced AD and her nondemented 47-year-old daughter, both dying from homicidal strangulation (591). While the mother showed fully-developed AD pathology, the daughter's brain revealed only perineuronal deposition of diffuse Aβ in cerebral cortex and abnormalities of the endosomal lysosomal system, without NFTs or glial changes, suggesting that amyloid deposition and endosomal-lysosomal changes are early events in late-onset AD that precede the onset of dementia. No genetic information about this AD family was available.

Elderly cognitively normal individuals had no or only few neocortical SPs or NFTs in limbic areas (Braak stages 0–2). While there was no significant relation between age at death and density of limbic or neocortical NFTs, the rate of cognitive change was correlated with NFT burden in the neocortex and to a lesser degree in limbic areas. NFT density decreased in order from the EC through amygdala, subiculum, and CA1, to infratemporal region. In patients who became demented, more severe NFT and SPs were seen (3).

These and data from the Vienna Prospective Dementia Study (mean age 81.7 ± 8.6 years) confirm the significant negative correlation between neuropsychological status and Braak stages in patients without other pathologies (509).

Neocortical Braak stages 5 and 6 were mainly, but not exclusively, seen in severely demented individuals, while limbic stages (2–4) were associated with a wide range between the cognitively normal to overt dementia (Fig. 2). Similar correlations have been observed in both younger (219,223,274,298) and older subjects (224,592,593), indicating a "gray" transitional zone of mild to moderate dementia showing a wide range of AD lesions (Fig. 3). These data support a continuum in which AD is infrequent in healthy, cognitively stable seniors, and preclinical pathology precedes cognitive impairment. All MCI patients had a tau pathology, but not necessarily Aβ pathology, whereas not all patients with tau pathology did not have MCI (219).

Among 11 MCI cases (mean age 89 years; CDR 0.5) five patients showed frequent NFTs and NTs in limbic regions and moderate DPs with sparse NPs and NFTs in neocortex, but were insufficient for the diagnosis of definite AD, while the others showed extensive tau pathology in the medial temporal lobe suggesting very early AD (594).

In the Religious Order Study (ROS) fewer NFTs and NTs in the parahippocampus were seen in cognitively unimpaired subjects compared to MCI and AD (10,295). NFT density within peri- and entorhinal cortex correlated with measures of episodic memory. NTs were not correlated with any cognitive ability. The NT burden increased from normal to MCI and then decreased in AD. Major findings were (1) that granulovacuolar lesions and NFTs correlated with measurements of episodic memory; (2) NTs precede NFTs that in turn precede

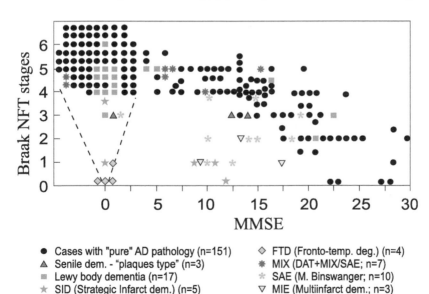

Figure 2 (*See color insert.*) Relationship between Mini-Mental State Examination (MMSE) and Braak neuritic Alzheimer's disease stages in 207 consecutive autopsies of aged individuals (mean age at death 81.4 ± 8.6 years).

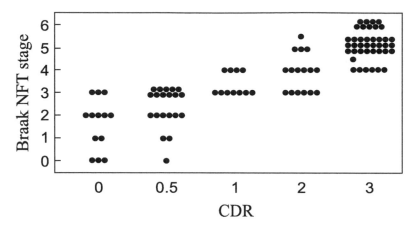

Figure 3 Column scatter plot of Braak stages versus Clinical Dementia Rating (CDR) scores in 100 oldest-old people (mean age at death 92.5 ± 2.5 years).

NPs; and (3) conformational tau changes emerged as a result of in situ reactivity to different antibodies, reflecting its structural status in NFTs that correlated with memory deficits (216). The authors presented a model for PHF degeneration beginning with NT formation, followed by NFT development and ending with appearance of NPs. Nondemented subjects showed the hierarchical pattern of NFTs, while the distribution of NPs varied among individuals. MCI cases had higher NFT densities than the cognitively normal in the medial temporal lobe, this being related to performance on memory tests, while amyloid SPs showed no correlation (11). It seems that the progression from Braak stages I and II to stage III, which may or may not be associated with signs and symptoms of mild AD or MCI, takes decades to occur and is presumably critical for developing AD.

The transition to clinical dementia (CDR ≥ 1) was associated with PHF-tau pathology in areas A9/10, A22, A23, and A39. A9/10 represents a prefrontal cortical network that provides "executive control" over complex goal-directed behaviors, while the other areas provide afferents to other frontal systems and have been implicated in early AD (595). Executive MCI in the absence of dementia has been suggested to be associated with decrease of soluble Aβ in the frontal cortex (596) and with frontal and anterior cingulate tau and Aβ load that may be early features of the frontal variant of AD (597).

Among 162 older Catholic clergy (mean age 75.8 years; 31 MCI, 57 cognitively unimpaired, and 53 clinical AD), nearly all brains had some AD pathology. Its average level in MCI was significantly higher than in controls and significantly lower than in AD. The occurrence of infarcts and LBs showed no difference between MCI and the two other groups. This suggests that patients with MCI show a level of Alzheimer type pathology that is significantly different from both AD and cognitively unimpaired individuals. LBs were usually not related to MCI (16), although MCI can evolve into DLB in some cases (598). Similar findings were reported recently from the ROS: among 180 participants (60 normal, 37 MCI, and 88 demented), nearly all had some AD pathology, cerebral infarctions were present in 35.3%, and 15.6% had DLB. Persons with MCI were intermittent in terms of Braak stage, CERAD, and NIA-RI neuropathologic criteria for AD compared to the other two groups, and the relationship between cognition and AD pathology did not significantly differ between the three groups which also showed intermediate levels of cerebral infarction, while only 8% had LB pathology (583).

In the Nun study, Braak stages 1 and 2 showed the greatest variation in cognitive profile, while in other reports stages 3 and 4 seemed to be the most diverse in terms of cognitive deterioration. Although stages 1 and 2 have been described as "clinically silent" (218), some subjects in these stages already had an identifiable cognitive impairment. Only cognitively unimpaired subjects were classified as either Braak stage 0 or 2–3, while those with MCI showed all Braak stages (24), but others found no or little pathological differences between persons with MCI and cognitively normal individuals (25), and between MCI and AD (216). Of the cognitively unimpaired individuals, 87% showed allocortical NFTs, only 37% displayed neocortical NPs, 19% had hippocampal NPs, and none exhibited neocortical NFTs, though the latter were not detected in 10% of AD brains or in nearly 50% of mild AD. Although NP and NFT density increased with dementia severity, significant differences emerged for NFTs alone. The increase in NPs and NFTs, in patients with even mild AD compared to normal controls, suggests that both lesions are associated with the earliest symptoms of AD (566a,599). Hence, NFT and NP pathology may constitute pathological substrates for memory loss in AD but also in normal aging and MCI.

However, demonstration of a distinct sequence of Aβ deposition suggests that nondemented individuals with Aβ or NPs may also represent early stages of AD (229). An asymptomatic prodromal stage appears to be associated with increasing Aβ in the brain. The initial symptoms of MCI may develop when a threshold level of neuronal and synaptic loss is reached in the EC and hippocampus concurrent with NFT formation and gliosis. Subsequent disease progression and conversion to clinical AD are associated with progressive neuronal and synaptic loss, and NFT formation on a background of elevated Aβ that reaches a "ceiling" early in the disease. NFT formation and synapse loss continue throughout the disease course (270). Dementia conversion rates increase as cognitive impairment increases, and the likelihood of subsequent conversion of MCI to dementia is usually related to the severity of local AD pathology (24), particularly in the ventromedial temporal lobe (566a).

In general, neuropathology data do not permit extrapolation in terms of prediction of progressive cognitive decline in individual cases. However, respondents with a final MMSE score in the "medium MMSE" group, analogous to but not identical with clinical MCI, show indices of AD pathology which appear intermediate between high and low performing groups: namely a paucity of neocortical tau pathology but with more advanced temporal lobe pathology than high performing patients.

The Role of Hippocampus in Early AD

The earliest clinical phase of AD, characterized by impairment of episodic memory and delayed recall, begins with subtle hippocampal synaptic dysfunction prior to frank neuronal degeneration, but their causes are unclear. Aβ deposition is associated with decreased hippocampal glucose metabolism and spatial memory impairment in APP/PSEN1 mice (600). Parahippocampal tau pathology was significantly less severe in cognitively normal individuals compared to MCI and/or full-blown AD, and the NFT density was significantly correlated with memory deficits but no other cognitive abilites. This indicates that tau pathology in the ventromedial temporal lobe develops prior to the onset of clinical dementia and is associated with cognitive impairment restricted to dysfunction of episodic memory. Substantial involvement of the hippocampus is often a key step for the transition from MCI to dementia, probably irrespective of the patient's age (601). Progression of the disease, especially beyond the boundaries of the limbic region, is associated with marked cognitive decline (602), and neuron number and volume measures significantly decline with increasing duration of AD. Tauopathy of the hippocampal formation in humans appears to be an age-related process that can be compensated for by some individuals and appears also to be independent of AD, but amplified by APP dysfunction (603).

Numerous primitive plaques and hippocampal alterations correlate with age-associated memory impairment, whereas substantial NFT formation in the neocortical temporal association areas is a prerequisite for the development of AD. No correlation was observed between SP densities and severity of dementia. Very old demented AD subjects had high NFT densities in the anterior CA1 field, but not in the entorhinal and anterior temporal cortices (2), while other authors considered the extent of NFT pathology in perforant pathway neurons to be a key determinant of dementia in the very old (592). Oldest-old AD patients showed decreased entorhinal PHF-tau lesions compared to younger ones, suggesting that it is not simply correlated with aging and that AD pathology may differ in the oldest age group (604). Thomas et al. (605) found a correlation between memory impairment, but not global cognitive impairment, and amyloid load particularly for Aβ42 and in the EC in AD and VaD but not in DLB. They conclude that the anatomic location of amyloid deposition is an important factor-specific item of memory impairment in AD and VaD.

Although the mesolimbic cortex and hippocampus are thought to be central in the integration of emotional responses, behavior, and intellect, neuritic SPs and NFTs in these areas do not appear to be a reliable predictor of dementia, as 20–100% of mentally intact elderly show neuritic lesions in these regions and cannot be clearly distinguished from demented persons (7,14). Early NFTs in layer II of the EC are present in normal aging (7,14,15,218,567,569,606). In nondemented elderly, Alz-50 immunoreactive neurons were found most frequently in the CA2 sector of hippocampus and only occasionally in layer II of the EC (607). In both nondemented elderly and late onset AD NFTs are frequently found in the CA1, and rarely in CA2 hippocampal area; their numbers increase with age in CA1, but not until the age of 90 years in the CA2 area (608). A heterogenous pathology of the hippocampus appears to be related to degeneration of the perforant pathway: NFT formation is restricted to CA2 related to the non-perforating route, while degeneration of the perforant pathway precedes NFT formation in pre-CA1 and presubiculum (609).

Aged cognitively unimpaired controls showed no changes in neuronal numbers in entorhinal and superior temporal cortices (589,610); MCI had a significant (32%) cell loss in EC, but none in superior temporal cortex, while in AD cell loss was 66% and 52%, respectively, and in entorhinal layer II was 60–90% (12). Others reported a substantial decrease (35%) in EC, 50% in layer II, and 46% in the CA1 in very mild AD (CDR 0.5), and a greater cell loss in CA1 in the severe AD group (589). MCI cases in layer II of the EC showed 65% of neurons compared to cognitively normal individuals; mild to moderate AD had 45% with 25% atrophy of layer II. Both lesions correlated with performance on MMSE, indicating that cell loss and atrophy of entorhinal layer II occur in elderly subjects with MCI before the onset of dementia (8). Memory impairment can occur in the presence of intact numbers of hippocampal neurons in non-AD dementias, while nerve cell loss in hippocampus might be characteristic of AD (611). Stereological studies gave evidence for persistence of viable neurons in the entorhinal layer II and the CA1 hippocampal field even in advanced stages of AD (612), and no significant loss of neurons in any other subdivisions of the hippocampus was seen in preclinical AD (613). There is a stage-dependent and sector-specific neuronal loss in AD hippocampus, with reduction of pyramidal cells in CA1 by 33–51%, in Braak stages 4 and 5 compared to stage I, while in the subiculum a 22% cell loss was seen only in stage 5 (614). Neuronal loss was higher than the numbers of NFTs with a relation of 10:1 (234), while there was no correlation with SP numbers. In stratum lacunosum moleculare, a subfield of the hippocampus regulating declarative memory function, elevated growth protein was positively correlated with the severity of AD, suggesting aberrant neuroplasticity (615), while hippocampal neurogenesis is apparently increased in AD (616). Functional magnetic resonance imaging (fMRI) studies suggest a phase of increased hippocampal activation in MCI, i.e., early in the course of prodromal AD, followed by a subsequent decrease as the disease progresses (617). In addition to increased glial fibrillary acidic protein (GFAP) expression due to astrogliosis, accumulation of specific GFAP isoforms have been observed in degenerating hippocampal neurons in AD brain, indicating probably a protective mechanism that remains to be elucidated (618).

Stereological studies fo the hippocampus showed significantly more severe loss of CA1 and CA2 neurons in AD compared with vascular ischemic dementia, without significant difference in neuron size. The number of CA1 neurons correlated with MRI-derived hippocampal volume and memory score, indicating that severity of cell loss shows correlations with structure and function across causative subtypes which have distinct pathologic correlates (619).

Analysis of AD-related pathology in 12 oldest-old individuals including assessment of total NFT, neuron numbers, and amyloid volume in EC, CA fields, and dentate gyrus showed that the progression of NFT numbers and amyloid volume across the different CDR groups was slower compared to younger cases. Although patients with mild and moderate dementia showed significantly lower mean neuron numbers compared to CDR 0–0.5 cases, there was a marked overlap in individual values among CDR groups. A modest proportion of the variability in CDR scores was explained by NFT numbers in the CA2 field (18.1%) and the dentate gyrus (17.3%), while neither neuron numbers nor total amyloid volume in the areas studied significantly predicted cognitive status. This indicates that the occurrence and progression of AD-related pathologic changes are not an unavoidable consequence of aging. The data also suggests that dementia in extreme age is dependent on damage to hippocampal subdivisions that normally show minimal pathology rather than on severe NFT formation and neuronal loss in the CA1 field and EC (620), while synaptic loss is an early event in AD (620a).

Alterations in the γ-aminobutyric acid (GABA) neurotransmitter and receptor systems contribute to vulnerability of hippocampal pyramidal neurons in AD. In control subjects (Braak I/II), the intensity of neuronal GABA receptor R1 protein (GBR1) immunoreactivity (IR) differed among hippocampal fields, being most prominent in the CA4 and CA3/2 fields, mild in the CA1 field, and very light in the dentate gyrus. AD cases with moderate NFT pathology (Braak III/IV) showed increased GBR1-IR, particularly in the CA4 and CA3 fields. In the CA1 field of the majority of AD cases, the numbers of GBR1-IR neurons were significantly reduced, despite the presence of neurons in this region. These data indicate that GBR1 expression changes with the progression of NFT in AD. At onset of hippocampal pathology, increased or stable expression of GBR1 could contribute to neuronal resistance to the disease process. Advanced hippocampal pathology appears to be associated with decreased neuronal GBR1 staining in the CA1 region, which precedes neuronal cell death. Thus, changes in hippocampal GBR1 may reflect alterations in the balance between excitatory and inhibitory neurotransmitter systems, which likely contributes to dysfunction of hippocampal circuitry in AD (621).

Synapsin I, a synaptic vesicle-associated protein participating in synapse formation, regulation of the synthesis of other synaptic vesicle proteins, and promotion of neurotransmitter release, is significantly decreased in the stratum radiatum of the CA1 subfield and the molecular layer of the dentate gyrus in AD brains, but was not reduced in the stratum pyramidale, where pretangles were observed (622). This indicates differential synaptic alterations in AD. Chromogranin B and secretoneurin, which are soluble constituents of large dense-core vesicles, were significantly reduced in the entorhinal and orbitofrontal cortex in AD, while chromogranin A was less reduced. This altered availability may be responsible for impaired transmission and reduced function of dense core vesicles (623,624). Loss of synaptophysin mRNA in NFT-bearing neurons in the hippocampus (625) and defects in expression of genes related to synaptic vesicle trafficking in frontal cortex of AD occur as well (626).

Caspase 3, a marker of apoptosis, is activated in the parahippocampal gyrus in subjects with MCI and low CERAD/intermediate Braak scores; caspase-like immunoreactiviy has a tangle-like appearance and co-evolved with PHF pathology in neurons, suggesting activation of apoptosis and of caspase-cleaved APP occurs very early in the medial temporal lobe in aging and AD (627,628). Mitochondrial defects in AD include COX-deficient hippocampal neurons that do not appear to be prone to apoptosis or directly participate in the overproduction of tau or Aβ. They are likely to contribute to the overall CNS dysfunction and possibly cause neurodegeneration via mechanisms other than apoptosis (629). Microarray analyses of hippocampal gene expression revealed a major transcriptional response comprising thousands of genes correlated with AD markers. There was up-regulation of many transcription factor/signalling genes regulating proliferation and differentiation, tumor suppressors, glial growth factors, protein kinase A modulators of adhesion, apoptosis, lipid metabolism, initial inflammation processes, and down-regulation of protein folding/transport, some energy metabolism, and signaling pathways. These findings suggest a new model of AD pathogenesis in which a genomically orchestrated up-regulation of tumor suppressor-mediated differentiation and involution processes induces the spread of pathology along myelinated axons (630).

The Cholinergic System in MCI and Early AD

The cholinergic neurons of the basal forebrain system provide a topographically organized input to all regions of the allo- and neocortex that is important for cortical activation. They not only influence their target neurons, but are also influenced by target-derived neurotrophic factors, such as nerve growth factor (NGF), which modulate cholinergic transmitter production and cellular structure (631). Depriving the cholinergic neurones of NGF-producing target cells in experimental animals causes pronounced cell atrophy. While neither aged animals nor AD patients show decline in cortical NGF production, both show evidence of disturbed retrograde transport of NGF (632). Precursor of NGF (proNGF) levels increase during the preclinical stage of AD—possibly an early biomarker for the onset of AD—and its accumulation in cerebral cortex correlates with loss of cognitive performance (633). Depending upon the cellular context these changes may result in increased pro-apoptotic signaling, cell survival, or a defect in retrograde transport mechanisms, the latter not being confirmed. Alterations in NGF and its receptors within the cholinotrophic basal forebrain system in early AD suggest that NGF-mediated cell signalling is required for the long-term survival of these neurons. Neurochemical and behavioral studies support the possibility that aging reveals the vulnerability of an abnormally regulated cortical cholinergic input system. Its decline and the decline in cognitive functions are further accelerated as a result of interactions with APP processing (634). Extracellular Aβ aggregation may affect cholinergic terminations prior to progression onto other neurotransmitter systems (635), and there may be relations between calbindin-D-28k, FADD expression, and phosphorylation of tau within the basal forebrain (636), but the interaction between cholinergic dysfunction and Aβ are not fully clarified (637,638).

Cognitively normal subjects and early stage AD (average Braak stage <2) in plaque-containing cases showed a significant decrease of ChAT activity (71–79.5%) compared to plaque-free cases, and in inferior temporal cortex, ChAT had an inverse correlation with Aβ concentration (639), suggesting a preclinical onset of the cholinergic deficit in AD (640). NFTs and AT8 immunoreactive neurons in the basal forebrain were seen even in cognitively unimpaired subjects, but the percentage of tau-positive basal forebrain neurons was greater in MCI cases and showed a significant correlation with memory scores (27). These results and reduction of cortical AChE activity (640a) indicate that the cholinergic deficit occurs at an early stage of AD before the onset of clinical symptoms. Whereas both the subicular cholinergic fibers and basal forebrain neurons were lost in AD, no cholinergic deficit was found in the temporal cortex in "pure" VaD (641), and subicular cholinergic fibers are unimpaired in Binswanger's disease (642).

Changes in some cholinergic basal forebrain markers, e.g., the high affinity TrkA receptor, but not others [e.g., cortical ChAT activity, the number of ChAT and vesicular acetylcholine (ACh) transporter-immunoreactive neurons], suggest specific phenotypical changes, but not the frontal neuronal degeneration that occurs early in cognitive decline. *APOE E4* and *E2* genotype, a predictor of cholinergic deficits (643), is accompanied by lower metabolic activity in the basal forebrain neurons in AD patients and also in aged controls as indicated by the size of the Golgi apparatus and may represent a risk factor for cognitive impairment (644). Others saw no correlation between *APOE E4* and *E2* and cholinergic decline (ChAT activity) in AD, while the presence of two *E4* alleles was an important determinant of both NP and NFT accumulation in the neocortex. By contrast, a strong relationship between *APOE E4* and *E2* alleles and decreased neocortical NP counts suggests a putative protective role for *E2* in AD (645). However, the fact that cholinergic neuron numbers and brain ChAT activity are not altered in MCI suggests that compensatory mechanisms occur in the remaining cholinergic perikarya that normalize cortical ChAT levels. Reductions of cortical TrkA in prodromal AD may be one of the earliest signs of subtle neurodegeneration in the basal forebrain system leading to the inability of this system to utilize NGF and may have important consequences for cholinergic basal forebrain function during the transition from MCI to AD (646). The accumulation of proNGF in the basal forebrain cholinergic target zones and the lack of retrograde signals are crucial for nuclear transcription of genes mediating cell survival. Increases in cell cycle proteins may be a response to the lack of cell survival signals, suggesting that basal forebrain neurons undergo degenerative events during the prodromal stages of AD (647). Progressive loss of cortical acetylcholinesterase (AChE) activity, indicating a progressive dysfunction of the ascending cholinergic system, correlated with cognitive decline (648). A significant reduction in the number of basal forebrain p75 neurotrophin receptor-immunoreactive neurons was seen in MCI (38%) and mild AD (43%). Its correlation with performance in the MMSE, some tests of working memory and attention, and other data lend support to the hypothesis that MCI is a preclinical stage of AD (649).

While strong correlations have been found between the density of NFTs in the hippocampus and neocortex with the degree of cholinergic pathology and dementia (650,651), many elderly subjects with MCI or early/very mild AD do not display deficits in ChAT activity (297,652), or show an upregulation in hippocampus and frontal cortex (9,647). A significant elevation of hippocampal ChAT in MCI was found selectively in the limbic (3/4) Braak stages which may reflect a compensatory response to the progressive denervation of the hippocampus by lost EC input (653). Hippocampal upregulation was no longer present in mild AD cases compared to cognitively unimpaired subjects, while severe AD showed markedly depleted ChAT levels. Cognitively normal individuals, MCI and mild-moderate AD, showed a positive correlation between hippocampal ChAT activity and progression of NP pathology in this area. In MCI and mild AD, ChAT activity was normal in inferior frontal, superior temporal, and anterior cingulate cortex (9). This suggests that earliest cognitive deficits, e.g., short-memory loss in MCI, do not involve cholinergic deficits, but more likely relate to disrupted entorhinal-hippocampus connectivity. Increased medial temporal NFT correlates strongly and better than hippocampal ChAT activity with impairment of episodic memory (654). Increased cholinergic activity during the early stages of AD may contribute to synaptic scaling, but the mechanisms of these changes are unknown (655). No changes in cortical or hippocampal levels of NGF were found in the brains of MCI individuals, and they did not correlate with an increase in ChAT activity in these regions, suggesting that brain NGF levels appear sufficient to support cholinergic plasticity (656). In vivo studies in mild to moderate AD showed significant reduction of ACh levels in amygdala and neocortex, whereas ACh activity and glucose metabolism appeared preserved or even increased in the basal forebrain. This suggests that changes in the cholinergic system are an early and leading event in AD rather than the consequence of neurodegeneration of basal nuclei (657). Cortical AChE activity is more robustly associated with functions of attention and working memory compared to performance on primary memory tests in AD (658).

While early-onset AD patients show a wide range of expression levels of the hippocampal cholinergic neurostimulating peptide (HCNP) precursor protein mRNA, in late-onset AD it is progressively decreased in hippocampus but not in the dentate gyrus (651). Since it stimulates the production of ChAT, this low expression in CA 1 may explain the downregulation of cholinergic neurons which show a progressive loss of synapsis and synaptic proteins in hippocampus and cortex even in early stages of AD (659).

Early Olfactory Involvement in AD and Other Neurodegenerating Diseases

Olfactory dysfunction (anosmia) is a common feature in old age and in AD (660–662), PD (663–668), DLB, and other neurodegenerative disorders (669,670), but not in vascular parkinsonism, PSP, and CBD (671). Anosmia is more frequent in DLB than in AD (672) and very common in LBV/AD (673). It also occurs in tg mice overexpressing human tau protein (674). NFTs and SPs in the olfactory system in AD have been reported previously (675–679), while LBs have been described in PD (306,680,681).

Recent studies indicate that the involvement of the olfactory bulb and tract is an early event in AD. Autopsy examination in elderly subjects showed degenerative olfactory changes in more than 84%, i.e., in all cases of definite AD and in 2/19 cognitively normal controls. NFTs and NTs appeared in the olfactory system as early as in the EC, and there was a statistical association between olfactory and olfactory system neocortical neuritic changes with respect to their frequency and severity (682), while others observed olfactory tau pathology in one-third of AD cases with Braak stage 2. They demonstrated that tau pathology in the olfactory system correlates with Braak stage and *APOE* ε4 and ε2 (683). These data suggest that olfactory dysfunction and *APOE* ε4 and ε2 are associated with a high risk of cognitive decline (660). Tau pathology in the olfactory bulb was common in AD and DLB, but minimal or absent in PSP, CBD, and controls, while AS-positive LBs were detected in most cases of DLB but absent in AD, PSP, and CBD. The severity of tau pathology also correlated with cortical and amygdala LBs, suggesting a possible synergistic effect between tau and AS, the main component of LBs, in the olfactory system in both pathological processes. In a personal consecutive autopsy study of 240 aged brains, tau pathology in the olfactory system was seen in all cases of definite AD (Braak stages 5 and 6), in 88% of Braak stage 4, 46% of Braak stage 3, and in 30% of MCI cases (Braak stage 2), while all NCI controls (Braak 0 and 1) were negative (684). Recently, hyposmia in PD was explained by increase of dopaminergic cells in the olfactory bulb (685).

Comparison Between Biopsy and Autopsy Findings in AD

Brain biopsy has an uncertain role in the diagnosis of dementia, although it may be of some value, when a treatable disease cannot be excluded by other means (686). Comparison of biopsy and autopsy findings in the same individuals provide opportunities to follow the disease process. Among four patients meeting the clinical criteria for AD who showed progressive deterioration from the time of biopsy to autopsy (nine to 11 years), three cases showed a striking increase in the density of SPs and NFTs in frontal cortex, and a significant increase of microglial activation in one. Severity of CAA varied significantly among patients (687). These findings contrasted with those of two other groups. Biopsies performed in five AD patients were compared with autopsies after AD duration of one to seven years (688). In all brains, density and nuclear volume of pyramidal neurons were significantly less than in controls and both measures fell significantly further from biopsy to autopsy, while NFT density either did not change or decreased. SP type in four brains was similar, and no increase in Aβ SPs was seen. Three brains showed no consistent changes in SP densities, while in one SP density increased only in layers I–III. In one brain density of SPs decreased at autopsy, while density of NFTs remained unchanged. Comparing autopsy findings in four patients with advanced AD (MMSE 2–20) who underwent biopsy one year after onset of symptoms and one to 47 years before death, despite marked decline in mental state, there was no consistent change in SP and NFT densities in the left frontal cortex. In one patient each, total SP count dropped and increased, while two cases showed little changes. NFT density in three brains dropped considerably and only in one case increased (689). These studies did not demonstrate an increase in Aβ density from biopsy to autopsy, which is in keeping with data indicating that amyloid burden does not correlate with duration of AD and that a dynamic balance exists between Aβ deposition and resolution (270,690).

In frontal cortical biopsy samples of autopsy-proven AD mean levels of ChAT activity were decreased to 36% of age-matched controls and were further, but not significantly, decreased in autopsied cases (691). The biopsy AD group showed a significant loss of synapses (35%), and a further loss in the autopsy AD group (692). These and comparable findings (693) indicated a continous decline of both ChAT activity and synapse density through the course of disease. Both changes correlated with the dementia score, cortical ChAT activity being considerably weaker than cortical synapse density.

Is Bioptic Demonstration of CAA a Dagnostic Tool for AD?

CAA is defined as deposition of congophilic material (Aβ) in the walls of meningeal and cerebral vessels (694–696). It is common in the brains of elderly demented and nondemented individuals; its incidence and severity increase with age (460,697–700), and it is associated with cerebral hemorrhages, infarcts, and WMLs (460,694,698,699,701–703). The prevalence of CAA in AD is 70–100% (460,696,704,705). In CAA, Aβ40 affects vessel walls more frequently and more severely than Aβ42, whereas in SPs, Aβ42 is predominant (696,706–708).

For the origin of Aβ in CAA three different mechanisms have been proposed (698): (1) derivation of Aβ from blood and/or cerebrospinal fluid (CSF) (709); (2) production by smooth muscle cells (SMC) within vessel walls and/or pericytes (710,711); or (3) derivation from the neuropil, i.e., SPs and NPs, in the course of its perivascular drainage (694,712–715). Aβ is present as globular deposits on the capillary wall and as thin layers in the pericapillary basement membrane, with dyshoric Aβ deposits in the adjacent neuropil (229,694,696, 714). This CapCAA is probably related to AD-associated Aβ deposition in the brain parenchyma, supporting the concept of its derivation from the neuropil, suggesting that transport across the BBB regulates brain Aβ (518).

The clinical diagnosis of "probable" CAA can be made in patients over age 60 years with multiple hemorrhages confined to lobar brain areas showing no other causes of hemorrhage. Over 50% of the patients develop new petechial hemorrhages within one to two years (716). Detection of small hemorrhages on MRI may be an efficient surrogate endpoint for pilot studies (717). Validation of the Boston criteria (Table 11) pathologically confirmed all 13 individuals diagnosed clinically with probable CAA (718). The frequency of cerebral infarctions and hemorrhages increased with the severity of CAA that was associated with the *APOE* ε4 and ε2 genotype (719). In brain biopsies CAA was seen in 13.1% of cases with cerebral infarcts, but only 3.7% Aβ in blood vessels of controls. CAA mainly involved large cortical vessels, while Aβ deposits in meningeal vessels were not different between infarct and control groups (701). This indicates that CAA, but not AP formation, is a risk factor for cerebral

Table 11   Boston Criteria for Diagnosis of Cerebral Amyloid Angiopathy–Related Hemorrhage

Definite CAA
  Full postmortem examination demonstrating:
    Lobar, cortical, or corticosubcortical hemorrhage
    Severe CAA with vasculopathy
    Absence of other diagnostic lesion
Probable CAA with supporting pathology
  Clinical data and pathologic tissue (evacuated hematoma or cortical biopsy)
      demonstrating:
    Lobar, cortical, or corticosubcortical hemorrhage
    Some degree of CAA in specimen
    Absence of other diagnostic lesion
Probable CAA
  Clinical data and MRI or CT demonstrating:
    Multiple hemorrhages restricted to lobar, cortical, or corticosubcortical regions
      (cerebellar hemorrhage allowed)
    Age ≥ 55 years
    Absence of other cause of hemorrhage
Possible CAA
  Clinical data and MRI or CT demonstrating:
    Single lobar, cortical, or corticosubcortical hemorrhage
    Age ≥ 55 years
    Absence of other cause of hemorrhage

Abbreviations: CAA, cerebral amyloid angiopathy; CT, computed tomography; MRI, magnetic resonance imaging.
Source: From Ref. 718.

infarction being significantly more common in elderly patients with cerebral infarction than in age-matched controls. While in nondemented subjects, the presence of CAA had no effect on cognitive ability, subjects with AD plus CAA had a lower test score than AD patients without CAA (720).

Recent studies reported both positive (229) and negative correlations between CAA and AD pathology (704,705). Neuritic AD pathology and CapCAA are highly correlated with only low correlations with general (non-capillary) CAA (696). Aβ42 deposits in capillaries, more precisely in the glia limitans, correlated highly with both Aβ42 plaques and morphological AD criteria, while only a low correlation with CAA was observed. Aβ40 deposits were significantly less frequent in both capillaries and plaques, and showed a low correlation with morphological AD criteria. These data suggest different pathomechanisms for both types of CAA, and a close relationship between CapCAA and AD pathology (721). Others observed different types of amyloid (Aβ42 and immunoglobulin-λ light chain amyloid) in CAA with spontaneous intracranial hemorrhage (722). Based on these findings, the demonstration of CAA in meningeal and superficial cortical vessels in brain biopsies may not indicate the presence of significant AD pathology and, therefore, may not be a reliable tool for diagnosing AD. This is illustrated by mildly to severely demented aged individuals who, at autopsy, showed severe general CAA, but no or only few cortical amyloid plaques and neuritic Braak stages 2 to 4, not fitting the morphological criteria of AD (722a,723), while other patients die showing clinical and pathological AD with virtually no Aβ within blood vessels (724). However, CAA, due to the effects of Aβ on cerebrovascular functions, may be an independent risk factor for vascular cognitive impairment (471,514).

EARLY MORPHOLOGICAL CHANGES IN DEMENTIA DISORDERS AND RELATION TO BIOMARKERS

Progress in our understanding of the molecular pathology and development of AD and its relationship to brain aging have provided clinically meaningful advances in the development of biomarkers, which may provide reasonable evidence for association with key mechanisms of pathogenesis and neurodegeneration. Emerging methods that are based on biochemical and imaging markers of disease specific pathology hold the potential to provide effective measures of early diagnosis, biological activity, disease outcome and markers of surrogate endpoints for their clinical use in diagnostic and preclinical purposes. Considerable progress has been made in the evaluation of biomarkers for AD. However, the nature of the majority of reported findings are still preliminary and most of them retrospective, and have been compared against a clinical rather than "gold standard" pathological diagnosis. Because clinical criteria lack specificity, particularly early in the disease course, quoted sensitivities and specificities for putative biomarkers are difficult to interpret.

Alzheimer's Disease

According to the guidelines of an international consensus group, a biomarker for AD should detect a manifestation of the fundamental neuropathology and be validated in morphologically confirmed cases. Its sensitivity for detecting AD and its specificity in differentiating AD and other dementias should exceed 80%. Ideally, a biomarker should also be reliable, reproducible, non-invasive, simple to perform, and inexpensive. Of particular interest is its ability to detect the disease at the earliest possible stage, i.e., before significant irreversible disease progression has occurred. Biomarkers are potentially useful to study disease pathogenesis in vivo and to study presymptomatic AD (725).

The relationship of functional neuroimaging to early morphological changes are reviewed in the respective chapters (see Chapters 6 and 8) (726). They appear superior to cognitive testing for early diagnosis of AD (727), but combined evaluation of neuropsychological, structural, and functional imaging offers greater predictive value (580). High resolution magnetic resonance imaging (MRI) showed that the volume of frontal grey matter was strongly associated with age, less with occipital grey and white matter, while the reduction in hippocampal volume (727a) was best modelled as a cubic regression model. Common changes in brain morphology as observed by cerebral MRI are associated with diminished cognitive functions in elderly individuals (728). Cerebral atrophy seems to closely parallel the distribution of neuritic pathology (and less the distribution of SPs). Significant correlations were observed between antemortem hippocampal volumes and both dementia severity and the density of hippocampal neurofibrillary tangles at autopsy. Total cerebral volumes, in contrast, were significantly correlated with the density of hippocampal SPs. This data suggests that hippocampal volume assessed in living subjects with probable AD is both a good marker of dementia severity and of the AD disease process (729). Voxel-based morphometry and automated brain volumetry showed a high discrimination accuracy between AD and controls, and could open up new possibilities for early diagnosis of AD (730,731). MRI shows differences in Braak stages and hippocampal volume between normal individuals and mild AD (601,732) with increased changes related to the duration of disease and may predict AD pathology (733). Early predictors of onset of AD in nondemented elderly subjects and of progression of amnestic MCI to AD include increased annual atrophy rate in the medial temporal lobe (734), inward deformation of the left hippocampal surface in a zone corresponding to the CA1 subfield (735), atrophy of the hippocampus (736), in particular of the EC (737), whole brain MRI spectroscopy (738), and reduced hippocampal metabolism (739–741). Findings from the Nun study indicated that both delayed recall measure and neuritic AD pathology in the CA1 region reflect associated hippocampal atrophy (742,743). Memory complaints in patients without any cognitive impairment were associated with smaller left hippocampal volumes and more depressive symptoms (744). As a result of neuron loss in the right amygdala-hippocampus complex it is correlated with declarative memory, in the left temporal-parietal region with performance in naming and praxia (745). Dementia severity is also reflected by reduced metabolism in posterior and frontal association areas in AD (746).

Morphological analysis in AD revealed severe atrophy in medial temporal lobe and in inferior temporal, superior, and middle frontal cortex. It was significantly greater for the fusiform gyrus, while the inferior frontal lobes were entirely spared. Atrophy of other cortical regions was less marked and not related to disease duration (747). Comparative volumetry revealed a strong relationship between neuron number and both hippocampal and brain volume in brains with and without AD (748). MRI volume measurements over time are valid biomarkers of AD progress (749–751). Higher atrophy rates in the EC than in the hippocampus are consistent with the view that AD pathology begins in the EC region (752,753) and are a good predictor of conversion from MCI to AD (754,755). Grey matter loss in the medial temporal lobe characterizes MCI, while in the parietal and cingulate cortex it may be a feature of AD (756). Increased activation of the medial temporal lobe, reflecting a compensatory response to accumulating AD pathology, may serve as a marker for impending clinical decline (757). Reduced medial temporal lobe N-acetylaspartate, together with reduced hippocampal gray matter values, may be early indicators for dementia-related pathology (758). Diffusion tensor MRI, helpful in quantifying MCI pathology to distinguish it from aged controls (759), can also detect differential vulnerability of anterior white matter with minimal acceleration in AD (760), while others show a similar distribution of WMLs in VaD, AD, and healthy aging, the frontal lesions correlating with MMSE scores (565). The pattern of hippocampus and corpus callosum atrophy in relation to dementia severity gives evidence for early neocortical degeneration in AD (761), and differs from VaD (762).

A novel amyloid-imaging PET tracer (see Chapter 10) showed marked consistence with the pattern of Aβ plaques in AD brain (188), and a combination of two imaging agents (IMPY and SB13); targeting APs may be useful to quantitate AP burden in the living AD patient, but not in tg mouse brains (763) while positron emission tomography (PET) imaging NFTs is under discussion (764,765). Increased [11C](R)-PK11195 binding in limbic and temporoparietal cortex in mild AD suggests early microglial activation (766), while regional cerebral blood flow patterns suggest that AD is a heterogenous disease (767).

A promising source of biomarkers is CSF which is in direct contact with the extracellular space of the CNS, where biochemical changes in the brain could potentially be reflected (see Chapter 3). However, CSF examination is not a "liquid biopsy." A growing body of literature has shown that total tau (t-tau), phosphorylated tau (p-tau), and Aβ42 in CSF and, in particular, combined measurement of tau and Aβ42 have reasonable specificity and sensitivity when differentiating AD from normal aging, to detect incipient AD and candidates for conversion of MCI to AD (768–781). Longitudinal CSF and MRI biomarkers may improve the diagnosis of MCI (782). One main criticism is that only three studies have compared CSF biomarkers and postmortem confirmation of diagnosis.

Large numbers of NPs were strongly associated with lower CSF Aβ42 levels that may reflect processes implicated in amyloid pathology (783). Studies in 106 patients with dementia and four NCI persons confirmed the association between elevated CSF p-tau premortem and the pathological hallmarks of AD, indicating that elevated CSF p-tau levels strongly support a diagnosis and may be helpful in distinguishing AD from other dementing disorders (784). A reduced ratio of Aβ42 to total Aβ in CSF of AD patients was consistent with previous clinical reports, but because of the broad range of Aβ values provided no meaningful additional diagnostic information when tau was elevated. Meta-analysis of CSF levels in a large number of AD cases (only 23% confirmed at autopsy) and controls showed significant decrease of Aβ42 and an increase of tau (785). A small autopsy cohort showed a significant decrease of postmortem CSF melatonin in aged individuals with early AD changes in the temporal cortex, suggesting that this may also be an early event in the development of AD (786). In view of diverging data between in vitro and postmortem CSF, this study awaits confirmation. Although CSF tau and Aβ42 may not be specific for AD, their evaluation combined with neuroimaging may improve diagnostic specifity (787). Quantitative proteomics of CSF from AD patients compared to age-matched cotrols, as well as from other neurodegenerative diseases, will allow us to generate a roster of proteins that may serve as specific biomarker panels for AD and other geriatric dementias (788).

With regard to plasma Aβ40 and Aβ42 levels, these may increase with age but are not specific for MCI or sporadic AD (789). Reports show these to have been elevated before and during the early stages of AD though then decline thereafter (790). These findings may be associated with *APOE E*4 (791) and may be a risk factor for microvascular damage (791a), although there are no reports of any neuropathological confirmation of this data. The same findings are evident for APP in platelets and other peripheral marker for sporadic AD (792). Morover, plasma Aβ42 levels are highly influenced by concomitant medications (793).

Salivary AChE activity may prove to be a useful marker of central cholinergic activity (794). It is important that any future studies on biomarkers are long-term prospective investigations with the aim of confirming the diagnosis pathologically (795).

PDD and DLB

Early morphological changes have been described and related to in vivo markers in PD and DLB. However, except for rare patients who died in early or preclinical stages of the disorder, the morphology of initial changes, beginning in the lower brainstem and olfactory system, with upward progression to the nigrostriatal dopaminergic system (306,307), is not available, and information depends on functional neuroimaging (652,796,797) and monitoring dopaminergic degeneration (798–802).

In DLB, determination of the loss of dopamine transporter as marker of striatonigral degeneration (803,804) and use of presynaptic and postsynaptic ligands may distinguish it from AD (805,806). A sensitivity of 83% and specificity of 100% have been reported for the association of an abnormal scan with an autopsy diagnosis in DLB (329). Regional correlation of dopaminergic functions in the striatum, using PET analysis, may be useful in distinguishing DLB from PD (807). Neuroimaging studies and their correlation with neuropathology may also be helpful in supporting the clinical diagnosis (808). Voxel-based morphometry (VBM) showing preservation of the medial temporal lobe, hippocampus, and amygdala in DLB was considered a potential antemortem marker in distinguishing it from AD (809). PD cases showed gray matter loss in prefrontal and limbic/paralimbic areas (810), and in PDD this extended to temporal and subcortical areas, with occipital atrophy in PDD being the only difference between the two groups, while no volumetric differences were observed between PDD and DLB (811). Diffuse glucose hypometabolism in the entire cortex including occipital cortex, only sparing the primary sensory-motor cortex, also seems to be a typical pattern for DLB distinct from AD (812–814). In vivo diffusion MRI showing selective involvement of parietal, frontal, and occipital lobe as well as subcortical abnormalities indicating nigrostriatal involvement in DLB and PD may be useful in the diagnosis of DLB (815).

Another possibility would be histological examination of biopsies of the olfactory epithelium (OE) showing prominent expression of AS and dystrophic neurites in patients with PD, DLB, multiple system atrophy (MSA), and AD (669). Further studies should validate the diagnostic sensitivity of olfactory mucosa biopsies.

No clinically useful tests have been reported using plasma and CSF analysis for the diagnosis of both PD and DLB (816). Some studies indicated that CSF p-tau may be lower in DLB than in AD, both showing decreased levels of Aβ (347,817,818), while others showed decreased Aβ42 in AD and a slight increase in DLB, but follow-up CSF analyses are of limited value for the differentiation of AD and DLB. This suggests that more specific markers have to be established for the differentiation and follow-up of these diseases (819). While the native form of AS was previously not found in CSF (820), recent studies demonstrated increased soluble AS in the blood and brain from familial PD with SNCA locus triplication (821).

Frontotemporal Dementias

Based on the severity of gross atrophy in FTD, four progressive stages were identified (822): stage 1: initial mild atrophy in the orbital and superior medial frontal regions, and hippocampus; stage 2: atrophy of the other anterior frontal regions, temporal cortices, and basal ganglia; stage 3: involvement of all remaining tissues on coronal slices; stage 4: marked atrophy in all brain areas. Severe atrophy of the frontal lobe, amygdala, and hippocampus in stage 2 suggests that they are among the earliest affected in FTD (823). Comparison of PID, DLDH, and FTD-MND found no differences in these subtypes, suggesting that disease stage rather than FTD subtype determines the pattern and extent of neuronal degeneration (824). This scheme provides the framework to determinate correlates relating to disease progression, e.g., with neuroimaging data (825–828).

FTD revealed elevated CSF tau (though lower than in AD), high *APOE E*4 and *E*2 frequency, and decreased Aβ42 levels (829). However, these values are in the intermediate range between FTD, AD, and other dementias, and are not useful for the diagnosis of FTD (830,831), and others showed significant reduction of t-tau levels in CSF (832). CSF t-tau was not increased in FTD patients with tau mutations (833), while p-tau 231 and p-tau 181 yielded excellent distinction between AD and FTD (834). It could be useful to develop techniques to study tau-isoform patterns in CSF, because they are disease specific when measured in brain homogenates (835). Unfortunately, none of these CSF studies was confirmed by postmortem studies, and a sensitive and a specific biomarker enabling differentiation of FTD from other conditions is still lacking.

Vascular Dementias

Previous neuroimaging studies in vascular cognitive impairment (VCI) have been partly contradictory (452,836). Independent correlates of post stroke dementia are the combination of infarct feature (volume of infarcts in middle cerebral artery, higher frequency of left-sided infarcts), extent of WMLs, medial temporal atrophy, and host factors (836). The volume of functional tissue loss may be more important than of total tissue because it also includes the effect of deafferented cortex (837,838). Absence of CVLs on CT and MRI is evidence against a vascular etiology of dementia, which is in agreement with neuropathological studies (460,461,477). Although the hippocampus is less affected by subcortical CVLs, dementia due to microvascular pathology showed significant hippocampal neuronal loss (478,839), and hippocampal atrophy may increase the development of post-stroke dementia (840). To date, however, it has not been possible to determine the specific amount of WML necessary to cause cognitive impairment, but it has been found that even relatively mild WMH can have deleterious effects on cognition (472). A standardized assessment of subcortical CVD on CT films can be combined into a unique score that is in good agreement with neuropathology. This supports the validity of the CT-based visual rating scale as a valid tool to detect subcortical vascular changes in elderly persons (841). MRI studies confirmed that infarcts located in strategic areas have a role in cognitive impairment, and their quantification correlates with neuropathological findings (842). There is a substantial overlap between cases classified as AD by NINCDS/ADRDA, and VaD by modified SCADDTC criteria. The substantial contribution of vascular disease would be missed without inclusion of MRI. Treatment of risk factors for VaD could have an important impact on the incidence of dementia (843).

Studies of cerebral blood flow (CBF) and metabolism, in general, failed to identify diagnostic features of VaD and to provide a robust, easily applicable diagnostic technique because of the heterogenous pathology underlying dementia.

WMLs usually have an independent correlation with VaD, while hyperperfusions and fronto-subcortical atrophy are substrates of mild cognitive deficits after stroke (844). They are often correlated with atrophy of the corpus callosum (845), supporting the role of disruption of white matter connections in the pathogenesis of cognitive impairment (846). WMLs are associated with reduced rCBV in the cerebral cortex, particularly in individuals with extensive hypertension (847).

Neurochemical markers, due to a wide range of levels, appear inconclusive for the diagnosis of VaD and its distinction from other dementing disorders (848). The diagnosis of VaD is difficult in epidemiologic studies because post-stroke dementia can be due to AD and evidence of VaD can be found in the MRI of dementia cases without clinical strokes. Whether the clinical progression is related to AD pathology or vascular disease is difficult to establish (450). Similar difficulties arise for the in vivo diagnosis of mixed type dementia.

CORRELATION OF CLINICAL AND PATHOLOGICAL CRITERIA

While recent studies clearly point to the importance of AD pathology in limbic areas for memory impairment, involvement of the neocortex is significantly correlated to the progress of dementia. According to most clinico-pathological studies, all demented patients had dystrophic neurites both free in the neuropil or surrounding SPs. The number of NFTs and, much less so, that of NTs usually correlated with the clinical severity of dementia, while even widespread Aβ deposition may be necessary but by itself is often insufficient for the development of dementia (298). Although there may be considerable overlap with isocortical Braak stages in cognitively normal individuals and MCI subjects (10,24,297), the only brain region in which NFT count is suggested to provide a significant marker for dementia is the association isocortex (223,650). Only up to 20% of aged cognitively normal subjects had no or only few AD changes, while all the others showed numerous AD lesions including 9% with isocortical Braak stags 5 or 6, indicating that some patients tolerate the insults of AD pathology, probably due to neurocognitive reserve or compensation (24,297). In other cohorts, 7–50% of individuals with no impairment or MCI met one or more of the morphological AD criteria or had tau pathology in the perforant path target zone and loss of entorhinal neurons, while only 10–20% were free of considerable AD-related lesions (10,24,238,599). About 29% of cases pathologically defined by CERAD criteria as AD do not have clinical dementia, whereas more than half of octogenarians without dementia meet CERAD criteria for pathologically confirmed AD (849). Therefore re-evaluation of the diagnostic criteria are necessary and require further development for reliable screening.

EFFECTS OF CONCURRENT PATHOLOGIES

Comorbidity in aged individuals may influence the clinical and morphological features of AD, and it is well established that AD patients frequently have other lesions (533). Among the most frequent coexisting pathologies are CVLs with an incidence of 18–80% (460,461,463,539,551,553,554), followed by LB pathology in 12–20% (275,540). Cortical LBs have been observed in 7–71% (334,335,850), and AS pathology in the amygdala and other brain areas in 15–60% of sporadic AD cases (275,332,338,339). The pathogenesis and clinico-pathological impact remains to be determined. While the *APOE* genotype usually shows no differences between AD and vascular disease, cerebral infarcts in regions typically destroyed by AD (e.g., limbic areas and the thalamus), and cortical LBs which frequently occur in both AD and DLB, all may exacerbate the clinical manifestations of AD and thus contribute to the heterogeneity of the disease (299,533).

NEUROPATHOLOGY OF AD AND CLINICAL RELEVANCE

AD is a heterogeneous disorder with variable clinical and pathological phenotypes. Current guidelines for the neuropathological diagnosis of AD are based on age-adapted (semi)quantitative assessment of plaques, either amyloid or dystrophic (279), neuritic plaques (CERAD), topographic spreading of neuritic AD pathology (218), and a combination of Braak and CERAD staging with probabilistic statement that dementia may be associated with AD. Khachaturian criteria may not be useful to differentiate between diffuse and neuritic plaques, and between AD cases and cognitively normal individuals. Neither CERAD nor NIA-RI guidelines discriminate AD from pathological aging in the absence of clinical findings. Braak staging does not correlate well with psychometric data in clincally nondemented subjects (297,851). Multivariate analysis of aged individuals revealed significant correlations between cognitive function assessed by the MMSE and Blessed test, and both the CERAD criteria and Braak staging, but much weaker correlations for both Tierney and Khachaturian criteria (289,291). High Braak stages and CERAD criteria identified 54% and 62% of demented individuals respectively, and eliminated 84% and 70% of non-demented individuals.

The major clinico-pathological correlates of AD can be summarized as follows:

1. Early, often preclinical involvement of the allocortex causes deafferentation of the hippocampus due to involvement of the (trans)-entorhinal region by alterations of synaptic function and neuronal degeneration due to cytoskeletal PHF changes and Aβ deposition clinically presenting as early cognition, olfactory, and amnestic deficits without overt dementia.
2. Spreading of AD pathology to the isocortex with hierarchic involvement of isocortical association areas cause the following syndromes:
    (*i*) *temporal isocortex* induces degeneration and disruption of cortico-cortical connections to prefrontal and parietal areas and causes visuospatial, speech, and auditory disorders.
    (*ii*) *frontal cortex*: high NFT- and Aβ-load in the frontal variant of AD with isolated executive impairment (597).

     (*iii*)   *orbito-frontal and cingulate pathology* often causes agitation.

     (*iv*)   *major NFT load in areas 7, 24, and CA1* induces spatial-temporal disorientation.

     (*v*)   *occipital cortex* induces rare visual variant of AD (852) recently referred to as progressive posterior cortical dysfunction involving selective visuospatial deficits (853).

     (*vi*)   *higher levels of AD pathology* are related to lower levels of implicit memory and conceptual but not to perceptual, proceeding resources (854).

     (*vii*)   *progressive degeneration of intracortical, cortico-cortical connections* causes global cortico-cortical discontinuation with loss of higher cortical functions and dementia.

3. Late spreading of AD pathology to subcortical areas cause degeneration of cortico-subcortical neuronal systems and induces primary sensory deafferentation with affective, extrapyramidal, and vegetative signs or symptoms.

CONCLUSIONS

In general, there is a good correlation between tau pathology and cognitive state as well as between the progress of both neuroimaging and the clinical manifestations of disease. These morphological markers (tau pathology, amyloidosis, and synaptic proteins as well as biochemical markers, i.e., ChAT and related mRNAs) usually identify cases with moderate to severe dementia. However, due to variable overlaps these changes often fail to distinguish between cognitively intact aged subjects from those with MCI/preclinical or mild AD. In particular these latter groups show a wide variety in the intensity and pattern of AD-related lesions. Although they often differ from "normal" aging, only a small proportion of cognitively intact aged individuals are free of AD pathology, while up to 50% may show various AD-related alterations or even definitive AD pathology. Additional difficulties arise from frequent coexistence with other pathologies that have a synergistic effect and may act by contributing to cognitive impairment.

    In view of these difficulties, further studies are needed to increase the diagnostic validity of current diagnostic criteria of AD and its distinction from "normal" aging and from other disorders causing dementia.

ABBREVIATIONS

3-R	3-repeat
ACh	acetylcholine
AChE	acetylcholinesterase
AD	Alzheimer's disease
ADDL	amyloid-ß derived diffusable ligand
ADRDA	Alzheimer's Disease and Related Disorders Association

AGD	argyrophilic grain disease
AP	amyloid plaque
APP	amyloid precursor protein
AS	α-synuclein
Aß	amyloid ß peptide
BBB	blood-brain barrier
BDNF	brain-derived neurotrophic factor
CAA	cerebral amyloid angiopathy
CBD	corticobasal degeneration
CDR	Clinical Dementia Rating Scale
CERAD	Consortium to Establish a Registry for Alzheimer's Disease
ChAT	choline acetyl transferase
CN	cognitively normal
CVD	cerebrovascular disease
CVL	cerebrovascular lesion
DLB	dementia with Lewy bodies
DLDH	dementia lacking distinctive histopathology
DP	diffuse plaque
EC	entorhinal cortex
ER	endoplasmic reticulum
FAD	familial AD
FTD	frontotemporal dementia
FTDP-17	frontotemporal dementia and parkinsonism related to chromosome 17
FTLD	frontotemporal lobe degeneration
FTLD-U	FTLD with Ub-only neuronal changes
GABA	γ-aminobutyric acid
GBR1	GABA receptor R1 protein
GFAP	glial fibrillary acidic protein
HHD	hypoperfusive hypoxic-ischemic dementia
HSD	hippocampal sclerosis dementia
HIS	Hachinski Ischemic Score
ICD	International Classification of Diseases
kDA	kilodalton
LB	Lewy body
LBD	Lewy body disease
LBV/AD	Lewy body variant of Alzheimer's disease
LVD	large vessel dementia
MAP	mitogen-activated protein
MBP	myelin basic protein
MCI	mild cognitive impairment
MD	mixed type dementia
MID	multiple-infarct dementia
MMSE	Mini-Mental State Examination

MND	motoneuron disease
MNDID	motor neuron disease inclusion dementia
MRI	magnetic resonance imaging
NAA	N-acetyl aspartate
NCDS	Neurological and Communicative Disorders and Stroke
NF	neurofilament
NFT	neurofibrillary tangle
NGF	nerve growth factor
NIA	National Institute for Aging
NINDS-AIREN	National Institutes of Neurological Diseases and Stroke
NP	neuritic plaque
NT	neuropil thread
OE	olfactory epithelium
OS	olfactory system
PD	Parkinson's disease
PDD	Parkinson's disease with dementia
p-PERK	phosphorylated pancreatic ER kinase
PHF	paired helical filaments
Pib	Pick body
PIB	Pittsburgh compound-B
PiD	Pick's disease
PSEN1	presenilin-1
PSD	post-stroke dementia
PSP	progressive supranuclear palsy
p-tau	phosphorylated tau protein
rCBF	Regional cerebral blood flow
RI	Ronald and Nancy Reagan Institute of the Alzheimer's Association
ROS	Religious Order Study
SCAA	severe CAA
SCADDTC	State of California Alzheimer's Disease Diagnostic and Treatment Center
SID	strategic infarct dementia
SNc	substantia nigra pars compacta
SP	senile plaque
SVD	small vessel disease
Tg	transgenic
t-tau	total tau protein
Ub	ubiquitin
UPR	unfolded protein response
VaD	vascular dementia
VID	vascular-ischemic dementia
VBM	voxel based morphometry

VCI   vascular cognitive impairment
WML   white matter lesion

ACKNOWLEDGMENTS

The study was supported by the Society for the Support of Research in Neurological Sciences, Vienna, Austria. Special thanks are due to Mr. E. Mitter-Ferstl, PhD, for secretarial and computer work.

REFERENCES

1. Dickson DW, Crystal HA, Bevona C, Honer W, Vincent I, Davies P. Correlations of synaptic and pathological markers with cognition of the elderly. Neurobiol Aging 1995; 16:285–298.
2. Giannakopoulos P, Hof PR, Michel JP, Guimon J, Bouras C. Cerebral cortex pathology in aging and Alzheimer's disease: a quantitative survey of large hospital-based geriatric and psychiatric cohorts. Brain Res Brain Res Rev 1997; 25:217–245.
3. Green MS, Kaye JA, Ball MJ. The Oregon brain aging study: neuropathology accompanying healthy aging in the oldest old. Neurology 2000; 54:105–113.
4. Purohit DP, Haroutunian V, Kapustin A, Marin D, Mohs R, Perl DP. Diffuse plaque formation in the cerebral cortex of non-demented elderly and individuals with mild to moderate dementia: a clinicopathological study of 88 cases (abstract). Neurobiol Aging 1998; 19:297.
5. Berg L, McKeel DW, Jr., Miller JP, Baty J, Morris JC. Neuropathological indexes of Alzheimer's disease in demented and nondemented persons aged 80 years and older. Arch Neurol 1993; 50:349–358.
6. Berg L, McKeel DW, Jr., Miller JP, et al. Clinicopathologic studies in cognitively healthy aging and Alzheimer's disease: relation of histologic markers to dementia severity, age, sex, and apolipoprotein E genotype. Arch Neurol 1998; 55:326–335.
7. Dickson DW, Crystal HA, Mattiace LA, et al. Identification of normal and pathological aging in prospectively studied nondemented elderly humans. Neurobiol Aging 1992; 13:179–189.
8. Kordower JH, Chu Y, Stebbins GT, et al. Loss and atrophy of layer II entorhinal cortex neurons in elderly people with mild cognitive impairment. Ann Neurol 2001; 49:202–213.
9. DeKosky ST, Ikonomovic MD, Styren SD, et al. Upregulation of choline acetyltransferase activity in hippocampus and frontal cortex of elderly subjects with mild cognitive impairment. Ann Neurol 2002; 51:145–155.
10. Mitchell TW, Mufson EJ, Schneider JA, et al. Parahippocampal tau pathology in healthy aging, mild cognitive impairment, and early Alzheimer's disease. Ann Neurol 2002; 51:182–189.
11. Guillozet AL, Weintraub S, Mash DC, Mesulam MM. Neurofibrillary tangles, amyloid, and memory in aging and mild cognitive impairment. Arch Neurol 2003; 60:729–736.

12. Gómez-Isla T, Hyman BT. Neuropathological changes in normal aging, mild cognitive impairment, and Alzheimer's disease. In: Petersen RC, ed. Cognitive Impairment—Aging to Alzheimer's Disease. Oxford: Oxford University Press, 2003:191–204.

13. Knopman DS. Alzheimer type dementia. In: Dickson DW, ed. Neurodegeneration. The Molecular Pathology of Dementia and Movement Disorders. Basel: ISN Neuropath Press, 2003:24–39.

14. Price JL, Davis PB, Morris JC, White DL. The distribution of tangles, plaques and related immunohistochemical markers in healthy aging and Alzheimer's disease. Neurobiol Aging 1991; 12:295–312.

15. Arriagada PV, Marzloff K, Hyman BT. Distribution of Alzheimer-type pathologic changes in nondemented elderly individuals matches the pattern in Alzheimer's disease. Neurology 1992; 42:1681–1688.

16. Bennett DA, Schneider JA, Bienias JL, Evans DA, Wilson RS. Neuropathology of mild cognitive impairment (abstract). Neurology 2004; 62:A87.

17. Agorogiannis EI, Agorogiannis GI, Papadimitriou A, Hadjigeorgiou GM. Protein misfolding in neurodegenerative diseases. Neuropathol Appl Neurobiol 2004; 30:215–224.

18. Bossy-Wetzel E, Schwarzenbacher R, Lipton SA. Molecular pathways to neurodegeneration. Nat Med 2004; 10:S2–S9.

19. Ross CA, Poirier MA. Protein aggregation and neurodegenerative disease. Nat Med 2004; 10:S10–S17.

20. Muchowski PJ, Wacker JL. Modulation of neurodegeneration by molecular chaperones. Nat Rev Neurosci 2005; 6:11–22.

21. Wacker JL, Zareie MH, Fong H, Sarikaya M, Muchowski PJ. Hsp70 and Hsp40 attenuate formation of spherical and annular polyglutamine oligomers by partitioning monomer. Nat Struct Mol Biol 2004; 11:1215–1222.

22. Bierer LM, Hof PR, Purohit DP, et al. Neocortical neurofibrillary tangles correlate with dementia severity in Alzheimer's disease. Arch Neurol 1995; 52:81–88.

23. Newell KL, Hyman BT, Growdon JH, Hedley-Whyte ET. Application of the National Institute on Aging (NIA)-Reagan Institute criteria for the neuropathological diagnosis of Alzheimer disease. J Neuropathol Exp Neurol 1999; 58:1147–1155.

24. Riley KP, Snowdon DA, Markesbery WR. Alzheimer's neurofibrillary pathology and the spectrum of cognitive function: findings from the Nun Study. Ann Neurol 2002; 51:567–577.

25. Morris JC, Storandt M, Miller JP, et al. Mild cognitive impairment represents early-stage Alzheimer disease. Arch Neurol 2001; 58:397–405.

26. Petersen RC, ed. Mild Cognitive Impairment: Aging to Alzheimer's Disease. Oxford: Oxford University Press, 2003.

27. Mesulam M, Shaw P, Mash D, Weintraub S. Cholinergic nucleus basalis tauopathy emerges early in the aging-MCI-AD continuum. Ann Neurol 2004; 55:815–828.

28. Petersen RC, Stevens JC, Ganguli M, Tangalos EG, Cummings JL, DeKosky ST. Practice parameter: early detection of dementia: mild cognitive impairment (an evidence-based review). Report of the Quality Standards Subcommittee of the American Academy of Neurology. Neurology 2001; 56:1133–1142.

29. Peng FC. Is dementia a disease? Gerontology 2003; 49:384–391.

30. Scheff SW, Price DA. Synaptic pathology in Alzheimer's disease: a review of ultrastructural studies. Neurobiol Aging 2003; 24:1029–1046.

31. Coleman P, Federoff H, Kurlan R. A focus on the synapse for neuroprotection in Alzheimer disease and other dementias. Neurology 2004; 63:1155–1162.

32. Duyckaerts C, Dickson DW. Neuropathology of Alzheimer's disease. In: Dickson DW, ed. Neurodegeneration. The Molecular Pathology of Dementia and Movement Disorders. Basel: ISN Neuropath Press, 2003:47–65.

33. Reddy PH, Mani G, Park BS, et al. Differential loss of synaptic proteins in Alzheimer's disease: Implications for synaptic dysfunction. J Alzheimers Dis 2005; 7:103–117.

34. Streit WJ. Microglia and Alzheimer's disease pathogenesis. J Neurosci Res 2004; 77:1–8.

35. Tuppo EE, Arias HR. The role of inflammation in Alzheimer's disease. Int J Biochem Cell Biol 2005; 37:289–305.

36. Francis PT. Neuroanatomy/pathology and the interplay of neurotransmitters in moderate to severe Alzheimer disease. Neurology 2005; 65:S5–S9.

37. Bayer TA, Wirths O, Majtenyi K, et al. Key factors in Alzheimer's disease: beta-amyloid precursor protein processing, metabolism and intraneuronal transport. Brain Pathol 2001; 11:1–11.

38. Rowan MJ, Klyubin I, Cullen WK, Anwyl R. Synaptic plasticity in animal models of early Alzheimer's disease. Philos Trans R Soc Lond B Biol Sci 2003; 358:821–828.

39. Selkoe DJ. Defining molecular targets to prevent Alzheimer disease. Arch Neurol 2005; 62:192–195.

40. Selkoe DJ, Schenk D. Alzheimer's disease: molecular understanding predicts amyloid-based therapeutics. Annu Rev Pharmacol Toxicol 2003; 43:545–584.

41. Kamenetz F, Tomita T, Hsieh H, et al. APP processing and synaptic function. Neuron 2003; 37:925–937.

42. Morgan C, Colombres M, Nunez MT, Inestrosa NC. Structure and function of amyloid in Alzheimer's disease. Prog Neurobiol 2004; 74:323–349.

43. Oddo S, Caccamo A, Smith IF, et al. A dynamic relationship between intracellular and extracellular pools of abeta. Am J Pathol 2006; 168:184–194.

44. Cuello AC. Intracellular and extracellular Abeta, a tale of two neuropathologies. Brain Pathol 2005; 15:66–71.

45. Tabaton M, Piccini A. Role of water-soluble amyloid-beta in the pathogenesis of Alzheimer's disease. Int J Exp Pathol 2005; 86:139–145.

46. Kokubo H, Kayed R, Glabe CG, Yamaguchi H. Soluble Abeta oligomers ultrastructurally localize to cell processes and might be related to synaptic dysfunction in Alzheimer's disease brain. Brain Res 2005; 1031:222–228.

47. Gandy S. The role of cerebral amyloid beta accumulation in common forms of Alzheimer disease. J Clin Invest 2005; 115:1121–1129.

48. LeVine H, III. The Amyloid hypothesis and the clearance and degradation of Alzheimer's beta-peptide. J Alzheimers Dis 2004; 6:303–314.

49. Arimon M, Diez-Perez I, Kogan MJ, et al. Fine structure study of Abeta1-42 fibrillogenesis with atomic force microscopy. FASEB J 2005.

50. Ehehalt R, Keller P, Haass C, Thiele C, Simons K. Amyloidogenic processing of the Alzheimer beta-amyloid precursor protein depends on lipid rafts. J Cell Biol 2003; 160:113–123.

51. Urano Y, Hayashi I, Isoo N, et al. Association of active {gamma}-secretase complex with lipid rafts. J Lipid Res 2005; 46:904–912.

52. Yu W, Zou K, Gong JS, Ko M, Yanagisawa K, Michikawa M. Oligomerization of amyloid beta-protein occurs during the isolation of lipid rafts. J Neurosci Res 2005; 80:114–119.

53. Gellermann GP, Appel TR, Tannert A, et al. Raft lipids as common components of human extracellular amyloid fibrils. Proc Natl Acad Sci USA 2005; 102:6297–6302.

54. Marchesi VT. An alternative interpretation of the amyloid Abeta hypothesis with regard to the pathogenesis of Alzheimer's disease. Proc Natl Acad Sci USA 2005; 102:9093–9098.

55. Barelli H, Lebeau A, Vizzavona J, et al. Characterization of new polyclonal antibodies specific for 40 and 42 amino acid-long amyloid beta peptides: their use to examine the cell biology of presenilins and the immunohistochemistry of sporadic Alzheimer's disease and cerebral amyloid angiopathy cases. Mol Med 1997; 3:695–707.

56. Ege C, Lee KY. Insertion of Alzheimer's A beta 40 peptide into lipid monolayers. Biophys J 2004; 87:1732–1740.

57. Bitan G, Kirkitadze MD, Lomakin A, Vollers SS, Benedek GB, Teplow DB. Amyloid beta-protein (Abeta) assembly: Abeta 40 and Abeta 42 oligomerize through distinct pathways. Proc Natl Acad Sci USA 2003; 100:330–335.

58. Benzing WC, Ikonomovic MD, Brady DR, Mufson EJ, Armstrong DM. Evidence that transmitter-containing dystrophic neurites precede paired helical filament and Alz-50 formation within senile plaques in the amygdala of nondemented elderly and patients with Alzheimer's disease. J Comp Neurol 1993; 334:176–191.

59. Irie K, Murakami K, Masuda Y, et al. Structure of beta-amyloid fibrils and its relevance to their neurotoxicity: Implications for the pathogenesis of Alzheimer's disease. J Biosci Bioengineering 2005; 99:437–447.

60. Nicoll JA, Yamada M, Frackowiak J, Mazur-Kolecka B, Weller RO. Cerebral amyloid angiopathy plays a direct role in the pathogenesis of Alzheimer's disease; Pro-CAA position statement. Neurobiol Aging 2004; 25:589–597.

61. Lazarov O, Lee M, Peterson DA, Sisodia SS. Evidence that synaptically released beta-amyloid accumulates as extracellular deposits in the hippocampus of transgenic mice. J Neurosci 2002; 22:9785–9793.

62. Sheng JG, Price DL, Koliatsos VE. Disruption of corticocortical connections ameliorates amyloid burden in terminal fields in a transgenic model of Abeta amyloidosis. J Neurosci 2002; 22:9794–9799.

63. Takahashi RH, Milner TA, Li F, et al. Intraneuronal Alzheimer abeta42 accumulates in multivesicular bodies and is associated with synaptic pathology. Am J Pathol 2002; 161:1869–1879.

64. Takahashi RH, Almeida CG, Kearney PF, et al. Oligomerization of Alzheimer's beta-amyloid within processes and synapses of cultured neurons and brain. J Neurosci 2004; 24:3592–3599.

65. Fernandez-Vizarra P, Fernandez AP, Castro-Blanco S, et al. Intra- and extracellular Abeta and PHF in clinically evaluated cases of Alzheimer's disease. Histol Histopathol 2004; 19:823–844.

66. Rebelo S, Henriques AG, da Cruz e Silva EF, da Cruz e Silva OA. Effect of cell density on intracellular levels of the Alzheimer's amyloid precursor protein. J Neurosci Res 2004; 76:406–414.

67. Heredia L, Lin R, Vigo FS, Kedikian G, Busciglio J, Lorenzo A. Deposition of amyloid fibrils promotes cell-surface accumulation of amyloid beta precursor protein. Neurobiol Dis 2004; 16:617–629.

68. Ruiz-Leon Y, Pascual A. Regulation of beta-amyloid precursor protein expression by brain-derived neurotrophic factor involves activation of both the Ras and phosphatidylinositide 3-kinase signalling pathways. J Neurochem 2004; 88:1010–1018.

69. Dawbarn D, Allen SJ. Neurotrophins and neurodegeneration. Neuropathol Appl Neurobiol 2003; 29:211–230.

70. Schmitz A, Schneider A, Kummer MP, Herzog V. Endoplasmic reticulum-localized amyloid beta-peptide is degraded in the cytosol by two distinct degradation pathways. Traffic 2004; 5:89–101.

71. D'Andrea MR, Nagele RG, Wang HY, Lee DH. Consistent immunohistochemical detection of intracellular beta-amyloid42 in pyramidal neurons of Alzheimer's disease entorhinal cortex. Neurosci Lett 2002; 333:163–166.

72. Gouras GK, Tsai J, Naslund J, et al. Intraneuronal Abeta42 accumulation in human brain. Am J Pathol 2000; 156:15–20.

73. Hartmann T, Bieger SC, Bruhl B, et al. Distinct sites of intracellular production for Alzheimer's disease A beta40/42 amyloid peptides. Nat Med 1997; 3:1016–1020.

74. Wirths O, Multhaup G, Czech C, et al. Intraneuronal Abeta accumulation precedes plaque formation in beta-amyloid precursor protein and presenilin-1 double-transgenic mice. Neurosci Lett 2001; 306:116–120.

75. Shie FS, LeBoeur RC, Jin LW. Early intraneuronal Abeta deposition in the hippocampus of APP transgenic mice. Neuroreport 2003; 14:123–129.

76. Lopez EM, Bell KF, Ribeiro-da-Silva A, Cuello AC. Early changes in neurons of the hippocampus and neocortex in transgenic rats expressing intracellular human a-beta. J Alzheimers Dis 2004; 6:421–431; discussion 443–449.

77. Echeverria V, Ducatenzeiler A, Alhonen L, et al. Rat transgenic models with a phenotype of intracellular Abeta accumulation in hippocampus and cortex. J Alzheimers Dis 2004; 6:209–219.

78. Redwine JM, Kosofsky B, Jacobs RE, et al. Dentate gyrus volume is reduced before onset of plaque formation in PDAPP mice: a magnetic resonance microscopy and stereologic analysis. Proc Natl Acad Sci USA 2003; 100:1381–1386.

79. Reilly JF, Games D, Rydel RE, et al. Amyloid deposition in the hippocampus and entorhinal cortex: quantitative analysis of a transgenic mouse model. Proc Natl Acad Sci USA 2003; 100:4837–4842.

80. Wu CC, Chawla F, Games D, et al. Selective vulnerability of dentate granule cells prior to amyloid deposition in PDAPP mice: digital morphometric analyses. Proc Natl Acad Sci USA 2004; 101:7141–7146.

81. Almeida CG, Tampellini D, Takahashi RH, et al. β-Amyloid accumulation in APP mutant neurons reduces PSD-95 and GluR1 in synapses. Neurobiol Dis 2005; 20:187–198.

82. Snyder EM, Nong Y, Almeida CG, et al. Regulation of NMDA receptor trafficking by amyloid-beta. Nat Neurosci 2005; 8:1051–1058.

83. Echeverria V, Cuello AC. Intracellular A-beta amyloid, a sign for worse things to come? Mol Neurobiol 2002; 26:299–316.

84. Moreira PI, Liu Q, Honda K, Smith MA, Santos MS, Oliveira CR. Is intraneuronal amyloid beta-peptide accumulation the trigger of Alzheimer's disease pathophysiology? J Alzheimers Dis 2004; 6:433–434 discussion 443–449.

85. Wirths O, Multhaup G, Bayer TA. A modified beta-amyloid hypothesis: intraneuronal accumulation of the beta-amyloid peptide—the first step of a fatal cascade. J Neurochem 2004; 91:513–520.

86. Davies P. Why is there a cholinergic deficit in Alzheimer's disease? 4th Ann. Meeting Int. College of Geriatric Psychoneuropharm. Basel, (Oct. 14-16): 2004 Abstract. 61.

87. Kim JH, Anwyl R, Suh YH, Djamgoz MB, Rowan MJ. Use-dependent effects of amyloidogenic fragments of (beta)-amyloid precursor protein on synaptic plasticity in rat hippocampus in vivo. J Neurosci 2001; 21:1327–1333.

88. Mucke L, Masliah E, Yu GQ, et al. High-level neuronal expression of abeta 1-42 in wild-type human amyloid protein precursor transgenic mice: synaptotoxicity without plaque formation. J Neurosci 2000; 20:4050–4058.

89. Lashuel HA, Hartley D, Petre BM, Walz T, Lansbury PT, Jr. Neurodegenerative disease: amyloid pores from pathogenic mutations. Nature 2002; 418(6895):291.

90. Ambroggio EE, Kim DH, Separovic F, et al. Surface behavior and lipid interaction of Alzheimer beta-amyloid peptide 1-42: a membrane-disrupting peptide. Biophys J 2005; 88:2706–2713.

91. Nixon RA. Endosome function and dysfunction in Alzheimer's disease and other neurodegenerative diseases. Neurobiol Aging 2005; 26:373–382.

92. Götz J, Chen F, van Dorpe J, Nitsch RM. Formation of neurofibrillary tangles in P301 l tau transgenic mice induced by Abeta 42 fibrils. Science 2001; 293:1491–1495.

93. Bonini NM, Fortini ME. Human neurodegenerative disease modeling using Drosophila. Annu Rev Neurosci 2003; 26:627–656.

94. Richardson JC, Kendal CE, Anderson R, et al. Ultrastructural and behavioural changes precede amyloid deposition in a transgenic model of Alzheimer's disease. Neuroscience 2003; 122:213–228.

95. Lewis J, Dickson DW, Lin WL, et al. Enhanced neurofibrillary degeneration in transgenic mice expressing mutant tau and APP. Science 2001; 293:1487–1491.

96. Oddo S, Caccamo A, Kitazawa M, Tseng BP, LaFerla FM. Amyloid deposition precedes tangle formation in a triple transgenic model of Alzheimer's disease. Neurobiol Aging 2003; 24:1063–1070.

97. Rutten BP, Wirths O, Van de Berg WD, et al. No alterations of hippocampal neuronal number and synaptic bouton number in a transgenic mouse model expressing the beta-cleaved C-terminal APP fragment. Neurobiol Dis 2003; 12:110–120.

98. Kelly BL, Vassar R, Ferreira A. {beta}-Amyloid-induced dynamin 1 depletion in hippocampal neurons: a potential mechanism for early cognitive decline in Alzheimer disease. J Biol Chem 2005; 280:31746–31753.

99. Irizarry MC, McNamara M, Fedorchak K, Hsiao K, Hyman BT. APPSw transgenic mice develop age-related A beta deposits and neuropil abnormalities, but no neuronal loss in CA1. J Neuropathol Exp Neurol 1997; 56:965–973.

100. Schwab C, Hosokawa M, McGeer PL. Transgenic mice overexpressing amyloid beta protein are an incomplete model of Alzheimer disease. Exp Neurol 2004; 188:52–64.

101. Trinchese F, Liu S, Battaglia F, Walter S, Mathews PM, Arancio O. Progressive age-related development of Alzheimer-like pathology in APP/PS1 mice. Ann Neurol 2004; 55:801–814.

102. Hartmann J, Erb C, Ebert U, et al. Central cholinergic functions in human amyloid precursor protein knock-in/presenilin-1 transgenic mice. Neuroscience 2004; 125:1009–1017.

103. Schmitz C, Rutten BP, Pielen A, et al. Hippocampal neuron loss exceeds amyloid plaque load in a transgenic mouse model of Alzheimer's disease. Am J Pathol 2004; 164:1495–1502.

104. Casas C, Sergeant N, Itier JM, et al. Massive CA1/2 neuronal loss with intraneuronal and N-terminal truncated Abeta42 accumulation in a novel Alzheimer transgenic model. Am J Pathol 2004; 165:1289–1300.

105. Ribe EM, Perez M, Puig B, et al. Accelerated amyloid deposition, neurofibrillary degeneration and neuronal loss in double mutant APP/tau transgenic mice. Neurobiol Dis 2005.

106. Rutten BP, Van der Kolk NM, Schafer S, et al. Age-related loss of synaptophysin immunoreactive presynaptic boutons within the hippocampus of APP751SL, PS1M146L, and APP751SL/PS1M146L transgenic mice. Am J Pathol 2005; 167:161–173.

107. Billings LM, Oddo S, Green KN, McGaugh JL, Laferla FM. Intraneuronal Abeta causes the onset of early Alzheimer's disease-related cognitive deficits in transgenic mice. Neuron 2005; 45:675–688.

108. Oddo S, Billings L, Kesslak JP, Cribbs DH, LaFerla FM. Abeta immunotherapy leads to clearance of early, but not late, hyperphosphorylated tau aggregates via the proteasome. Neuron 2004; 43:321–332.

109. Lewis J, McGowan E, Rockwood J, et al. Neurofibrillary tangles, amyotrophy and progressive motor disturbance in mice expressing mutant (P301L) tau protein. Nat Genet 2000; 25:402–405.

110. Grateau G, Verine J, Delpech M, Ries M. Amyloidosis: a model of misfolded protein disorder. Med Sci (Paris) 2005; 21:627–633.

111. Walsh DM, Klyubin I, Fadeeva JV, et al. Naturally secreted oligomers of amyloid beta protein potently inhibit hippocampal long-term potentiation in vivo. Nature 2002; 416:535–539.

112. Bucciantini M, Calloni G, Chiti F, et al. Prefibrillar amyloid protein aggregates share common features of cytotoxicity. J Biol Chem 2004; 279:31374–31382.

113. MacRaild CA, Stewart CR, Mok YF, et al. Non-fibrillar components of amyloid deposits mediate the self-association and tangling of amyloid fibrils. J Biol Chem 2004; 279:21038–21045.

114. Wang HW, Pasternak JF, Kuo H, et al. Soluble oligomers of beta amyloid (1-42) inhibit long-term potentiation but not long-term depression in rat dentate gyrus. Brain Res 2002; 924:133–140.

115. Hoshi M, Sato M, Matsumoto S, et al. Spherical aggregates of beta-amyloid (amylospheroid) show high neurotoxicity and activate tau protein kinase I/glycogen synthase kinase-3beta. Proc Natl Acad Sci USA 2003; 100:6370–6375.

116. Klein WL, Stine WB, Jr., Teplow DB. Small assemblies of unmodified amyloid beta-protein are the proximate neurotoxin in Alzheimer's disease. Neurobiol Aging 2004; 25:569–580.

117. Lacor PN, Buniel MC, Chang L, et al. Synaptic targeting by Alzheimer's-related amyloid beta oligomers. J Neurosci 2004; 24:10191–10200.

118. Gouras GK, Almeida CG, Takahashi RH. Intraneuronal Abeta accumulation and origin of plaques in Alzheimer's disease. Neurobiol Aging 2005; 26:1235–1244.

119. Zhu X, Mei M, Lee HG, et al. P38 activation mediates amyloid-beta cytotoxicity. Neurochem Res 2005; 30:791–796.

120. Klein WL. Synaptic targeting by Aβ oligomeres (ADDLs) as a basis for memory loss in early Alzheimer's disease. Alzheimer's and Dementia 2006; 2:43–55.

121. Gong Y, Chang L, Viola KL, et al. Alzheimer's disease-affected brain: presence of oligomeric A beta ligands (ADDLs) suggests a molecular basis for reversible memory loss. Proc Natl Acad Sci USA 2003; 100:10417–10422.

122. Lue LF, Kuo YM, Roher AE, et al. Soluble amyloid beta peptide concentration as a predictor of synaptic change in Alzheimer's disease. Am J Pathol 1999; 155:853–862.

123. Bucciantini M, Giannoni E, Chiti F, et al. Inherent toxicity of aggregates implies a common mechanism for protein misfolding diseases. Nature 2002; 416:507–511.

124. Hoozemans JJ, Veerhuis R, Van Haastert ES, et al. The unfolded protein response is activated in Alzheimer's disease. Acta Neuropathol (Berl) 2005.

125. Gylys KH, Fein JA, Yang F, Wiley DJ, Miller CA, Cole GM. Synaptic changes in Alzheimer's disease: increased amyloid-beta and gliosis in surviving terminals is accompanied by decreased PSD-95 fluorescence. Am J Pathol 2004; 165:1809–1817.

126. Dodart JC, Bales KR, Gannon KS, et al. Immunization reverses memory deficits without reducing brain Abeta burden in Alzheimer's disease model. Nat Neurosci 2002; 5:452–457.

127. Verdier Y, Zarandi M, Penke B. Amyloid beta-peptide interactions with neuronal and glial cell plasma membrane: binding sites and implications for Alzheimer's disease. J Pept Sci 2004; 10:229–248.

128. Tsai J, Grutzendler J, Duff K, Gan WB. Fibrillar amyloid deposition leads to local synaptic abnormalities and breakage of neuronal branches. Nat Neurosci 2004; 7:1181–1183.

129. Lu DC, Shaked GM, Masliah E, Bredesen DE, Koo EH. Amyloid beta protein toxicity mediated by the formation of amyloid-beta protein precursor complexes. Ann Neurol 2003; 54:781–789.

130. Sudo H, Hashimoto Y, Niikura T, et al. Secreted Abeta does not mediate neurotoxicity by antibody-stimulated amyloid precursor protein. Biochem Biophys Res Commun 2001; 282:548–556.

131. Hashimoto M, Rockenstein E, Crews L, Masliah E. Role of protein aggregation in mitochondrial dysfunction and neurodegeneration in Alzheimer's and Parkinson's diseases. Neuromolecular Med 2003; 4:21–36.

132. Cardoso SM, Santana I, Swerdlow RH, Oliveira CR. Mitochondria dysfunction of Alzheimer's disease cybrids enhances Abeta toxicity. J Neurochem 2004; 89:1417–1426.

133. Butterfield DA. Amyloid beta-peptide [1-42]-associated free radical-induced oxidative stress and neurodegeneration in Alzheimer's disease brain: mechanisms and consequences. Curr Med Chem 2003; 10:2651–2659.

134. Butterfield DA, Boyd-Kimball D. Amyloid beta-peptide(1-42) contributes to the oxidative stress and neurodegeneration found in Alzheimer disease brain. Brain Pathol 2004; 14:426–432.

135. Butterfield DA. Proteomics: a new approach to investigate oxidative stress in Alzheimer's disease brain. Brain Res 2004; 1000:1–7.

136. Zhu X, Raina AK, Lee HG, Casadesus G, Smith MA, Perry G. Oxidative stress signalling in Alzheimer's disease. Brain Res 2004; 1000:32–39.

137. Watt JA, Pike CJ, Walencewicz-Wasserman AJ, Cotman CW. Ultrastructural analysis of beta-amyloid-induced apoptosis in cultured hippocampal neurons. Brain Res 1994; 661:147–156.

138. Gentile MT, Vecchione C, Maffei A, et al. Mechanisms of soluble beta-amyloid impairment of endothelial function. J Biol Chem 2004; 279:48135–48142.

139. Zlokovic BV, Deane R, Sallstrom J, Chow N, Miano JM. Neurovascular pathways and Alzheimer amyloid beta-peptide. Brain Pathol 2005; 15:78–83.

140. Selznick LA, Zheng TS, Flavell RA, Rakic P, Roth KA. Amyloid beta-induced neuronal death is bax-dependent but caspase-independent. J Neuropathol Exp Neurol 2000; 59:271–279.

141. Takuma H, Tomiyama T, Kuida K, Mori H. Amyloid beta peptide-induced cerebral neuronal loss is mediated by caspase-3 in vivo. J Neuropathol Exp Neurol 2004; 63:255–261.

142. Onyango IG, Tuttle JB, Bennett JP, Jr. Altered intracellular signaling and reduced viability of Alzheimer's disease neuronal cybrids is reproduced by beta-amyloid peptide acting through receptor for advanced glycation end products (RAGE). Mol Cell Neurosci 2005; 29:333–343.

143. Markesbery WR, Krysclo RJ, Lovell MA, et al. Lipid peroxidation is an early event in the brain in amnestic mild cognitive impairment. Ann Neurol 2005; 58:730–735.

144. Boyd-Kimball D, Castegna A, Sultana R, et al. Proteomic identification of proteins oxidized by Abeta(1-42) in synaptosomes: implications for Alzheimer's disease. Brain Res 2005; 1044:206–215.

145. Pamplona R, Dalfo E, Ayala V, et al. Proteins in human brain cortex are modified by oxidation, glycoxidation, and lipoxidation. Effects of Alzheimer disease and identification of lipoxidation targets. J Biol Chem 2005; 280:21522–21530.

146. Pratico D, Uryu K, Leight S, Trojanoswki JQ, Lee VM. Increased lipid peroxidation precedes amyloid plaque formation in an animal model of Alzheimer amyloidosis. J Neurosci 2001; 21:4183–4187.

147. Lin H, Bhatia R, Lal R. Amyloid beta protein forms ion channels: implications for Alzheimer's disease pathophysiology. FASEB J 2001; 15:2433–2444.

148. Pierrot N, Ghisdal P, Caumont AS, Octave JN. Intraneuronal amyloid-beta1-42 production triggered by sustained increase of cytosolic calcium concentration induces neuronal death. J Neurochem 2004; 88:1140–1150.

149. Dougherty JJ, Wu J, Nichols RA. Beta-amyloid regulation of presynaptic nicotinic receptors in rat hippocampus and neocortex. J Neurosci 2003; 23:6740–6747.

150. Dickson DW. Apoptotic mechanisms in Alzheimer neurofibrillary degeneration: cause or effect? J Clin Invest 2004; 114:23–27.

151. Howlett DR. Neurotoxicity of the Alzheimer's β-amyloid peptide. In: Broderick PA, Rahni DN, Kolodny EH, eds. Bioimaging in Neurodegeneration. Totowa, NJ: Humana Press, 2005:61–74.

152. Yang Y, Geldmacher DS, Herrup K. DNA replication precedes neuronal cell death in Alzheimer's disease. J Neurosci 2001; 21:2661–2668.
153. Takuma K, Yan SS, Stern DM, Yamada K. Mitochondrial dysfunction, endoplasmic reticulum stress, and apoptosis in Alzheimer's disease. J Pharmacol Sci 2005; 97:312–316.
154. Raff MC, Barres BA, Burne JF, Coles HS, Ishizaki Y, Jacobson MD. Programmed cell death and the control of cell survival: lessons from the nervous system. Science 1993; 262:695–700.
155. Ohyagi Y, Asahara H, Chui DH, et al. Intracellular Abeta42 activates p53 promoter: a pathway to neurodegeneration in Alzheimer's disease. FASEB J 2005; 19:255–257.
156. Cardoso SM, Oliveira CR. The role of calcineurin in amyloid-beta-peptides-mediated cell death. Brain Res 2005; 1050:1–7.
157. Cotman CW, Anderson AJ. A potential role for apoptosis in neurodegeneration and Alzheimer's disease. Mol Neurobiol 1995; 10:19–45.
158. Gervais FG, Xu D, Robertson GS, et al. Involvement of caspases in proteolytic cleavage of Alzheimer's amyloid-beta precursor protein and amyloidogenic A beta peptide formation. Cell 1999; 97:395–406.
159. Rohn TT, Head E, Su JH, et al. Correlation between caspase activation and neurofibrillary tangle formation in Alzheimer's disease. Am J Pathol 2001; 158:189–198.
160. Cribbs DH, Poon WW, Rissman RA, Blurton-Jones M. Caspase-mediated degeneration in Alzheimer's disease. Am J Pathol 2004; 165:353–355.
161. Guo H, Albrecht S, Bourdeau M, Petzke T, Bergeron C, LeBlanc AC. Active caspase-6 and caspase-6-cleaved tau in neuropil threads, neuritic plaques, and neurofibrillary tangles of Alzheimer's disease. Am J Pathol 2004; 165:523–531.
162. Graeber MB, Moran LB. Mechanisms of cell death in neurodegenerative diseases: fashion, fiction, and facts. Brain Pathol 2002; 12:385–390.
163. Jellinger KA. Apoptosis vs. nonapoptotic mechanisms in neurodegeneration. In: Wood PL, ed. Mechanisms and Management, 2nd ed. Totowa, NJ: Humana Press Inc., 2003:29–88.
164. Roth KA. Caspases, apoptosis, and Alzheimer disease: causation, correlation, and confusion. J Neuropathol Exp Neurol 2001; 60:829–838.
165. Johnstone M, Gearing AJ, Miller KM. A central role for astrocytes in the inflammatory response to beta-amyloid; chemokines, cytokines and reactive oxygen species are produced. J Neuroimmunol 1999; 93:182–193.
166. D'Andrea MR. Evidence linking neuronal cell death to autoimmunity in Alzheimer's disease. Brain Res 2003; 982:19–30.
167. D'Andrea MR, Cole GM, Ard MD. The microglial phagocytic role with specific plaque types in the Alzheimer disease brain. Neurobiol Aging 2004; 25:675–683.
168. Hashimoto M, Masliah E. Cycles of aberrant synaptic sprouting and neurodegeneration in Alzheimer's and dementia with Lewy bodies. Neurochem Res 2003; 28:1743–1756.
169. Tanzi RE. The synaptic Abeta hypothesis of Alzheimer disease. Nat Neurosci 2005; 8:977–979.
170. Bishop GM, Robinson SR. The amyloid paradox: amyloid-beta-metal complexes can be neurotoxic and neuroprotective. Brain Pathol 2004; 14:448–452.
171. Maynard CJ, Bush AI, Masters CL, Cappai R, Li QX. Metals and amyloid-beta in Alzheimer's disease. Int J Exp Pathol 2005; 86:147–159.

172. Akiyama H, Mori H, Saido T, Kondo H, Ikeda K, McGeer PL. Occurrence of the diffuse amyloid beta-protein (Abeta) deposits with numerous A beta-containing glial cells in the cerebral cortex of patients with Alzheimer's disease. Glia 1999; 25:324–331.

173. Thal DR, Schultz C, Dehghani F, Yamaguchi H, Braak H, Braak E. Amyloid beta-protein (Abeta)-containing astrocytes are located preferentially near N-terminal-truncated Abeta deposits in the human entorhinal cortex. Acta Neuropathol (Berl) 2000; 100:608–617.

174. Yamaguchi H, Sugihara S, Ogawa A, Oshima N, Ihara Y. Alzheimer beta amyloid deposition enhanced by apoE ε4 gene precedes neurofibrillary pathology in the frontal association cortex of nondemented senior subjects. J Neuropathol Exp Neurol 2001; 60:731–739.

175. Yamaguchi H, Sugihara S, Ogawa A, Saido TC, Ihara Y. Diffuse plaques associated with astroglial amyloid beta protein, possibly showing a disappearing stage of senile plaques. Acta Neuropathol (Berl) 1998; 95:217–222.

176. Rossner S. New players in old amyloid precursor protein-processing pathways. Int J Dev Neurosci 2004; 22:467–474.

177. Koistinaho M, Lin S, Wu X, et al. Apolipoprotein E promotes astrocyte colocalization and degradation of deposited amyloid-beta peptides. Nat Med 2004; 10:719–726.

178. Nagele RG, D'Andrea MR, Lee H, Venkataraman V, Wang HY. Astrocytes accumulate A beta 42 and give rise to astrocytic amyloid plaques in Alzheimer disease brains. Brain Res 2003; 971:197–209.

179. Nagele RG, Wegiel J, Venkataraman V, Imaki H, Wang KC. Contribution of glial cells to the development of amyloid plaques in Alzheimer's disease. Neurobiol Aging 2004; 25:663–674.

180. Paradisi S, Sacchetti B, Balduzzi M, Gaudi S, Malchiodi-Albedi F. Astrocyte modulation of in vitro beta-amyloid neurotoxicity. Glia 2004; 46:252–260.

181. Stern EA, Bacskai BJ, Hickey GA, Attenello FJ, Lombardo JA, Hyman BT. Cortical synaptic integration in vivo is disrupted by amyloid-beta plaques. J Neurosci 2004; 24:4535–4540.

182. Parvathy S, Davies P, Haroutunian V, et al. Correlation between Abetax-40-, Abetax-42-, and Abetax-43-containing amyloid plaques and cognitive decline. Arch Neurol 2001; 58:2025–2032.

183. Fonte J, Miklossy J, Atwood C, Martins R. The severity of cortical Alzheimer's type changes is positively correlated with increased amyloid-beta levels: resolubilization of amyloid-beta with transition metal ion chelators. J Alzheimers Dis 2001; 3:209–219.

184. Funato H, Yoshimura M, Kusui K, et al. Quantitation of amyloid beta-protein (A beta) in the cortex during aging and in Alzheimer's disease. Am J Pathol 1998; 152:1633–1640.

185. Naslund J, Haroutunian V, Mohs R, et al. Correlation between elevated levels of amyloid beta-peptide in the brain and cognitive decline. JAMA 2000; 283:1571–1577.

186. Vehmas AK, Kawas CH, Stewart WF, Troncoso JC. Immune reactive cells in senile plaques and cognitive decline in Alzheimer's disease. Neurobiol Aging 2003; 24:321–331.

187. Iijima K, Liu HP, Chiang AS, Hearn SA, Konsolaki M, Zhong Y. Dissecting the pathological effects of human Abeta40 and Abeta42 in Drosophila: a potential model for Alzheimer's disease. Proc Natl Acad Sci USA 2004; 101:6623–6628.

188. Klunk WE, Engler H, Nordberg A, et al. Imaging brain amyloid in Alzheimer's disease with Pittsburgh Compound-B. Ann Neurol 2004; 55:306–319.

189. Lockhart A, Ye L, Judd DB, et al. Evidence for the presence of three distinct binding sites for the thioflavin T class of Alzheimer's disease PET imaging agents on beta-amyloid peptide fibrils. J Biol Chem 2005; 280:7677–7684.

190. Plant LD, Boyle JP, Smith IF, Peers C, Pearson HA. The production of amyloid beta peptide is a critical requirement for the viability of central neurons. J Neurosci 2003; 23:5531–5535.

191. Bishop GM, Robinson SR. Physiological roles of amyloid-beta and implications for its removal in Alzheimer's disease. Drugs Aging 2004; 21:621–630.

192. Koudinov AR, Berezov TT. Alzheimer's amyloid-beta (A beta) is an essential synaptic protein, not neurotoxic junk. Acta Neurobiol Exp 2004; 64:71–79.

193. Lee HG, Casadesus G, Zhu X, Takeda A, Perry G, Smith MA. Challenging the amyloid cascade hypothesis: senile plaques and amyloid-beta as protective adaptations to Alzheimer disease. Ann NY Acad Sci 2004; 1019:1–4.

194. Avila J, Lucas JJ, Perez M, Hernandez F. Role of tau protein in both physiological and pathological conditions. Physiol Rev 2004; 84:361–384.

195. Bancher C, Brunner C, Lassmann H, et al. Accumulation of abnormally phosphorylated tau precedes the formation of neurofibrillary tangles in Alzheimer's disease. Brain Res 1989; 477:90–99.

196. Braak E, Braak H, Mandelkow EM. A sequence of cytoskeleton changes related to the formation of neurofibrillary tangles and neuropil threads. Acta Neuropathol (Berl) 1994; 87:554–567.

197. Mitchell TW, Nissanov J, Han LY, et al. Novel method to quantify neuropil threads in brains from elders with or without cognitive impairment. J Histochem Cytochem 2000; 48:1627–1638.

198. Perry G, Kawai M, Tabaton M, et al. Neuropil threads of Alzheimer's disease show a marked alteration of the normal cytoskeleton. J Neurosci 1991; 11:1748–1755.

199. Togo T, Akiyama H, Iseki E, et al. Immunohistochemical study of tau accumulation in early stages of Alzheimer-type neurofibrillary lesions. Acta Neuropathol (Berl) 2004; 107:504–508.

200. Schmidt ML, Murray JM, Trojanowski JQ. Continuity of neuropil threads with tangle-bearing and tangle-free neurons in Alzheimer disease cortex. A confocal laser scanning microscopy study. Mol Chem Neuropathol 1993; 18:299–312.

201. Goedert M, Spillantini MG, Potier MC, Ulrich J, Crowther RA. Cloning and sequencing of the cDNA encoding an isoform of microtubule-associated protein tau containing four tandem repeats: differential expression of tau protein mRNAs in human brain. Embo J 1989; 8:393–399.

202. Sergeant N, David JP, Goedert M, et al. Two-dimensional characterization of paired helical filament-tau from Alzheimer's disease: demonstration of an additional 74-kDa component and age-related biochemical modifications. J Neurochem 1997; 69:834–844.

202a. Kitamura T, Sugimori K, Sudo S, Kobayashi K. Relationship between microtubule-binding repeats and morphology of neurofibrillary tangle in Alzheimer's disease. Acta Neurol Scand 2005; 112:327–334.

203. Iqbal K, Alonso ADC, Chen S, et al. Tau pathology in Alzheimer disease and other tauopathies. Biochim Biophys Acta-Mol Basis Dis 2005; 1739:198–210.

204. Gong CX, Liu F, Grundke-Iqbal I, Iqbal K. Post-translational modifications of tau protein in Alzheimer's disease. J Neural Transm 2005; 112:813–838.

205. Binder LI, Guillozet-Bongaarts AL, Garcia-Sierra F, Berry RW. Tau, tangles, and Alzheimer's disease. Biochim Biophys Acta 2005; 1739:216–223.

206. Boutajangout A, Boom A, Leroy K, Brion JP. Expression of tau mRNA and soluble tau isoforms in affected and non-affected brain areas in Alzheimer's disease. FEBS Lett 2004; 576:183–189.

207. Hyman BT, Augustinack JC, Ingelsson M. Transcriptional and conformational changes of the tau molecule in Alzheimer's disease. Biochim Biophys Acta 2005; 1739:150–157.

208. Liu Q, Smith MA, Avila J, et al. Alzheimer-specific epitopes of tau represent lipid peroxidation-induced conformations. Free Radic Biol Med 2005; 38:746–754.

209. Guillozet-Bongaarts AL, Garcia-Sierra F, Reynolds MR, et al. Tau truncation during neurofibrillary tangle evolution in Alzheimer's disease. Neurobiol Aging 2005; 28:1013–1022.

210. Nakano H, Kobayashi K, Sugimori K, et al. Regional analysis of differently phosphorylated tau proteins in brains from patients with Alzheimer's disease. Dement Geriatr Cogn Disord 2004; 17:122–131.

211. Katsuno T, Morishima-Kawashima M, Saito Y, et al. Independent accumulations of tau and amyloid beta-protein in the human entorhinal cortex. Neurology 2005; 64:687–692.

212. SantaCruz K, Lewis J, Spires T, et al. Tau suppression in a neurodegenerative mouse model improves memory function. Science 2005; 309:476–481.

213. Trojanowski JQ, Lee VM. Pathological tau: a loss of normal function or a gain in toxicity? Nat Neurosci 2005; 8:1136–1137.

214. Andorfer C, Acker CM, Kress Y, Hof PR, Duff K, Davies P. Cell-cycle reentry and cell death in transgenic mice expressing nonmutant human tau isoforms. J Neurosci 2005; 25:5446–5454.

215. Lee HG, Perry G, Moreira PI, et al. Tau phosphorylation in Alzheimer's disease: pathogen or protector? Trends Mol Med 2005; 11:164–169.

216. Ghoshal N, Garcia-Sierra F, Wuu J, et al. Tau conformational changes correspond to impairments of episodic memory in mild cognitive impairment and Alzheimer's disease. Exp Neurol 2002; 177:475–493.

217. Garcia-Sierra F, Ghoshal N, Quinn B, Berry RW, Binder LI. Conformational changes and truncation of tau protein during tangle evolution in Alzheimer's disease. J Alzheimers Dis 2003; 5:65–77.

218. Braak H, Braak E. Neuropathological stageing of Alzheimer-related changes. Acta Neuropathol (Berl) 1991; 82:239–259.

219. Delacourte A, David JP, Sergeant N, et al. The biochemical pathway of neurofibrillary degeneration in aging and Alzheimer's disease. Neurology 1999; 52:1158–1165.

220. Hyman BT, Van Hoesen GW, Kromer LJ, Damasio AR. Perforant pathway changes and the memory impairment of Alzheimer's disease. Ann Neurol 1986; 20:472–481.
221. Mizutani T, Kasahara M. Degeneration of the intrahippocampal routes of the perforant and alvear pathways in senile dementia of Alzheimer type. Neurosci Lett 1995; 184:141–144.
222. Delatour B, Blanchard V, Pradier L, Duyckaerts C. Alzheimer pathology disorganizes cortico-cortical circuitry: direct evidence from a transgenic animal model. Neurobiol Dis 2004; 16:41–47.
223. Gertz HJ, Xuereb J, Huppert F, et al. Examination of the validity of the hierarchical model of neuropathological staging in normal aging and Alzheimer's disease. Acta Neuropathol (Berl) 1998; 95:154–158.
224. Gold G, Bouras C, Kovari E, et al. Clinical validity of Braak neuropathological staging in the oldest-old. Acta Neuropathol (Berl) 2000; 99:579–582.
225. Perl DP, Purohit DP, Haroutunian V. Clinicopathological correlations of the Alzheimer disease staging system introduced by Braak and Braak. J Neuropathol Exp Neurol 1997; 56:577.
226. Jellinger KA. Neuropathological staging of Alzheimer-related lesions: The challenge of establishing relations to age (commentary). Neurobiol Aging 1997; 18:369–375.
227. Bussiere T, Giannakopoulos P, Bouras C, Perl DP, Morrison JH, Hof PR. Progressive degeneration of nonphosphorylated neurofilament protein-enriched pyramidal neurons predicts cognitive impairment in Alzheimer's disease: stereologic analysis of prefrontal cortex area 9. J Comp Neurol 2003; 463:281–302.
228. Haroutunian V, Purohit DP, Perl DP, et al. Neurofibrillary tangles in nondemented elderly subjects and mild Alzheimer disease. Arch Neurol 1999; 56:713–718.
229. Thal DR, Rub U, Orantes M, Braak H. Phases of A beta-deposition in the human brain and its relevance for the development of AD. Neurology 2002; 58:1791–1800.
230. Meyer-Luehmann M, Stalder M, Herzig MC, et al. Extracellular amyloid formation and associated pathology in neural grafts. Nat Neurosci 2003; 6:370–377.
231. Delacourte A, Sergeant N, Champain D, et al. The biochemical spreading of tau and amyloid beta precursor protein pathologies in aging and sporadic Alzheimer's disease. Brain Aging 2001; 1:33–42.
232. Dickson TC, Vickers JC. The morphological phenotype of beta-amyloid plaques and associated neuritic changes in Alzheimer's disease. Neuroscience 2001; 105:99–107.
233. Kraszpulski M, Soininen H, Helisalmi S, Alafuzoff I. The load and distribution of beta-amyloid in brain tissue of patients with Alzheimer's disease. Acta Neurol Scand 2001; 103:88–92.
234. Gomez-Isla T, Hollister R, West H, et al. Neuronal loss correlates with but exceeds neurofibrillary tangles in Alzheimer's disease. Ann Neurol 1997; 41:17–24.
235. Ingelsson M, Fikumoto H, Newell K, Hyman BT, Irizarry MC. Lack of correlation between biochemical and neuropathological amyloid measures in the Alzheimer brain. In: Iqbal K, Winblad B, eds. Alzheimer's Disease and Related Disorders. Bucharest, Romania: Ana Aslan Intl Acad of Aging, 2003:193–201.

236. Knowles RB, Gomez-Isla T, Hyman BT. Abeta associated neuropil changes: correlation with neuronal loss and dementia. J Neuropathol Exp Neurol 1998; 57:1122–1130.
237. Morris JC, Storandt M, McKeel DW, Jr., et al. Cerebral amyloid deposition and diffuse plaques in "normal" aging: Evidence for presymptomatic and very mild Alzheimer's disease. Neurology 1996; 46:707–719.
238. Price JL, Morris JC. Tangles and plaques in nondemented aging and "preclinical" Alzheimer's disease. Ann Neurol 1999; 45:358–368.
239. Mena R, Wischik CM, Novak M, Milstein C, Cuello AC. A progressive deposition of paired helical filaments (PHF) in the brain characterizes the evolution of dementia in Alzheimer's disease. An immunocytochemical study with a monoclonal antibody against the PHF core. J Neuropathol Exp Neurol 1991; 50:474–490.
240. Bussiere T, Gold G, Kovari E, et al. Stereologic analysis of neurofibrillary tangle formation in prefrontal cortex area 9 in aging and Alzheimer's disease. Neuroscience 2003; 117:577–592.
241. Morishima-Kawashima M, Ihara Y. Alzheimer's disease: beta-Amyloid protein and tau. J Neurosci Res 2002; 70:392–401.
242. Mudher A, Lovestone S. Alzheimer's disease-do tauists and baptists finally shake hands? Trends Neurosci 2002; 25:22–26.
243. Hardy J, Selkoe DJ. The amyloid hypothesis of Alzheimer's disease: progress and problems on the road to therapeutics. Science 2002; 297:353–356.
244. Götz J, Schild A, Hoerndli F, Pennanen L. Amyloid-induced neurofibrillary tangle formation in Alzheimer's disease: insight from transgenic mouse and tissue-culture models. Int J Dev Neurosci 2004; 22:453–465.
245. Ramsden M, Kotilinek L, Forster C, et al. Age-dependent neurofibrillary tangle formation, neuron loss, and memory impairment in a mouse model of human tauopathy (P301L). J Neurosci 2005; 25:10637–10647.
246. Kitazawa M, Yamasaki TR, Laferla FM. Microglia as a potential bridge between the amyloid {beta}-peptide and tau. Ann NY Acad Sci 2004; 1035:85–103.
247. Perez M, Cuadros R, Benitez MJ, Jimenez JS. Interaction of Alzheimer's disease amyloid beta peptide fragment 25-35 with tau protein, and with a tau peptide containing the microtubule binding domain. J Alzheimers Dis 2004; 6:461–467.
248. Delacourte A, Sergeant N, Champain D, et al. Nonoverlapping but synergetic tau and APP pathologies in sporadic Alzheimer's disease. Neurology 2002; 59:398–407.
249. Delacourte A, Sergeant N, Wattez A, et al. Tau aggregation in the hippocampal formation: an ageing or a pathological process? Exp Gerontol 2002; 37:1291–1296.
250. Esteban JA. Living with the enemy: a physiological role for the beta-amyloid peptide. Trends Neurosci 2004; 27:1–3.
251. Cotman CW, Poon WW, Rissman RA, Blurton-Jones M. The role of caspase cleavage of tau in Alzheimer disease neuropathology. J Neuropathol Exp Neurol 2005; 64:104–112.
252. Rohn TT, Rissman RA, Davis MC, Kim YE, Cotman CW, Head E. Caspase-9 activation and caspase cleavage of tau in the Alzheimer's disease brain. Neurobiol Dis 2002; 11:341–354.

253. Rohn TT, Rissman RA, Head E, Cotman CW. Caspase activation in the Alzheimer's disease brain: tortuous and torturous. Drug News Perspect 2002; 15:549–557.
254. Rissman RA, Poon WW, Blurton-Jones M, et al. Caspase-cleavage of tau is an early event in Alzheimer disease tangle pathology. J Clin Invest 2004; 114:121–130.
255. Gamblin TC, Chen F, Zambrano A, et al. Caspase cleavage of tau: linking amyloid and neurofibrillary tangles in Alzheimer's disease. Proc Natl Acad Sci USA 2003; 100:10032–10037.
256. Newman J, Rissman RA, Sarsoza F, et al. Caspase-cleaved tau accumulation in neurodegenerative diseases associated with tau and alpha-synuclein pathology. Acta Neuropathol (Berl) 2005; 110:135–144.
257. Rametti A, Esclaire F, Yardin C, Terro F. Linking alterations in tau phosphorylation and cleavage during neuronal apoptosis. J Biol Chem 2004; 279:54518–54528.
258. Rapoport M, Dawson HN, Binder LI, Vitek MP, Ferreira A. Tau is essential to beta -amyloid-induced neurotoxicity. Proc Natl Acad Sci USA 2002; 99:6364–6369.
259. Braak H, Braak E. Frequency of stages of Alzheimer-related lesions in different age categories. Neurobiol Aging 1997; 18:351–357.
260. Duyckaerts C, Hauw JJ. Prevalence, incidence and duration of Braak's stages in the general population: can we know? Neurobiol Aging 1997; 18:362–369, discussion 389–392.
261. Mandelkow EM, Stamer K, Vogel R, Thies E, Mandelkow E. Clogging of axons by tau, inhibition of axonal traffic and starvation of synapses. Neurobiol Aging 2003; 24:1079–1085.
262. Guzik BW, Goldstein LS. Microtubule-dependent transport in neurons: steps towards an understanding of regulation, function and dysfunction. Curr Opin Cell Biol 2004; 16:443–450.
263. Roy S, Zhang B, Lee VM, Trojanowski JQ. Axonal transport defects: a common theme in neurodegenerative diseases. Acta Neuropathol (Berl) 2005; 109:5–13.
264. Stokin GB, Lillo C, Falzone TL, et al. Axonopathy and transport deficits early in the pathogenesis of Alzheimer's disease. Science 2005; 307:1282–1288.
265. Ferrari A, Hoerndli F, Baechi T, Nitsch RM, Gotz J. beta-Amyloid induces paired helical filament-like tau filaments in tissue culture. J Biol Chem 2003; 278:40162–40168.
265a. Ribe EM, Perez M, Puig B, et al. Accelerated amyloid deposition, neurofibrillary degeneration and neuronal loss in double mutant APP/tau transgenic mice. Neurobiol Dis 2005; 20:814–822.
266. Metsaars WP, Hauw JJ, van Welsem ME, Duyckaerts C. A grading system of Alzheimer disease lesions in neocortical areas. Neurobiol Aging 2003; 24:563–572.
267. Coria F, Moreno A, Rubio I, Garcia MA, Morato E, Mayor F, Jr. The cellular pathology associated with Alzheimer beta-amyloid deposits in non-demented aged individuals. Neuropathol Appl Neurobiol 1993; 19:261–268.

268. Schonheit B, Zarski R, Ohm TG. Spatial and temporal relationships between plaques and tangles in Alzheimer-pathology. Neurobiol Aging 2004; 25:697–711.

269. Eckert A, Marques CA, Keil U, Schussel K, Muller WE. Increased apoptotic cell death in sporadic and genetic Alzheimer's disease. Ann NY Acad Sci 2003; 1010:604–609.

270. Ingelsson M, Fukumoto H, Newell KL, et al. Early Abeta accumulation and progressive synaptic loss, gliosis, and tangle formation in AD brain. Neurology 2004; 62:925–931.

271. Bennett DA, Schneider JA, Wilson RS, Bienias JL, Arnold SE. Neurofibrillary tangles mediate the association of amyloid load with clinical Alzheimer disease and level of cognitive function. Arch Neurol 2004; 61:378–384.

272. Dickson TC, Chuckowree JA, Chuah MI, West AK, Vickers JC. alpha-Internexin immunoreactivity reflects variable neuronal vulnerability in Alzheimer's disease and supports the role of the beta-amyloid plaques in inducing neuronal injury. Neurobiol Dis 2005; 18:286–295.

273. Duyckaerts C. Looking for the link between plaques and tangles. Neurobiol Aging 2004; 25:735–739, discussion 743–746.

274. Haroutunian V, Perl DP, Purohit DP, et al. Regional distribution of neuritic plaques in the nondemented elderly and subjects with very mild Alzheimer disease. Arch Neurol 1998; 55:1185–1191.

275. Jellinger KA. Alpha-synuclein pathology in Parkinson's and Alzheimer's disease brain: incidence and topographic distribution—a pilot study. Acta Neuropathol (Berlin) 2003; 106:191–201.

276. Jellinger KA. Prevalence of vascular lesions in dementia with Lewy bodies. A postmortem study. J Neural Transm 2003; 110:771–778.

277. Jellinger KA. Neuropathology of Alzheimer disease and clinical relevance. In: Iqbal K, Winblad B, eds. Alzheimer's Disease and Related Disorders: Research Advances. Bucharest, Romania: Ana Aslan Intl Acad of Aging, 2003:152–169.

278. Bartzokis G, Sultzer D, Luc PH, Nuechterlein KH, Mintz J, Cummings JL. Heterogeneous age-related breakdown of white matter structural integrity: implications for cortical "disconnection" in aging and Alzheimer's disease. Neurobiol Aging 2004; 25:843–851.

279. Khachaturian ZS. Diagnosis of Alzheimer's disease. Arch Neurol 1985; 42:1097–1105.

280. Tierney MC, Fisher RH, Lewis AJ, et al. The NINCDS-ADRDA work Group criteria for the clinical diagnosis of probable Alzheimer's disease: a clinicopathologic study of 57 cases. Neurology 1988; 38:359–364.

281. Mirra SS, Heyman A, McKeel D, et al. The Consortium to Establish a Registry for Alzheimer's Disease (CERAD). Part II. Standardization of the neuropathologic assessment of Alzheimer's disease. Neurology 1991; 41:479–486.

282. The National Institute on Aging, and Reagan Institute Working Group on Diagnostic Criteria for the Neuropathological Assessment of Alzheimer's Disease. Consensus recommendations for the postmortem diagnosis of Alzheimer's disease. Neurobiol Aging 1997; 18:S1–S2.

283. McKeel DW, Price JL, Miller JP, et al. Neuropathologic criteria for diagnosing Alzheimer disease in persons with pure dementia of Alzheimer type. J Neuropathol Exp Neurol 2004; 63:1028–1037.

284. Hibbard LS, Arnicar-Sulze TL, McKeel DW, Jr., Burrell LD. Computed detection and quantitative morphometry of Alzheimer senile plaques. J Neurosci Methods 1994; 52:175–189.

285. Hyman BT, Trojanowski JQ. Consensus recommendations for the postmortem diagnosis of Alzheimer disease from the National Institute on Aging and the Reagan Institute Working Group on diagnostic criteria for the neuropathological assessment of Alzheimer disease. J Neuropathol Exp Neurol 1997; 56:1095–1097.

286. Terry RD, Hansen LA, DeTeresa R, Davies P, Tobias H, Katzman R. Senile dementia of the Alzheimer type without neocortical neurofibrillary tangles. J Neuropathol Exp Neurol 1987; 46:262–268.

287. Tiraboschi P, Sabbagh MN, Hansen LA, et al. Alzheimer disease without neocortical neurofibrillary tangles: "a second look". Neurology 2004; 62:1141–1147.

288. Jellinger KA. Plaque-predominant and tangle-predominant variants of Alzheimer's disease. In: Dickson DW, ed. Neurodegeneration: The Molecular Pathology of Dementia and Movement Disorders. Basel: ISN Neuropath Press, 2003:66–68.

289. Jellinger KA, Bancher C. Neuropathology of Alzheimer's disease: a critical update. J Neural Transm Suppl 1998; 54:77–95.

290. Hansen L, Salmon D, Galasko D, et al. The Lewy body variant of Alzheimer's disease: a clinical and pathologic entity. Neurology 1990; 40:1–8.

291. Nagy Z, Esiri MM, Joachim C, et al. Comparison of pathological diagnostic criteria for Alzheimer disease. Alzheimer Dis Assoc Disord 1998; 12:182–189.

292. Mirra SS, Hyman BT. Aging and dementia. In: Graham DI, Lantos PL, eds. Greenfield's Neuropathology, 7th ed. London: E. Arnold, 2002:195–271.

293. Paulus W, Bancher C, Jellinger K. Interrater reliability in the neuropathologic diagnosis of Alzheimer's disease. Neurology 1992; 42:329–332.

294. Halliday G, Ng T, Rodriguez M, et al. Consensus neuropathological diagnosis of common dementia syndromes: testing and standardising the use of multiple diagnostic criteria. Acta Neuropathol (Berl) 2002; 104:72–78.

295. Cochran EJ, Schneider JA, Bennett DA, et al. Application of NIA/Reagan Institute Working Group Criteria for diagnosis of Alzheimer's disease to members of the Religious Orders Study (abstract). J Neuropathol Exp Neurol 1998; 57:508.

296. Harding AJ, Lakay B, Halliday GM. Selective hippocampal neuron loss in dementia with Lewy bodies. Ann Neurol 2002; 51:125–128.

297. Davis DG, Schmitt FA, Wekstein DR, Markesbery WR. Alzheimer neuropathologic alterations in aged cognitively normal subjects. J Neuropathol Exp Neurol 1999; 58:376–388.

298. McKee AC, Kowall NW, Au R. Topography of neurofibrillary tangles distinguishes aging from Alzheimer disease (abstract). J Neuropathol Exp Neurol 2002; 61:488.

299. Bowler JV, Munoz DG, Merskey H, Hachinski V. Fallacies in the pathological confirmation of the diagnosis of Alzheimer's disease. J Neurol Neurosurg Psychiatry 1998; 64:18–24.

300. Ince PG, McKeith IG. Dementia with Lewy bodies. In: Dickson DW, ed. Neurodegeneration: The Molecular Pathology of Dementia and Movement Disorders. Basel: ISN Neuropath Press, 2003:188–199.

301. Mosimann UP, McKeith IG. Dementia with Lewy bodies and Parkinson's disease dementia - two synucleinopathies. ACNR 2003; 3:8–16.
302. Heidebrink JL. Is dementia with Lewy bodies the second most common cause of dementia? J Geriatr Psych Neurol 2002; 15:182–187.
303. Takao M, Ghetti B, Yoshida H, et al. Early-onset Dementia with Lewy Bodies. Brain Pathol 2004; 14:137–147.
304. Duda JE. Pathology and neurotransmitter abnormalities of dementia with Lewy bodies. Dement Geriatr Cogn Disord 2004; 1:3–14.
305. McKeith IG, Galasko D, Kosaka K, et al. Consensus guidelines for the clinical and pathologic diagnosis of dementia with Lewy bodies (DLB): report of the consortium on DLB international workshop. Neurology 1996; 47:1113–1124.
306. Braak H, Del Tredici K, Rub U, de Vos RA, Jansen Steur EN, Braak E. Staging of brain pathology related to sporadic Parkinson's disease. Neurobiol Aging 2003; 24:197–211.
307. Saito Y, Ruberu NN, Sawabe M, et al. Lewy body-related alpha-synucleinopathy in aging. J Neuropathol Exp Neurol 2004; 63:742–749.
308. Jellinger KA. Lewy body-related alpha-synucleinopathy in the aged human brain. J Neural Transm 2004; 111:219–235.
309. Iseki E. Dementia with Lewy bodies: reclassification of pathological subtypes and boundary with Parkinson's disease or Alzheimer's disease. Neuropathology 2004; 24:72–78.
310. Tsuboi Y, Dickson DW. Dementia with Lewy bodies and Parkinson's disease with dementia: are they different? Parkinsonism Relat Disord 2005; 1:S47–S51.
310a. Apaydin H, Ahiskog JE, Parisi JE, et al. Parkinson disease neuropathology: later-developing dementia and loss of the levodopa response. Arch Neurol 2002; 59:102–112.
311. Brown DF, Dababo MA, Bigio EH, et al. Neuropathologic evidence that the Lewy body variant of Alzheimer disease represents coexistence of Alzheimer disease and idiopathic Parkinson disease. J Neuropathol Exp Neurol 1998; 57:39–46.
312. Harding AJ, Halliday GM. Simplified neuropathological diagnosis of dementia with Lewy bodies. Neuropathol Appl Neurobiol 1998; 24:195–201.
313. Jellinger KA, Seppi K, Wenning GK. Clinical and neuropathological correlates of Lewy body disease. Acta Neuropathol (Berl) 2003; 106:188–189.
314. Hansen LA, Daniel SE, Wilcock GK, Love S. Frontal cortical synaptophysin in Lewy body diseases: relation to Alzheimer's disease and dementia. J Neurol Neurosurg Psychiatry 1998; 64:653–656.
315. Lee JM. Functional status of cortical M1 cholinergic receptors in Alzheimer's disease and the Lewy body variant of Alzheimer's disease (abstract). J Neuropathol Exp Neurol 2004; 63:552.
316. Imamura K, Hishikawa N, Ono K, et al. Cytokine production of activated microglia and decrease in neurotrophic factors of neurons in the hippocampus of Lewy body disease brains. Acta Neuropathol 2004; 109:141–150.
317. Imamura K, Hishikawa N, Sawada M, et al. Distribution of major histocompatibility complex class II-positive microglia and cytokine profile of Parkinson's disease brains. Acta Neuropathol (Berl) 2003; 106:518–526.
318. Merdes AR, Hansen LA, Jeste DV, et al. Influence of Alzheimer pathology on clinical diagnostic accuracy in dementia with Lewy bodies. Neurology 2003; 60:1586–1590.

319. Sabbagh MN, Corey-Bloom J, Tiraboschi P, Thomas R, Masliah E, Thal LJ. Neurochemical markers do not correlate with cognitive decline in the Lewy body variant of Alzheimer disease. Arch Neurol 1999; 56:1458–1461.

320. Ballard CG, Jacoby R, Del Ser T, et al. Neuropathological substrates of psychiatric symptoms in prospectively studied patients with autopsy-confirmed dementia with lewy bodies. Am J Psychiatry 2004; 161:843–849.

321. Kenny RA, Shaw FE, O'Brien JT, Scheltens PH, Kalaria R, Ballard C. Carotid sinus syndrome is common in dementia with Lewy bodies and correlates with deep white matter lesions. J Neurol Neurosurg Psychiatry 2004; 75:966–971.

322. Kraybill ML, Larson EB, Tsuang DW, et al. Cognitive differences in dementia patients with autopsy-verified A.D., Lewy body pathology, or both. Neurology 2005; 64:2069–2073.

323. Gomez-Isla T, Growdon WB, McNamara M, et al. Clinicopathologic correlates in temporal cortex in dementia with Lewy bodies. Neurology 1999; 53:2003–2009.

324. Sahin HA, Emre M, Ziabreva I, Perry E, Celasun B, Perry R. The distribution pattern of pathology and cholinergic deficits in amygdaloid complex in Alzheimer's disease and dementia with Lewy bodies. Acta Neuropathol 2006 [Epub ahead of print]: PMID: 16468020.

325. Klucken J, McLean PJ, Gomez-Tortosa E, Ingelsson M, Hyman BT. Neuritic alterations and neural system dysfunction in Alzheimer's disease and dementia with Lewy bodies. Neurochem Res 2003; 28:1683–1691.

326. Aarsland D, Ballard CG, Halliday G. Are Parkinson's disease with dementia and dementia with Lewy bodies the same entity? J Geriatr Psychiatry Neurol 2004; 17:137–145.

327. Marui W, Iseki E, Kato M, Akatsu H, Kosaka K. Pathological entity of dementia with Lewy bodies and its differentiation from Alzheimer's disease. Acta Neuropathol (Berl) 2004; 108:121–128.

328. Burn DJ. Cortical Lewy body disease. J Neurol Neurosurg Psychiatry 2004; 75:175–178.

329. Perneczky R, Mosch D, Neumann M, et al. The Alzheimer variant of Lewy body disease: a pathologically confirmed case-control study. Dement Geriatr Cogn Disord 2005; 20:89–94.

330. O'Brien J, Ames D, McKeith I, et al. Dementia with Lewy bodies and Parkinson's disease dementia. London: Taylor & Francis, 2006.

331. Deramecourt V, Bombois S, Maurage CA, et al. Biochemical staging of synucleinopathy and amyloidopathy in dementia with Lewy bodies. Neurology 2006; in press.

332. Dickson DW. Alpha-synuclein and the Lewy body disorders. Curr Opin Neurol 2001; 14:423–432.

333. Popescu A, Lippa CF, Lee VM, Trojanowski JQ. Lewy bodies in the amygdala: increase of alpha-synuclein aggregates in neurodegenerative diseases with tau-based inclusions. Arch Neurol 2004; 61:1915–1919.

334. Trembath Y, Rosenberg C, Ervin JF, et al. Lewy body pathology is a frequent co-pathology in familial Alzheimer's disease. Acta Neuropathol (Berl) 2003; 105:484–488.

335. Lippa CF. Lewy bodies in conditions other than disorders of alpha-synuclein. In: Dickson DW, ed. Neurodegeneration: The Molecular Pathology of Dementia and Movement Disorders. Basel: ISN Neuropath Press, 2003:200–202.

336. Arai Y, Yamazaki M, Mori O, Muramatsu H, Asano G, Katayama Y. Alpha-synuclein-positive structures in cases with sporadic Alzheimer's disease: morphology and its relationship to tau aggregation. Brain Res 2001; 888:287–296.

337. Tsuang DW, Wilson RK, Lopez OL, et al. Genetic association between the APOE*4 allele and Lewy bodies in Alzheimer disease. Neurology 2005; 64:509–513.

338. Parkkinen L, Soininen H, Alafuzoff I. Regional distribution of alpha-synuclein pathology in unimpaired aging and Alzheimer disease. J Neuropathol Exp Neurol 2003; 62:363–367.

339. Saito Y, Kawashima A, Ruberu NN, et al. Accumulation of phosphorylated alpha-synuclein in aging human brain. J Neuropathol Exp Neurol 2003; 62:644–654.

340. Ishizawa T, Mattila P, Davies P, Wang D, Dickson DW. Colocalization of tau and alpha-synuclein epitopes in Lewy bodies. J Neuropathol Exp Neurol 2003; 62:389–397.

341. Iseki E, Togo T, Suzuki K, et al. Dementia with Lewy bodies from the perspective of tauopathy. Acta Neuropathol (Berl) 2003; 105:265–270.

342. Maries E, Dass B, Collier TJ, Kordower JH, Steece-Collier K. The role of alpha-synuclein in Parkinson's disease: insights from animal models. Nat Rev Neurosci 2003; 4:727–738.

343. Neumann M, Muller V, Gorner K, Kretzschmar HA, Haass C, Kahle PJ. Pathological properties of the Parkinson's disease-associated protein DJ-1 in alpha-synucleinopathies and tauopathies: relevance for multiple system atrophy and Pick's disease. Acta Neuropathol (Berl) 2004; 107:489–496.

344. Giasson BI, Forman MS, Higuchi M, et al. Initiation and synergistic fibrillization of tau and alpha-synuclein. Science 2003; 300:636–640.

345. Lee VM, Giasson BI, Trojanowski JQ. More than just two peas in a pod: common amyloidogenic properties of tau and alpha-synuclein in neurodegenerative diseases. Trends Neurosci 2004; 27:129–134.

346. Pletnikova O, West N, Lee MK, et al. Abeta deposition is associated with enhanced cortical alpha-synuclein lesions in Lewy body diseases. Neurobiol Aging 2005; 26:1183–1192.

347. Gomez-Tortosa E, Gonzalo I, Fanjul S, et al. Cerebrospinal fluid markers in dementia with Lewy bodies compared with Alzheimer disease. Arch Neurol 2003; 60:1218–1222.

348. Harding AJ, Halliday GM. Cortical Lewy body pathology in the diagnosis of dementia. Acta Neuropathol (Berl) 2001; 102:355–363.

349. Kertesz A, Munoz DG, Hillis A. Preferred terminology. Ann Neurol 2003; 5:S3–S6.

350. Neary D, Snowden JS, Gustafson L, et al. Frontotemporal lobar degeneration: a consensus on clinical diagnostic criteria. Neurology 1998; 51:1546–1554.

351. Ikeda M, Ishikawa T, Tanabe H. Epidemiology of frontotemporal lobar degeneration. Dement Geriatr Cogn Disord 2004; 17:265–268.

352. Hodges JR, Davies RR, Xuereb JH, et al. Clinicopathological correlates in frontotemporal dementia. Ann Neurol 2004; 56:399–406.

353. McKhann GM, Albert MS, Grossman M, Miller B, Dickson D, Trojanowski JQ. Clinical and pathological diagnosis of frontotemporal dementia: report of the Work Group on Frontotemporal Dementia and Pick's Disease. Arch Neurol 2001; 58:1803–1809.

354. Knopman DS, Boeve BF, Parisi JE, et al. Antemortem diagnosis of frontotemporal lobar degeneration. Ann Neurol 2005; 57:480–488.

355. Seeley WW, Bauer AM, Miller BL, et al. The natural history of temporal variant frontotemporal dementia. Neurology 2005; 64:1384–1390.

356. Munoz DG. Histopathology. In: Bowler JV, Hachinski V, eds. Vascular Cognitive Impairment. Preventable Dementia. Oxford: Oxford University Press, 2003:57–75.

357. Broe M, Kril J, Halliday GM. Astrocytic degeneration relates to the severity of disease in frontotemporal dementia. Brain 2004; 127:2214–2220.

358. Constantinidis J. Pick dementia. Anatomoclinical correlations and pathophysiological considerations. In: Rose FC, ed. In: Modern approaches to the dementias. Part, I., Etiology and pathophysiology, interdisciplinary topics in gerontology, Vol. 19. Basel: Karger, 1985:72–97.

359. Bergeron C, Morris HR, Rossor M. Pick's disease. In: Dickson DW, ed. Neurodegeneration. Basel: ISN Neuropathol Press, 2003:124–131.

360. Knopman DS, Mastri AR, Frey WH, II, Sung JH, Rustan T. Dementia lacking distinctive histologic features: a common non-Alzheimer degenerative dementia. Neurology 1990; 40:251–256.

361. Trojanowski JQ, Dickson D. Update on the neuropathological diagnosis of frontotemporal dementias. J Neuropathol Exp Neurol 2001; 60:1123–1126.

362. Mott RT, Dickson DW, Trojanowski JQ, et al. Neuropathologic, biochemical, and molecular characterization of the frontotemporal dementias. J Neuropathol Exp Neurol 2005; 64:420–428.

363. Bigio EH, Lipton AM, White CL, III, Dickson DW, Hirano A. Frontotemporal and motor neurone degeneration with neurofilament inclusion bodies: additional evidence for overlap between FTD and ALS. Neuropathol Appl Neurobiol 2003; 29:239–253.

364. Davies RR, Hodges JR, Kril JJ, Patterson K, Halliday GM, Xuereb JH. The pathological basis of semantic dementia. Brain 2005; 128:1984–1995.

365. Cairns NJ, Brannstrom T, Khan MN, Rossor MN, Lantos PL. Neuronal loss in familial frontotemporal dementia with ubiquitin-positive, tau-negative inclusions. Exp Neurol 2003; 181:319–326.

366. Kertesz A, Kawarai T, Rogaeva E, et al. Familial frontotemporal dementia with ubiquitin-positive, tau-negative inclusions. Neurology 2000; 54:818–827.

367. Rosso SM, Kamphorst W, de Graaf B, et al. Familial frontotemporal dementia with ubiquitin-positive inclusions is linked to chromosome 17q21-22. Brain 2001; 124:1948–1957.

368. Bigio EH, Johnson NA, Rademaker AW, et al. Neuronal ubiquitinated intranuclear inclusions in familial and non-familial frontotemporal dementia of the motor neuron disease type associated with amyotrophic lateral sclerosis. J Neuropathol Exp Neurol 2004; 63:801–811.

369. Yaguchi M, Okamoto K, Nakazato Y. Frontotemporal dementia with cerebral intraneuronal ubiquitin-positive inclusions but lacking lower motor neuron involvement. Acta Neuropathol (Berl) 2003; 105:81–85.

370. Josephs KA, Holton JL, Rossor MN, et al. Frontotemporal lobar degeneration and ubiquitin immunohistochemistry. Neuropathol Appl Neurobiol 2004; 30:369–373.

371. Rosso SM, Donker Kaat L, Baks T, et al. Frontotemporal dementia in The Netherlands: patient characteristics and prevalence estimates from a population-based study. Brain 2003; 126:2016–2022.

372. Mackenzie IR, Feldman H. Neuronal intranuclear inclusions distinguish familial FTD-MND type from sporadic cases. Dement Geriatr Cogn Disord 2004; 17:333–336.

373. Dickson DW, Bergeron C, Chin SS, et al. Office of Rare Diseases neuropathologic criteria for corticobasal degeneration. J Neuropathol Exp Neurol 2002; 61:935–946.

374. Boeve BF, Lang AE, Litvan I. Corticobasal degeneration and its relationship to progressive supranuclear palsy and frontotemporal dementia. Ann Neurol 2003; 5:S15–S19.

375. Arai T, Ikeda K, Akiyama H, et al. Identification of amino-terminally cleaved tau fragments that distinguish progressive supranuclear palsy from corticobasal degeneration. Ann Neurol 2004; 55:72–79.

376. Poorkaj P, Grossman M, Steinbart E, et al. Frequency of tau gene mutations in familial and sporadic cases of non-Alzheimer dementia. Arch Neurol 2001; 58:383–387.

377. Johnson J, Ostojic J, Lannfelt L, et al. No evidence for tau duplications in frontal temporal dementia families showing genetic linkage to the tau locus in which tau mutations have not been found. Neurosci Lett 2004; 363:99–101.

378. Lee VM, Goedert M, Trojanowski JQ. Neurodegenerative tauopathies. Annu Rev Neurosci 2001; 24:1121–1159.

379. Schofield E, Kersaitis C, Shepherd CE, Kril JJ, Halliday GM. Severity of gliosis in Pick's disease and frontotemporal lobar degeneration: tau-positive glia differentiate these disorders. Brain 2003; 4:827–840.

380. Zhukareva V, Shah K, Uryu K, et al. Biochemical analysis of tau proteins in argyrophilic grain disease. Alzheimer's disease, and Pick's disease: a comparative study. Am J Pathol 2002; 161:1135–1141.

381. Morris HR, Baker M, Yasojima K, et al. Analysis of tau haplotypes in Pick's disease. Neurology 2002; 59:443–445.

382. Dermaut B, Kumar-Singh S, Engelborghs S, et al. A novel presenilin 1 mutation associated with Pick's disease but not beta-amyloid plaques. Ann Neurol 2004; 55:617–626.

383. Pickering-Brown SM, Baker M, Nonaka T, et al. Frontotemporal dementia with Pick-type histology associated with Q336R mutation in the tau gene. Brain 2004; 127:1415–1426.

384. Kobayashi K, Hayashi M, Kidani T, et al. Pick's disease pathology of a missense mutation of S305N of frontotemporal dementia and parkinsonism linked to chromosome 17: another phenotype of S305N. Dement Geriatr Cogn Disord 2004; 17:293–297.

385. Zhukareva V, Vogelsberg-Ragaglia V, Van Deerlin VM, et al. Loss of brain tau defines novel sporadic and familial tauopathies with frontotemporal dementia. Ann Neurol 2001; 49:165–175.

386. Chang HT, Cortez S, Vonsattel JP, Stopa EG, Schelper RL. Familial frontotemporal dementia: a report of three cases of severe cerebral atrophy with rare inclusions that are negative for tau and synuclein, but positive for ubiquitin. Acta Neuropathol (Berl) 2004; 108:10–16.

387. Hutton M, Lendon CL, Rizzu P, et al. Association of missense and 5(-splice-site mutations in tau with the inherited dementia FTDP-17. Nature 1998; 393:702–705.

388. Sobrido MJ, Miller BL, Havlioglu N, et al. Novel tau polymorphisms, tau haplotypes, and splicing in familial and sporadic frontotemporal dementia. Arch Neurol 2003; 60:698–702.

389. Stanford PM, Brooks WS, Teber ET, et al. Frequency of tau mutations in familial and sporadic frontotemporal dementia and other tauopathies. J Neurol 2004; 251:1098–1104.

390. Yancopoulou D, Crowther RA, Chakrabarti L, Gydesen S, Brown JM, Spillantini MG. Tau protein in frontotemporal dementia linked to chromosome 3 (FTD-3). J Neuropathol Exp Neurol 2003; 62:878–882.

391. Gydesen S, Brown JM, Brun A, et al. Chromosome 3 linked frontotemporal dementia (FTD-3). Neurology 2002; 59:1585–1594.

392. Ghetti B, Hutton ML, Wszolek ZK. Frontotemporal dementia and parkinsonism linked to chromosome 17 associated with tau gene mutations (FTDP-17T). In: Dickson DW et al, ed. Neurodegeneration. Basel: ISN Neuropathol Press, 2003:85–102.

393. Spillantini MG, Yoshida H, Rizzini C, et al. A novel tau mutation (N296N) in familial dementia with swollen achromatic neurons and corticobasal inclusion bodies. Ann Neurol 2000; 48:939–943.

394. Schraen-Maschke S, Dhaenens CM, Delacourte A, Sablonniere B. Microtubule-associated protein tau gene: a risk factor in human neurodegenerative diseases. Neurobiol Dis 2004; 15:449–460.

395. Vitali A, Piccini A, Borghi R, et al. Soluble amyloid beta-protein is increased in frontotemporal dementia with tau gene mutations. J Alzheimers Dis 2004; 6:45–51.

396. Wilhelmsen KC, Forman MS, Rosen HJ, et al. 17q-linked frontotemporal dementia-amyotrophic lateral sclerosis without tau mutations with tau and alpha-synuclein Inclusions. Arch Neurol 2004; 61:398–406.

397. Taniguchi S, McDonagh AM, Pickering-Brown SM, et al. The neuropathology of frontotemporal lobar degeneration with respect to the cytological and biochemical characteristics of tau protein. Neuropathol Appl Neurobiol 2004; 30:1–18.

398. Lipton AM, White CL, III, Bigio EH. Frontotemporal lobar degeneration with motor neuron disease-type inclusions predominates in 76 cases of frontotemporal degeneration. Acta Neuropathol 2004; 108:379–385.

399. Paviour DC, Lees AJ, Josephs KA, et al. Frontotemporal lobar degeneration with ubiquitin-only-immunoreactive neuronal changes: broadening the clinical picture to include progressive supranuclear palsy. Brain 2004; 11:2441–2451.

400. Procter AW, Qurne M, Francis PT. Neurochemical features of frontotemporal dementia. Dement Geriatr Cogn Disord 1999; 10:80–84.

401. Huey ED, Putnam KT, Grafman J. A Systematic review of neurotransmitter deficits and treatments in frontotemporal dementia. Neurology 2006; 66:17–22.

402. Munoz DG, Dickson DW, Bergeron C, Mackenzie IR, Delacourte A, Zhukareva V. The neuropathology and biochemistry of frontotemporal dementia. Ann Neurol 2003; 5:S24–S28.

403. Cairns NJ, Uryu K, Bigio EH, et al. alpha-Internexin aggregates are abundant in neuronal intermediate filament inclusion disease (NIFID) but rare in other neurodegenerative diseases. Acta Neuropathol (Berl) 2004.

404. Lee VM, Kenyon TK, Trojanowski JQ. Transgenic animal models of tauopathies. Biochim Biophys Acta 2005; 1739:251–259.

405. Cairns NJ, Grossman M, Arnold SE, et al. Clinical and neuropathologic variation in neuronal intermediate filament inclusion disease. Neurology 2004; 63:1376–1384.

406. Ala TA, Beh GO, Frey WH. II. Pure hippocampal sclerosis: a rare cause of dementia mimicking Alzheimer's disease. Neurology 2000; 54:843–848.

407. Troncoso JC, Kawas CH, Chang CK, Folstein MF, Hedreen JC. Lack of association of the apoE4 allele with hippocampal sclerosis dementia. Neurosci Lett 1996; 204:138–140.

408. Corey-Bloom J, Sabbagh MN, Bondi MW, et al. Hippocampal sclerosis contributes to dementia in the elderly. Neurology 1997; 48:154–160.

409. Dickson DW, Davies P, Bevona C, et al. Hippocampal sclerosis: a common pathological feature of dementia in very old (>or=80 years of age) humans. Acta Neuropathol (Berl) 1994; 88:212–221.

410. Leverenz JB, Agustin CM, Tsuang D, et al. Clinical and neuropathological characteristics of hippocampal sclerosis: a community-based study. Arch Neurol 2002; 59:1099–1106.

411. Rasmusson DX, Brandt J, Steele C, Hedreen JC, Troncoso JC, Folstein MF. Accuracy of clinical diagnosis of Alzheimer disease and clinical features of patients with non-Alzheimer disease neuropathology. Alzheimer Dis Assoc Disord 1996; 10:180–188.

412. Kuslansky G, Verghese J, Dickson D, Katz M, Buschke H, Lipton R. Hippocampal sclerosis: cognitive consequences and contributions to dementia (abstract). Neurology 2004; 62:A128–A129.

413. Beach TG, Sue L, Scott S, et al. Hippocampal sclerosis dementia with tauopathy. Brain Pathol 2003; 13:263–278.

414. Crystal HA, Dickson D, Davies P, Masur D, Grober E, Lipton RB. The relative frequency of "dementia of unknown etiology" increases with age and is nearly 50% in nonagenarians. Arch Neurol 2000; 57:713–719.

415. Vinters HV, Ellis WG, Zarow C, et al. Neuropathologic substrates of ischemic vascular dementia. J Neuropathol Exp Neurol 2000; 59:931–945.

416. Clark AW, White CL, III, Manz IM. Primary degenerative dementia without Alzheimer pathology. Can J Neurol Sci 1986; 13:462–470.

417. Blass DM, Hatanpaa KJ, Brandt J, et al. Dementia in hippocampal sclerosis resembles frontotemporal dementia more than Alzheimer disease. Neurology 2004; 63:492–497.

418. Josephs KA, Jones AG, Dickson DW. Hippocampal sclerosis and ubiquitin-positive inclusions in dementia lacking distinctive histopathology. Dement Geriatr Cogn Disord 2004; 17:342–345.

419. Hatanpaa KJ, Blass DM, Pletnikova O, et al. Most cases of dementia with hippocampal sclerosis may represent frontotemporal dementia. Neurology 2004; 63:538–542.

420. Ishizawa T, Ko LW, Cookson N, Davias P, Espinoza M, Dickson DW. Selective neurofibrillary degeneration of the hippocampal CA2 sector is associated with four-repeat tauopathies. J Neuropathol Exp Neurol 2002; 61:1040–1047.

421. Braak H, Braak E. Argyrophilic grain disease: frequency of occurrence in different age categories and neuropathological diagnostic criteria. J Neural Transm 1998; 105:801–819.

422. Tolnay M, Clavaguera F. Argyrophilic grain disease: a late-onset dementia with distinctive features among tauopathies. Neuropathology 2004; 24:269–283.

423. Jicha GA, Petersen RC, Johnson KA, et al. Argyrophilic grain disease in mild cognitive impairment progressing to dementia. J Neuropathol Exp Neurol 2003;62.

424. Thal DR, Schulte C, Botez G, et al. The impact of argyrophilic grain disease on the development of dementia and its relationship to concurrent Alzheimer's disease-related pathology. Neuropathol Appl Neurobiol 2005; 31:270–279.

425. Ishihara K, Araki S, Ihori N, et al. Argyrophilic grain disease presenting with frontotemporal dementia: a neuropsychological and pathological study of an autopsied case with presenile onset. Neuropathology 2005; 25:165–170.

426. Togo T, Sahara N, Yen SH, et al. Argyrophilic grain disease is a sporadic 4-repeat tauopathy. J Neuropathol Exp Neurol 2002; 61:547–556.

427. Fujino Y, Wang DS, Thomas N, Espinoza M, Davies P, Dickson DW. Increased frequency of argyrophilic grain disease in Alzheimer disease with 4R tau-specific immunohistochemistry. J Neuropathol Exp Neurol 2005; 64:209–214.

428. Tolnay M, Sergeant N, Ghestem A, et al. Argyrophilic grain disease and Alzheimer's disease are distinguished by their different distribution of tau protein isoforms. Acta Neuropathol (Berl) 2002; 104:425–434.

429. Miserez AR, Clavaguera F, Monsch AU, Probst A, Tolnay M. Argyrophilic grain disease: molecular genetic difference to other four-repeat tauopathies. Acta Neuropathol (Berl) 2003; 106:363–366.

430. Saito Y, Ruberu NN, Sawabe M, et al. Staging of argyrophilic grains: an age-associated tauopathy. J Neuropathol Exp Neurol 2004; 63:911–918.

431. Conrad C, Vianna C, Schultz C, et al. Molecular evolution and genetics of the Saitohin gene and tau haplotype in Alzheimer's disease and argyrophilic grain disease. J Neurochem 2004; 89:179–188.

432. Dib M. Methodological issues and therapeutic perspectives in vascular dementia: a review. Arch Gerontol Geriatr 2001; 33:71–80.

433. Román GC. Clinical forms of vascular dementia. In: Paul RH, Cohen R, Ott BR, Salloway S, eds. Vascular Dementia: Cerebrovascular Mechanisms and Clinical Management. Totowa, NJ: Humana Press Inc., 2005:7–21.

434. Erkinjuntti T. Vascular cognitive impairment and dementia. In: Mohr JP, Choi DW, Grotta JC, Weir B, Wolf PA, eds. In: Stroke: Pathophysiology, Diagnosis, and Management. Philadelphia: Churchill Livingstone, 2004:648–660.

435. Hebert R, Lindsay J, Verreault R, Rockwood K, Hill G, Dubois MF. Vascular dementia: incidence and risk factors in the Canadian study of health and aging. Stroke 2000; 31:1487–1493.

436. Meyer JS, Rauch GM, Lechner H, Loeb C, eds. Vascular Dementia. Armonk, NY: Futura Publishing, 2001.

437. World Health Organization. ICD-10 Classification of Mental and Behavioural Disorders: Diagnostic Criteria for Research. Geneva: WHO, 1993.

438. American Psychiatric Association. Diagnostic and Statistical Manual of Mental Disorders, 4th ed. Washington, DC: American Psychiatric Association, 1994.

439. Chui HC, Victoroff JI, Margolin D, Jagust W, Shankle R, Katzman R. Criteria for the diagnosis of ischemic vascular dementia proposed by the state of California Alzheimer's disease diagnostic and treatment centers. Neurology 1992; 42:473–480.

440. Román GC, Tatemichi TK, Erkinjuntti T, et al. Vascular dementia: diagnostic criteria for research studies. Report of the NINDS-AIREN international workshop. Neurology 1993; 43:250–260.

441. Hachinski VC, Iliff L, Zihlka E, et al. Cerebral blood flow in dementia. Arch Neurol 1975; 32:632–637.

442. Small GW. Revised Ischemic Score for diagnosing multi-infarct dementia. J Clin Psychiatry 1985; 46:514–517.

443. Gold G, Giannakopoulos P, Montes-Paixao C, Jr., et al. Sensitivity and specificity of newly proposed clinical criteria for possible vascular dementia. Neurology 1997; 49:690–694.

444. Knopman DS, Rocca WA, Cha RH, Edland SD, Kokmen E. Incidence of vascular dementia in Rochester, Minn, 1985–1989. Arch Neurol 2002; 59:1605–1610.

445. Moroney JT, Bagiella E, Desmond DW, et al. Meta-analysis of the hachinski ischemic score in pathologically verified dementias. Neurology 1997; 49:1096–1105.

446. Rocca WA, Knopman DS. Prevalence and incidence patterns of vascular dementia, in vascular cognitive impairment. In: Bowler JV, Hachinski V, eds. Preventable Dementia. Oxford: Oxford University Press, 2003:21–32.

447. Tang WK, Chan SS, Chiu HF, et al. Impact of applying NINDS-AIREN criteria of probable vascular dementia to clinical and radiological characteristics of a stroke cohort with dementia. Cerebrovasc Dis 2004; 18:98–103.

448. Ballard CG, Burton EJ, Barber R, et al. NINDS AIREN neuroimaging criteria do not distinguish stroke patients with and without dementia. Neurology 2004; 63:983–988.

449. van Straaten EC, Scheltens P, Knol DL, et al. Operational definitions for the NINDS-AIREN criteria for vascular dementia: an interobserver study. Stroke 2003; 34:1907–1912.

450. Lopez OL, Kuller LH, Becker JT, et al. Classification of vascular dementia in the cardiovascular health study cognition study. Neurology 2005; 64:1539–1547.

451. Price CC, Jefferson AL, Merino JG, Heilman KM, Libon DJ. Subcortical vascular dementia: integrating neuropsychological and neuroradiologic data. Neurology 2005; 65:376–382.

452. Bowler JV, Hachinski V. Current criteria for vascular dementia—a critical appraisal, in vascular cognitive impairment. In: Bowler JV, Hachinski V, eds. Preventable Dementia. Oxford: Oxford University Press, 2003:1–11.

453. O'Brien JT, Erkinjuntti T, Reisberg B, et al. Vascular cognitive impairment. Lancet Neurol 2003; 2:89–98.

454. Román GC, Sachdev P, Royall DR, et al. Vascular cognitive disorder: a new diagnostic category updating vascular cognitive impairment and vascular dementia. J Neurol Sci 2004; 226:81–87.

455. Merino JG, Hachinski V. diagnosis of vascular dementia In: Paul RH, Cohen R, Ott Br, Salloway S, eds. Vascular Dementia Cerebrovascular Mechanisms and Clinical Management. Totowa, NJ: Humana Press Inc, 2005:57–71.

456. Garcia JH, Brown GG. Vascular dementia: neuropathologic alterations and metabolic brain changes. J Neurol Sci 1992; 109:121–131.

457. Jellinger JA. The neuropathologic substrates of vascular-ischemic dementia. In: Paul RH, Cohen R, Ott BR, Salloway S, eds. Cerebrovascular Mechanisms and Clinical Management. Totowa, NJ: Human Press Inc, 2004:23–57.

458. Jellinger KA. Pathology and pathophysiology of vascular cognitive impairment. A critical update. Panminerva Med 2004; 46:217–226.

459. Ince P. Acquired forms of vascular dementia. In: Kalimo H, et al. ed. Cerebrovascular Diseases. Basel: ISN Neuropath Press, 2005:316–323.

460. Jellinger KA. Alzheimer disease and cerebrovascular pathology: an update. J Neural Transm 2002; 109:813–836.

461. Jellinger KA. The pathology of ischemic-vascular dementia: an update. J Neurol Sci 2002; 203-204:153–157.

462. Jellinger KA. Understanding the pathology of vascular cognitive impairment. J Neurol Sci 2005; 229-230:57–63.

463. Jellinger KA. Vascular-ischemic dementia: an update. J Neural Transm Suppl 2002; 62:1–23.

464. Ward N, Brown MM Cerebral blood flow and metabolism in vascular dementia, in vascular cognitive impairment. In: Bowler JV, Hachinski V, eds. Preventable Dementia. London: Oxford University Press, 2003:192–207.

465. Stys PK. White matter injury mechanisms. Curr Mol Med 2004; 4:113–130.

466. Farkas E, Donka G, De Vos RA, Mihaly A, Bari F, Luiten PG. Experimental cerebral hypoperfusion induces white matter injury and microglial activation in the rat brain. Acta Neuropathol (Berl) 2004; 108:57–64.

467. Englund E. White matter pathology of vascular dementia. In: O'Brien J, Ames D, Gustafson L, Foctin M, Chui E, eds. Vascular Dementi. London: M. Dunitz, 2004: 117–130.

468. Mungas D. Contributions of subcortical lacunar infarcts to cognitive impairment in older persons. In: Paul RH, Cohen R, Ott BR, Salloway S, eds. Cerebrovascular Mechanisms and Clinical Management. Totowa, NJ: Humana Press Inc: 2005:211–222.

469. Wardlaw JM. What causes lacunar stroke? J Neurol Neurosurg Psychiatry 2005; 76:617–619.

470. Andin U, Gustafson L, Passant U, Brun A. A clinico-pathological study of heart and brain lesions in vascular dementia. Dement Geriatr Cogn Disord 2005; 19:222–228.

471. Fernando MS, Ince PG. Vascular pathologies and cognition in a population-based cohort of elderly people. J Neurol Sci 2004; 226:13–17.

472. Moser DJ, Kanz JE, Garrett KD. White matter hyperintensities and cognition. In: Paul RH, Cohen R, Ott BR, eds. Cerebrovascular Mechanisms and Clinical Management. Totowa, NJ: Humana Press Inc, 2005:223–229.

473. D'Abreu A, Ott BR. Poststroke dementia: the role of strategic infarcts. In: Paul RH, Cohen R, Ott BR, Salloway S, eds. Cerebrovascular Mechanisms and Clinical Management. Totowa, NJ: Human Press Inc, 2005:231–241.

474. Liebetrau M, Steen B, Hamann GF, Skoog I. Silent and symptomatic infarcts on cranial computerized tomography in relation to dementia and mortality: a population-based study in 85-year-old subjects. Stroke 2004; 35:1816–1820.

475. Ballard CG, Morris CM, Rao H, et al. APOE ε4 and cognitive decline in older stroke patients with early cognitive impairment. Neurology 2004; 63:1399–1402.

476. Tomlinson BE, Blessed G, Roth M. Observations on the brains of demented old people. J Neurol Sci 1970; 11:205–242.

477. Markesbery WR. Vascular dementia. In: Markesbery W, ed. Neuropathology of Dementing Disorders 1998:293–311.

478. Kril JJ, Patel S, Harding AJ, Halliday GM. Patients with vascular dementia due to microvascular pathology have significant hippocampal neuronal loss. J Neurol Neurosurg Psychiatry 2002; 72:747–751.

479. Pantoni L. Subtypes of vascular dementia and their pathogenesis: a critical overview. In: Bowler JV, Hachinski V, eds. Vascular Cognitive Impairment— Preventable Dementia. New York: Oxford University Press, 2003:217–229

480. Markesbery WR. Overview of vascular dementia. In: Iqbal K, Sisodia S, Winblad B, eds. Alzheimer Disease: Advances in Etiology, Pathogenetics and Therapy. Paris: John Wiley & Sons, 2001:205–220.

481. Zhou DH, Wang JY, Li J, Deng J, Gao C, Chen M. Study on frequency and predictors of dementia after ischemic stroke. The Chongqing stroke study. J Neurol 2004; 251:421–427.

482. Srikanth VK, Anderson JF, Donnan GA, et al. Progressive dementia after first-ever stroke: a community-based follow-up study. Neurology 2004; 63:785–792.

483. Ivan CS, Seshadri S, Beiser A, et al. Dementia after stroke: the Framingham study. Stroke 2004; 35:1264–1268.

484. Bakker FC, Klijn CJM, van der Grond J, Kappelle LJ, Jennekens-Schinkel A. Cognition and quality of life in patients with carotid artery occlusion. A follow-up study. Neurology 2004; 62:2230–2235.

485. Johnston SC, O'Meara ES, Manolio TA, et al. Cognitive impairment and decline are associated with carotid artery disease in patients without clinically evident cerebrovascular disease. Ann Intern Med 2004; 140:237–247.

486. Talelli P, Ellul J, Terzis G, et al. Common carotid artery intima media thickness and post-stroke cognitive impairment. J Neurol Sci 2004; 223:129–134.

487. Leys D, Henon H. Many patients with dementia identified after stroke already had dementia present before. J Neurol 2004; 251:609–610.

488. Mackowiak-Cordoliani MA, Bombois S, Memin A, Henon H, Pasquier F. Poststroke dementia in the elderly. Drugs Aging 2005; 22:483–493.

489. Altieri M, Di Piero V, Pasquini M, et al. Delayed poststroke dementia: a 4-year follow-up study. Neurology 2004; 62:2193–2197.

490. Appelros P, Samuelsson M, Lindell D. Lacunar infarcts: functional and cognitive outcomes at five years in relation to MRI findings. Cerebrovasc Dis 2005; 20:34–40.

491. de Mendonca A, Ribeiro F, Guerreiro M, Palma T, Garcia C. Clinical significance of subcortical vascular disease in patients with mild cognitive impairment. Eur J Neurol 2005; 12:125–130.

492. Artero S, Tiemeier H, Prins ND, Sabatier R, Breteler MM, Ritchie K. Neuroanatomical localisation and clinical correlates of white matter lesions in the elderly. J Neurol Neurosurg Psychiatry 2004; 75:1304–1308.

493. Schmidt R, Scheltens P, Erkinjuntti T, et al. White matter lesion progression: a surrogate endpoint for trials in cerebral small-vessel disease. Neurology 2004; 63:139–144.

494. Schmidt R, Ropele S, Enzinger C, et al. White matter lesion progression, brain atrophy, and cognitive decline: the Austrian stroke prevention study. Ann Neurol 2005; 58:610–616.

495. Garde E, Lykke Mortensen E, Rostrup E, Paulson OB. Decline in intelligence is associated with progression in white matter hyperintensity volume. J Neurol Neurosurg Psychiatry 2005; 76:1289–1291.

496. Rasquin SM, Verhey FR, van Oostenbrugge RJ, Lousberg R, Lodder J. Demographic and CT scan features related to cognitive impairment in the first year after stroke. J Neurol Neurosurg Psychiatry 2004; 75:1562–1567.

497. Tullberg M, Fletcher E, DeCarli C, et al. White matter lesions impair frontal lobe function regardless of their location. Neurology 2004; 63:246–253.

498. Du A-T, Schuff N, Chao LL, et al. White matter lesions are associated with cortical atrophy more than entorhinal and hippocampal atrophy. Neurobiol Aging 2005; 26:553–559.

499. Prins ND, van Dijk EJ, den Heijer T, et al. Cerebral white matter lesions and the risk of dementia. Arch Neurol 2004; 61:1531–1534.

500. Wen HM, Mok VC, Fan YH, et al. Effect of white matter changes on cognitive impairment in patients with lacunar infarcts. Stroke 2004; 35:1826–1830.

501. Reed BR, Eberling JL, Mungas D, Weiner M, Kramer JH, Jagust WJ. Effects of white matter lesions and lacunes on cortical function. Arch Neurol 2004; 61:1545–1550.

502. van der Flier WM, van Straaten EC, Barkhof F, et al. Small vessel disease and general cognitive function in nondisabled elderly: the LADIS study. Stroke 2005; 36:2116–2120.

503. de Mendonca A, Guerreiro M, Ribeiro F, Mendes T, Garcia C. Mild cognitive impairment: focus on diagnosis. J Mol Neurosci 2004; 23:143–148.

504. Fernando MS, O'Brien JT, Perry RH, et al. Comparison of the pathology of cerebral white matter with post-mortem magnetic resonance imaging (MRI) in the elderly brain. Neuropathol Appl Neurobiol 2004; 30:385–395.

505. Masterman DL, Cummings JL. Frontal-subcortical circuits: the anatomic basis of executive, social and motivated behaviors. J Psychopharmacol 1997; 11:107–114.

506. Nagga K, Radberg C, Marcusson J. CT brain findings in clinical dementia investigation–underestimation of mixed dementia. Dement Geriatr Cogn Disord 2004; 18:59–66.

507. Emery VO, Gillie EX, Smith JA. Noninfarct vascular dementia and Alzheimer dementia spectrum. J Neurol Sci 2005; 229-230:27–36.

508. Bowler J, Hachinski V. Vascular dementia. In: Ginsberg M, Bogousslavsky J, eds. Cerebrovascular Disease. II: Pathophysiology, Diagnosis and Management. Oxford: Blackwell Science, 1998:1126–1144.

509. Jellinger KA. Is Alzheimer's disease a vascular disorder? J Alzheimers Dis 2003; 5:247–250.

510. de la Torre JC. Alzheimer's disease is a vasocognopathy: a new term to describe its nature. Neurol Res 2004; 26:517–524.

511. Gorelick PB. Risk factors for vascular dementia and Alzheimer disease. Stroke 2004; 35:2620–2622.

512. de la Torre JC. Is Alzheimer's disease a neurodegenerative or a vascular disorder? Data, dogma, and dialectics. Lancet Neurol 2004; 3:184–190.

513. Kalback W, Esh C, Castano EM, et al. Atherosclerosis, vascular amyloidosis and brain hypoperfusion in the pathogenesis of sporadic Alzheimer's disease. Neurol Res 2004; 26:525–539.

514. Greenberg SM, Gurol ME, Rosand J, Smith EE. Amyloid angiopathy-related vascular cognitive impairment. Stroke 2004; 35:2616–2619.

515. Vinters HV, Farag ES. Amyloidosis of cerebral arteries. Adv Neurol 2003; 92:105–112.

516. Farkas E, Luiten PG. Cerebral microvascular pathology in aging and Alzheimer's disease. Prog Neurobiol 2001; 64:575–611.

517. Bailey TL, Rivara CB, Rocher AB, Hof PR. The nature and effects of cortical microvascular pathology in aging and Alzheimer's disease. Neurol Res 2004; 26:573–578.

518. Zlokovic BV. Clearing amyloid through the blood-brain barrier. J Neurochem 2004; 89:807–811.

519. Deane R, Wu Z, Sagare A, et al. LRP/amyloid beta-peptide interaction mediates differential brain efflux of Abeta isoforms. Neuron 2004; 43:333–344.

520. Zlokovic BV. Neurovascular mechanisms of Alzheimer's neurodegeneration. Trends Neurosci 2005; 28:202–208.

521. Yip AG, McKee AC, Green RC, et al. APOE, vascular pathology, and the AD brain. Neurology 2005; 65:259–265.

522. Weller RO, Cohen NR, Nicoll JAR. Cerebrovascular disease and the pathophysiology of Alzheimer's disease. Implications for therapy. Panminerva Med 2004; 47:239–251.

523. Koistinaho M, Koistinaho J. Interactions between Alzheimer's disease and cerebral ischemia–focus on inflammation. Brain Res Brain Res Rev 2005; 48:240–250.

524. Bowler JV, Eliasziw M, Steenhuis R, et al. Comparative evolution of Alzheimer disease, vascular dementia, and mixed dementia. Arch Neurol 1997; 54:697–703.

525. Esiri MM, Nagy Z, Smith MZ, Barnetson L, Smith AD. Cerebrovascular disease and threshold for dementia in the early stages of Alzheimer's disease. Lancet 1999; 354:919–920.

526. Jellinger KA. Small concomitant cerebrovascular lesions are not important for cognitive decline in severe Alzheimer disease. Arch Neurol 2001; 58:520–521.

527. Snowdon DA, Greiner LH, Mortimer JA, Riley KP, Greiner PA, Markesbery WR. Brain infarction and the clinical expression of Alzheimer disease. The Nun Study. JAMA 1997; 277:813–817.

528. Rockwood K, Wentzel C, Hachinski V, Hogan DB, MacKnight C, McDowell I. Prevalence and outcomes of vascular cognitive impairment. Vascular cognitive impairment investigators of the Canadian study of health and aging. Neurology 2000; 54:447–451.

529. Cohen CI, Araujo L, Guerrier R, Henry KA. Mixed dementia: adequate or antiquated? A critical review. Am J Geriatr Psychiatry 1997; 5:279–283.

530. Rockwood K. Lessons from mixed dementia. Int Psychogeriatr 1997; 9:245–249.

531. Gunstad J, Browndyke J. Understanding incidence and prevalence rates in mixed dementia, in vascular dementia. In: Paul RH, Cohen R, Ott B/R, Salloway S, eds. Cerebrovascular Mechanisms and Clinical Management. Totowa, NJ: Humana Press Inc, 2005:245–255.

532. Ince PG, McArthur FK, Bjertness E, Torvik A, Candy JM, Edwardson JA. Neuropathological diagnoses in elderly patients in Oslo: Alzheimer's disease, Lewy body disease, vascular lesions. Dementia 1995; 6:162–168.

533. Nagy Z, Esiri MM, Jobst KA, et al. The effects of additional pathology on the cognitive deficit in Alzheimer disease. J Neuropathol Exp Neurol 1997; 56:165–170.

534. Gearing M, Mirra SS, Hedreen JC, Sumi SM, Hansen LA, Heyman A. The consortium to establish a registry for Alzheimer's disease (CERAD), part X: neuropathology confirmation of the clinical diagnosis of Alzheimer's disease. Neurology 1995; 45:461–466.

535. Vermeer SE, Prins ND, den Heijer T, Hofman A, Koudstaal PJ, Breteler MM. Silent brain infarcts and the risk of dementia and cognitive decline. N Engl J Med 2003; 348:1215–1222.

536. Corbett A, Bennett H, Kos S. Cognitive dysfunction following subcortical infarction. Arch Neurol 1994; 51:999–1007.

537. Heyman A, Fillenbaum GG, Welsh-Bohmer KA, et al. Cerebral infarcts in patients with autopsy-proven Alzheimer's disease: CERAD, part XVIII. Consortium to establish a registry for Alzheimer's disease. Neurology 1998; 51:159–162.

538. Del Ser T, Hachinski V, Merskey H, Munoz DG. Alzheimer's disease with and without cerebral infarcts. J Neurol Sci 2005; 231:3–11.

539. Neuropathology Group. Pathological correlates of late-onset dementia in a multicentre community-based population in England and Wales. Neuropathology Group of the Medical Research Council Cognitive Function and Ageing Study (MRC CFAS). Lancet 2001; 357:169–175.

540. Lim A, Tsuang D, Kukull W, et al. Clinico-neuropathological correlation of Alzheimer's disease in a community-based case series. J Am Geriatr Soc 1999; 47:564–569.

541. Petrovich H, Ross GW, Steinhorn SC, et al. AD lesions and infarcts in demented and no-demented Japanese-American men. Ann Neurol 2005; 57:98–103.

542. Honig LS, Kukull W, Mayeux R. Atherosclerosis and AD: analysis of data from the U.S. National Alzheimer's Coordinating Center. Neurology 2005; 64:494–500.

543. de la Torre JC. Alzheimer disease as a vascular disorder: nosological evidence. Stroke 2002; 33:1152–1162.

544. Price JM, Hellermann A, Hellermann G, Sutton ET. Aging enhances vascular dysfunction induced by the Alzheimer's peptide beta-amyloid. Neurol Res 2004; 26:305–311.

545. Iadecola C. Neurovascular regulation in the normal brain and in Alzheimer's disease. Nat Rev Neurosci 2004; 5:347–360.

546. Zekry D, Duyckaerts C, Belmin J, Geoffre C, Moulias R, Hauw JJ. Cerebral amyloid angiopathy in the elderly: vessel walls changes and relationship with dementia. Acta Neuropathol (Berl) 2003; 106:367–373.

547. Olichney JM, Ellis RJ, Katzman R, Sabbagh MN, Hansen L. Types of cerebrovascular lesions associated with severe cerebral amyloid angiopathy in Alzheimer's disease. Ann N Y Acad Sci 1997; 826:493–497.

548. Haglund M, Sjobeck M, Englund E. Severe cerebral amyloid angiopathy characterizes an underestimated variant of vascular dementia. Dement Geriatr Cogn Disord 2004; 18:132–137.

549. Petrovitch H, White LR, Izmirilian G, et al. Midlife blood pressure and neuritic plaques, neurofibrillary tangles, and brain weight at death: the HAAS. Honolulu-Asia aging study. Neurobiol Aging 2000; 21:57–62.
550. Sparks DL, Scheff SW, Liu H, et al. Increased density of senile plaques (SP), but not neurofibrillary tangles (NFT), in non-demented individuals with the apolipoprotein E4 allele: comparison to confirmed Alzheimer's disease patients. J Neurol Sci 1996; 138:97–104.
551. Crystal H, Dickson D. Cerebral infarcts in patients with autopsy proven Alzheimer's disease (abstract). Neurobiol Aging 2002; 23:207.
552. Jellinger KA, Attems J. Prevalence and pathogenic role of cerebrovascular lesions in Alzheimer's disease. J Neurol Sci 2005; 229-230:37–41.
553. Jellinger KA, Attems J. Incidence of cerebrovascular lesions in Alzheimer's disease: a postmortem study. Acta Neuropathol (Berl) 2003; 105:14–17.
554. Jellinger KA, Mitter-Ferstl E. The impact of cerebrovascular lesions in Alzheimer disease. A comparative autopsy study. J Neurol 2003; 250:1050–1055.
555. Etiene D, Kraft J, Ganju N, et al. Cerebrovascular pathology contributes to the heterogeneity of Alzheimer's disease. J Alzheimers Dis 1998; 1:119–134.
556. Sadowski M, Pankiewicz J, Scholtzova H, et al. Links between the pathology of Alzheimer's disease and vascular dementia. Neurochem Res 2004; 29:1257–1266.
557. Schneider JA, Wilson RS, Bienias JL, Evans DA, Bennett DA. Cerebral infarctions and the likelihood of dementia from Alzheimer disease pathology. Neurology 2004; 62:1148–1155.
558. Honig LS, Tang MX, Albert S, et al. Stroke and the risk of Alzheimer disease. Arch Neurol 2003; 60:1707–1712.
559. Lee JH, Olichney JM, Hansen LA, Hofstetter CR, Thal LJ. Small concomitant vascular lesions do not influence rates of cognitive decline in patients with Alzheimer disease. Arch Neurol 2000; 57:1474–1479.
560. Frisoni GB, Geroldi C. Cerebrovascular disease affects noncognitive symptoms in Alzheimer disease. Arch Neurol 2001; 58:1939–1940.
561. Capizzano AA, Acion L, Bekinschtein T, et al. White matter hyperintensities are significantly associated with cortical atrophy in Alzheimer's disease. J Neurol Neurosurg Psychiatry 2004; 75:822–827.
562. Kono I, Mori S, Nakajima K, et al. Do white matter changes have clinical significance in Alzheimer's disease? Gerontology 2004; 50:242–246.
563. van der Flier WM, Middelkoop HA, Weverling-Rijnsburger AW, et al. Interaction of medial temporal lobe atrophy and white matter hyperintensities in AD. Neurology 2004; 62:1862–1864.
564. Kovari E, Gold G, Herrmann FR, et al. Cortical microinfarcts and demyelination significantly affect cognition in brain aging. Stroke 2004; 35:410–414.
565. van den Heuvel DM, ten Dam VH, de Craen AJ, et al. Increase in periventricular white matter hyperintensities parallels decline in mental processing speed in a non-demented elderly population. J Neurol Neurosurg Psychiatry 2006; 77:149–153.
566. Jellinger KA. What is new in degenerative dementia disorders? Wien Klin Wochenschr 1999; 111:682–704.
566a. Markesbery WR, Schmitt FA, Kryscio RJ, et al. Neuropathologic substrate of mild cognitive impairment. Arch Neurol 2006; 63:38–46.

567. Jellinger KA. Morphology of the aging brain and relation to Alzheimer's disease, in advances in research on neurodegeneration. In: Calne DB, Horowski R, Mizuno Y, eds. Definition, Clinical Features and Morphology. Boston, Basel, Berlin: Birkhäuser, 1993:107–137.

568. Mann DM, Brown AM, Prinja D, Jones D, Davies CA. A morphological analysis of senile plaques in the brains of non-demented persons of different ages using silver, immunocytochemical and lectin histochemical staining techniques. Neuropathol Appl Neurobiol 1990; 16:17–25.

569. McKee AC, Kosik KS, Kowall NW. Neuritic pathology and dementia in Alzheimer's disease. Ann Neurol 1991; 30:156–165.

570. Kazee AM, Eskin TA, Lapham LW, Gabriel KR, McDaniel KD, Hamill RW. Clinicopathologic correlates in Alzheimer disease: assessment of clinical and pathologic diagnostic criteria. Alzheimer Dis Assoc Disord 1993; 7:152–164.

571. Troncoso JC, Martin LJ, Dal Forno G, Kawas CH. Neuropathology in controls and demented subjects from the Baltimore Longitudinal study of aging. Neurobiol Aging 1996; 17:365–371.

572. Schmitt FA, Davis DG, Wekstein DR, Smith CD, Ashford JW, Markesbery WR. "Preclinical" AD revisited: neuropathology of cognitively normal older adults. Neurology 2000; 55:370–376.

573. Morris JC, Price JL, McKeel DW, Jr., Higdon R, Buckles VD. The neuropathology of nondemented aging. Neurobiol Aging 2004; 25:S137.

574. Knopman DS, Parisi JE, Salviati A, et al. Neuropathology of cognitively normal elderly. J Neuropathol Exp Neurol 2003; 62:1087–1095.

575. Jungwirth S, Weissgram S, Zehetmayer S, Tragl KH, Fischer P. VITA: subtypes of mild cognitive impairment in a community-based cohort at the age of 75 years. Int J Geriatr Psychiatry 2005; 20:452–458.

576. Geslani DM, Tierney MC, Herrmann N, Szalai JP. Mild cognitive impairment: an operational definition and its conversion rate to Alzheimer's disease. Dement Geriatr Cogn Disord 2005; 19:383–389.

577. Petersen RC. Mild cognitive impairment as a diagnostic entity. J Intern Med 2004; 256:183–194.

578. Winblad B, Palmer K, Kivipelto M, et al. Mild cognitive impairment–beyond controversies, towards a consensus: report of the international working group on mild cognitive impairment. J Intern Med 2004; 256:240–246.

579. Grundman M, Petersen RC, Ferris SH, et al. Mild cognitive impairment can be distinguished from Alzheimer disease and normal aging for clinical trials. Arch Neurol 2004; 61:59–66.

580. Nestor PJ, Scheltens P, Hodges JR. Advances in the early detection of Alzheimer's disease. Nat Rev Neurosci 2004:S34–S41.

581. Ganguli M, Dodge HH, Shen C, DeKosky ST. Mild cognitive impairment, amnestic type: an epidemiologic study. Neurology 2004; 63:115–121.

582. Visser PJ, Scheltens P, Verhey FR. Do MCI criteria in drug trials accurately identify subjects with predementia Alzheimer's disease? J Neurol Neurosurg Psychiatry 2005; 76:1348–1354.

583. Bennett DA, Schneider JA, Bienias JL, Evans DA, Wilson RS. Mild cognitive impairment is related to Alzheimer disease pathology and cerebral infarctions. Neurology 2005; 64:834–841.

584. DeCarli C, Mungas D, Harvey D, et al. Memory impairment, but not cerebrovascular disease, predicts progression of MCI to dementia. Neurology 2004; 63:220–227.

585. Borrie M, Smith MA, Wells J. Mild cognitive impairment: functional predictors of progression to Alzheimer disease. Brain Aging 2004; 4:21–25.

586. Petersen RC, Bennett D. Mild cognitive impairment: is it Alzheimer's disease or not? J Alzheimers Dis 2005; 7:241–245.

587. Morris JC, Cummings J. Mild cognitive impairment (MCI) represents early-stage Alzheimer's disease. J Alzheimers Dis 2005; 7:235–239.

588. Backman L, Jones S, Berger AK, Laukka EJ, Small BJ. Cognitive impairment in preclinical Alzheimer's disease: a meta-analysis. Neuropsychology 2005; 19:520–531.

589. Price JL, Ko AI, Wade MJ, Tsou SK, McKeel DW, Morris JC. Neuron number in the entorhinal cortex and CA1 in preclinical Alzheimer disease. Arch Neurol 2001; 58:1395–1402.

590. Hulette CM, Welsh-Bohmer KA, Murray MG, Saunders AM, Mash DC, McIntyre LM. Neuropathological and neuropsychological changes in normal aging: evidence for preclinical Alzheimer disease in cognitively normal individuals. J Neuropathol Exp Neurol 1998; 57:1168–1174.

591. Troncoso JC, Cataldo AM, Nixon RA, et al. Neuropathology of preclinical and clinical late-onset Alzheimer's disease. Ann Neurol 1998; 43:673–676.

592. Garcia-Sierra F, Hauw JJ, Duyckaerts C, Wischik CM, Luna-Munoz J, Mena R. The extent of neurofibrillary pathology in perforant pathway neurons is the key determinant of dementia in the very old. Acta Neuropathol (Berl) 2000; 100:29–35.

593. Jellinger KA. Clinical validity of Braak staging in the oldest-old. Acta Neuropathol 2000; 99:583–584.

594. Parisi JE, Dickson DW, Johnson KA, et al. Neuropathologic features in subjects with mild cognitive impairment. Brain Pathol 2000; 10:S620.

595. Royall DR, Palmer R, Mulroy AR, et al. Pathological determinants of the transition to clinical dementia in Alzheimer's disease. Exp Aging Res 2002; 28:143–162.

596. Wang L, Swank JS, Glick IE, et al. Changes in hippocampal volume and shape across time distinguish dementia of the Alzheimer type from healthy aging. Neuroimage 2003; 20:667–682.

597. Johnson JK, Vogt BA, Kim R, Cotman CW, Head E. Isolated executive impairment and associated frontal neuropathology. Dement Geriatr Cogn Disord 2004; 17:360–367.

598. Boeve BF, Ferman TJ, Smith GE, et al. Mild cognitive impairment preceding dementia with Lewy bodies (abstract). Neurology 2004; 62:A86–A87.

599. Tiraboschi P, Hansen LA, Thal LJ, Corey-Bloom J. The importance of neuritic plaques and tangles to the development and evolution of AD. Neurology 2004; 62:1984–1989.

600. Sadowski M, Pankiewicz J, Scholtzova H, et al. Amyloid-β deposition is associated with decreased hippocampal glucose metabolism and spatial memory impairment in APP/PS1 mice. J Neuropathol Exp Neurol 2004; 63:418–428.

601. Wolf H, Hensel A, Kruggel F, et al. Structural correlates of mild cognitive impairment. Neurobiol Aging 2004; 25:913–924.

602. Nagy Z, Hindley NJ, Braak H, et al. The progression of Alzheimer's disease from limbic regions to the neocortex: clinical, radiological and pathological relationships. Dement Geriatr Cogn Disord 1999; 10:115–120.

603. Delacourte A. Alzheimer's disease: A true tauopathy fueled by amyloid precursor protein dysfunction. In: Hanin I, Cacabelos R, Fisher A, eds. Progress in Alzheimer's and Parkinson's. London, New York: Taylor & Francis, 2005:301–307

604. Ringman JM, Kawas CH, Corrada MM, Kim RC, Head E. Decreased entorhinal paired helical filament pathology in oldest old Alzheimer's disease cases (abstract). Neurology 2003; 60:A209.

605. Thomas A, Ballard C, Kenny RA, O'Brien J, Oakley A, Kalaria R. Correlation of entorhinal amyloid with memory in Alzheimer's and vascular but not Lewy body dementia. Dement Geriatr Cogn Disord 2005; 19:57–60.

606. Morris JC, McKeel DW, Jr., Storandt M, et al. Very mild Alzheimer's disease: informant-based clinical, psychometric, and pathologic distinction from normal aging. Neurology 1991; 41:469–478.

607. Brady DR, Mufson EJ. Alz-50 immunoreactive neuropil differentiates hippocampal complex subfields in Alzheimer's disease. J Comp Neurol 1991; 305:489–507.

608. Fukutani Y, Kobayashi K, Nakamura I, Watanabe K, Isaki K, Cairns NJ. Neurons, intracellular and extracellular neurofibrillary tangles in subdivisions of the hippocampal cortex in normal ageing and Alzheimer's disease. Neurosci Lett 1995; 200:57–60.

609. Takayama N, Iseki E, Yamamoto T, Kosaka K. Regional quantitative study of formation process of neurofibrillary tangles in the hippocampus of non-demented elderly brains: comparison with late-onset Alzheimer's disease brains. Neuropathology 2002; 22:147–153.

610. Gomez-Isla T, Price JL, McKeel DW, Jr., Morris JC, Growdon JH, Hyman BT. Profound loss of layer II entorhinal cortex neurons occurs in very mild Alzheimer's disease. J Neurosci 1996; 16:4491–4500.

611. Korbo L, Amrein I, Lipp HP, et al. No evidence for loss of hippocampal neurons in non-Alzheimer dementia patients. Acta Neurol Scand 2004; 109:132–139.

612. Hof PR, Bussiere T, Gold G, et al. Stereologic evidence for persistence of viable neurons in layer II of the entorhinal cortex and the CA1 field in Alzheimer disease. J Neuropathol Exp Neurol 2003; 62:55–67.

613. West MJ, Kawas CH, Stewart WF, Rudow GL, Troncoso JD. Hippocampal neurons in pre-clinical Alzheimer's disease. Neurobiol Aging 2004; 25:1205–1212.

614. Rosler N, Wichart I, Jellinger KA. Current clinical neurochemical diagnosis of Alzheimer disease. J Lab Med 2002; 26:139–148.

615. Rekart JL, Quinn B, Mesulam MM, Routtenberg A. Subfield-specific increase in brain growth protein in postmortem hippocampus of Alzheimer's patients. Neuroscience 2004; 126:579–584.

616. Jin K, Peel AL, Mao XO, et al. Increased hippocampal neurogenesis in Alzheimer's disease. Proc Natl Acad Sci USA 2004; 101:343–347.

617. Dickerson BC, Salat DH, Greve DN, et al. Increased hippocampal activation in mild cognitive impairment compared to normal aging and AD. Neurology 2005; 65:404–411.

618. Hol EM, Roelofs RF, Moraal E, et al. Neuronal expression of GFAP in patients with Alzheimer pathology and identification of novel GFAP splice forms. Mol Psychiatry 2003; 8:786–796.

619. Zarow C, Vinters HV, Ellis WG, et al. Correlates of hippocampal neuron number in Alzheimer's disease and ischemic vascular dementia. Ann Neurol 2005; 57:896–903.

620. von Gunten A, Kovari E, Rivara CB, Bouras C, Hof PR, Giannakopoulos P. Stereologic analysis of hippocampal Alzheimer's disease pathology in the oldest-old: evidence for sparing of the entorhinal cortex and CA1 field. Exp Neurol 2005; 193:198–206.

620a. Scheff SW, Price DA, Schmitt FA, et al. Hippocampal synaptic loss in early Alzheimer's disease and mild cognitive impairment Epub ahead of pint: PMID: 16289476 Neurobiol Aging 2005.

621. Iwakiri M, Mizukami K, Ikonomovic MD, et al. Changes in hippocampal GABABR1 subunit expression in Alzheimer's patients: association with Braak staging. Acta Neuropathol (Berl) 2005; 109:467–474.

622. Qin S, Hu XY, Xu H, Zhou JN. Regional alteration of synapsin I in the hippocampal formation of Alzheimer's disease patients. Acta Neuropathol (Berl) 2004; 107:209–215.

623. Lechner T, Adlassnig C, Humpel C, et al. Chromogranin peptides in Alzheimer's disease. Exp Gerontol 2004; 39:101–113.

624. Marksteiner J, Kaufmann WA, Gurka P, Humpel C. Synaptic proteins in Alzheimer's disease. J Mol Neurosci 2002; 18:53–63.

625. Callahan LM, Vaules WA, Coleman PD. Progressive reduction of synaptophysin message in single neurons in Alzheimer disease. J Neuropathol Exp Neurol 2002; 61:384–395.

626. Yao PJ, Zhu M, Pyun EI, et al. Defects in expression of genes related to synaptic vesicle trafficking in frontal cortex of Alzheimer's disease. Neurobiol Dis 2003; 12:97–109.

627. Gastard MC, Troncoso JC, Koliatsos VE. Caspase activation in the limbic cortex of subjects with early Alzheimer's disease. Ann Neurol 2003; 54:393–398.

628. Zhao M, Su J, Head E, Cotman CW. Accumulation of caspase cleaved amyloid precursor protein represents an early neurodegenerative event in aging and in Alzheimer's disease. Neurobiol Dis 2003; 14:391–403.

629. Cottrell DA, Borthwick GM, Johnson MA, Ince PG, Turnbull DM. The role of cytochrome c oxidase deficient hippocampal neurones in Alzheimer's disease. Neuropathol Appl Neurobiol 2002; 28:390–396.

630. Blalock EM, Geddes JW, Chen KC, Porter NM, Markesbery WR, Landfield PW. Incipient Alzheimer's disease: microarray correlation analyses reveal major transcriptional and tumor suppressor responses. Proc Natl Acad Sci USA 2004; 101:2173–2178.

631. Counts SE, Mufson EJ. The role of nerve growth factor receptors in cholinergic basal forebrain degeneration in prodromal Alzheimer disease. J Neuropathol Exp Neurol 2005; 64:263–272.

632. Sofroniew MV. Nerve growth factor, ageing and Alzheimer's disease. Alzheimer's Res 1996; 2:7–14.

633. Peng SY, Wuu J, Mufson EJ, Fahnestock M. Increased proNGF levels in subjects with mild cognitive impairment and mild Alzheimer disease. J Neuropathol Exp Neurol 2004; 63:641–649.

634. Sarter M, Bruno JP. Developmental origins of the age-related decline in cortical cholinergic function and associated cognitive abilities. Neurobiol Aging 2004; 25:1127–1139.

635. Hu L, Wong TP, Cote SL, Bell KF, Cuello AC. The impact of Abeta-plaques on cortical cholinergic and non-cholinergic presynaptic boutons in alzheimer's disease-like transgenic mice. Neuroscience 2003; 121:421–432.

636. Wu CK, Thal L, Pizzo D, Hansen L, Masliah E, Geula C. Apoptotic signals within the basal forebrain cholinergic neurons in Alzheimer's disease. Exp Neurol 2005; 195:484–496.

637. Yan Z, Feng J. Alzheimer's disease: interactions between cholinergic functions and beta-amyloid. Curr Alzheimer Res 2004; 1:241–248.

638. Schliebs R. Basal forebrain cholinergic dysfunction in Alzheimer's disease—interrelationship with beta-amyloid, inflammation and neurotrophin signaling. Neurochem Res 2005; 30:895–908.

639. Beach TG, Kuo YM, Spiegel K, et al. The cholinergic deficit coincides with Abeta deposition at the earliest histopathologic stages of Alzheimer disease. J Neuropathol Exp Neurol 2000; 59:308–313.

640. Potter P, Pandya Y, Poston M, et al. Cortical cholinergic deficit is associated with plaque development at preclinical stages of Alzheimer's disease. Neurobiol Aging 2004; 25:S79.

640a. Herholz K, Weisenbach S, Kalbe E, et al. Cerebral acetylcholine asterase activity in mild cognitive impairment. Neuroreport 2005; 16:1431–1434.

641. Perry E, Ziabreva I, Perry R, Aarsland D, Ballard C. Absence of cholinergic deficits in pure vascular dementia. Neurology 2005; 64:132–133.

642. Tomimoto H, Ohtani R, Shibata M, Nakamura N, Ihara M. Loss of cholinergic pathways in vascular dementia of the binswanger type. Dement Geriatr Cogn Disord 2005; 19:282–288.

643. Poirier J, Delisle MC, Quirion R, et al. Apolipoprotein E4 allele as a predictor of cholinergic deficits and treatment outcome in Alzheimer disease. Proc Natl Acad Sci USA 1995; 92:12260–12264.

644. Dubelaar EJ, Verwer RW, Hofman MA, Van Heerikhuize JJ, Ravid R, Swaab DE. ApoE ε4 genotype is accompanied by lower metabolic activity in nucleus basalis of Meynert neurons in Alzheimer patients and controls as indicated by the size of the Golgi apparatus. J Neuropathol Exp Neurol 2004; 63:159–169.

645. Tiraboschi P, Hansen LA, Masliah E, Alford M, Thal LJ, Corey-Bloom J. Impact of APOE genotype on neuropathologic and neurochemical markers of Alzheimer disease. Neurology 2004; 62:1977–1983.

646. Counts SE, Nadeem M, Wuu J, Ginsberg SD, Saragovi HU, Mufson EJ. Reduction of cortical TrkA but not p75(NTR) protein in early-stage Alzheimer's disease. Ann Neurol 2004; 56:520–531.

647. Mufson EJ, Ginsberg SD, Ikonomovic MD, DeKosky ST. Human cholinergic basal forebrain: chemoanatomy and neurologic dysfunction. J Chem Neuroanat 2003; 26:233–242.

648. Shinotoh H, Namba H, Fukushi K, et al. Progressive loss of cortical acetylcholinesterase activity in association with cognitive decline in

Alzheimer's disease: a positron emission tomography study. Ann Neurol 2000; 48:194–200.

649. Mufson EJ, Ma SY, Dills J, et al. Loss of basal forebrain P75(NTR) immunoreactivity in subjects with mild cognitive impairment and Alzheimer's disease. J Comp Neurol 2002; 443:136–153.

650. Geula C, Mesulam MM, Saroff DM, Wu CK. Relationship between plaques, tangles, and loss of cortical cholinergic fibers in Alzheimer disease. J Neuropathol Exp Neurol 1998; 57:63–75.

651. Maki M, Matsukawa N, Yuasa H, et al. Decreased expression of hippocampal cholinergic neurostimulating peptide precursor protein mRNA in the hippocampus in Alzheimer disease. J Neuropathol Exp Neurol 2002; 61:176–185.

652. Rinne JO, Kaasinen V, Jarvenpaa T, et al. Brain acetylcholinesterase activity in mild cognitive impairment and early Alzheimer's disease. J Neurol Neurosurg Psychiatry 2003; 74:113–115.

653. Ikonomovic MD, Mufson EJ, Wuu J, Cochran EJ, Bennett DA, DeKosky ST. Cholinergic plasticity in hippocampus of individuals with mild cognitive impairment: correlation with Alzheimer's neuropathology. J Alzheimers Dis 2003; 5:39–48.

654. DeKosky ST, Mufson EJ, Bennett DA, Wuu J, Ikonomovic MD. Episodic memory function correlates with neurofibrillary pathology but not cholinergic enzyme changes in the hippocampus of normal elderly and subjects with mild cognitive impairment. Neurobiol Aging 2004; 25:S75.

655. Small DH. Do acetylcholinesterase inhibitors boost synaptic scaling in Alzheimer's disease? Trends Neurosci 2004; 27:245–249.

656. Mufson EJ, Ikonomovic MD, Styren SD, et al. Preservation of brain nerve growth factor in mild cognitive impairment and Alzheimer disease. Arch Neurol 2003; 60:1143–1148.

657. Herholz K, Weisenbach S, Zundorf G, et al. In vivo study of acetylcholine esterase in basal forebrain, amygdala, and cortex in mild to moderate Alzheimer disease. Neuroimage 2004; 21:136–143.

658. Bohnen NI, Kaufer DI, Hendrickson R, et al. Cognitive correlates of alterations in acetylcholinesterase in Alzheimer's disease. Neurosci Lett 2005; 380:127–132.

659. Masliah E, Mallory M, Alford M, et al. Altered expression of synaptic proteins occurs early during progression of Alzheimer's disease. Neurology 2001; 56:127–129.

660. Graves AB, Bowen JD, Rajaram L, et al. Impaired olfaction as a marker for cognitive decline: interaction with apolipoprotein E ε 4 status. Neurology 1999; 53:1480–1487.

661. Kesslak JP, Cotman CW, Chui HC, et al. Olfactory tests as possible probes for detecting and monitoring Alzheimer's disease. Neurobiol Aging 1988; 9:399–403.

662. Nores JM, Biacabe B, Bonfils P. [Olfactory disorders in Alzheimer's disease and in Parkinson's disease. Review of the literature]. Ann Med Interne (Paris) 2000; 151:97–106.

663. Doty RL, Stern MB, Pfeiffer C, Gollomp SM, Hurtig HI. Bilateral olfactory dysfunction in early stage treated and untreated idiopathic Parkinson's disease. J Neurol Neurosurg Psychiatry 1992; 55:138–142.

664. Henderson JM, Lu Y, Wang S, Cartwright H, Halliday GM. Olfactory deficits and sleep disturbances in Parkinson's disease: a case-control survey. J Neurol Neurosurg Psychiatry 2003; 74:956–958.

665. Liberini P, Parola S, Spano PF, Antonini L. Olfaction in Parkinson's disease: methods of assessment and clinical relevance. J Neurol 2000; 247:88–96.

666. Ponsen MM, Stoffers D, Booij J, Van Eck-Smit BL, Wolters E, Berendse HW. Idiopathic hyposmia as a preclinical sign of Parkinson's disease. Ann Neurol 2004; 56:173–181.

667. Muller A, Mungersdorf M, Reichmann H, Strehle G, Hummel T. Olfactory function in Parkinsonian syndromes. J Clin Neurosci 2002; 9:521–524.

668. Hawkes C. Olfactory testing in parkinsonism. Lancet Neurol 2004; 3:393–394.

669. Duda JE, Shah U, Arnold SE, Lee VM, Trojanowski JQ. The expression of alpha-, beta-, and gamma-synucleins in olfactory mucosa from patients with and without neurodegenerative diseases. Exp Neurol 1999; 160:515–522.

670. Mesholam RI, Moberg PJ, Mahr RN, Doty RL. Olfaction in neurodegenerative disease: a meta-analysis of olfactory functioning in Alzheimer's and Parkinson's diseases. Arch Neurol 1998; 55:84–90.

671. Katzenschlager R, Lees AJ. Olfaction and Parkinson's syndromes: its role in differential diagnosis. Curr Opin Neurol 2004; 17:417–423.

672. McShane RH, Nagy Z, Esiri MM, et al. Anosmia in dementia is associated with Lewy bodies rather than Alzheimer's pathology. J Neurol Neurosurg Psychiatry 2001; 70:739–743.

673. Olichney JM, Murphy C, Hofstetter CR, et al. Anosmia is very common in the Lewy body variant of Alzheimer's disease. J Neurol Neurosurg Psychiatry 2005; 76:1342–1347.

674. Macknin JB, Higuchi M, Lee VM, Trojanowski JQ, Doty RL. Olfactory dysfunction occurs in transgenic mice overexpressing human tau protein. Brain Res 2004; 1000:174–178.

675. Esiri MM, Wilcock GK. The olfactory bulbs in Alzheimer's disease. J Neurol Neurosurg Psychiatry 1984; 47:56–60.

676. Hyman BT, Arriagada PV, Van Hoesen GW. Pathologic changes in the olfactory system in aging and Alzheimer's disease. Ann N Y Acad Sci 1991; 640:14–19.

677. Kovacs T, Cairns NJ, Lantos PL. Beta-amyloid deposition and neurofibrillary tangle formation in the olfactory bulb in ageing and Alzheimer's disease. Neuropathol Appl Neurobiol 1999; 25:481–491.

678. Ohm TG, Braak H. Olfactory bulb changes in Alzheimer's disease. Acta Neuropathol (Berl) 1987; 73:365–369.

679. Serby M, Larson P, Kalkstein D. The nature and course of olfactory deficits in Alzheimer's disease. Am J Psychiatry 1991; 148:357–360.

680. Pearce RK, Hawkes CH, Daniel SE. The anterior olfactory nucleus in Parkinson's disease. Mov Disord 1995; 10:283–287.

681. Del Tredici K, Rub U, De Vos RA, Bohl JR, Braak H. Where does Parkinson disease pathology begin in the brain? J Neuropathol Exp Neurol 2002; 61:413–426.

682. Christen-Zaech S, Kraftsik R, Pillevuit O, et al. Early olfactory involvement in Alzheimer's disease. Can J Neurol Sci 2003; 30:20–25.

683. Tsuboi Y, Wszolek ZK, Graff-Radford NR, Cookson N, Dickson DW. Tau pathology in the olfactory bulb correlates with Braak stage. Lewy body pathology and apolipoprotein ε4. Neuropathol Appl Neurobiol 2003; 29:503–510.

684. Attems J, Lintner F, Jellinger KA. Olfactory involvement in aging and Alzheimer's disease: an autopsy study. J Alzheimers Dis 2005; 7:149–157.

685. Huisman E, Uylings HB, Hoogland PV. A 100% increase of dopaminergic cells in the olfactory bulb may explain hyposmia in Parkinson's disease. Mov Disord 2004; 19:687–692.

686. Warren JD, Schott JM, Fox NC, et al. Brain biopsy in dementia. Brain 2005; 128:2016–2025.

687. Di Patre PL, Read SL, Cummings JL, et al. Progression of clinical deterioration and pathological changes in patients with Alzheimer disease evaluated at biopsy and autopsy. Arch Neurol 1999; 56:1254–1261.

688. Mann DM, Marcyniuk B, Yates PO, Neary D, Snowden JS. The progression of the pathological changes of Alzheimer's disease in frontal and temporal neocortex examined both at biopsy and at autopsy. Neuropathol Appl Neurobiol 1988; 14:177–195.

689. Bennett DA, Cochran EJ, Saper CB, Leverenz JB, Gilley DW, Wilson RS. Pathological changes in frontal cortex from biopsy to autopsy in Alzheimer's disease. Neurobiol Aging 1993; 14:589–596.

690. Hyman BT, Marzloff K, Arriagada PV. The lack of accumulation of senile plaques or amyloid burden in Alzheimer's disease suggests a dynamic balance between amyloid deposition and resolution. J Neuropathol Exp Neurol 1993; 52:594–600.

691. DeKosky ST, Harbaugh RE, Schmitt FA, et al. Cortical biopsy in Alzheimer's disease: diagnostic accuracy and neurochemical, neuropathological, and cognitive correlations. Intraventricular Bethanecol Study Group. Ann Neurol 1992; 32:625–632.

692. DeKosky ST, Scheff SW. Synapse loss in frontal cortex biopsies in Alzheimer's disease: correlation with cognitive severity. Ann Neurol 1990; 27:457–464.

693. Davies CA, Mann DM, Sumpter PQ, Yates PO. A quantitative morphometric analysis of the neuronal and synaptic content of the frontal and temporal cortex in patients with Alzheimer's disease. J Neurol Sci 1987; 78:151–164.

694. Preston SD, Steart PV, Wilkinson A, Nicoll JA, Weller RO. Capillary and arterial cerebral amyloid angiopathy in Alzheimer's disease: defining the perivascular route for the elimination of amyloid beta from the human brain. Neuropathol Appl Neurobiol 2003; 29:106–117.

695. Vinters HV, Secor DL, Pardridge WM, Gray F. Immunohistochemical study of cerebral amyloid angiopathy. III. Widespread Alzheimer A4 peptide in cerebral microvessel walls colocalizes with gamma trace in patients with leukoencephalopathy. Ann Neurol 1990; 28:34–42.

696. Attems J, Jellinger KA. Only cerebral capillary amyloid angiopathy correlates with Alzheimer pathology—a pilot study. Acta Neuropathol (Berl) 2004; 107:83–90.

697. Chalmers K, Wilcock GK, Love S. APOE ε 4 influences the pathological phenotype of Alzheimer's disease by favouring cerebrovascular over parenchymal accumulation of a beta protein. Neuropathol Appl Neurobiol 2003; 29:231–238.

698. Revesz T, Ghiso J, Lashley T, et al. Cerebral amyloid angiopathies: a pathologic, biochemical, and genetic view. J Neuropathol Exp Neurol 2003; 62:885–898.

699. Revesz T, Holton JL, Lashley T, et al. Sporadic and familial cerebral amyloid angiopathies. Brain Pathol 2002; 12:343–357.

700. Xu D, Yang C, Wang L. Cerebral amyloid angiopathy in aged Chinese: a clinico-neuropathological study. Acta Neuropathol (Berl) 2003; 106:89–91.

701. Cadavid D, Mena H, Koeller K, Frommelt RA. Cerebral beta amyloid angiopathy is a risk factor for cerebral ischemic infarction. A case control study in human brain biopsies. J Neuropathol Exp Neurol 2000; 59:768–773.

702. Oide T, Takahashi H, Yutani C, Ishihara T, Ikeda S. Relationship between lobar intracerebral hemorrhage and leukoencephalopathy associated with cerebral amyloid angiopathy: clinicopathological study of 64 Japanese patients. Amyloid 2003; 10:136–143.

703. Olichney JM, Hansen LA, Hofstetter CR, Grundman M, Katzman R, Thal LJ. Cerebral infarction in Alzheimer's disease is associated with severe amyloid angiopathy and hypertension. Arch Neurol 1995; 52:702–708.

704. Tian J, Shi J, Bailey K, Mann DM. Negative association between amyloid plaques and cerebral amyloid angiopathy in Alzheimer's disease. Neurosci Lett 2003; 352:137–140.

705. Tian J, Shi J, Bailey K, Mann DM. Relationships between arteriosclerosis, cerebral amyloid angiopathy and myelin loss from cerebral cortical white matter in Alzheimer's disease. Neuropathol Appl Neurobiol 2004; 30:46–56.

706. Iwatsubo T, Saido TC, Mann DM, Lee VM, Trojanowski JQ. Full-length amyloid-beta (1-42(43)) and amino-terminally modified and truncated amyloid-beta 42(43) deposit in diffuse plaques. Am J Pathol 1996; 149:1823–1830.

707. Love S. Contribution of cerebral amyloid angiopathy to Alzheimer's disease. J Neurol Neurosurg Psychiatry 2004; 75:1–4.

708. Wilson CA, Doms RW, Lee VM. Intracellular APP processing and A beta production in Alzheimer disease. J Neuropathol Exp Neurol 1999; 58:787–794.

709. Mackic JB, Weiss MH, Miao W, et al. Cerebrovascular accumulation and increased blood-brain barrier permeability to circulating Alzheimer's amyloid beta peptide in aged squirrel monkey with cerebral amyloid angiopathy. J Neurochem 1998; 70:210–215.

710. Natte R, de Boer WI, Maat-Schieman ML, et al. Amyloid beta precursor protein-mRNA is expressed throughout cerebral vessel walls. Brain Res 1999; 828:179–183.

711. Alonzo NC, Hyman BT, Rebeck GW, Greenberg SM. Progression of cerebral amyloid angiopathy: accumulation of amyloid β-40 in affected vessels. J Neuropathol Exp Neurol 1998; 57:353–359.

712. Calhoun ME, Burgermeister P, Phinney AL, et al. Neuronal overexpression of mutant amyloid precursor protein results in prominent deposition of cerebrovas-cular amyloid. Proc Natl Acad Sci USA 1999; 96:14088–14093.

713. Roher AE, Kuo YM, Esh C, et al. Cortical and leptomeningeal cerebrovascular amyloid and white matter pathology in Alzheimer's disease. Mol Med 2003; 9:112–122.

714. Weller RO, Massey A, Newman TA, Hutchings M, Kuo YM, Roher AE. Cerebral amyloid angiopathy: amyloid beta accumulates in putative interstitial fluid drainage pathways in Alzheimer's disease. Am J Pathol 1998; 153:725–733.

715. Weller RO, Nicoll JA. Cerebral amyloid angiopathy: pathogenesis and effects on the ageing and Alzheimer brain. Neurol Res 2003; 25:611–616.

716. Greenberg SM. Cerebral amyloid angiopathy: prospects for clinical diagnosis and treatment. Neurology 1998; 51:690–694.

717. Greenberg SM, Rosand J. Outcome markers for clinical trials in cerebral amyloid angiopathy. Amyloid 2001; 8:56–60.
718. Knudsen KA, Rosand J, Karluk D, Greenberg SM. Clinical diagnosis of cerebral amyloid angiopathy: validation of the Boston criteria. Neurology 2001; 56:537–539.
719. Olichney JM, Hansen LA, Hofstetter CR, Lee JH, Katzman R, Thal LJ. Association between severe cerebral amyloid angiopathy and cerebrovascular lesions in Alzheimer disease is not a spurious one attributable to apolipoprotein E4. Arch Neurol 2000; 57:869–874.
720. Pfeifer LA, White LR, Ross GW, Petrovitch H, Launer LJ. Cerebral amyloid angiopathy and cognitive function: the HAAS autopsy study. Neurology 2002; 58:1629–1634.
721. Attems J, Lintner F, Jellinger KA. Amyloid beta peptide 1-42 highly correlates with capillary cerebral amyloid angiopathy and Alzheimer disease pathology. Acta Neuropathol (Berl) 2004; 107:283–291.
722. Galuske RAW, Drach LM, Nichtweiß M, et al. Colocalization of different types of amyloid in the walls of cerebral blood vessels of patients suffering from cerebral amyloid angiopathy and spontaneous intracranial hemorrhage: a report of 5 cases. Clin Neuropathol 2004; 23:113–119.
722a. Attems J. Sporadic cerebral amyloid angiopathy: pathology, clinical implications, and possible pathomechanisms. Acta Neuropathol (Berl) 2005; 110:345–359.
723. Vidal R, Calero M, Piccardo P, et al. Senile dementia associated with amyloid beta protein angiopathy and tau perivascular pathology but not neuritic plaques in patients homozygous for the APOE-ε4 allele. Acta Neuropathol (Berl) 2000; 100:1–12.
724. Castellani RJ, Smith MA, Perry G, Friedland RP. Cerebral amyloid angiopathy: major contributor or decorative response to Alzheimer's disease pathogenesis. Neurobiol Aging 2004; 25:599–602.
725. Morris JC, Quald KA, Holtzman DM, et al. Role of biomarkers in studies of presymptomatic Alzheimer's disease. Alzheimer's & Dementia 2005; 1:145–151.
726. Lee BC, Mintun M, Buckner RL, Morris JC. Imaging of Alzheimer's disease. J Neuroimaging 2003; 13:199–214.
727. Zamrini E, De Santi S, Tolar M. Imaging is superior to cognitive testing for early diagnosis of Alzheimer's disease. Neurobiol Aging 2004; 25:685–691.
727a. Allen JS, Bruss J, Brown CK, et al. Normal neuroanatomical variation due to age: the major lobes and a parcellation of the temporal region. Neurobiol Aging 2005; 26:1245–1260.
728. Mosley TH, Jr., Knopman DS, Catellier DJ, et al. Cerebral MRI findings and cognitive functioning: the atherosclerosis risk in communities study. Neurology 2005; 64:2056–2062.
729. Csernansky JG, Hamstra J, Wang L, et al. Correlations between antemortem hippocampal volume and postmortem neuropathology in AD subjects. Alzheimer Dis Assoc Disord 2004; 18:190–195.
730. Hirata Y, Matsuda H, Nemoto K, et al. Voxel-based morphometry to discriminate early Alzheimer's disease from controls. Neurosci Lett 2005; 382:269–274.

731. Mega MS, Dinov ID, Mazziotta JC, et al. Automated brain tissue assessment in the elderly and demented population: construction and validation of a sub-volume probabilistic brain atlas. Neuroimage 2005; 26:1009–1018.

732. Jack CR, Jr., Dickson DW, Parisi JE, et al. Antemortem MRI findings correlate with hippocampal neuropathology in typical aging and dementia. Neurology 2002; 58:750–757.

733. Silbert LC, Quinn JF, Moore MM, et al. Changes in premorbid brain volume predict Alzheimer's disease pathology. Neurology 2003; 61:487–492.

734. Rusinek H, Endo Y, De Santi S, et al. Atrophy rate in medial temporal lobe during progression of Alzheimer disease. Neurology 2004; 63:2354–2359.

735. Csernansky JG, Wang L, Swank J, et al. Preclinical detection of Alzheimer's disease: hippocampal shape and volume predict dementia onset in the elderly. Neuroimage 2005; 25:783–792.

736. Kantarci K, Petersen RC, Boeve BF, et al. DWI predicts future progression to Alzheimer disease in amnestic mild cognitive impairment. Neurology 2005; 64:902–904.

737. Stoub TR, Bulgakova M, Leurgans S, et al. MRI predictors of risk of incident Alzheimer disease: a longitudinal study. Neurology 2005; 64:1520–1524.

738. Falini A, Bozzali M, Magnani G, et al. A whole brain MR spectroscopy study from patients with Alzheimer's disease and mild cognitive impairment. Neuroimage 2005; 26:1159–1163.

739. Mosconi L, Tsui WH, De Santi S, et al. Reduced hippocampal metabolism in MCI and AD: automated FDG-PET image analysis. Neurology 2005; 64:1860–1867.

740. Ackl N, Ising M, Schreiber YA, Atiya M, Sonntag A, Auer DP. Hippocampal metabolic abnormalities in mild cognitive impairment and Alzheimer's disease. Neurosci Lett 2005; 384:23–28.

741. Rapport SI. Stages of brain functional failure in Alzheimer's disease. In: Broderick PA, Rahni DN, Kolodny EH, eds. Bioimaging in Neurodegeneration. Totowa, NJ: Humana Press, 2005:107–124.

742. Mortimer JA, Gosche KM, Riley KP, Markesbery WR, Snowdon DA. Delayed recall, hippocampal volume and Alzheimer neuropathology: findings from the nun study. Neurology 2004; 62:428–432.

743. Gosche KM, Mortimer JA, Smith CD, Markesbery WR, Snowdon DA. Hippocampal volume as an index of Alzheimer neuropathology: findings from the nun study. Neurology 2002; 58:1476–1482.

744. van der Flier WM, Van Buchem MA, Weverling-Rijnsburger AW, et al. Memory complaints in patients with normal cognition are associated with smaller hippocampal volumes. J Neurol 2004; 251:671–675.

745. Pantel J, Schonknecht P, Essig M, Schroder J. Distribution of cerebral atrophy assessed by magnetic resonance imaging reflects patterns of neuropsychological deficits in Alzheimer's dementia. Neurosci Lett 2004; 361:17–20.

746. Salmon E, Lespagnard S, Marique P, et al. Cerebral metabolic correlates of four dementia scales in Alzheimer's disease. J Neurol 2005.

747. Halliday GM, Double KL, Macdonald V, Kril JJ. Identifying severely atrophic cortical subregions in Alzheimer's disease. Neurobiol Aging 2003; 24:797–806.

748. Kril JJ, Hodges J, Halliday G. Relationship between hippocampal volume and CA1 neuron loss in brains of humans with and without Alzheimer's disease. Neurosci Lett 2004; 361:9–12.

749. Jack CR, Jr., Shiung MM, Gunter JL, et al. Comparison of different MRI brain atrophy rate measures with clinical disease progression in AD. Neurology 2004; 62:591–600.

750. Kantarci K, Jack CR, Jr. Quantitative magnetic resonance techniques as surrogate markers of Alzheimer's disease. NeuroRX 2004; 1:196–205.

751. Schott JM, Price SL, Frost C, Whitwell JL, Rossor MN, Fox NC. Measuring atrophy in Alzheimer disease: a serial MRI study over 6 and 12 months. Neurology 2005; 65:119–124.

752. Killiany RJ, Hyman BT, Gomez-Isla T, et al. MRI measures of entorhinal cortex vs hippocampus in preclinical AD. Neurology 2002; 58:1188–1196.

753. Du AT, Schuff N, Kramer JH, et al. Higher atrophy rate of entorhinal cortex than hippocampus in AD. Neurology 2004; 62:422–427.

754. deToledo-Morrell L, Stoub TR, Bulgakova M, et al. MRI-derived entorhinal volume is a good predictor of conversion from MCI to AD. Neurobiol Aging 2004; 25:1197–1203.

755. Korf ES, Wahlund LO, Visser PJ, Scheltens P. Medial temporal lobe atrophy on MRI predicts dementia in patients with mild cognitive impairment. Neurology 2004; 63:94–100.

756. Karas GB, Scheltens P, Rombouts SA, et al. Global and local gray matter loss in mild cognitive impairment and Alzheimer's disease. Neuroimage 2004; 23:708–716.

757. Dickerson BC, Salat DH, Bates JF, et al. Medial temporal lobe function and structure in mild cognitive impairment. Ann Neurol 2004; 56:27–35.

758. Chao LL, Schuff N, Kramer JH, et al. Reduced medial temporal lobe N-acetylaspartate in cognitively impaired but nondemented patients. Neurology 2005; 64:282–289.

759. Fellgiebel A, Wille P, Muller MJ, et al. Ultrastructural hippocampal and white matter alterations in mild cognitive impairment: a diffusion tensor imaging study. Dement Geriatr Cogn Disord 2004; 18:101–108.

760. Head D, Buckner RL, Shimony JS, et al. Differential vulnerability of anterior white matter in nondemented aging with minimal acceleration in dementia of the Alzheimer type: evidence from diffusion tensor imaging. Cereb Cortex 2004; 14:410–423.

761. Teipel SJ, Bayer W, Alexander GE, et al. Regional pattern of hippocampus and corpus callosum atrophy in Alzheimer's disease in relation to dementia severity: evidence for early neocortical degeneration. Neurobiol Aging 2003; 24:85–94.

762. Tomimoto H, Lin JX, Matsuo A, et al. Different mechanisms of corpus callosum atrophy in Alzheimer's disease and vascular dementia. J Neurol 2004; 251:398–406.

763. Klunk WE, Lopresti BJ, Ikonomovic MD, et al. Binding of the position emission tomography tracer Pittsburgh compound-B reflects the amount of amyloid-beta in Alzheimer's disease brain but not in transgenic mouse brain. J Neurosci 2005; 25:10598–10606.

764. Mathis CA, Wang Y, Klunk WE. Imaging beta-amyloid plaques and neurofibrillary tangles in the aging human brain. Curr Pharm Des 2004; 10:1469–1492.

765. Small GW, Ercoli LM, Silverman DH, et al. Cerebral metabolic and cognitive decline in persons at genetic risk for Alzheimer's disease. Proc Natl Acad Sci USA 2000; 97:6037–6042.

766. Cagnin A, Brooks DJ, Kennedy AM, et al. In-vivo measurement of activated microglia in dementia. Lancet 2001; 358:461–467.
767. Warkentin S, Ohlsson M, Wollmer P, Edenbrandt L, Minthon L. Regional cerebral blood flow in Alzheimer's disease: classification and analysis of heterogeneity. Dement Geriatr Cogn Disord 2004; 17:207–214.
768. Blennow K, Hampel H. CSF markers for incipient Alzheimer's disease. Lancet Neurol 2003; 2:605–613.
769. Blennow K. CSF biomarkers in Alzheimer disease. In: Iqbal K, Winblad B, eds. Research Advances in Alzheimer Disease and Related Disorders 2004. Chicago, IL: Alzheimer's Association, 2005:36–45.
770. Buerger K, Hampel H. Evolution of phosphorylated tauprotein as a core biomarker of Alzheimer disease. In: Iqbal K, Winblad B, eds. Research Advances in Alzheimer Disease and Related Disorders 2004. Chicago, IL: Alzheimer's Association, 2005:46–58.
771. Blennow K. CSF biomarkers for mild cognitive impairment. J Intern Med 2004; 256:224–234.
772. Wiltfang J, Lewczuk P, Riederer P, et al. Consensus paper of the WFSBP task force on biological markers of dementia: the role of CSF and blood analysis in the early and differential diagnosis of dementia. World J Biol Psychiatry 2005; 6:69–84.
773. Maccioni RB, Lavados M, Maccioni CB, Mendoza-Naranjo A. Biological markers of Alzheimer's disease and mild cognitive impairment. Curr Alzheimer Res 2004; 1:307–314.
774. Maruyama M, Matsui T, Tanji H, et al. Cerebrospinal fluid tau protein and periventricular white matter lesions in patients with mild cognitive impairment: implications for 2 major pathways. Arch Neurol 2004; 61:716–720.
775. Schoonenboom NS, Pijnenburg YA, Mulder C, et al. Amyloid beta(1-42) and phosphorylated tau in CSF as markers for early-onset Alzheimer disease. Neurology 2004; 62:1580–1584.
776. Hampel H, Mitchell A, Blennow K, et al. Core biological marker candidates of Alzheimer's disease—perspectives for diagnosis, prediction of outcome and reflection of biological activity. J Neural Transm 2004; 111:247–272.
777. Sobow T, Flirski M, Liberski PP. Amyloid-beta and tau proteins as biochemical markers of Alzheimer's disease. Acta Neurobiol Exp 2004; 64:53–70.
778. Blennow K. Cerebrospinal fluid protein biomarkers for Alzheimer's disease. NeuroRX 2004; 1:213–225.
779. Moonis M, Swearer JM, Dayaw MP, et al. Familial Alzheimer disease: decreases in CSF Abeta42 levels precede cognitive decline. Neurology 2005; 65:323–325.
780. Lavados M, Farias G, Rothhammer F, et al. ApoE alleles and tau markers in patients with different levels of cognitive impairment. Arch Med Res 2005; 36:474–479.
781. Vanderstichele H, De Meyer G, Andreasen N. Amino-truncated {beta}-amyloid42 peptides in cerebrospinal fluid and prediction of progression of mild cognitive impairment. Clin Chem 2005; 51:1650–1660.
782. de Leon MJ, Desanti S, Zinkowski R, et al. Longitudinal CSF and MRI biomarkers improve the diagnosis of mild cognitive impairment. Neurobiol Aging 2006; 27:394–401.

783. Strozyk D, Blennow K, White LR, Launer LJ. CSF Abeta 42 levels correlate with amyloid-neuropathology in a population-based autopsy study. Neurology 2003; 60:652–656.

784. Clark CM, Xie S, Chittams J, et al. Cerebrospinal fluid tau and beta-amyloid: how well do these biomarkers reflect autopsy-confirmed dementia diagnoses? Arch Neurol 2003; 60:1696–1702.

785. Sunderland T, Linker G, Mirza N, et al. Decreased beta-amyloid1-42 and increased tau levels in cerebrospinal fluid of patients with Alzheimer disease. JAMA 2003; 289:2094–2103.

786. Zhou JN, Liu RY, Kamphorst W, Hofman MA, Swaab DF. Early neuropathological Alzheimer's changes in aged individuals are accompanied by decreased cerebrospinal fluid melatonin levels. J Pineal Res 2003; 35:125–130.

787. de Leon MJ, DeSanti S, Zinkowski R, et al. MRI and CSF studies in the early diagnosis of Alzheimer's disease. J Intern Med 2004; 256:205–223.

788. Zhang J, Goodlett DR, Quinn JF, et al. Quantitative proteomics of cerebrospinal fluid from patients with Alzheimer disease. J Alzheimers Dis 2005; 7:125–133.

789. Fukumoto H, Tennis M, Locascio JJ, Hyman BT, Growdon JH, Irizarry MC. Age but not diagnosis is the main predictor of plasma amyloid beta-protein levels. Arch Neurol 2003; 60:958–964.

790. Mayeux R, Honig LS, Tang MX, et al. Plasma A[beta]40 and A[beta]42 and Alzheimer's disease: relation to age, mortality, and risk. Neurology 2003; 61:1185–1190.

791. Prince JA, Zetterberg H, Andreasen N, Marcusson J, Blennow K. APOE ε4 allele is associated with reduced cerebrospinal fluid levels of Abeta42. Neurology 2004; 62:2116–2118.

791a. Gurol ME, Irizarry MC, Smith EE, et al. Plasma beta-amyloid and white matter lesions in AD, MCI, and cerebral amyloid angiopathy. Neurol 2006; 66:23–29.

792. Irizarry MC. Biomarkers of Alzheimer disease in plasma. NeuroRX 2004; 1:226–234.

793. Blasko I, Kemmler G, Krampla W, et al. Plasma amyloid beta protein 42 in non-demented persons aged 75 years: effects of concomitant medication and medial temporal lobe atrophy. Neurobiol Aging 2005; 26:1135–1143.

794. Sayer R, Law E, Connelly PJ, Breen KC. Association of a salivary acetylcholinesterase with Alzheimer's disease and response to cholinesterase inhibitors. Clin Biochem 2004; 37:98–104.

795. Burkhard PR, Fournier R, Mermillod B, Krause KH, Bouras C, Irminger I. Cerebrospinal fluid tau and Abeta42 concentrations in healthy subjects: delineation of reference intervals and their limitations. Clin Chem Lab Med 2004; 42:396–407.

796. Rinne JO, Nurmi E, Ruottinen HM, Bergman J, Eskola O, Solin O. [F-18]FDOPA and [F-18]CFT are both sensitive PET markers to detect presynaptic dopaminergic hypofunction in early Parkinson disease. Synapse 2001; 40:193–200.

797. Nurmi E, Bergman J, Eskola O, et al. Progression of dopaminergic hypofunction in striatal subregions in Parkinson's disease using [18F]CFT PET. Synapse 2003; 48:109–115.

798. Winogrodzka A, Bergmans P, Booij J, van Royen EA, Stoof JC, Wolters EC. [(123)I]beta-CIT SPECT is a useful method for monitoring dopaminergic

degeneration in early stage Parkinson's disease. J Neurol Neurosurg Psychiatry 2003; 74:294–298.

799. Prunier C, Bezard E, Montharu J, et al. Presymptomatic diagnosis of experimental Parkinsonism with 123I-PE2I SPECT. Neuroimage 2003; 19:810–816.

800. Marshall V, Grosset D. Role of dopamine transporter imaging in routine clinical practice. Mov Disord 2003; 18:1415–1423.

801. Prunier C, Payoux P, Guilloteau D, et al. Quantification of dopamine transporter by 123I-PE2I SPECT and the noninvasive Logan graphical method in Parkinson's disease. J Nucl Med 2003; 44:663–670.

802. Nutt JG, Carter JH, Sexton GJ. The dopamine transporter: importance in Parkinson's disease. Ann Neurol 2004; 55:766–773.

803. Ransmayr G, Seppi K, Donnemiller E, et al. Striatal dopamine transporter function in dementia with Lewy bodies and Parkinson's disease. Eur J Nucl Med 2001; 28:1523–1528.

804. O'Brien JT, Colloby S, Fenwick J, et al. Dopamine transporter loss visualized with FP-CIT SPECT in the differential diagnosis of dementia with Lewy bodies. Arch Neurol 2004; 61:919–925.

805. Colloby SJ, Fenwick JD, Williams ED, et al. A comparison of (99m)Tc-HMPAO SPET changes in dementia with Lewy bodies and Alzheimer's disease using statistical parametric mapping. Eur J Nucl Med Mol Imaging 2002; 29:615–622.

806. Gilman S, Koeppe RA, Little R, et al. Decreased striatal monoaminergic presynaptic terminals detected with PET in DLB but not AD. Ann Neurol 2004; 56:774–780.

807. Walker Z, Costa DC, Walker RW, et al. Striatal dopamine transporter in dementia with Lewy bodies and Parkinson disease: a comparison. Neurology 2004; 62:1568–1572.

808. Small GW. Neuroimaging as a diagnostic tool in dementia with Lewy bodies. Dement Geriatr Cogn Disord 2004; 17:25–31.

809. Burton EJ, Karas G, Paling SM, et al. Patterns of cerebral atrophy in dementia with Lewy bodies using voxel-based morphometry. Neuroimage 2002; 17:618–630.

810. Nagano-Saito A, Washimi Y, Arahata Y, et al. Cerebral atrophy and its relation to cognitive impairment in Parkinson disease. Neurology 2005; 64:224–229.

811. Burton EJ, McKeith IG, Burn DJ, Williams ED, O'Brien JT. Cerebral atrophy in Parkinson's disease with and without dementia: a comparison with Alzheimer's disease, dementia with Lewy bodies and controls. Brain 2004; 127:791–800.

812. Lobotesis K, Fenwick JD, Phipps A, et al. Occipital hypoperfusion on SPECT in dementia with Lewy bodies but not AD. Neurology 2001; 56:643–649.

813. Imamura T, Ishii K, Hirono N, et al. Occipital glucose metabolism in dementia with Lewy bodies with and without Parkinsonism: a study using positron emission tomography. Dement Geriatr Cogn Disord 2001; 12:194–197.

814. Mirzaei S, Rodrigues M, Koehn H, Knoll P, Bruecke T. Metabolic impairment of brain metabolism in patients with Lewy body dementia. Eur J Neurol 2003; 10:573–575.

815. Bozzali M, Falini A, Cercignani M, et al. Brain tissue damage in dementia with Lewy bodies: an in vivo diffusion tensor MRI study. Brain 2005; 128:1595–1604.

816. Michell AW, Lewis SJ, Foltynie T, Barker RA. Biomarkers and Parkinson's disease. Brain 2004; 127:1693–1705.

817. Buerger K, Zinkowski R, Teipel SJ, et al. Differential diagnosis of Alzheimer disease with cerebrospinal fluid levels of tau protein phosphorylated at threonine 231. Arch Neurol 2002; 59:1267–1272.

818. Parnetti L, Lanari A, Amici S, Gallai V, Vanmechelen E, Hulstaert F. CSF phosphorylated tau is a possible marker for discriminating Alzheimer's disease from dementia with Lewy bodies. Phospho-Tau International Study Group. Neurol Sci 2001; 22:77–78.

819. Mollenhauer B, Bibl M, Trenkwalder C, et al. Follow-up investigations in cerebrospinal fluid of patients with dementia with Lewy bodies and Alzheimer's disease. J Neural Transm 2005; 112:933–948.

820. Jakowec MW, Petzinger GM, Sastry S, Donaldson DM, McCormack A, Langston JW. The native form of alpha-synuclein is not found in the cerebrospinal fluid of patients with Parkinson's disease or normal controls. Neurosci Lett 1998; 253:13–16.

821. Miller DW, Hague SM, Clarimon J, et al. Alpha-synuclein in blood and brain from familial Parkinson disease with SNCA locus triplication. Neurology 2004; 62:1835–1838.

822. Broe M, Hodges JR, Schofield E, Shepherd CE, Kril JJ, Halliday GM. Staging disease severity in pathologically confirmed cases of frontotemporal dementia. Neurology 2003; 60:1005–1011.

823. Kril JJ, Halliday GM. Clinicopathological staging of frontotemporal dementia severity: correlation with regional atrophy. Dement Geriatr Cogn Disord 2004; 17:311–315.

824. Kersaitis C, Halliday GM, Kril JJ. Regional and cellular pathology in frontotemporal dementia: relationship to stage of disease. Acta Neuropathol 2004; 108:515–523.

825. Rosen HJ, Gorno-Tempini ML, Goldman WP, et al. Patterns of brain atrophy in frontotemporal dementia and semantic dementia. Neurology 2002; 58:198–208.

826. Boccardi M, Sabattoli F, Laakso MP, et al. Frontotemporal dementia as a neural system disease. Neurobiol Aging 2005; 26:37–44.

827. Diehl J, Grimmer T, Drzezga A, Riemenschneider M, Forstl H, Kurz A. Cerebral metabolic patterns at early stages of frontotemporal dementia and semantic dementia. A PET study. Neurobiol Aging 2004; 25:1051–1056.

828. Rombouts SA, van Swieten JC, Pijnenburg YA, Goekoop R, Barkhof F, Scheltens P. Loss of frontal fMRI activation in early frontotemporal dementia compared to early AD. Neurology 2003; 60:1904–1908.

829. Verbeek MM, Pijnenburg YA, Schoonenboom NS, et al. Cerebrospinal fluid tau levels in frontotemporal dementia. Ann Neurol 2005; 58:656–657.

830. Pijnenburg YA, Schoonenboom NS, Scheltens P. Tau and Abeta42 protein in CSF of patients with frontotemporal degeneration. Neurology 2003; 60:353–354.

831. Pijnenburg YA, Schoonenboom NS, Rosso SM, et al. CSF tau and Abeta42 are not useful in the diagnosis of frontotemporal lobar degeneration. Neurology 2004; 62:1649.

832. Grossman M, Farmer J, Leight S, et al. Cerebrospinal fluid profile in frontotemporal dementia and Alzheimer's disease. Ann Neurol 2005; 57:721–729.

833. Rosso SM, van Herpen E, Pijnenburg YA, et al. Total tau and phosphorylated tau 181 levels in the cerebrospinal fluid of patients with frontotemporal dementia due to P301L and G272V tau mutations. Arch Neurol 2003; 60:1209–1213.

834. Hampel H, Teipel SJ. Total and phosphorylated tau proteins: evaluation as core biomarker candidates in frontotemporal dementia. Dement Geriatr Cogn Disord 2004; 17:350–354.

835. Buée L, Bussiere T, Buee-Scherrer V, Delacourte A, Hof PR. Tau protein isoforms, phosphorylation and role in neurodegenerative disorders. Brain Res Brain Res Rev 2000; 33:95–130.

836. Erkinjuntti T, Pohjasvaara T. Anatomical imaging, in vascular cognitive impairment. In: Bowler JV, Hachinski V, eds. Preventable Dementia. London: Oxford Univ. Press, 2003:176–191.

837. Mielke R, Herholz K, Grond M, Kessler J, Heiss WD. Severity of vascular dementia is related to volume of metabolically impaired tissue. Arch Neurol 1992; 49:909–913.

838. Mielke R, Pietrzyk U, Jacobs A, et al. HMPAO SPET and FDG PET in Alzheimer's disease and vascular dementia: comparison of perfusion and metabolic pattern. Eur J Nucl Med 1994; 21:1052–1060.

839. Kril JJ, Patel S, Harding AJ, Halliday GM. Neuron loss from the hippocampus of Alzheimer's disease exceeds extracellular neurofibrillary tangle formation. Acta Neuropathol (Berl) 2002; 103:370–376.

840. Cordoliani-Mackowiak MA, Henon H, Pruvo JP, Pasquier F, Leys D. Poststroke dementia: influence of hippocampal atrophy. Arch Neurol 2003; 60:585–590.

841. Rossi R, Joachim C, Geroldi C, Esiri MM, Smith AD, Frisoni GB. Pathological validation of a CT-based scale for subcortical vascular disease. The OPTIMA study. Dement Geriatr Cogn Disord 2005; 19:61–66.

842. Zekry D, Duyckaerts C, Belmin J, et al. The vascular lesions in vascular and mixed dementia: the weight of functional neuroanatomy. Neurobiol Aging 2003; 24:213–219.

843. Kuller LH, Lopez OL, Jagust WJ, et al. Determinants of vascular dementia in the cardiovascular health cognition study. Neurology 2005; 64:1548–1552.

844. Burton E, Ballard C, Stephens S, et al. Hyperintensities and fronto-subcortical atrophy on MRI are substrates of mild cognitive deficits after stroke. Dement Geriatr Cogn Disord 2003; 16:113–118.

845. Meguro K, Constans JM, Courtheoux P, Theron J, Viader F, Yamadori A. Atrophy of the corpus callosum correlates with white matter lesions in patients with cerebral ischaemia. Neuroradiology 2000; 42:413–419.

846. O'Sullivan M, Morris RG, Huckstep B, Jones DK, Williams SC, Markus HS. Diffusion tensor MRI correlates with executive dysfunction in patients with ischaemic leukoaraiosis. J Neurol Neurosurg Psychiatry 2004; 75:441–447.

847. Wen W, Sachdev P, Shnier R, Brodaty H. Effect of white matter hyperintensities on cortical cerebral blood volume using perfusion MRI. Neuroimage 2004; 21:1350–1356.

848. Sjogren M, Blennow K, Wallin A. Neurochemical markers, in vascular cognitive impairment. In: Bowler JV, Hachinski V, eds. Preventable Dementia. London: Oxford Univ. Press, 2003:208–216.

849. Polvikoski T, Sulkava R, Myllykangas L, et al. Prevalence of Alzheimer's disease in very elderly people: a prospective neuropathological study. Neurology 2001; 56:1690–1696.

850. Hamilton RL. Lewy bodies in Alzheimer's disease: a neuropathological review of 145 cases using alpha-synuclein immunohistochemistry. Brain Pathol 2000; 10:378–384.

851. Geddes JW, Tekirian TL, Soultanian NS, Ashford JW, Davis DG, Markesbery WR. Comparison of neuropathologic criteria for the diagnosis of Alzheimer's disease. Neurobiol Aging 1997; 18:S99–S105.

852. Nestor PJ, Caine D, Fryer TD, Clarke J, Hodges JR. The topography of metabolic deficits in posterior cortical atrophy (the visual variant of Alzheimer's disease) with FDG-PET. J Neurol Neurosurg Psychiatry 2003; 74:1521–1529.

853. Renner JA, Burns JM, Hou CE, McKeel DW, Jr., Storandt M, Morris JC. Progressive posterior cortical dysfunction: a clinicopathologic series. Neurology 2004; 63:1175–1180.

854. Fleischman DA, Wilson RS, Gabrieli JD, Schneider JA, Bienias JL, Bennett DA. Implicit memory and Alzheimer's disease neuropathology. Brain 2005; 128:2006–2015.

12

Guideline and Perspective

Karl Herholz

*Wolfson Molecular Imaging Centre, University of Manchester, Manchester,
U.K., and Department of Neurology, University of Cologne,
Cologne, Germany*

Daniela Perani

*Departments of Neuroscience and Nuclear Medicine, Vita-Salute
San Raffaele University and San Raffaele Scientific Institute, Milan, Italy*

Chris Morris

*Wolfson Unit of Clinical Pharmacology, Chemical Hazards and Poisons
Division–Newcastle, Health Protection Agency, and School of Neurology,
Neurobiology, and Psychiatry, The Medical School, University of Newcastle
upon Tyne, Newcastle upon Tyne, Tyne and Wear, U.K.*

INTRODUCTION

Early diagnosis of dementia has many aspects. There is no, and probably will not
be any, diagnostic measure that can be expected to suit all diagnostic situations
equally well and therefore a differentiated approach is necessary. Three gross
scenarios can be distinguished: (1) diagnosis of mild dementia that is clinically
manifest, (2) diagnosis of a dementing disease in a subject who has cognitive
impairment but is not yet demented, and (3) detection of a dementing disease in
an asymptomatic individual.

   In addition to these diagnostic aspects, new methods may play an important
role in clinical trials, e.g., by defining efficient inclusion criteria particularly at a
presymptomatic stage, or by providing pathophysiological insights into treatment
effects that have not been available in the past. In this context, imaging and
biomarkers are expected to play an increasing role. A list of criteria for such
markers to be clinically acceptable has been defined by a joint working group of

the Ronald and Nancy Reagan Research Institute of the Alzheimer's Association and the National Institute on Aging (1):

1. There should be at least two independent studies that specify the biomarker's sensitivity, specificity, and positive and negative predictive values
2. Sensitivity and specificity should be no less than 80%; positive predictive value should approach 90%
3. The studies should be well powered, conducted by investigators with expertise to conduct such studies, and the results published in peer-reviewed journals
4. The studies should specify type of control subjects, including normal subjects and those with a dementing illness but not Alzheimer's disease (AD)
5. Once a marker is accepted, follow-up data should be collected and disseminated to monitor its accuracy and diagnostic value.

Some imaging techniques now appear to fulfill or come close to these requirements, although the request for 90% positive prediction obviously depends on the selection of subjects. Even excellent biomarkers providing more than 95% specificity in selected samples would fall short of that goal in the context of population screening. It can be achieved only in subjects who have been selected on the grounds that their clinical symptoms already include dementia or at least a severe memory deficit.

DIAGNOSIS OF MILD MANIFEST DEMENTIA

Quite frequently under standard health care in most countries, even clinically manifest dementia is diagnosed only at a late stage of the illness, or sometimes not at all. There are several possible reasons for this including a reluctance to seek medical help on the patient's part, and to make a specific diagnosis of dementia on the part of the physician. Patients may not feel impaired to a degree where they would ask for treatment or they may be simply unaware of their deficits and their severity as a consequence of dementia. But even when recognizing the deficits and possibly complaining about them, they may not expect effective treatment and may be afraid of being diagnosed with dementia and therefore avoid medical advice. Such fears are probably not entirely unfounded since a diagnosis of dementia may mean a loss of self-esteem and personal and financial independence, and may lead to social isolation and perhaps even discrimination. Only with adequate and unconditional support from friends, relatives, caregivers, and social institutions can an early diagnosis of dementia help in maintaining self-esteem and smooth the transition to dependency, thereby improving the situation of the affected individual rather than deteriorating it. Thus, early diagnosis touches many ethical issues, and it is therefore mandatory that seeking early diagnosis needs to be a decision of the affected individual rather than a requirement from other perhaps (but not necessarily always) well-meaning people. The situation changes as soon as dementia is severe enough that patients endanger other people or themselves by hazardous actions or neglect, and social and legal actions are then required for protection—yet, it is at this stage that we have left the arena of early diagnosis that is treated in this book.

Physicians and nurses may also be reluctant to diagnose dementia at an early stage, perhaps because they may feel that such a diagnosis is not in their patient's interest. Since there is currently no effective treatment that prevents progression of disease, the quest for an early diagnosis may be seen as an unwarranted action that incurs costs to cover diagnostic procedures but provides little benefit. Health care systems may explicitly or implicitly discourage early diagnosis of dementia, most likely for economic reasons. Standard diagnostic criteria are also imprecise and do not correspond with each other entirely at the very mild stages of dementia, causing objective difficulties in obtaining a reliable diagnosis. Nevertheless, N. Foster provides many good reasons in chapter 1 why, even in the current situation, obtaining an early diagnosis is important and worthwhile, and the urgency of that will of course increase enormously once drug treatments become available that are either highly effective in ameliorating symptoms, or may even delay or prevent progression of dementia. There is already limited albeit controversial evidence for this with currently used drugs; therefore, even small advances in treatment possibilities will cause an enormous demand for better diagnosis to avoid under, or inappropriate treatment.

Diagnosis of early dementia has two components: revealing the clinical syndrome of dementia and distinguishing between dementing diseases, such as AD, frontotemporal dementia, dementia with Lewy bodies, and vascular dementia (VaD). Obviously, the distinction between diseases is more demanding than detecting the dementia syndrome. Many studies that deal with issues of sensitivity and specificity only address the discrimination of one dementia type (most frequently AD, of course) from normal individuals. Thus, they often are validated against the clinical standard of comprehensive assessment using neuropsychological test batteries and exclusion of other diseases by clinical examination, computed tomography (CT) or magnetic resonance imaging (MRI), and standard laboratory tests. Thus, it is difficult to judge whether there is any additional benefit to be had by using new tests beyond those that are the clinical standard, especially when implemented optimally as part of a multidisciplinary dementia or memory clinic.

Comprehensive neuropsychological assessment is a demanding procedure with respect to expertise of the examiner, time needed, and patient cooperation. However, several compact cognitive batteries have been designed which show considerable promise for dementia screening in the earliest phase of AD (2–5). A wide range of cognitive functions appear to decline in persons who are diagnosed with AD, including memory, attention, language, visuospatial skill, perceptual speed, and executive functioning. There is sufficient evidence to recommend specific tests or cut-off scores. Daniela Perani makes the case for using certain neuropsychological tests for the detection of the earliest stages of dementia, though these may only be able to detect individuals with certain types of dementia amnestic mild cognitive impairment (MCI). While requiring longitudinal validation, the application of such tests should in the future provide much simplified diagnosis. Thus, in a clinical setting, the degree of impairment can be assessed neuropsychologically, but fulfillment of different dementia criteria is ultimately determined through clinical judgement using information from these tests within a framework that includes other tools. New biomarkers probably could not reasonably aim at replacing the detection of dementia by clinical judgement, but should always be seen as part of that process.

Claims for the more ambitious goal of an early distinction between dementing diseases are difficult to verify because the appropriate gold standard for this is histopathological postmortem examination and, as pointed out by Jellinger (see Chapter 11), these standards are lacking at the earliest stages of dementing diseases. Thus, only longitudinal studies that cover the five to 10 years that may pass between onset of dementia and death with definitive pathological diagnosis could have a chance to achieve this. The lack of such studies, though, demonstrates an urgent scientific need for carefully designed longitudinal studies that include modern diagnostic procedures that assess specific pathophysiological processes. Particularly in very elderly individuals with dementia, they should also address the issue of how various pathophysiological processes interact, such as cytoskleletal and synaptic changes, deposition of amyloid, tau protein, and α-synuclein with vascular pathology, and especially during the progression of dementia. Such studies are costly and difficult to organize, but the payoff is likely to be enormous.

Somewhat less firm evidence can be gathered when comparing new diagnostic procedures against each other and against standard clinical criteria. From the correspondence of diagnostic classifications, we can at least get an upper estimate of their accuracy and, by considering their pathophysiological rationale and closeness to purported core pathophysiological events, an idea of their potential. Most of the studies that are available today fall into this category and guide our ideas about their relative merits and perspectives.

Qualitative judgment of atrophy on CT and MRI is already in common use as part of clinical assessment. Progress is to be expected by using age-adjusted quantitative measures or, at least, standardised performance and reading of scans, as described by Frisoni and Filippini (see Chapter 6), but the specificity of using simple measures of atrophy will probably remain low. New techniques, e.g., diffusion-weighted imaging and magnetisation transfer techniques, could be added relatively easily to the standard clinical test batteries in use and show some promise in improving diagnostic specificity. Molecular laboratory blood tests could be integrated easily, but none with high predictive power is currently available. Cerebrospinal fluid (CSF) testing is less likely to be adopted widely due to its invasiveness. Functional imaging by single photon emission computed tomography (SPECT) (see Chapter 7) and ^{18}F-2-fluoro-2-deoxy-D-glucose

(FDG) positron emission tomography (PET) (see Chapter 8) can be a component of the clinical workup where the necessary technical equipment, expertise in performing scans and reading results, and financial resources are available, but more standardisation and proof of efficacy is required to allow implementation as a standard procedure. Molecular tracers, especially for amyloid imaging, may potentially make a major contribution once the remaining open issues about their diagnostic specificity, costs, and availability have been solved. Genetic testing has a clear role in familial disease (see Chapter 4), but its efficacy is still too low in sporadic disease to be of much clinical value.

NONDEMENTED SUBJECTS WITH COGNITIVE IMPAIRMENT

Subjects with progressive cognitive impairment who are not demented, which essentially means that cognitive impairment is not severe enough to impair activities of daily living, are at increased risk of becoming demented. This would be the primary target population for a drug or other intervention that could prevent dementia. The degree of risk at which that intervention was effective would depend on its efficiency, cost, and side effects. A drug with moderate efficiency but significant side effects or high cost probably should be reserved for individuals at very high risk, whereas a cheap drug without significant side effects could be given to a much more broadly defined at risk population.

In this context, a major difficulty exists with diagnostic classification. There is a widely accepted operational definition for MCI based on clinical and neuropsychological examination (6), and it is well documented that individuals with predominant severe memory impairment (amnesic MCI) are at particular risk of developing AD and this risk increases steeply with age. However, when applying the criteria on a population basis, most studies found that specificity is low and up to 50% of individuals fulfilling the criteria do not develop AD within the next few years (7). For example, in the PAQUID study, while MCI was found to be a good predictor of dementia with a conversion rate of approximately 8%, over 40% of those diagnosed with MCI did not convert to dementia over a five-year period. In contrast, conversion rates of MCI to dementia (either AD or VaD) of 44% were found in a clinic-based study with half of the MCI patients remaining cognitively impaired but dementia free and with a very small (<5%) proportion being free of dementia at follow up. The suggestion has been made that the discrepancy for these results may be due to selection bias in clinic-based studies, participants having more severe cognitive impairment and therefore being more likely to present and also to progress to dementia. In population based studies, MCI may not simply represent prodromal AD but may be due to a variety of factors including late onset depression and be of a milder nature.

Neuropsychological tools for early detection of dementia that are sensitive enough to differentiate among incipient dementia, normal aging, and other brain disorders that can mimic dementia, in particular depression (8) have been proposed. The evaluation of memory is the basis for the differential diagnosis of a dementia in its early stages and cognitive changes related to normal aging. The availability of proper normative data, however, represents a current challenge that requires a solution. In the last few years, specific criteria for the diagnosis of memory deficits in elderly have been proposed. The criteria for "age-associated memory deficit" and for the nosographic picture of MCI underline that, in the two conditions, the diagnosis is based on very different psychometric criteria of memory performance. In MCI an impairment on tests of episodic memory is generally the most predictive measure (6), but also tests of many different cognitive capacities have been shown to be predictive of a future diagnosis of AD among memory-impaired subjects (9–11).

The results from a general practice study of cognitive impairment have suggested guidelines for the detection of MCI (12). The role of the general practitioner in the diagnosis of MCI and the potential feasibility of general practice screening is particularly relevant. It may be possible for the family practitioner to verify cognitive complaints and to screen for MCI with a high degree of accuracy using a brief test battery derived from empirical observations in population studies. Neuropsychological tests with the highest predictive value for dementia conversion and suitable for use in general practice comprise three tests (delayed auditory verbal recall, verbal fluency, and visuospatial construction), giving a specificity of 99% and sensitivity of 73%. In addition, MCI detection should not be limited to cognitive performance alone. Proxy observations of behavioral change and information relating to loss of ability to perform activities of daily living should also be used to improve sensitivity and also to provide information needed in patient management. However, the assessment of specific domains of complex instrumental activities of daily living that might be impaired in MCI need to be determined.

There is a consensus that cognitive and functional abilities need to be considered in the evaluation of MCI. Individual slopes of decline in both functional and cognitive performance may be better measures than deficits assessed according to age-specific norms. However, a true consensus can only be achieved after longitudinal studies establish the age-specific levels of cognitive functioning, as well as normal rates of cognitive decline over specific time periods.

Thus, there is a substantial need for improvement in detection by means of more reliable diagnostic methods. We are also lacking appropriate diagnostic terms to label individuals who present clinically as MCI with additional evidence that this is early AD. Even when the histopathological signs of AD are found at postmortem examination, standard diagnostic criteria require evidence of dementia during life to diagnose AD since the presence of some plaques and tangles is quite common in cognitively intact elderly subjects and the correlation between these changes and cognitive status is not very close. Quite obviously, the issue of whether those individuals with histopathological signs of AD but no dementia would eventually have become demented cannot be clarified based on postmortem research because it cannot be done longitudinally. We can, however, longitudinally follow subjects who are asymptomatic or who present with MCI and show significant amyloid deposition based on PET images, to clarify whether this is indeed an indicator of incipient AD (see Chapter 10).

If a reliable predictor of AD was found, the situation would become somewhat similar to how it is in Huntington's disease today. Before onset of chorea in that disorder, there is a stage when unspecific motor symptoms and psychiatric symptoms may be present. Prediction of manifestation of this autosomal dominant disease with complete penetrance can be made on the basis of genetic testing, and the degree of caudate atrophy provides additional clues to predict time until onset quite accurately (13). Thus, an optimum time window for entry into prevention trials with development of clinical symptoms as outcome parameter can be defined in order to achieve high trial power.

Since AD is a multifactorial disorder, it is unlikely that the same degree of predictive accuracy as in Huntington's disease can be achieved. A scientifically appropriate approach to the problem of quantifying risk is studying dementia-free survival, this probably being best achieved by using a proportional hazards model. This approach has been used to determine the predictive utility of *APOE* genotyping for AD in MCI patients (14) demonstrating that its predictive power is higher at age 70 to 85 than below age 70. Dementia-free survival curves have also been plotted for different degrees of hippocampal atrophy on MRI by Jack et al. (15), demonstrating that the risk is more significant than that associated with age or *APOE* status. The application of novel statistical methods based on Bayesian theory has been applied in conjunction with *APOE* genotype to at risk families with AD, though even here margins of error are perhaps larger than are needed for application in a clinical setting. Methods such as these may though in future be applied to give the higher sensitivity and specificity required for clinical use. There is therefore a need to perform larger studies with statistical analyses including other biomarkers to obtain a more complete and reliable picture.

Since for practical purposes medicine requests diagnostic categories, we should find a consensus to define a new diagnostic category for cognitively impaired individuals at very high risk to develop AD within the next two years. As a suggestion for a suitable term we would like to put forward MCI-AD as an abbreviation for "MCI, at high risk for AD." This group would be a prime target for clinical trials of neuroprotective agents. Some authors suggest that this is already possible by careful patient selection based on careful clinical and extended neuropsychological examination (16), but that involves a substantial degree of subjective clinical judgement that should be overcome by better objective tests. Memory loss alone rarely predicts AD, whereas multiple mild deficits do, especially if reported or confirmed by informants (17,18). Deficits not only in memory but also in problem solving, slowed psychomotor performance, and depressive features are further clinical predictors of dementia in old age (19). To achieve reasonable specificity, it is also important to exclude reversible conditions that can cause memory impairment by appropriate medical tests (see Chapter 1) (20,21). Visser and colleagues achieved 80% specificity and a positive predictive value of 77% for AD within five years using a combination of neuropsychological testing, assessment of hippocampal atrophy, and *APOE* genotyping in an MCI sample drawn from a memory clinic (22). Some studies indicate that combining targeted neuropsychology testing with MRI volumetry (23) or with PET (24), combining MRI with SPECT (25), or CSF testing with SPECT (26) may reach a prediction accuracy very close to 90%. Hampel and Burger (Chapter 3) show that newer in vitro tests for MCI may provide high sensitivity for detecting those individuals which progress to AD on the basis of reductions in CSF β-amyloid (Aβ) and elevations in phosphorylated tau. Similarly, Klunk and colleagues (Chapter 10) demonstrate the possibility of detecting MCI-AD using Aβ-specific PET imaging agents where Aβ plays a significant part in the etiology of the dementia. With a combination of tests it may therefore be possible in the near future be able to identify individuals with MCI who are at high risk of AD (MCI-AD) who are candidates for early therapeutic intervention, and trials of such combination tests are currently underway. These very promising results, however, still have to be confirmed in larger studies before current practice guidelines that rely on clinical judgement and neuropsychological testing (27) should be revised substantially.

ASYMPTOMATIC SUBJECTS

On a population basis, early diagnosis may mean screening of asymptomatic individuals who may be at increased risk of AD because they are old or have a relative with AD and carry a common risk factor such as the *APOE* epsilon 4 allele. In the current situation without proven interventions that could prevent onset of dementia, there is usually little reason to perform such screening other than for the purpose of epidemiologic studies, but individuals may still be worried and seek advice (28).

Genetic counselling is usually recommended for subjects who have multiple (typically three or more) family members who developed early onset AD, especially when age of onset was at 55 years or younger. Up to 70% of such families may have mutations in the amyloid precursor protein (*APP*), presenilin-1 (*PSEN1*), or presenilin-2 (*PSEN2*) genes that can be identified by comprehensive genetic screening (29). Yet, even in such cases, genetic testing may not provide a conclusive answer in some families (30). In those rare families where mutations in *APP, PSEN1,* or *PSEN2* are identified, or in other families where there is a clear indication of genetically defined autosomal dominant dementia, there are good reasons to consider predictive testing in at risk family members since, in the vast majority of cases, the presence of a mutation indicates a high likelihood of developing dementia (see Chapter 4). This, however, brings with it certain ethical issues particularly since there are currently no disease slowing therapies. As with other neurodegenerative disorders with a clearly defined genetic basis, prior to any genetic testing, support in the form of counselling should be provided to family members prior to any specific testing, and regimes and guidelines recommended for Huntington's are strongly recommended. Individuals are then free to make any life choices and undertake testing if they wish. If an individual agrees to undergo testing or not, there is also a need to provide support and counselling for a prolonged period after the initial stages of counselling, and this is particularly the case where a mutation is found, where systems should be in place for monitoring and supporting the individual (32). There is now a consensus in most countries that genetic testing should be offered for adults asking for it only on the background of professional genetic counselling that addresses and deals with the psychological and social implications (31).

The presence of the *APOE* E4 allele is currently the strongest and most consistent indicator of genetic risk for "sporadic" AD. The remaining lifetime risk at age 65 of developing AD for *APOE* E4 homozygotes is about four times, and for heterozygotes about twice that of non-carriers (where it is 4.6% in men and 9.3% in women) (30). With advancing age, however, the influence of *APOE* E4 status gradually weakens, and for individuals living beyond 90 years of age where the prevalence of dementia is higher than 30%, dementia is largely independent of *APOE* E4 status. Some of the new techniques presented in this book might provide additional evidence to adjust that risk individually, though one should keep in mind that providing an individual prognosis before age 65 will be fraught with a significant number of false positive predictions because at low baseline prevalence, even 90% specificity of a test (currently most in vivo tests provide less than that and there is little that achieves much beyond that) implies a low positive predictive value, and many people will not live long enough to develop dementia. Thus, there is a very real danger of worrying and thus reducing the quality of life of a significant number of healthy individuals. This in our opinion should lead to a policy of not providing any new diagnostic procedures to individuals who are at a risk that is so low as to imply that testing would lead to more false than correct positive findings. Most recommendations of professional organizations agree that the predictive value of *APOE* testing or other diagnostic procedures at an asymptomatic stage in subjects who do not have a clear family history of early-onset AD is too low to justify the burdens of testing (32,33).

MONITORING TREATMENT

The traditional approach for assessment of treatment outcome involves clinical endpoints that are directly related to symptoms of the disease under investigation, and this is the approach required by drug licensing agencies, such as the United States Food and Drug Administration, for approval of drugs. For dementia, these endpoints are usually based on clinical ratings and neuropsychological test scores to demonstrate an improvement of symptoms (34). It is much more difficult to prove a reduction in progression of the underlying disease by clinical trials, but that could perhaps be achieved by the use of a biomarker that is closely linked to disease pathophysiology (35,36).

In a recent trial with Aβ immunization that was stopped because some patients developed meningoencephalitis, a decline in CSF tau was observed in antibody responders compared to placebo controls (37). In a trial of the cholesterol-lowering drug simvastatin, CSF alpha-sAPP and CSF beta-sAPP were significantly reduced, but the CSF levels of tau, phosphorylated tau (p-tau), and Aβ (42) and the plasma levels of Aβ (42) were unchanged after 12 weeks of treatment (38). Thus, molecular analysis of CSF appears useful in order to obtain some insight into possible mechanisms of drug action, but because of the invasive nature of CSF sampling and a lack of a clear association with clinical benefits, it is unlikely to be useful as a surrogate marker to determine drug efficacy.

Imaging proposals have been put forward for measurement of atrophy progression by MRI (39), although it is still difficult to achieve consistency of measurements across scanners and centres. Nutrition and hydration status may also have an influence on brain volume (40), but they are unlikely to influence specifically local mesial temporal atrophy that is typical of AD. Feasibility of quantitative PET analysis has been demonstrated in multi-center studies (41,42). Tools for efficient quantitative regional image analysis have been developed for multi-center trials that are now underway (43).

Measurement of the progression of hippocampal atrophy by MRI appears to have some face validity as a marker of degenerative disease progression and is beginning to be used in drug trials (44). Analysis of the recent immunization trial, however, has suggested that under certain circumstances there may be a dissociation between clinical scores and progression of atrophy, e.g., if volume changes were due to amyloid removal and associated cerebral fluid shifts (45).

Measurement of functional changes in the brain in therapeutic trials have been accomplished with SPECT (46–48) and PET (49) (see Chapter 8 for further citations), and also more recently with magnetic resonance spectroscopy (MRS) (44,50) and functional magnetic resonance imaging (fMRI) (51). In these studies, there was generally a good correlation between clinical response and an increase in regional blood flow and glucose metabolism. Such data suggests that functional imaging techniques have the potential to be used as a surrogate endpoint in clinical trials although a number of limitations such as the technical variability across centers and a clear definition of reproducible functional conditions during studies still applies (35).

Molecular tracers also permit measurement of specific drug effects. The degree of acetylcholinesterase (AChE) inhibition in the brain of AD patients has been measured by PET (52,53), demonstrating that cognitive effects are related to local drug activity which varies among patients and may not be very well predicted by preclinical studies (54). Amyloid imaging tracers are likely to provide the most direct in vivo evidence of whether new drugs are actually able to reduce Aβ deposition in the brain and whether that is related to clinical benefits (see Chapter 10). In addition, drug companies are increasingly likely to study human regional pharmacokinetics and receptor binding using PET and SPECT at the preclinical and early clinical phase of drug development (55).

CONCLUSION

A large number of new tools have been developed in recent years for the improved early diagnosis of AD. New neuropsychological screening tools facilitate diagnosis of MCI as a condition with substantially increased risk for developing AD. Functional imaging methods and MRI volumetry have demonstrated usefulness in identifying subgroups of MCI patients with a very high likelihood of developing AD within a few years. Molecular CSF tests and imaging techniques even hold the promise for the early distinction of AD from other disorders that lead to dementia prior to its onset, and new molecular techniques for identifying new diagnostic targets may provide improved methods of detection. Genetic counselling is recommended in early-onset familial AD, where specific monogenetic mutations may play a causative role. In the future we should see integration of these new possibilities into longitudinal and therapeutic intervention studies that should lead to more effective development of drugs to slow progression or even prevent development of dementia.

REFERENCES

1. The Ronald and Nancy Reagan Research Institute of the Alzheimer's Association and NIoAWG. Consensus report of the working group on: "molecular and biochemical markers of Alzheimer's disease". Neurobiol Aging 1998; 19:109–116.
2. Darby D, Maruff P, Collie A, McStephen M. Mild cognitive impairment can be detected by multiple assessments in a single day. Neurology 2002; 59:1042–1046.
3. Kalbe E, Kessler J, Calabrese P, et al. DemTect: a new, sensitive cognitive screening test to support the diagnosis of mild cognitive impairment and early dementia. Int J Geriatr Psychiatry 2004; 19:136–143.
4. Nasreddine ZS, Phillips NA, Bedirian V, et al. The montreal cognitive assessment, MoCA: a brief screening tool for mild cognitive impairment. J Am Geriatr Soc 2005; 53:695–699.
5. Shankle WR, Romney AK, Hara J, et al. Methods to improve the detection of mild cognitive impairment. Proc Natl Acad Sci USA 2005; 102:4919–4924.
6. Petersen RC, Doody R, Kurz A, et al. Current concepts in mild cognitive impairment. Arch Neurol 2001; 58:1985–1992.
7. Gauthier S, Touchon J. Mild cognitive impairment is not a clinical entity and should not be treated. Arch Neurol 2005; 62:1164–1166 discussion 1167.
8. Blackwell AD, Sahakian BJ, Vesey R, Semple JM, Robbins TW, Hodges JR. Detecting dementia: novel neuropsychological markers of preclinical Alzheimer's disease. Dement Geriatr Cogn Disord 2004; 17:42–48.

9. Chen P, Ratcliff G, Belle SH, Cauley JA, DeKosky ST, Ganguli M. Cognitive tests that best discriminate between presymptomatic AD and those who remain nondemented. Neurology 2000; 55:1847–1853.

10. Estevez-Gonzalez A, Garcia-Sanchez C, Boltes A, et al. Semantic knowledge of famous people in mild cognitive impairment and progression to Alzheimer's disease. Dement Geriatr Cogn Disord 2004; 17:188–195.

11. Albert MS, Moss MB, Tanzi R, Jones K. Preclinical prediction of AD using neuropsychological tests. J Int Neuropsychol Soc 2001; 7:631–639.

12. Artero S, Ritchie K. The detection of mild cognitive impairment in the general practice setting. Aging Ment Health 2003; 7:251–258.

13. Aylward EH, Sparks BF, Field KM, et al. Onset and rate of striatal atrophy in preclinical Huntington disease. Neurology 2004; 63:66–72.

14. Devanand DP, Pelton GH, Zamora D, et al. Predictive utility of Apolipoprotein E genotype for Alzheimer disease in outpatients with mild cognitive impairment. Arch Neurol 2005; 62:975–980.

15. Jack CR, Jr., Petersen RC, Xu YC, et al. Prediction of AD with MRI-based hippocampal volume in mild cognitive impairment. Neurology 1999; 52:1397–1403.

16. Petersen RC. Mild cognitive impairment clinical trials. Nat Rev Drug Discov 2003; 2:646–653.

17. Bozoki A, Giordani B, Heidebrink JL, Berent S, Foster NL. Mild cognitive impairments predict dementia in nondemented elderly patients with memory loss. Arch Neurol 2001; 58:411–416.

18. Tabert MH, Albert SM, Borukhova-Milov L, et al. Functional deficits in patients with mild cognitive impairment: prediction of AD. Neurology 2002; 58:758–764.

19. Galvin JE, Powlishta KK, Wilkins K, et al. Predictors of preclinical Alzheimer disease and dementia: a clinicopathologic study. Arch Neurol 2005; 62:758–765.

20. Dubois B, Albert ML. Amnestic MCI or prodromal Alzheimer's disease? Lancet Neurol 2004; 3:246–248.

21. Petersen RC, Morris JC. Mild cognitive impairment as a clinical entity and treatment target. Arch Neurol 2005; 62:1160–1163 discussion 1167.

22. Visser PJ, Verhey FR, Scheltens P, et al. Diagnostic accuracy of the Preclinical AD Scale (PAS) in cognitively mildly impaired subjects. J Neurol 2002; 249:312–319.

23. Killiany RJ, Gomez-Isla T, Moss M, et al. Use of structural magnetic resonance imaging to predict who will get Alzheimer's disease. Ann Neurol 2000; 47:430–439.

24. Anchisi D, Borroni B, Franceschi M, et al. Heterogeneity of glucose brain metabolism in mild cognitive impairment predicts clinical progression to Alzheimer's disease. Arch Neurol 2005; 62:1728–1733.

25. El Fakhri G, Kijewski MF, Johnson KA, et al. MRI-guided SPECT perfusion measures and volumetric MRI in prodromal Alzheimer disease. Arch Neurol 2003; 60:1066–1072.

26. Okamura N, Arai H, Maruyama M, et al. Combined analysis of CSF Tau levels and [(123)I]Iodoamphetamine SPECT in mild cognitive impairment: implications for a novel predictor of Alzheimer's disease. Am J Psychiatry 2002; 159:474–476.

27. Petersen RC, Stevens JC, Ganguli M, Tangalos EG, Cummings JL, DeKosky ST. Practice parameter: early detection of dementia: mild cognitive impairment (an evidence-based review). Report of the quality standards subcommittee of the American academy of neurology. Neurology 2001; 56:1133–1142.

28. Roberts JS, LaRusse SA, Katzen H, et al. Reasons for seeking genetic susceptibility testing among first-degree relatives of people with Alzheimer disease. Alzheimer Dis Assoc Disord 2003; 17:86–93.

29. Campion D, Dumanchin C, Hannequin D, et al. Early-onset autosomal dominant Alzheimer disease: prevalence, genetic heterogeneity, and mutation spectrum. Am J Hum Genet 1999; 65:664–670.

30. Liddell MB, Lovestone S, Owen MJ. Genetic risk of Alzheimer's disease: advising relatives. Br J Psychiatry 2001; 178:7–11.

31. Meiser B, Dunn S. Psychological impact of genetic testing for Huntington's disease: an update of the literature. J Neurol Neurosurg Psychiatry 2000; 69:574–578.

32. McConnell LM, Koenig BA, Greely HT, Raffin TA. Genetic testing and Alzheimer disease: recommendations of the Stanford program in genomics, ethics, and society. Genet Test 1999; 3:3–12.

33. Hall WD, Morley KI, Lucke JC. The prediction of disease risk in genomic medicine. EMBO Rep 2004; 5:S22–S26.

34. Caban-Holt A, Bottiggi K, Schmitt FA. Measuring treatment response in Alzheimer's disease clinical trials. Geriatrics 2005; S3–S8.

35. Katz R. Biomarkers and surrogate markers: an FDA perspective. NeuroRx 2004; 1:189–195.

36. Dickerson BC, Sperling RA. Neuroimaging biomarkers for clinical trials of disease-modifying therapies in Alzheimer's disease. NeuroRx 2005; 2:348–360.

37. Gilman S, Koller M, Black RS, et al. Clinical effects of Abeta immunization (AN1792) in patients with AD in an interrupted trial. Neurology 2005; 64:1553–1562.

38. Sjogren M, Gustafsson K, Syversen S, et al. Treatment with simvastatin in patients with Alzheimer's disease lowers both alpha- and beta-cleaved amyloid precursor protein. Dement Geriatr Cogn Disord 2003; 16:25–30.

39. Fox NC, Cousens S, Scahill R, Harvey RJ, Rossor MN. Using serial registered brain magnetic resonance imaging to measure disease progression in Alzheimer disease: power calculations and estimates of sample size to detect treatment effects. Arch Neurol 2000; 57:339–344.

40. Swayze VW, II, Andersen A, Arndt S, et al. Reversibility of brain tissue loss in anorexia nervosa assessed with a computerized Talairach 3-D proportional grid. Psychol Med 1996; 26:381–390.

41. Herholz K, Salmon E, Perani D, et al. Discrimination between Alzheimer dementia and controls by automated analysis of multicenter FDG PET. Neuroimage 2002; 17:302–316.

42. Ito H, Kanno I, Kato C, et al. Database of normal human cerebral blood flow, cerebral blood volume, cerebral oxygen extraction fraction and cerebral metabolic rate of oxygen measured by positron emission tomography with 15O-labelled carbon dioxide or water, carbon monoxide and oxygen: a multicentre study in Japan. Eur J Nucl Med Mol Imaging 2004; 31:635–643.

43. Mega MS, Dinov ID, Mazziotta JC, et al. Automated brain tissue assessment in the elderly and demented population: construction and validation of a sub-volume probabilistic brain atlas. Neuroimage 2005; 26:1009–1018.

44. Krishnan KR, Charles HC, Doraiswamy PM, et al. Randomized, placebo-controlled trial of the effects of donepezil on neuronal markers and hippocampal volumes in Alzheimer's disease. Am J Psychiatry 2003; 160:2003–2011.

45. Fox NC, Black RS, Gilman S, et al. Effects of A{beta} immunization (AN1792) on MRI measures of cerebral volume in Alzheimer disease. Neurology 2005.
46. van Dyck CH, Lin CH, Robinson R, et al. The acetylcholine releaser linopirdine increases parietal regional cerebral blood flow in Alzheimer's disease. Psychopharmacology (Berl) 1997; 132:217–226.
47. Lojkowska W, Ryglewicz D, Jedrzejczak T, et al. The effect of cholinesterase inhibitors on the regional blood flow in patients with Alzheimer's disease and vascular dementia. J Neurol Sci 2003; 216:119–126.
48. Nobili F, Koulibaly M, Vitali P, et al. Brain perfusion follow-up in Alzheimer's patients during treatment with acetylcholinesterase inhibitors. J Nucl Med 2002; 43:983–990.
49. Tuszynski MH, Thal L, Pay M, et al. A phase 1 clinical trial of nerve growth factor gene therapy for Alzheimer disease. Nat Med 2005.
50. Frederick B, Satlin A, Wald LL, Hennen J, Bodick N, Renshaw PF. Brain proton magnetic resonance spectroscopy in Alzheimer disease: changes after treatment with xanomeline. Am J Geriatr Psychiatry 2002; 10:81–88.
51. Goekoop R, Rombouts SARB, Jonker C, et al. Challenging the cholinergic system in mild cognitive impairment: a pharmacological fMRI study. Neuroimage 2004; 23:1450–1459.
52. Kaasinen V, Nagren K, Jarvenpaa T, et al. Regional effects of donepezil and rivastigmine on cortical acetylcholinesterase activity in Alzheimer's disease. J Clin Psychopharmacol 2002; 22:615–620.
53. Bohnen NI, Kaufer DI, Hendrickson R, et al. Degree of inhibition of cortical acetylcholinesterase activity and cognitive effects by donepezil treatment in Alzheimer's disease. J Neurol Neurosurg Psychiatry 2005; 76:315–319.
54. Herholz K. Action of cholinesterase inhibitors in patients' brains. J Neurol Neurosurg Psychiatry 2005; 76:305.
55. Halldin C, Gulyas B, Farde L. PET for drug development. Ernst Schering Res Found Workshop 2004; 48:95–109.

Index

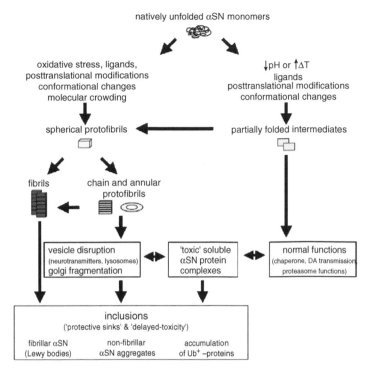

natively unfolded αSN monomers

oxidative stress, ligands,
posttranslational modifications
conformational changes
molecular crowding

↓pH or ↑ΔT
ligands
posttranslational modifications
conformational changes

spherical protofibrils ← partially folded intermediates

fibrils

chain and annular
protofibrils

vesicle disruption
(neurotransmitters, lysosomes)
golgi fragmentation

'toxic' soluble
αSN protein
complexes

normal functions
(chaperone, DA transmission,
proteasome functions)

inclusions
('protective sinks' & 'delayed-toxicity')

| fibrillar αSN | non-fibrillar | accumulation |
| (Lewy bodies) | αSN aggregates | of Ub⁺ –proteins |

Figure 4.5 Molecular pathophysiology of α-synuclein (αSN) monomers converting into partially folded, toxic, and/or aggregated forms. (*See page 128.*)

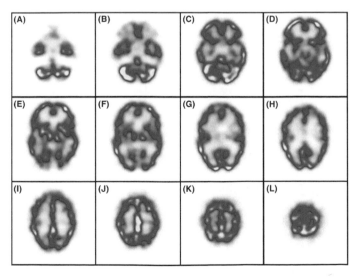

Figure 7.1 Tc99m HMPAO SPECT scan of a healthy volunteer (MMSE = 30). (*See page 200.*)

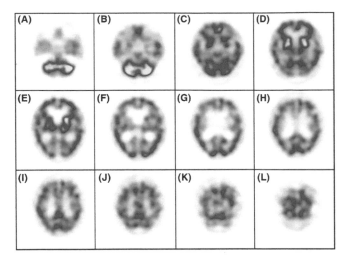

Figure 7.2 Tc99m HMPAO SPECT scan of Alzheimer's disease (MMSE = 22). (*See page 201.*)

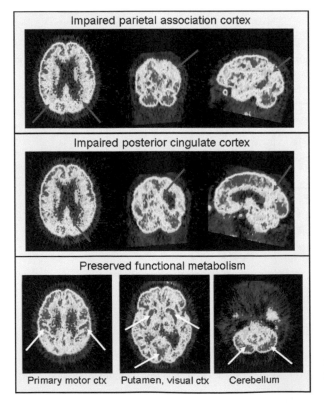

Impaired parietal association cortex

Impaired posterior cingulate cortex

Preserved functional metabolism

Primary motor ctx   Putamen, visual ctx   Cerebellum

Figure 8.1 Typical findings with FDG PET in Alzheimer's disease. (*See page 232.*)

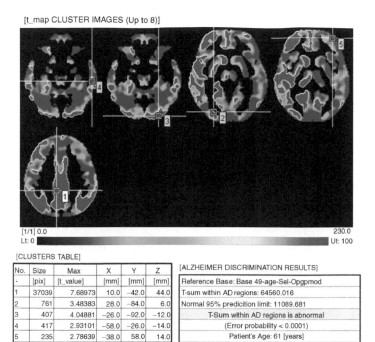

[t_map CLUSTER IMAGES (Up to 8)]

[1/1] 0.0   230.0
Lt: 0   Ut: 100

[CLUSTERS TABLE]

No.	Size	Max	X	Y	Z
-	[pix]	[t_value]	[mm]	[mm]	[mm]
1	37039	7.68973	10.0	−42.0	44.0
2	761	3.48383	28.0	−84.0	6.0
3	407	4.04881	−26.0	−92.0	−12.0
4	417	2.93101	−58.0	−26.0	−14.0
5	235	2.78639	−38.0	58.0	14.0

[ALZHEIMER DISCRIMINATION RESULTS]

Reference Base: Base 49-age-Sel-Opgpmod
T-sum within AD regions: 64560.016
Normal 95% predicition limit: 11089.681
T-Sum within AD regions is abnormal
(Error probability < 0.0001)
Patient's Age: 61 [years]

Figure 8.2 Automatic detection of abnormal metabolism, including correction for age. (*See page 233.*)

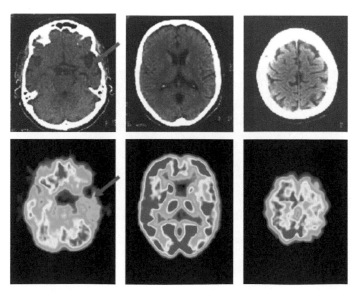

Figure 8.3 Asymmetric frontotemporal atrophy and metabolic impairment in frontotemporal dementia. (*See page 239.*)

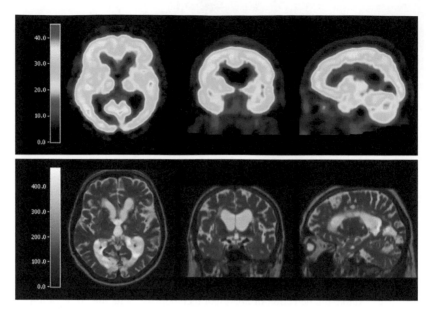

Figure 8.4 Global reduction of cerebral glucose metabolism in vascular dementia. (*See page 241.*)

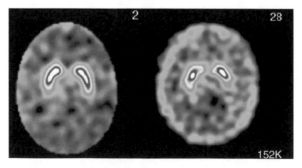

Figure 9.1 Loss of dopamine transporters with age. (*See page 256.*)

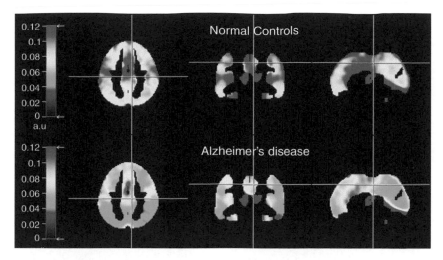

Figure 9.3 Acetylcholinesterase activity in the central nervous system evaluated with C11-MP4A. (*See page 262.*)

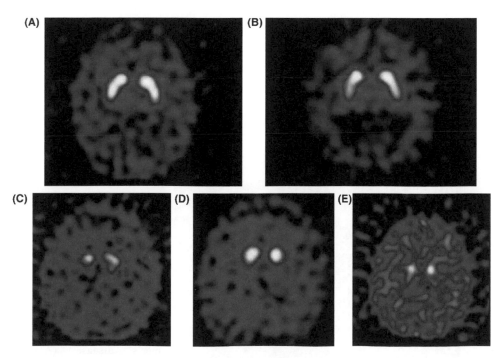

Figure 9.4 Dopamine transporter loss visualized with FP-CIT SPECT in the differential diagnosis of dementia with Lewy bodies (DLB). (*See page 267.*)

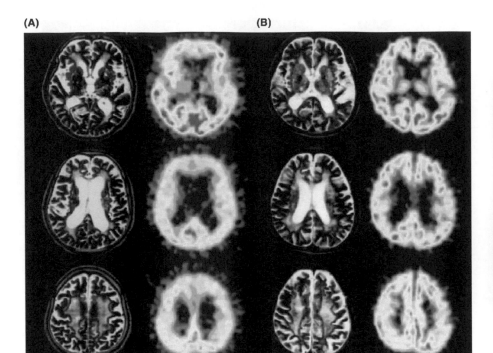

Figure 9.5 Differences in cortical GABA$_A$ receptor density between patients with leukoaraiosis and dementia (**A**) and patients with leukoaraiosis without dementia (**B**). (*See page 269.*)

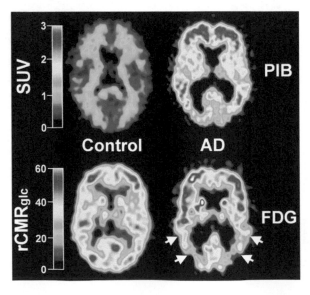

Figure 10.2 Pittsburgh compound-B (PIB) standard uptake value (SUV) images demonstrate a marked difference between PIB retention in Alzheimer's disease (AD) patients and HC subjects. (*See page 289.*)

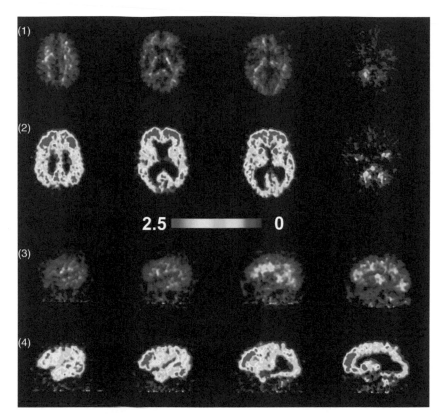

Figure 10.3 Serial planes demonstrate the topography of Pittsburgh compound-B (PIB) retention. (*See page 290.*)

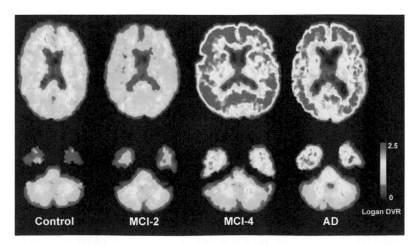

Figure 10.6 Examples of Pittsburgh compound-B (PIB) Logan distribution volume ratio (DVR) images. (*See page 295.*)

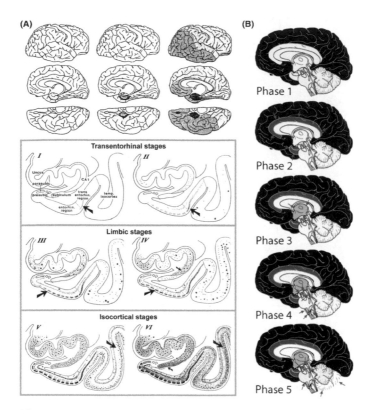

Figure 11.1 Spreading pattern of (**A**) cytoskeletal/tau pathology and (**B**) of Aβ deposition. (*See page 325.*)

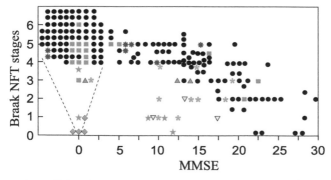

Figure 11.2 Relationship between Mini-Mental State Examination (MMSE) and Braak neuritic Alzheimer's disease stages in 207 consecutive autopsies of aged individuals (mean age at death 81.4 ± 8.6 years). (*See page 355.*)

● Cases with "pure" AD pathology (n=151)
▲ Senile dem. - "plaques type" (n=3)
■ Lewy body dementia (n=17)
★ SID (Strategic Infarct dem.) (n=5)
◆ FTD (Fronto-temp. deg.) (n=4)
✳ MIX (DAT+MIX/SAE; n=7)
✦ SAE (M. Binswanger; n=10)
▽ MIE (Multiinfarct dem.; n=3)